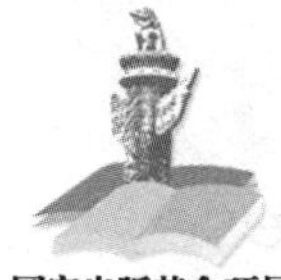

An Intensively Compiled Practical English-Chinese Library of Traditional Chinese Medicine

(英汉对照)精编实用中医文库

Chief General Compilers CHEN Kaixian LI Qizhong(Executive) HE Xinghai
总主编 陈凯先 李其忠(执行) 何星海
Chief General Translators SHI Jianrong HU Hongyi XU Yao(Executive)
总主译 施建蓉 胡鸿毅 徐 瑶(执行)

Ophthalmology and Otorhinolaryngology of Traditional Chinese Medicine

中医眼耳鼻咽喉科学

Chief Compilers HUANG Ping MIAO Wanhong ZHANG Zhijun
Chief Translator XU Yao
主编 黄 平 缪晚虹 张治军
主译 徐 瑶

上海浦江教育出版社(原上海中医药大学出版社)
Shanghai Pujiang Education Press (Former Shanghai University of TCM Press)

An Intensively Compiled Practical English-Chinese Library of Traditional Chinese Medicine

Compilation Board of the Library

Chief General Compilers CHEN Kaixian LI Qizhong(Executive) HE Xinghai

Members(Listed in the order of the number of strokes in the Chinese names)

MA Lieguang	HE Jiancheng	YU Xiaoping	SHEN Xueyong
ZHANG Tingting	CHEN Hongfeng	CHEN Dexing	ZHAO Yi
GUO Xin	HUANG Ping	YU Jian'er	ZHAN Hongsheng
MIAO Wanhong			

Compilation and Translation Committee of the Library

Chief General Translators SHI Jianrong HU Hongyi XU Yao(Executive)

Translators(Listed in the order of the number of strokes in the Chinese names)

ZHU Aixiu	YANG Yu	XIAO Yuanchun	ZHANG Yiping
ZHU Jianmin	HUANG Guoqi	DONG Jing	HAN Chouping

Ophthalmology and Otorhinolaryngology of Traditional Chinese Medicine

Chief Compilers HUANG Ping MIAO Wanhong ZHANG Zhijun

Chief Translator Xu Yao

《(英汉对照)精编实用中医文库》

编纂委员会

总　主　编　陈凯先　李其忠(执行)　何星海
编　　　委(按姓氏笔画为序)
马烈光　何建成　余小萍　沈雪勇
张婷婷　陈红风　陈德兴　赵　毅
郭　忻　黄　平　虞坚尔　詹红生
缪晚虹

编译委员会

总　主　译　施建蓉　胡鸿毅　徐　瑶(执行)
编　译　者(按姓氏笔画为序)
朱爱秀　杨　渝　肖元春　张忆萍
诸建民　黄国琪　董　晶　韩丑萍

《中医眼耳鼻咽喉科学》

主　　　编　黄　平　缪晚虹　张治军
主　　　译　徐　瑶

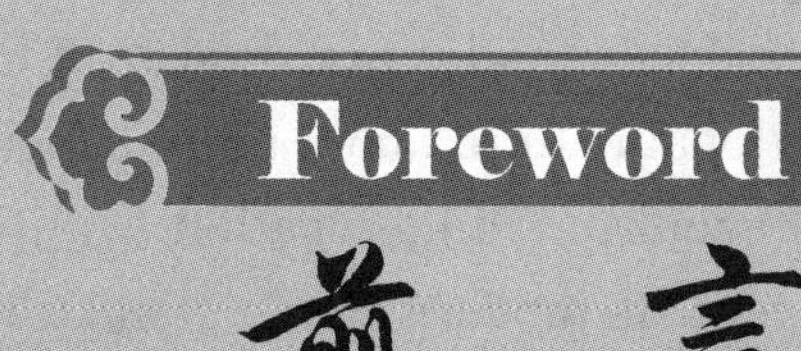

Foreword
前言

With the traditional medical philosophy and clinical experience as the principal body, the science of Traditional Chinese Medicine (TCM) is a comprehensive subject to study the rules of life activities and the disease prevention, diagnosis, treatment, rehabilitation as well as healthcare. The science of TCM has a long history of development and belongs to a summary of experiences that Chinese nation has fought against diseases for over several thousand years, is also an important component part of Chinese outstanding traditional culture and has contributed greatly to the healthcare undertaking and development of Chinese nation.

By increasing enhancement of modern living standard, change of living modes and acceleration of ageing process, the chronic diseases represented by tumors, cardiovascular diseases and diabetes become gradually the important factors in impacting the health of mankind, but TCM presents the better therapeutic effects. Nowadays, the modern medical mode of "society-psychology-biology" has been advocated in medical science, changing from the medical idea of "disease treatment" to "health promotion". The more and more patients in China and abroad have chosen natural and low side-effect Chinese herbal medicine for their problems. With the changes in medicine modes and in spectrum of diseases in the recent several dozens of years, TCM has increasingly been concerned by the medical experts and ordinary people in China and abroad, and the global " TCM upsurge" keeps rising. In order to meet the growing needs of the domestic and international professionals in learning the knowledge of TCM, we have edited particularly the series books of *An Intensively Compiled Practical English-Chinese Library of Traditional Chinese Medicine*.

The scientific, systematic and practical features have been emphasized in the series books. Based upon the full absorption of new progress in teaching and research achievements of TCM , the series books highlight the academic essentials of TCM, with precise exposition of medical philosophy and down-to-earth clinical practice, to introduce the "original and authentic" TCM to the readers. The series books introduce the commonly used therapeutic methods and clinical skills in Chinese medicine, by the clinically encountered and frequently seen diseases and the relevant ailments predominantly effective by Chinese medical therapies.By studying the series books, the readers can learn the knowledge and techniques of TCM on gradual progress and become proficient gradually in TCM.

The series books highlight "the precise features in three aspects"—capable in authors, refined in contents and accurate in translation. The majority of the authors of the series books are senior experts from the related faculties of Shanghai University of Traditional Chinese Medicine. The translator team is composed of the senior teachers with plentiful expertise in translation of TCM from international education college and foreign language center of Shanghai University of Traditional Chinese Medicine. In order to meet the needs of the readers in China and abroad, the basic and clinical core contents are selected and the latest research achievements are consulted based upon the principle "to seek its essentials but its completion" in the series books.

The series books can satisfy the beginners with certain knowledge of English language in studying TCM systematically and can also be used as the textbooks for education of TCM and pharmacy for foreign students. We sincerely hope the publication of the series books plays its promoting role for TCM going to the world.

Editors

June, 2017

中医学是以传统医学理论与实践经验为主体，研究人体生命活动规律和疾病预防、诊断、治疗、康复以及保健的一门综合性学科。中医学历史悠久，源远流长，是中华民族几千年来同疾病作斗争的经验总结，也是中国传统文化的重要组成部分，长期以来为中国人民的健康保健事业和民族繁衍作出了巨大的贡献。

随着现代生活水平的不断提高、生活方式的改变以及老龄化进程的加快，以肿瘤、心血管疾病和糖尿病等为代表的慢性病日渐成为影响人类健康的重要因素，而中医药显示了良好的治疗效果。当今的医学倡导“社会—心理—生物”的现代医学模式，医学理念从“疾病治疗”向“健康促进”转变，国内外越来越多的患者选择天然、毒副作用低的中医药治疗疾病。近几十年来，随着医学模式的转变和疾病谱的改变，中医学日益引起越来越多的海内外医学专家和普通民众的关注，全球性的“中医热”正在持续升温。为了满足海内外人士日益高涨的学习中医学知识的需求，我们特地编撰了《（英汉对照）精编实用中医文库》丛书。

本丛书注重“三性”——科学性、系统性、实用性。丛书在充分吸取近年中医教学、科研进展的基础上，突出中医学术精华，理论阐述准确、临床切合实际，向读者介绍“原汁原味”的中医学；丛书介绍中医学常用的治疗方法和临床技能，所涉及的病证均为临床常见病、多发病和中医优势病种。丛书的13个分册涵盖了中医基础与临床的主干课程，通过阅读本丛书，读者可以由浅入深、循序渐进地学习中医药知识和技能。

本丛书突出“三精”——作者精干、内容精炼、翻译精准。丛书的中文作者绝大部分为上海中医药大学各相关教研室的资深专家，翻译团队由上海中医药大学国际教育学院和外语中心具有丰富的中医药学翻译经验的骨干教师组成。为了适合海内外读者的需求，丛书本着“求其精而不求其全”的原则，选取了基础和临床的核心内容，翻译上参考了最新的研究成果。

本丛书既可满足具有一定英语水平的初学中医者系统学习中医所用，也可供中医药留学生教育作为教材使用，衷心希望本丛书的出版在中医药走向海外进程中发挥应有的推动作用。

编者

2017年6月

Note for Compilation
编写说明

This book includes two major parts of "Ophthalmology of Traditional Chinese Medicine" and "Otorhinolaryngology of Traditional Chinese Medicine", and each part is also divided into the general introduction and specific introduction.

The part of general introduction in "Ophthalmology of Traditional Chinese Medicine" is composed of three chapters, respectively explaining the relationship between the eyes and Zangfu organs, etiology and pathogenesis of eye diseases, the diagnostic and therapeutic essentials of eye diseases by Chinese medical philosophy. The part of specific introduction is divided into the five chapters of cytoplasm, two canthus, white of eye, black of eye and pupil, respectively introducing TCM diagnostic and therapeutic modalities for 27 types of the commonly and frequently-encountered eye diseases, and summarizing the diagnostic and therapeutic steps and essentials by "speculative map", in order for the readers to enhance their comprehension.

The part of the general introduction in "Otorhinolaryngology of Traditional Chinese Medicine" is composed of four chapters, respectively introducing the relationship of the ear, nose and throat with Zangfu organs, the commonly used inspection methods of otorhinolaryngology, and pattern identification and TCM therapeutic modalities for otorhinolaryngological diseases. The part of specific introduction is divided into otology, rhinology and pharynx and larynx, respectively introducing TCM diagnostic and therapeutic modalities for 32 types of the commonly and frequently encountered eye diseases.

The contents in this book are close to the actual clinical situation and practical by referring to both conventional medicine and Chinese medicine. But, "Not everything can be explained in one book". With the development of the clinical disciplines, the theories and clinical skills in the otorhinolaryngology of traditional Chinese medicine are being constantly updated. We would like to continuously follow the development of those clinical disciplines and update the relevant contents in time. We also hope the readers would offer us their opinions and suggestions for revising the book in the republication.

本书包括“中医眼科学”和“中医耳鼻咽喉科学”两大部分，每一部分又分为总论和各论。

“中医眼科学”的总论共 3 章，分别介绍眼与脏腑的关系、眼病的病因病机、中医对眼病的诊断和诊疗概要；各论分胞睑、两眦、白睛、黑睛和瞳神 5 章，介绍 27 种眼科常见病、多发病的中医诊治方法，并对每种疾病都以“思辨导图”总结诊治步骤与要点，以便读者加深理解。

“中医耳鼻咽喉科学”的总论共 4 章，分别介绍耳鼻咽喉与脏腑经络的关系、耳鼻咽喉科常用检查方法、耳鼻咽喉科疾病的辨证方法和中医治法；各论分耳科、鼻科、咽喉科介绍 32 种常见病、多发病的中医诊治方法。

本书内容紧贴临床实际、衷中参西，较为实用。但是，“书不尽言”，随着学科的发展，中医眼耳鼻咽喉科学的理论与临床也在不断更新，我们将不断关注学科发展动态，及时更新相关内容，也希望读者向我们提出意见、建议，以便再版时修改。

General Contents

总目录

Ophthalmology of Traditional Chinese Medicine

中医眼科学

Chief Compiler MAIO Wanhong

Chief Translator Xu Yao

主编 缪晚虹

主译 徐 瑶

Contents

General Introduction

Specific Introduction

目　　录

总　　论

各　　论

General Introduction

总　论

Chapter 1 Relationships between Eyes and Zang-Fu Organs

第1章 眼与脏腑的关系

Section 1 Theory of five wheels

第1节 五轮学说

The theory of five wheels of ophthalmology in traditional Chinese medicine is originated from Chapter 80, On Big Perplexing Questions, *Spiritual Pivot* (Ling Shu): "The Jing (Essential) Qi of five zang organs and six fu organs flows upwards and enters into the eyes, to generate the vision. The organ of vision is called the eyes. The Jing (Essential) Qi of the bones generates the pupil, the Jing (Essential) Qi of the tendons generates the eye black, the Jing (Essential) Qi of the blood generates the blood vessels, the Jing (Essential) Qi of the lung generates the eye white, and that of the muscles generates the eyelids. The Jing (Essential) Qi of tendons, bones, blood and qi travels with the collaterals, to form up the eye system, which belongs to the brain in the upper and reaches to the surface of the nape." The term of "five wheels" was first seen in *Liu Hao's Verses of Standards on Eyes* (Liu Hao Yan Lun Zhun Di Ge) in late Tang Dynasty (618—907). The relationships between the five wheels and five zang or-

中医眼科五轮学说源于《灵枢·大惑论》:"五脏六腑之精气皆上注于目而为之精,精之窠为眼,骨之精为瞳子,筋之精为黑眼,血之精为络,其窠气之精为白眼,肌肉之精为约束,裹撷筋骨血气之精而与脉并为系,上属于脑,后出项中。"五轮之名最早见于晚唐《刘皓眼论准的歌》。而轮脏对应详见于明末医家傅仁宇所著《审视瑶函》卷一"五轮所属论"谓:"……上下眼胞,属乎脾土……脾主肉,故曰肉轮……目又有两锐角,为目大小眦,属心火……心主血,故曰血轮……其内白睛,则属肺金……肺主气,故曰气轮。白睛内之青睛,则属肝木……

gans were illustrated in Volume 1, On Attribution of Five Wheels, *Complete Survey on Ophthalmology* (Shen Shi Yao Han) by Fu Ren-yu, a physician in late Ming Dynasty (1368—1644): "The upper and lower eyelids, attributive to the spleen-earth which dominates the muscles, are so called the muscle wheel. The outer and inner canthi, attributive to the heart-fire which dominates the blood, are so called the blood wheel. The eye white, attributive to the lung-metal which dominates qi, is so called the qi wheel. The eye black, attributive to the liver-wood which dominates the wind, is so called the wind wheel. The pupil, attributive to the kidney-water which dominates the water, is so called the water wheel." It is also said: "The five wheels are activated by the essence of the five zang organs. The so-called wheels mean the motions." It is said in General Introduction to Five Wheels and Eight Contours, *Silver Sea's Essentials* (Yin Hai Jing Wei): "The liver, attributive to the wood and called the wind wheel, dominates the eye black. The heart, attributive to the fire and called the blood wheel, dominates the outer and inner canthi of the eye. The spleen, attributive to the earth and called the muscle wheel, dominates the upper and lower eyelids. The lung, attributive to the metal and called the qi wheel, dominates the eye white. The kidney, attributive to the water and called the water wheel, dominates to the pupil."

肝木主风,故曰风轮;青睛之内一点黑莹者,则为瞳神,属乎肾水……肾主水,故曰水轮。"并曰:"五轮者,皆五脏之精华所发,名之曰轮,其像如车轮,运动之意也。"《银海精微・五轮八廓总论》曰:"肝属木,曰风轮,在眼为乌睛;心属火,曰血轮,在眼为二眦;脾属土,曰肉轮,在眼为上下胞睑;肺属金,曰气轮,在眼为白轮;肾属水,曰水轮,在眼为瞳人。"

The reason why the eyes can see all things clearly and identify different colors, is the nourishment of the Jing (Essential) Qi of five zang organs and six fu organs. It is said in Chapter 80, On Big Perplexing Questions, *Spiritual Pivot* (Ling Shu):

眼之能够明视万物,辨别颜色,是赖五脏六腑精气的滋养,如《灵枢・大惑论》谓"五脏六腑之精气皆上注于目而为之精"。而脏腑功

"The Jing (Essential) Qi of five zang organs and six fu organs flows upwards and enters into the eyes, to generate the vision." Therefore, the dysfunction of zang-fu organs may cause various eye diseases.

能失调则可致眼病。

Section 2 Relationships between eyes and zang-fu organs

第2节 眼与脏腑的关系

1 Relationships between the eyes and the heart and small intestine

1 眼与心和小肠的关系

1.1 The heart dominates the blood and vessels, while all vessels reach the eyes

The heart dominates the blood and vessels of whole body. The blood, promoted by the heart qi, circulates inside the vessels, reaches the whole body and travels upwards to the eyes. Only when they are nourished by the blood, can the eyes maintain the vision.

1.1 心主血脉,诸脉属目

心主全身血脉,脉中血液受心气推动,循环全身,上输于目,目受血养,才能维持视觉。

1.2 The heart houses the Shen (Spirit and Mind), while the eyes are the messenger of the heart

The heart is the house of the Shen (Spirit and Mind). The spirit and mind are dominated by the heart, but manifested in the eyes, which are so called the messenger of the heart. It is said by the ancient physicians: "The heart spirit is manifested in the eyes and called the spiritual light. The kidney-water and spiritual light locate deeply inside the center of pupil, acting to make eyes see all things."

1.2 心主藏神,目为心使

因心为神之舍,精神虽统于心,而外用则在目,故目为心之使。古代医家谓:"心神在目,发为神光,肾水、神光深居瞳神之中,才能明视万物。"

1.3 The relationship between eyes and small intestine

The water and grain are digested in the small

1.3 眼与小肠的关系

水谷经小肠分清别浊,

intestine by its function to separate the clear from the turbid. The clear is transmitted all over the body through the spleen, so the eyes are nourished. Furthermore, the heart and small intestine are exteriorly-interiorly related, so that the normal function of the small intestine is related to the heart and also to the eyes as well.

清者由脾转输全身，从而使目受到滋养。此外，心与小肠相表里，小肠功能是否正常，既关系到心，也影响到眼。

2 Relationships between the eyes and the liver and gallbladder

2 眼与肝和胆的关系

2.1 The liver opens into the eyes

The eyes are the superficial orifice to connect the liver with the external reaction. The essential substance stored in the liver is transmitted to eyes to nourish the eyes, so as to maintain the vision of the eyes.

2.1 肝开窍于目

目为肝与外界联系的窍道。故肝所受藏的精微物质能输送至眼，使眼受到滋养，从而维持其视觉功能。

2.2 The eyes are the superficial orifice of the liver and nourished by the liver blood

It is said in Chapter 10, Birth and Growth of Five Zang Organs, *Essential Questions* (Su Wen): "When the liver is filled with blood, the eyes can see."

2.2 肝受血而能视

目为肝之窍，尤以肝血的濡养为重要，故《素问·五藏生成》曰："肝受血而能视。"

2.3 The liver qi reaches the eyes

The blood and body fluid that supply the eyes are based upon the promoting function of qi. The normal qi activity of human body is closely related to the draining and dispersing function of liver. It is said in Chapter 17, Length of Meridians, *Spiritual Pivot* (Ling Shu): "The liver qi reaches the eyes. If the liver is harmonious, the eyes can differentiate five colors."

2.3 肝气通于目

供给眼部的血液、津液，依赖气的推动，而人体气机是否调畅，又与肝的疏泄功能密切相关，故《灵枢·脉度》曰："肝气通于目，肝和则目能辨五色矣。"

2.4 The Liver Meridian connects with the eye system

Among the twelve regular meridians of human

2.4 肝脉连目系

人体十二经脉中，唯有

body, the Liver Meridian is the only one which travels upwards to connect the eye system directly. The Liver Meridians plays a communicating role between the liver and eyes, to connect the surface with the internal and to circulate qi and blood to the eyes.

肝脉是本经直接上连于目系的。肝脉在眼与肝之间起着沟通表里、联络眼与肝脏、为之运行气血的作用。

2.5 The relationship between the eyes and gallbladder

2.5 眼与胆的关系

The surplus of the liver qi flows into the gallbladder to transform into the essence of gallbladder, the bile. The secretion and excretion of bile is influenced by the draining and dispersing function of the liver. The bile is very important to the eyes. It is said in Chapter 54, Natural Life Span, *Spiritual Pivot* (Ling Shu): "At the age of fifty, the liver qi starts to decline, the liver lobe starts to be thin, the bile starts to decrease, and the vision of eyes starts to be blurred." It is raised a point in *Standards of Diagnosis and Treatment* (Zheng Zhi Zhun Sheng) that the essential bile of gallbladder is accumulated into a kind of spiritual extract to nourish the eye black.

肝之余气溢入于胆，聚而成精，乃为胆汁。胆汁的分泌和排泄，受肝的疏泄功能的影响。胆汁于眼，十分重要。如《灵枢·天年》曰："五十岁，肝气始衰，肝叶始薄，胆汁始减，目始不明。"《证治准绳》进一步提出了胆之精汁积成珠内神膏，膏涵养瞳神之说。

3 Relationships between the eyes and spleen and stomach

3 眼与脾和胃的关系

3.1 The spleen transports the Jing (Essence) Qi upwards to the eyes

3.1 脾输精气，上贯于目

It is said in Chapter 19, On Jade Instruments and True Organ Pulses, *Essential Questions* (Su Wen): The deficiency of spleen "may cause obstruction of nine orifices". It implies that the spleen deficiency may cause eye diseases. The spleen qi flows upwards to transport the essential substances upwards to the eyes, so that the eyes are warmed and nourished by the pure yang and qi and can see things

《素问·玉机真藏论》论脾之虚实曰："其不及，则令人九窍不通。"即包含脾虚能致眼病。脾气上升，才能将精微物质上运于目，目得清阳之气的温养则视物清明。

clearly.

3.2 The spleen controls the blood which nourishes the eyes

The reason why the blood can circulate inside the eye collaterals without spilling over is the controlling and checking function of the spleen qi. If the spleen qi is deficient and loses its controlling and checking function, there can be ocular bleeding.

3.2 脾主统血，血养目窍

血液行于眼络中不外溢，赖于脾气的统摄。若脾气虚衰，失去统摄能力，可引起眼部的出血。

3.3 The spleen dominates the muscles and controls the opening and closing of eyelids

It is said in Chapter 44, On Wei (Flaccidity) Pattern, *Essential Questions* (Su Wen): "The spleen dominates the muscles of whole body." The spleen dominates transportation and transformation, to transport the essence of water and grain to nourish the muscles. If the muscles of eyelids are nourished, they can open and close freely.

3.3 脾主肌肉，睑能开合

《素问・痿论》曰："脾主身之肌肉。"脾主运化水谷之精，以养肌肉。胞睑肌肉得养则开合自如。

3.4 The relationship between the eyes and stomach

The spleen and stomach are exteriorly-interiorly related, as "the acquired basis" of human body. It is said in On Transference and Progression of Deficiency and Excess of Spleen and Stomach, *On Spleen and Stomach* (Pi Wei Lun): "The nine orifices are dominated by the five zang organs. The five zang organs can function normally when they are nourished by the stomach qi." It is also pointed out that "if the stomach qi is deficient, the ears, eyes, mouth and nose are all sick". Furthermore, it is said in Chapter 5, Great Treatise on Yin-Yang Classifications of Natural Phenomena, *Essential Questions* (Su Wen): "The clear yang flows to the orifices in the upper, while the turbid yin flows to the orifices in the lower." The spleen uplifts the

3.4 眼与胃的关系

脾胃互为表里，为"后天之本"。《脾胃论・脾胃虚实传变论》曰："九窍者，五脏主之，五脏皆得胃气乃能通利。"并指出"胃气一虚，耳目口鼻俱为之病"。此外，《素问・阴阳应象大论》曰："清阳出上窍，浊阴出下窍。"脾主升清，胃主降浊，二者升降正常，则清浊分明，浊阴从下窍出，不致上犯清窍。

clear, while the stomach subdues the turbid. If their uplifting and subduing functions are normal, the clear and the turbid can be separated. If the turbid yin flows to the orifices in the lower, it will not attack the clear orifices in the upper.

4 Relationships between the eyes and the lung and large intestine

4 眼与肺和大肠的关系

4.1 The lung is the dominator of qi, and the eyes are brightened if qi is harmonious

4.1 肺为气主,气和目明

The lung collects all the vessels, and it dominates qi of whole body. Qi promotes the blood circulation, so that both qi and blood flow parallel to the whole body and to warm and nourish the eyes. If the lung qi is harmonious, qi and blood circulate smooth, the Jing (Essence) Qi and yang qi of five zang organs and six fu organs may infuse into the eyes, which can see things clearly. If the lung qi is insufficient and fails to nourish the eyes, the vision of eyes becomes blurred.

肺朝百脉,主一身之气,气能推动血行,气血并行于全身,目受其温煦濡养,又肺气调和,气血流畅,五脏六腑精阳之气皆能注入于目,故目视精明。若肺气不足,以致目失所养,则昏暗不明。

4.2 The lung dominates dispersing and descending, so the eye collaterals are unblocked

4.2 肺主宣降,眼络通畅

If the dispersing and descending function of lung is normal, the blood vessels are unblocked, and the Wei (Defensive) Qi and body fluid can warm, moisturize and nourish the eyes. If the Wei (Defensive) Qi is normal and can protect the body surface, the turbid subdues and does not attack the upper, so the eyes are not sick.

肺之宣降正常,则血脉通利,目得卫气和津液的温煦濡养,卫外有权,且浊物下降,不得上犯,目不易病。

4.3 The relationship between the eyes and large intestine

4.3 眼与大肠关系

The small intestine sends the turbid downwards to the large intestine and transform the turbid into

小肠浊物下注大肠,化为粪便,有赖肺气肃降,以推

feces. The large intestine relies on the descending function of lung qi to discharge the feces. If there is accumulated heat in large intestine, it is blocked and the descending function of lung qi is disturbed, leading to the eye diseases due to stagnation of qi, blood or body fluid at the eyes.

送其排出体外。若大肠积热，腑气不通，影响肺之肃降，导致有眼部因气血津液壅滞而发病。

5 Relationships between the eyes and the kidney and bladder

5 眼与肾和膀胱的关系

5.1 If the kidney essence is sufficient, the eyes can see things clearly

5.1 肾精充足，目视精明

The reason why the eyes can see things is the moisture and nourishment of the Jing (Essence) Qi. It is said in Chapter 1, On Heavenly Truth of Ancient Times, *Essential Questions* (Su Wen): "The kidney dominates the water and stores the Jing (Essence) Qi of five zang organs and six fu organs." Therefore, the eyes are closely related to the kidney essence.

眼之所以能视物，有赖于充足的精气濡养。《素问·上古天真论》强调"肾者主水，受五脏六腑之精气而藏之"，故眼与肾精关系密切。

5.2 The kidney produces the brain marrows, and the eye system belongs to the brain

5.2 肾生脑髓，目系属脑

It is said in traditional Chinese medicine that "the kidney produces marrows", and "the brain is termed as the sea of marrows". Furthermore, the eye system "belongs to the brain in the upper and reaches to the surface of the nape". The brain marrow is transformed from the kidney essence, while the eye system is connected with the brain, so that the eyes are related to the kidney's functions in storing essence and in producing brain marrow. If the kidney essence is sufficient, the sea of marrow is full and rich, so the eyes are flashing. If the kidney essence is deficient, the sea of marrow is empty, so as to cause dizziness, tinnitus and poor vision.

中医学有"肾生骨髓""脑为髓海"之说，而且目系"上输于脑。后出于项中"。脑和髓异名同类，都由肾精生化，而目之系连于脑，也就与肾藏精生脑髓功能相关。故肾精充沛，髓海丰满，则目光敏锐，若肾精亏虚，髓海不足则脑转耳鸣，目无所见。

5.3 The kidney dominates the body fluid, which flows upward to moisturize the eyes

The kidney dominates the body fluid, and "the body fluid of all five zang organs and six fu organs flows upwards to permeate into the eyes". The body fluid flows to the eyes to transform into the tear which moisturizes the borders of eyes, and to transform into the spiritual water which nourishes the eyes.

5.3 肾主津液,上润于目

肾主津液,"五脏六腑之津液,尽上渗于目"。津液在目化为泪,则为目外润泽之水,化为神水,则为眼内充养之液。

5.4 The relationship between the eyes and bladder

The transforming function of the bladder qi relies on the sufficient kidney qi. If the kidney qi is insufficient, or if the damp-heat is accumulated in the bladder, the transforming function of the bladder qi is disturbed, leading to retention of water. The pathogenic water-damp may flow upwards to eyes to cause eye diseases. Furthermore, the bladder is attributive to the Taiyang Meridians, which dominate the body surface. So the attack of the exogenous pathogens on the body surface may cause eye diseases.

5.4 眼与膀胱关系

膀胱的气化作用主要取决于肾气的盛衰。若肾气不足,或湿热蕴结,引起膀胱气化失常,水液潴留,可致水湿上泛于目。此外,膀胱属太阳经,主一身之表,易遭外邪侵袭,常引起眼病。

6 Relationships between the eyes and the triple energizer

The triple energizer, an isolate fu organ, acts as a passage to circulate the Yuan (Primary) Qi and essence of water and grain and functions to dredge the water passage. If the triple energizer's function is disturbed, it may cause the disturbance or dysfunction in digesting, absorbing, distributing and discharging the essence of water and grain, so that the eyes are not moisturized and nourished. If the water passage of triple energizer is blocked, there

6 眼与三焦的关系

三焦为孤腑,主通行元气与运行水谷,疏通水道的功能。若三焦功能失常,致使水谷精微之消化、吸收、输布、排泄紊乱或发生障碍,则目失濡养。若三焦水道不利,致使水液潴留,水液上犯于目,引起眼病。

can be retention of water. The pathogenic water-damp may flow upwards to eyes to cause eye diseases.

The relationships between the eyes and the five zang organs and six fu organs are distinctive with different degrees of closeness. These relationships are mutually associated and mutually dependent in physiology, and mutually influenced and mutually transferring and progressing in pathology.

眼与五脏六腑之间的关系,各自具备特点,其密切程度不同,他们在生理上是相互协调,相互依存的;在病理上是相互影响,相互传变的。

Chapter 2 Etiology and Pathogenesis in Ophthalmology

第2章 眼病的病因病机

Etiology refers to all factors to cause diseases in both internal and external environments. Pathogenesis refers to the important method in traditional Chinese medicine to understand ophthalmologic diseases, by exploring the local or overall etiological regulations in the whole pathogenic process and their mutual relationships and transferences.

病因是指一切内外环境中可以导致疾病的原因，探索病因在致病过程中局部或整体出现的规律，及其相互间的联系和转化是中医认识眼科疾病的重要方法。

Section 1 Exogenous factors

第1节 外因

1 Six Exogenous Pathogens

1 六淫

1.1 Pathogenic wind

1.1 风淫

(1) The wind is featured by lightness and flying and easy to attack the yang parts. The pathogenic wind has the characteristics of ascending, dispersing, upward moving and outward moving, and of attacking the eyes. It is the most common exogenous factor of circumocular diseases.

（1）风性轻扬、易袭阳位：风邪具有升发、向上、向外的特点，易犯目窍，在外障眼病中为最常见病因。

(2) The wind is featured by constantly moving and rapidly changing, so the eye diseases are characterized by quick onset and fast change.

（2）善行而速变：引起眼病发病迅速、变化快。

(3) The wind is featured by leading other pathogens, such as cold, heat, summer-heat, damp,

（3）风性裹挟：风邪常与其他病因如寒、热、暑、湿、

dryness and fire, to cause diseases. The eye diseases caused by singular pathogenic wind are rare.

燥、火相合为患，风邪单独致病者较少。

1.2 Pathogenic fire

1.2 火淫

(1) The fire is featured by scorching and flaming upwards. As a yang pathogen, the pathogenic fire is characterized by ascending and rising, and rushing the head and eyes to cause eye diseases. It is said in *Confucians' Duties for Their Patients* (Ru Men Qin Shi): "The eyes are not sick without fire."

(1) 火性炎上：火为阳邪，其性升腾，易上冲头目，引起眼疾。《儒门事亲》中有“目不因火则不病”的说法。

(2) The fire is featured by urgency. The eye diseases caused by the pathogenic fire are characterized by quick onset and severe reaction, manifested by local redness, swelling, hotness, pain, ulcer and purulence of local tissues.

(2) 火性急迫：病势凶猛，外障眼病起病急、反应重，常造成局部组织红肿热痛，酿脓溃破。

(3) The fire is easy to burn and damage the vessels. The pathogenic fire makes the blood flowing recklessly, so the blood spills over the vessels to cause hemorrhagic eye diseases.

(3) 易迫血妄行，血溢脉外造成出血性眼病。

(4) The fire is easy to consume the body fluid. In the late stage of eye diseases caused by pathogenic fire, there are the manifestations of body fluid consumption.

(4) 眼病后期，常表现为津液耗损的现象。

1.3 Pathogenic damp

1.3 湿淫

(1) The damp is featured by stickiness and stagnation. The pathogenic damp attacks the eyes to cause diseases, which are long and lingering in progression with repeated attacks.

(1) 湿性黏滞：湿邪侵犯目窍犯病，病程缠绵，反复发作。

(2) The pathogenic damp is dirty and sticky. The eye diseases caused by pathogenic damp are characterized by erosion and dirtiness of local tissues.

(2) 湿邪污腻：湿邪为患，局部组织常有糜烂污浊感。

(3) The damp is a yin pathogen, easy to block the qi activity. The pathogenic damp disturbs the ascending and descending of qi activity at eyes,

(3) 湿为阴邪，易阻遏气机：可致眼部气机升降失调，经脉不畅。

leading to obstruction of local meridians.

1.4 Pathogenic cold

(1) The cold is featured by congealing and stagnation. The pathogenic cold is a yin pathogen to cause the eye diseases with the manifestations of preference for warmth and pressure, dull pain and thin and clear tears.

(2) The cold is featured by constriction and contraction. The pathogenic cold causes contraction of tendons and vessels and stays between meridians and collaterals and between tendons and muscles, leading to spasm of tendons and vessels. The vessels of the eyes are very thin, so the pathogenic cold attacks the vessels to cause redness, purple and distension of vessels.

1.5 Pathogenic summer-heat

(1) The summer-heat is a yang pathogen. As a seasonal pathogen in summer, the pathogenic summer-heat causes the eye diseases with yang-heat symptoms at eyes.

(2) The summer-heat often attacks body together with the damp. The pathogenic summer-heat leads the pathogenic damp to cause diseases.

1.6 Pathogenic dryness

The dryness is featured by consuming the body fluid. The pathogenic dryness often causes the eye diseases with symptoms of dryness.

2 Li (Epidemic) Qi

The physicians in ancient times regarded the infectious diseases occurring at the same time with similar symptoms for men and women of all ages as the diseases caused by the Li (Epidemic) Qi. The Li (Epidemic) Qi is characterized by the sudden onset

1.4 寒淫

（1）寒性凝滞：为阴邪，病患喜暖喜按，隐隐作痛，泪液清稀。

（2）筋脉不舒，脉络凝滞，客于经络筋肉之间，常引起筋脉挛急。眼部血管脉络较细，寒邪凝滞脉络常可致赤脉紫胀。

1.5 暑淫

（1）暑为阳邪：暑为夏令主气，眼部多出现阳热症状。

（2）暑多挟湿：常挟湿共为患。

1.6 燥淫

燥易耗伤津液：常与眼部干燥性疾病有关。

2 疠气

疠气，又称“戾气”“疫疠”“天行”“时气”等。古医将同期患病，形症相同，病状相似，不分老幼，触之即染视为疠气所致。戾气致病迅

of severe and risky diseases with similar symptoms, high infection and strong epidemic. It is the major pathogenic factor of infectious diseases in ophthalmology, such as acute infectious conjunctivitis, acute catarrhal and allergic conjunctivitis, etc.

速、来势凶猛、流行广泛，是眼科传染性疾病，如天行赤眼、暴风客热等的主要发病原因。

3 Traumatic injury

The eyes are the visual organs which are fine in structure, fragile and sensitive, so the eye is easy to be injured by an outside foreign body. In the mild injury of eye by an outside foreign body, such as sand, dust, etc., the skin, muscle, tendon or vessel of eye may be injured, to cause injury of eye white or injury of eye black. In the severe injury of eye by an outside foreign body, such as blunt power, sharp instrument, etc., the optic bulb may be injured, to cause impairment of visual acuity, even blindness. After the eye is injured, there can be qi stagnation and blood stasis of the eye, or the attack of pathogenic wind, heat or toxin, to make the eye injury more serious. If the eyeball is injured, the healthy eye can be influenced, to cause sympathetic ophthalmia.

3 外伤

眼为构造精细、脆弱敏感的器官，极易受外界损伤。眼被外物所伤，轻者皮肉筋脉损伤，如沙尘、异物入目造成白睛、黑睛破损；重则血络神明破损，如钝力、锐器伤目造成晶珠破损，严重损害视力，甚至失明，且受损者皆有气血瘀滞之患，或并受风热邪毒，乘隙害目变化尤堪。眼珠破损者甚或影响健眼，出现交感性眼炎。

Section 2 Endogenous factors

第2节 内因

1 Seven emotional factors

The seven emotional factors are joy, anger, melancholy, worry, grief, fear and fright. The seven emotions are the normal emotional responses of the body to the external stimuli, pertaining to the normal psychological activities, and do not normally cause diseases. The abrupt, severe or continuous oc-

1 七情

人之七情，喜、怒、忧、思、悲、恐、惊，本为个体正常的精神活动，持续强烈的刺激超出个体所能调适的范围，致脏腑气机失衡，气血津液逆乱而致病。正所谓“衡

curring emotional stimuli, however, which surpass the regulative adaptability of the human body, will cause the disturbance of qi activities, the disharmony between yin and yang and between qi and blood of zang-fu organs, resulting in the occurrence of diseases. It is said that "the harmony makes healthy, while the disturbance leads to sick". The eye diseases caused by the seven emotional factors are often theintraocular diseases. The impaired qi activity, obstruction of vessels and collaterals, or blockage of the clear apertures may cause the eye diseases with sudden decrease of vision, such as glaucoma, sudden blindness, etc. The unsmooth flow of qi and blood or dysfunction of zang-fu organs may make the essence of zang-fu organs fail to go upwards to the eyes, which lose the nourishment, to cause the eye diseases with gradual decrease of vision, such as glaucoma, bluish glaucoma, etc.

则健，乱则病”。七情所致眼病以内障眼病为多见。气机运行不利，脉络瘀滞，清窍闭塞，产生视力急剧下降的眼病，如绿风内障、络阻暴盲；气血不畅，脏腑功能失调，五脏六腑精华无法上乘于目，目失濡养，日渐昏矇，如青盲、青风内障等。

2 Improper diet

The intake of unclean food, the intake of inordinate food or overindulgence in particular foods may damage the spleen and stomach, which fail to transport and transform qi and blood, so the eyes lose the nourishment of qi and blood. The over-full state of food intake may cause food retention in intestines and stomach, becoming damp-heat which causes the eye diseases with redness or ulcer of eyes. The over-hungry state of food intake may cause spleen and stomach deficiency and malnutrition, so as to lead to dystrophic eye diseases.

2 饮食失调

饮食不洁不节、偏嗜，致脾胃受损，气血生化无源，目失所养。饮食过饱则食滞肠胃，郁而化热，纵生湿热性眼病如睑眩赤烂。少食、偏食则营养不良，脾胃虚弱，可致营养不良性眼病。

3 Overstrain and fatigue

Overstrain includes eye overstrain, heart overstrain, spiritual overstrain, sexual overstrain, etc.

3 劳倦

包括眼劳、心劳、神劳、房劳过度等。劳倦过度可导

Overstrain and fatigue may consume qi and blood to cause dysfunction of zang-fu organs, such as the liver blood deficiency, the liver and kidney insufficiency, the disharmony between heart and kidney, etc., further leading to the eye diseases as blurring of vision, dry sensation of eyes, etc.

致气血耗伤、肝血亏耗、肝肾不足、心肾不交等脏腑功能紊乱，从而引发视瞻昏渺、目涩不舒等眼症。

Section 3 Miscellaneous factors

第3节 不内外因

The senile factor, the genetic factor, the congenital eye diseases and the drug-induced eye disease all pertain to the category of miscellaneous factors. Retinal pigment degeneration, viviparous cataract, farsightedness, high myopia and astigmatism are all closely related to the insufficiency of natural endowment. From the age of fifty, qi and blood start to be deficient gradually, and the eye diseases such as presbyopia, cataract, macular degeneration, etc. occur. The application some medicines for long time, such as steroids, quinine, etc. may cause the eye diseases, as cataract, bluish glaucoma, glaucoma, etc.

衰老、遗传、与生俱来之眼病、药物所致眼病等都归于不内外因中。高风雀目、胎生内障、远视、高度近视、散光皆与先天禀赋不足密切相关。人至五十脏气始衰，气血渐弱如花眼，圆翳内障、黄斑退变均将不期而至。长期使用某些药物，如激素、奎宁等可造成圆翳内障、青风内障、青盲等目系疾病。

According to the philosophy of pattern identification originating from traditional Chinese medicine, the mechanism of occurrence, development, transference and progression of the diseases is called pathogenesis. The pathogenesis of ophthalmologic diseases in traditional Chinese medicine refers to disharmony of qi and blood, of yin and yang and of zang-fu organs which lead to the eye diseases, and then further influence their development and progression under the roles of exogenous factors, en-

源于中医学理论体系的辨证思维阐述疾病发生发展变化转归的机理称为病机，中医眼科的病机是指在外因、内因、不内外因作用下气血阴阳、脏腑功能的失调导致的眼疾，进而影响其发展、变化的过程。所谓“正气存内，邪不可干”“邪之所凑，其气必虚”。揭示了疾病发生

dogenous factors and miscellaneous factors. It is said that "if the Zheng (Anti-Pathogenic) Qi exists inside, the Xie (Pathogenic) Qi will never attack", and that "why the Xie (Pathogenic) Qi invades, it is because the Zheng (Anti-Pathogenic) Qi is deficient". These quotations reveal the nature of the disease occurrence. Only when the human body is abnormal, can any of the pathogenic factors cause diseases. The occurrence and development of the ophthalmologic diseases are determined by the result of the conflict between the Zheng (Anti-Pathogenic) Qi and Xie (Pathogenic) Qi. The causes of pathological changes are nothing more than functional disharmony of qi and blood, of body fluid, of meridians and collaterals, or of zang-fu organs, leading to disequilibrium of yin and yang, so as to cause various diseases of eyes.

的本质:任何致病原因只有在人体机能失常的情况下才能致病。眼病的发生发展取决于正邪双方的斗争结果,造成的病理变化不外乎气血、津液、经络、脏腑功能失调,阴阳失衡,从而表现于眼部的各种病证。

Chapter 3 Essentials of Diagnostics in Ophthalmology

第3章 诊断概要

Section 1 Four diagnostic methods in ophthalmology

第1节 眼科四诊

The four diagnostic methods in ophthalmology are inspection, auscultation-olfaction, inquiry and palpation in traditional Chinese medicine, but the inquiry and inspection are the major methods.

眼科四诊应遵循中医望闻问切,但以问诊、望诊为主。

1 Inquiry

1 问诊

As for the patients of ophthalmologic diseases, besides the symptoms of whole body, it is stressed on the inquiry of the symptoms related to eyes.

对于眼科患者,除询问其全身症状外,应着重问眼部症状。

1.1 Blurring of vision

1.1 视物模糊

Blurring of vision refers to failure to see clearly in the distance, or failure to see clearly in the near, or both. Blurring of vision is one of the most common causes of consultation. In the inquiry, it is necessary to pay attention to the time, degree and status of blurred vision and then to make a record, such as sudden occurrence, occasional occurrence, transient blurred vision, continuous blurred vision, fluctuant blurred vision, or progressive blurred vision, and any other secondary symptoms which may

视物模糊是指看远不得,或看近不清,或兼而有之。视物模糊是最常见的就诊原因之一,临床医生在接诊时通过询问,一定要关注视物模糊的时间与程度、状态并记录,比如:突然发现、偶尔发现、短暂模糊、持续模糊、波动模糊、渐进模糊;有无兼症作为临证提供鉴别的

provide basis for differential diagnosis. Generally, the sudden occurrence indicates that the course of disease is short and the case history is traceable, the occasional occurrence indicates that the course of disease is unpredictable, and transient blurred vision refers that the vision can be recovered in 24 hours.

依据。通常突然发现，提示疾病病程短，可追踪病史；偶然发现，提示病程的不可预知性；短暂视物模糊指可在24小时内恢复。

1.2 Black shadow waving before eyes

The black shadow waving before eyes refers that there are black shadows of different shapes are moving irregularly before eyes along with the eye movement. This symptom is more obvious under the bright light. For example, the cloud and mist in the nature can be thick or thin, and changeable. There are many vivid descriptions, such as "cloud moving before eyes", "flowering vision when standing up", or "sparks flying before eyes". The essential cause is the decrease of vitreous opacity inside the eye cavity, so that the projection is formed on the retina under the proper light condition. The symptom is gradually worsened along with age. Generally, it is physiological, but the fundus examination with mydriasis is needed if the black shadow occurs suddenly or increases obviously. It indicates the pathological change of the vitreous body. The common causes are posterior vitreous detachment, vitreous hemorrhage, uveitis and retinitis. It can also be the premonitory symptom of retinal tear and retinal detachment. Therefore, it is necessary to great attention in the exclusive diagnosis, so as to avoid the misdiagnosis.

1.2 眼前黑影飘动

眼前黑影飘动是指眼前有形态各异的黑影随着眼球的运动而发生无规律的移动。通常在明亮的光线下特别明显，如自然界的云雾，可浓可淡，变化多端，中医文献上有很多形象的描述"云雾移睛""坐起生花""萤星满目"。本质上是因为眼球腔内的玻璃体的透明度下降，在适度的光照条件下在视网膜上形成的投影，一般随着年龄增长会逐步加重，大部分属于生理性的，但是黑影突然发生或明显增多时提示玻璃体出现病理性改变，需要散瞳做眼底详查，最常见的原因是：玻璃体后脱离、玻璃体出血、葡萄膜炎、视网膜炎，也可以是视网膜撕裂、视网膜脱离的前驱症状。因而临证时要有高度的警觉性，需要一一加以排除，以免误诊。

1.3 Rainbow vision

The rainbow vision refers to the rainbow ring formed periphery when the patient fixes his gaze on

1.3 虹视

虹视是指患者在注视光源时外围形成的彩虹环。其

the light source. The cause is the diffraction effect of the eye ocular media (the eye black and the crystalline lens) on the light entering in the eye. It indicates the possibility of glaucoma. Due to the high intraocular pressure, edema occurs at the pupil which is bright originally, so as to make the light diffraction, leading to the symptom. In a fewer cases, the discharge of the eye black surface may also cause the symptom, so it is identified by wiping away the discharge. In some cases of cataract of early stage, the irregular turbidity of the crystalline lens may also cause this phenomenon. It is necessary to make the differential diagnosis.

原因是眼的主要屈光介质(黑睛、晶珠)对射入眼内光线的衍射效应,特征性地提示青光眼可能。原本透亮的黑睛在高眼压的作用下出现水肿而使光线出现了衍射而形成的症状,少部分黑睛表面的分泌物也可以造成,拭去分泌物可作鉴别,另有部分早期白内障,晶珠的不规则混浊也可以出现这个现象。临证需要假以识别。

1.4 Double vision

The double vision refers to phenomenon of "two objects occurring when watching one". Some of the patients describe "blurring of vision" as "double vision", so it is necessary to confirm the examination by using a pen or a finger. It can be known that if the double vision occurring in one eye or both eyes by covering one eye. The double vision of one eye occurs in refractive errors and senile cataract. The double vision of both eyes indicates ocular muscle motor incoordination, such as convergence insufficiency, ophthalmoplegia, orbital space-occupying lesion, thyroid dysfunction, or the sixth, the third or the fourth cranial nerve paralysis. It is necessary to make the differential diagnosis.

1.4 复视

复视是指"视一为二"的现象。部分患者会把视物模糊现象描述为复视,在临证时需要医生加以确认,如用笔或手指测试。遮盖一眼即可分辨复视发生在单眼还是双眼。单眼的复视在屈光不正、圆翳内障过程中会出现,双眼的复视提示眼肌运动的不协调,如:辐辏不足、眼肌麻痹、眼眶占位、甲状腺功能异常;或者第 6、第 3、第 4 脑神经麻痹。需要临床医师逐一排查。

1.5 Multiple-shadow vision

It refers the phenomenon that the image does not form a single focus on the retina when watching an object, occurring in refractive errors, senile cataract and retinal diseases, or in functional injury of cerebral visual cortex.

1.5 视物多影

视物时影像在视网膜上未形成单一焦点,出现多影,在屈光不正、圆翳内障、视网膜病变中可出现,也可因大脑视皮层功能受损导致。

1.6 Distorted vision

The distorted vision refers to phenomenon of "a bent object occurring when watching a straight one". It can be found in the early stage of visual change for those whose visual changes are more sensitive. The cause of the symptom is the morphological change due to the abnormal array of the macular cells in the visual sensitive area, leading to imaging abnormalities, such as macular edema, exudation, hemorrhage, macular detachment, macular holes, vitreomacular traction syndrome, epiretinal membrane, retinal or choroid neovascularization, the big drusen at pigment epithelium layer retina (retinal drusen, a colloid transparent body, a kind of allergic disease happened at the choroid semisolid membrane, caused by the abnormal deposition of metabolic product of retinal epithelial cells on the semisolid membrane). It can also happen in retinal detachment surgery, because the reset retina has not completely repaired morphologically. It is necessary to distinguish the complaint of line tilt occurring in some people with high astigmatism.

1.6 视物变形

视物变形是指"视直为曲"的现象。对视觉改变较为敏锐的人,可以在视觉变化的早期发现,原因在于视觉敏感区的黄斑部细胞排列异常形成形态学上的改变而导致成像的异常。如:黄斑水肿、渗出、出血以及黄斑脱离、黄斑孔、玻璃体黄斑牵引综合征、黄斑前膜以及黄斑部视网膜内或脉络膜新生血管,视网膜色素上皮层大的Drusen(玻璃膜疣,是胶样或透明的小体,是一种发生在脉络膜玻璃膜的一种变性疾病,是视网膜上皮细胞代谢产物在玻璃膜上的异常沉积所致)。视网膜脱离术后因为复位的视网膜在形态学上尚未完全修复也可发生。而部分高度散光的人所出现的线条倾斜的主诉需要加以鉴别。

1.7 Flashing-light sensation

The flashing-light sensation refers to a lightning light that transiently flash over eyes of the patient. Such a phenomenon was described in the ancient classics of traditional Chinese medicine as "heavenly light appearing automatically". The cause is that the retinal visual cells are stimulated by vitreous body traction. In clinical diagnosis, it is necessary to take the mydriasis examination, so as to confirm if the retinal tear holes exist. If the posterior vitreous de-

1.7 闪光感

闪光感是指患者感觉眼前闪电样的亮光短暂掠过,中医古籍把这种无法解释的现象喻为"神光自现"。原因在于视网膜密布的感光细胞受到玻璃体牵拉的刺激,临证时需要引起重视并散瞳详查有无视网膜撕裂孔的存在,存在玻璃体后脱离则需

tachment exists, it is advisable to tell the patient to decrease strenuous exercise and to take a follow-up visit all times.

要告诫患者减少剧烈活动并及时随访。

1.8 Night blindness

It refers to the vision decrease in the dark environment, or different vision from normal people (prolonged dark adaptation). The rod cells around the retina are responsible for the scotopic vision, so the symptom is caused by the rod cell injury in those with high myopia, glaucoma, retinal pigment degeneration, etc.

1.8 夜盲

夜盲是指在暗环境下视力下降,或者异于正常人(暗适应延长)。因视网膜周边的视杆细胞负责暗视力,而高度近视、青光眼、视网膜色素变性等患者周边视细胞受损所致。

1.9 Discomfort

It refers to a kind strange sensation that is not comfortable but cannot be described precisely. It indicates the circumocular diseases, often accompanied by other symptoms, so it is advisable to ask some accompanied symptoms, so as to judge the cause.

1.9 眼不适

眼不适是指眼不舒服又不能准确描述的轻微异样感,提示外障眼病。通常会伴随其他症状,临证时要询问一些伴随症状以判断原因。

1.10 Itching

It refers to the itching sensation at the eyelid or inner eyelid, a common symptom of the circumocular diseases, which caused by the invasion of pathogenic wind. Itching with pain afterwards pertains to the excess pattern, caused by pathogenic wind leading fire to attack. Sporadic itching without accompanied symptoms pertains to the deficiency pattern. Intolerable itching with accompanied symptoms indicates allergic conjunctivitis, vernal conjunctivitis, palpebral dermatitis, palpebral allergy, insect-bites on eyelid or process of wound healing.

1.10 痒

痒是指眼胞睑皮层或内层的瘙痒感觉,属外障眼病最常见症状,中医学认为因风邪侵袭所致。可先痒后痛,风携火邪多为实证;若忽痒而无兼症为虚;若奇痒难忍必有兼症,提示为过敏性结膜炎、春季卡他性结膜炎、眼睑皮炎、眼睑过敏、眼睑虫咬,伤口愈合中也可出现瘙痒。

1.11 Foreign-body sensation

It refers that the patient feels some foreign body inside the eye, described as "blockage and dryness" in traditional Chinese medicine. It happens in one eye or both eyes, a symptom occurring in the

1.11 异物感

异物感是指患者感觉眼内有异物,中医学有"碜涩"的描述,可发于单眼或双眼,结膜炎症、眼结膜囊内异物

circumocular diseases, such as conjunctivitis, foreign body or stone in eye conjunctival sac, trichiasis, blockage of meibomian gland, injury of corneal epithelium, xerophthalmia, etc.

或结石、倒睫、睑板腺阻塞、角膜上皮受损、干眼症等外障眼病都有类似症状。

1.12 Photophobia

It refers that the patient feels the light is dazzling and cannot open the eyes at ease. It indicates stimulation of cornea or ciliary muscle, such as keratitis, iridocyclitis, glaucoma, traumatic injury or postoperation.

1.12 畏光

畏光是指自觉光线刺眼，不能从容睁眼。提示角膜、睫状肌受刺激，如角膜炎、虹膜睫状体炎、青光眼、外伤或手术后。

1.13 Lacrimation

It refers to the increase of tear secretion due to infectious stimulation in circumocular diseases. In traditional Chinese medicine, "hot tear as water" pertains to pathogenic heat attacking eyes, often accompanied by other symptoms. Watery tear in infants and children without other symptoms pertains to blockage of lower portion of nasolacrimal duct or congenital glaucoma. "Tear dropping now and then" or "tear dropping in wind" occurring in old people pertains to the deficiency pattern. It is necessary to identify lacrimal point obstruction, lower eyelid flabby, facial paralysis, obstruction of lacrimal duct, etc. Transient lacrimation may occur in lacrimal gland lesions and traumatic injury.

1.13 流泪

外障眼病时因炎症刺激使泪液分泌增加，中医学以“热泪如汤”名之，属邪热犯目，必兼有他症；婴幼儿无恙而泪多为鼻泪管下端膜闭或先天性青光眼；老年者久现“不时泪下”或“迎风泪出”以虚证辨之，需分辨泪点闭塞、下胞睑松弛、面瘫、泪道阻塞等；泪腺病变、外伤也可一过性流泪。

1.14 Heavy eyelids

It refers to the tired eyelids, failure to open eyes for long time and preference for closing eyes all the time. It occurs in the circumocular diseases, such as visual fatigue, eyelid spasm, myasthenia gravis, trachoma, vesiculated dermatitis of eyelid, etc., accompanied by other symptoms.

1.14 眼睑沉重

眼睑沉重指胞睑困乏，不能长久睁开，总想闭合的证候。可见于视疲劳、胞睑痉挛、重症肌无力、椒疮、风赤疮痍等外障眼病。

1.15 Visual fatigue

It refers to the sensation of soreness, distension

1.15 视疲劳

视疲劳指使用目力后感

and discomfort after using eyes, accompanied by supraorbital pain, unwilling to watch things for long time and will be improved after rest. The essential cause is over-tesion and dysregulation occurring when the ocular muscle and extraocular muscle are mutually assisting to watch things. It often occurs after watching at a near distance for long time. In the application of eyes at a near distance, the ocular muscle is to regulate the focus and the extraocular muscle is to assist to set convergence. The symptom occurs in those with refractive errors or merging disturbance.

觉酸胀不适，同时伴有眉棱骨痛，不愿长久视物，休息后有所好转。本质是由于眼内、外肌在协助视物时出现的过度紧张和调节不济。多发生在近距离久视之后。近距离用眼时眼内肌需要调节聚焦，眼外肌需要协同集合辐辏。有屈光不正及(或)融合障碍者即可出现症状。

1.16 Eye pain

It may occur in both the circumocular and intraocular diseases. The eyelid pain occurs in the circumocular diseases, such as hordeolum, erysipelas of eyelid, dacryocystitis and vesiculated dermatitis of eyelid. The orbital pain occurs in orbital abscess, orbital space-occupying lesions, supraorbital neuralgia and paranasal sinusitis. The eyeball pain occurs in eye black injury or infection, glaucoma and contracted pupil. The oculomotor pain often indicates optic nerve disease or extraocular muscle disease. In traditional Chinese medicine, it is advisable to determine the deficiency or excess pattern according to the degrees of pain. The severe pain pertains to the excess pattern, while the mild pain to the deficiency pattern. The pain which is worsened by pressure pertains to the excess of Xie (Pathogenic) Qi, while the pain which is relieved by pressure to the deficiency of Zheng (Anti-Pathogenic) Qi. Furthermore, it is described in the ancient classics that the nature of pain determines yin or yang, the position of pain determines the meridian, and the accompa-

1.16 目痛

内外障眼病均可出现。胞睑疼痛见于外障眼病，如麦粒肿、眼丹、漏睛、风赤疮痍；眼眶疼痛见于眼眶脓肿、占位、眶神经痛、副鼻窦炎症；眼珠疼痛见于黑睛损伤或炎症，绿风内障，瞳神紧小；眼球转动疼痛常提示视神经或眼外肌疾病。中医临床以疼痛轻重定虚实：剧痛为实、缓痛为虚；拒按为邪实、喜按为正虚；古籍有以疼痛性质定阴阳，以疼痛部位定经络，以伴随症状定脏腑。

nied symptoms determine the zang-fu organs.

1.17 Headache

It is necessary to confirm if the headache is of eye diseases. The headache caused by eye diseases are featured by ① eye pain first inducing headache, such as in the attack of glaucoma when the continuous high intraocular pressure causes headache; ② application of eyes inducing headache, often related to using eyes at a near distance. It is necessary to know the details of the patient's age, life habit, application of eyes in job, frequency and time of headache occurrence, and to apply the refractive adjustment examination, so as to confirm the cause.

1.18 Dizziness

It refers to the sensation of outside object rotation which causes the failure to open eyes. The ocular dizziness is more obvious in double vision due to external ophthalmoplegia, or in disharmony of internal and external rotators. It is featured by shielding one eye to relieve the symptom.

2 Inspection

Inspection in ophthalmology includes the observation by the physician's naked eyes and the observation by equipments, such as microscopy. The former is introduced in this section, while the latter is introduced in Section 3 of this chapter.

2.1 Eye discharge

It is the most common symptom in inflammation of eye white. The watery discharge indicates viral infection, sticky discharge indicates allergy, and purulent discharge indicates bacterial infection. In traditional Chinese medicine, it is to identify the discharge into the pathogenic wind, pathogenic heat

1.17 头痛

临证需要确认是否眼源性，由眼部疾病引发的头痛需符合以下特点：先眼痛后引发头痛，如青光眼发作时因持续的高眼压导致头痛；用眼后诱发头痛，通常与近距离使用目力有关，需详细了解患者年龄，生活、工作用眼状态，以及眼痛出现的频率、时间，辅助屈光调节的检查方可确定原因。

1.18 眩晕

眩晕是指感觉外界物体旋转而不敢睁眼的状态。眼源性眩晕在眼外肌麻痹导致的复视尤其是内外旋肌失衡时尤其明显，遮挡一眼即缓解为其特征。

2 望诊

眼科望诊包括通过医师的肉眼观察和借助显微镜等设备观察两大部分，本节仅介绍前者，后者见本章第 3 节。

2.1 眼分泌物

眼分泌物为白睛炎症的最常见症状，水样分泌物提示病毒感染；黏性分泌物提示过敏性；脓性分泌物提示细菌性感染。中医学对分泌物的稀稠性状依次辨识为风

and pathogenic fire according to the thickness and nature of discharge.

邪、热邪、火邪。

2.2 Redness of eye

It refers to the redness of eye white, as the most major symptom in the circumocular diseases. There are also accompanied symptoms except subconjunctival hemorrhage. It is necessary to inquire the length of the disease course (to determine if the disease is acute, or chronic, or lacunar), the location of redness of eye (to determine if it is localized or diffuse), the nature of the accompanied discharge, if there is pain or not, accompanied other discomforts (sharp-stabbing pain, soreness and distension, itching, dryness, burning-heat, or foreign body sensation), and if the vision decreases or not. In children, it is mostly the symptom of inflammation of eye white. In young people, the acute and painless redness of eye mostly pertains to inflammation of eye white and is identified according to the features of discharge. Redness and itching of eye are mostly of allergy. In old people, slight redness and discomfort of eyes are mostly of ocular surface problems, such as xerophthalmia, meibomian glad dysfunction, conjunctivochalasis, etc. It is necessary in diagnosis of painful redness of eye to exclude eye black disease or pupil disease. Usually the eye black disease or pupil disease is accompanied by visual disturbance. In the patient of hyperthyroidism, there can be redness of eye and exophthalmos.

2.2 眼红

眼红是指白睛发红，属外障眼病中最主要的症状，除外球结膜下出血都会有伴随症状。需要询问病程的长短（确定急性或慢性；时有时无为间隙性）；眼红的位置（局限的或弥漫的）；伴随的分泌物状态；有无疼痛；伴随的其他不适（刺痛、酸胀、瘙痒、干涩、灼热、异物感）视力是否下降等对眼红进行逐一排查。儿童多为白睛炎症；年轻人急性无痛性眼红以白睛炎症为多，需按分泌物特征甄别，红而痒者过敏反应居多；老年微红不适者考虑眼表问题如：干眼、睑板腺功能异常、结膜松弛。痛性眼红首先要排除黑睛或瞳神疾病；黑睛、瞳神疾病多伴视力障碍。甲亢患者也会出现眼红及突眼改变。

2.3 Ptosis of upper eyelid

It is divided into congenital and acquired types. It is mostly of congenital type in children, while it is mostly of acquired type in old people. It can also be pseudo-ptosis of upper eyelid caused by blepharoch-

2.3 上胞下垂

上胞下垂可有先天、后天之别：儿童多为先天性，老人多为后天性，亦有胞睑皮肤松垂、胞睑痉挛或外伤所

alasis, eyelid twitch or traumatic injury.

致假性下垂。

2.4 Spasm of eyelid

It is mostly caused by stimulating factors, often seen in the circumocular diseases of eyelid, conjunctiva and cornea. The idiopathic factors may lead to spasm of eyelid or facial muscle.

2.4 胞睑痉挛

胞睑痉挛多因刺激性原因导致，常见于胞睑、结膜、角膜等外障眼病；特发性原因导致胞睑或面部肌肉痉挛。

2.5 Blink

It is mostly caused by discomforts in eye diseases. In children, the facial muscle spasm may lead to frequent blink.

2.5 眨眼

眨眼多由患眼不适所致，儿童亦有因面部肌肉痉挛而至频繁眨眼。

2.6 Eyelid twitching

It refers to involuntary twitch of eyelid in occasion or in continuity, often caused by fatigue, insomnia or mental stress. In traditional Chinese medicine, the blood deficiency of heart and spleen may induce wind, so as to cause twitching of eyelid.

2.6 眼睑瞤动

胞睑常不由自主跳动，可偶尔或持续，多为疲劳、失眠、精神紧张导致，心脾血虚，久致生风而振跳。

2.7 Trichiasis

Congenitally, it is often accompanied by entropion. Acquired factors of trachoma, traumatic injury or surgery may cause scar, accompanied by entropion or ectropion. It is mostly seen in spasmodic entropion in the old people. It may also be caused by facial muscle flaccidity or blepharochalasis, or by paralysis.

2.7 倒睫

先天性倒睫见于小儿合并胞睑内翻；后天性由瘢痕导致如沙眼、外伤、手术等原因，可胞睑合并内外翻；老年性多见痉挛性胞睑内翻；也有面肌或胞睑肌松弛或麻痹。

2.8 Squint

It refers to sensation of frowning, preference for closing eyes and dislike of opening eyes. It is often caused by refractive error or eye fatigue, and caused by eyelid twitching occasionally.

2.8 迷眼

迷眼表现为眉头紧锁、愿闭不睁。多为屈光不正、眼疲劳。偶见胞睑痉挛。

2.9 Eyelids

It is necessary to examine the color, luster and motor state of eyelid, to find out if there is defect, scar, lump or edema or not, to examine the size of

2.9 胞睑

需要详查其色泽与运动状态，是否有缺损、瘢痕、肿块、水肿；睑裂的大小，睑缘

palpebral fissure, the location and state of eyelid margin, and the mutual relation between eyelid margin and eyelashes.

的位置、状态、睑缘与睫毛的相互关系等等。

2.10 Eyelid lump

The eyelid lump accompanied by redness of eyes is caused by eyelid furuncle, acute dacryocystitis or eyelid erysipelas. The eyelid lump without redness of eyes is caused by chalazion, dacryocystitis, tumor or chronic dacryocystitis. These diseases can be identified by determining the location of the lump. It is judge preliminarily the nature of the eyelid lump according to the size, property, hardness and relation to the nearby tissues by palpation. The skin of eyelid is the extension of the skin of face, but the skin of eyelid is thinner than the skin of other parts of body. The skin, due to inflammatory stimulation, becomes reddish. The localized edema at the diseased area occurs in the inflammatory effusion of the subcutaneous loose connective tissues. The cellulites may involve the whole eyelid. The symptoms of these circumocular diseases are caused by the invasion of the exogenous wind, heat, damp or toxin in traditional Chinese medicine. The ecchymosis may occur due to subcutaneous hemorrhage. The different colour changes may occur in vascular nevus, pigmented nevus, vitiligo or xanthoma.

(1) Various skin lesions may occur at the eyelid skin, such as the changes of red rash, blister, wheal, erosion or diabrosis.

(2) The orbicular muscle and levator muscle of upper eyelid inside the eyelid dominate the opening and closing of the eyelid. The ptosis of upper eye-

2.10 伴有眼红的胞睑肿块

伴有眼红的眼睑肿块有胞睑疖、漏睛疮、眼丹、(急性泪腺炎);不伴有眼红的胞睑肿块有胞生痰核、漏睛、肿瘤、慢性泪腺炎等;确认肿块的位置可作分辨。通过触摸分辨肿块的大小、质地、软硬度以及与相邻组织的关系,作出对肿块性质的初步判断,胞睑的皮肤面是脸部皮肤的延伸,只是胞睑的皮肤较全身其他部位更薄,皮肤的色泽会因为炎症刺激皮肤充血呈现局部发红,皮下疏松的结缔组织在炎症渗出时出现不同病变位置的局限性水肿,蜂窝织炎时可弥散累及整个胞睑。这些外障病变的证候在中医辨证中被认为由风、热、湿毒邪外袭所致。也可因皮下出血而呈现瘀斑。胞睑的血管痣、色素痣、白癜风、黄色瘤而出现不同的色泽改变。

(1) 胞睑皮肤还可出现各种皮损:红疹、水疱、风团、糜烂、溃破等改变。

(2) 胞睑内层的轮匝肌、提上睑肌控制胞睑的开合,上胞下垂、胞睑痉挛、内翻倒

lid, eyelid twitching, entropion and trichiasis are related to them.

(3) The palpebral margin structure refers to the free margin of tarso, and the juncture of the eyelash follicles and the skin. It is the outlet of the tarso secretion studded inside the tarso, and needed to observe carefully under the microscope. The flush, scale, erosion, festering and incrustation of the palpebral margin indicted the exogenous pathogens of wind, dryness, damp or toxin.

(4) The most inner layer of the eyelid is mucous membrane (palpebral conjunctiva). It is possible to observe the colour of the eyelid by naked eyes in flip of eyelid. Its normal structure should be the transparent and smooth membrane, through which the vessel texture and the light-yellow longitudinal meibomian gland can be seen clearly. In the abnormal condition, this tissue becomes chorionic reddish, and the vessel texture and meibomian gland cannot be seen clearly. In severe condition, its surface becomes rough and unsmooth. It indicates a kind of inflammatory state. The filling state of blood vessels can be identified exactly under the microscope. Another type of reaction state of the palpebral conjunctiva, such as that of papilla (vascular proliferation reaction), that of follicle (lymphocytic infiltration), etc., indicates a kind of specific chronic inflammation. In the inflammation, it is necessary to identify the membrane from the pseudomembrane according to the condition in which if there is the effusion on the tarso surface or not. Besides, the stone, scar, granuloma, cyst, hemangioma, foreign body, etc., can be found in the examination. And the meibomian gland obstruction can be identified

睫均与此相关。

（3）睑缘结构指睑板的游离缘、睫毛毛囊与皮肤黏膜的交界处，是睑板内密布的睑板腺分泌的出口，需要在显微镜下细细观察。睑缘处的潮红、鳞屑、糜烂以及溃脓、结痂提示风、燥、湿、毒之外邪。

（4）胞睑的最内层是黏膜（睑结膜），翻转胞睑可以肉眼观其色泽，正常的结构应该是透明、光滑的薄膜，透见清晰的血管纹理和其下淡黄色的纵形睑板腺。异常情况可发现该层组织呈绒毯状发红、血管条纹不清，更无法透见下面的睑板腺结构，甚至表面粗糙不平，提示一种炎症状态，显微镜下可以确切地分辨出血管的充盈状态，而睑结膜的另一种反应状态，乳头（血管增生反应）、滤泡（淋巴细胞浸润）等提示了一种特定的慢性炎症。炎症时依据睑板表面的渗出是否易于去除分辨膜与伪膜；另外结石、瘢痕、肉芽肿、囊肿、血管瘤、异物等都可以在检查时被发现，显微镜下还能分辨出睑板腺的阻塞。

under the microscope.

2.11 Eye white (bulbar conjunctiva and sclera)

Under the bright light, apply the thumb and index finger to open the eyelids and ask the patient to move the eyeball to all directions. It is possible to observe by the naked eyes the transparent bulbar conjunctiva and the inner sclera, the so-called the eye white in traditional Chinese medicine. It is necessary to identify the redness of eye white (bulbar congestion) from the redness of circum-eyeball (ciliary congestion), or the concurrence of the both.

(1) Congestion of eye white: It is more obvious if it is closer to the formix. The colour of blood is fresh red. It is moveable by pushing and squeezing the bulbar conjunctiva. Morphologically, the branches of the superficial conjunctival blood vessels can be seen clearly. It can be relieved temporarily by one drop of adrenalin hydrochloride. It is the symptom of conjunctivitis.

(2) Edema of eye white: The exudation of blood vessels occurs due to inflammation. The exudates accumulate under the bulbar conjunctiva of the superficial layer of the eye white, to cause an obvious prominence, called chemosis conjunctiva. It indicates the blood vessel reaction or the backflow obstruction of blood vessels. In traditional Chinese medicine, it is diagnosed as the pathogenic damp attacking eyes or as the abnormality of qi activity. The small transparent nodules of 1 to 2 mm in size occurring at the bulbar conjunctiva can be caused by the lymphocytes accumulation or the lymphatic backflow obstruction.

(3) Tumor of eye white: It refers to the prominent plaque at the eye white, or the conjunctival de-

2.11 白睛(球结膜及巩膜)

在明亮的光线下,用拇食指撑开胞睑,嘱患者眼球各方向转动,用肉眼即可观察到透明的球结膜和里层的巩膜,即中医学所说的白睛,首先必须区分的是白睛红赤(球结膜充血)与抱轮红赤(睫状充血),但也可见两者混合出现。

(1) 白睛充血:其特征为在部位上愈近穹隆部愈明显;出血颜色为鲜红色;推挤球结膜可随之移动;在形态上浅层结膜血管可明显看到分支;滴 1‰盐酸肾上腺素液可使之暂时消退。其病为结膜炎症。

(2) 白睛水肿:白睛的血管因炎症而渗出,渗出液聚积在白睛表层的球结膜下而显著隆起称为结膜水肿。这种提示血管性反应或血管回流受阻的状况在中医证候辨识为湿邪犯目或气机失常。球结膜上出现透明的 1～2 毫米的小结节可由淋巴细胞的聚积或淋巴管的回流受阻引起。

(3) 白睛肿物:在白睛隆起的斑块抑或仅是结膜的变

generation (pinguecula). It is called pterygium if it is close to the side of the nose. It can be more clearly seen under the microscope the depth of the tumor head entering the eye black and thickness of the tumor. The microsurgery has an obvious advantage in decreasing the recurrence. The tumor of eye white, according to its color, can be divided into dermoid cyst, hemangioma, melanoma and plasmacytoma. The diagnosis can be further confirmed in virtue of lab examinations.

性(睑裂斑)。在鼻侧近眦部的为胬肉,在显微镜下可以更明确地发现头部渐入黑睛的深度及体部的厚度。尤其在手术治疗时显微操作减少复发的优势更为明显。白睛肿物依据色泽分辨为皮样囊肿、血管瘤、黑色素瘤、浆细胞瘤,可借助实验室检验进一步明确。

(4) Discoloration, hemorrhage, black nevus or jaundice of eye white may lead to red-colored, black-colored or yellow-colored state.

(4) 白睛色变、出血、黑痣、黄疸而呈现红、黑、黄色。

2.12 Eye black (cornea)

The transparent cornea overlaps the dark-brown iris in Asian, so it is so-called the eye black in the ancient classics. The cornea is actually the transparent lens 0.5 to 1 mm in thickness. The curvature of its anterior and posterior surfaces ensures the cornea's refraction rate of 48.21 D to the parallel rays, while the superficial lacrimal film ensures the smoothness and crystal clear of the cornea. The fine change of the diseased eye black can be identified clearly in virtue of microscope in the clinic diagnosis.

2.12 黑睛(角膜)

全透明的角膜因透见的是亚洲人暗棕色的虹膜,因而被古医学称为黑睛。角膜实际上是厚度为 0.5～1 毫米的全透明的透镜,其前后表面的曲率确保了角膜对平行光线具有 48.21D 的屈光能力,而表面的泪膜层保证了角膜平滑而晶莹透亮。病变的黑睛细微改变,在眼科临症时必须借助于显微设备的观察才能对症候有明确的辨识。

(1) Epithelial defects of eye black: Epithelial defects of eye black is caused by invasion of pathogen on the surface of the eye black, or by sheltering loss of the eyelid, or by lack of protection of the lacrimal film. A small amount of epithelial defects of eye black do not influence the vision. A large amount of epithelial defects of eye black may cause

(1) 黑睛上皮的缺损:黑睛表面遭受病原体的侵袭;亦或缺少眼睑的遮挡抑或表面泪膜的保护,皆会造成上皮的缺损。黑睛少量上皮缺损并不影响视力,上皮较大范围的不完整在外观上显示

decrease of the eye black transparency apparently and influence the vision. Clinically, 1% fluorescein is applied to stain, and the stained fluorescein in different shapes and sizes can be seen under the slit lamp corneal microscope. The description and record of these changes are the necessary method in the follow-up observation. In traditional Chinese medicine, the disease is diagnosed as invasion of pathogenic wind, heat or toxin according to the accompanied symptoms of photophobia, lacrimation, pain, etc.

的是黑睛透明度的下降,可影响视力,临症用1%的荧光素染色,在裂隙灯显微镜下可见不同形态或大小的荧光着染,描绘和记录这些改变是随访观察的必要方法。中医依据伴随的畏光、流泪、疼痛等自我描述性症状审因为风、热、毒邪。

(2) Inflammatory nubecula of eye black: The local white colour and decrease of transparency can be seen by naked eyes at the eye black. Under the slit lamp, it is clearer to observe the local grey-white nubecula focus, called the corneal infiltration. The nubecula focus of eye black varies in depth. According to the different shapes and different properties of necrotic tissue (the congealed fat), it can be identified into infection of bacteria or fungus. In traditional Chinese medicine, the major involved organs are the liver and gallbladder, and the exogenous pathogens are the heat-toxin or the damp-heat. The multiple nebulas or the singular nubecula without necrotic tissue are often caused by viral infection. According to its symptomatic features of abrupt onset, photophobia and lacrimation, it indicates the invasion of pathogenic wind-heat. If the nubecula progressively develops from the periphery of eye black, or if it locates in the deep layer of eye black, it is immunogenic. It is caused by the endogenous pathogens, diagnosed as disequilibrium of zang-fu organs.

(2) 黑睛炎性混浊:肉眼或可见黑睛局部发白,透明度下降,而裂隙灯下更明确地观察到局限性灰白色浑浊灶,称为角膜浸润。黑睛混浊病灶可深浅不一,依据不同形状、伴有不同性状的坏死组织覆盖(凝脂),分辨为细菌或真菌感染。中医内因责之脏腑以肝胆为主。外因强调热毒或湿热所致。多个星翳或单个混浊不伴有坏死组织常为病毒感染引起。根据其起病急、畏光流泪的症状特点,常提示风热之邪。混浊自黑睛周边进行性发展或位于黑睛深层,常为免疫源性。内因为主,脏腑失衡为要。

(3) Non-inflammatory nubecula of eye black:

(3) 黑睛非炎性混浊:不

The nubecula without accompanied stimulating symptoms of redness, pain, photophobia, lacrimation, etc. is often called non-inflammatory nubecula. It is the most commonly seen in corneal tissue degeneration, or scars left by diseases or traumatic injuries.

伴有红、痛、畏光、流泪等角膜刺激症状的混浊多为非炎性混浊。角膜组织变性或疾病、外伤遗留下的瘢痕最为常见。

(4) Morphological change of eye black: The corneal topography method is the specific examination measure to observe the curvature change of eye black. It is necessary to observe if there are any wounds in traumatic injury of eye. It is helpful to identify it in virtue of stained fluorescein to observe the leakage.

(4) 黑睛形态的改变:角膜地形图是观察黑睛曲率改变的特异性检查手段。在眼外伤时应注意黑睛有无破损,用荧光素染色观察渗漏可有助于分辨。

(5) Tumor of eye black: There are no blood vessels in the eye black, but there are the rich blood vessels at the juncture (the corneal limbus) of the eye black and eye white. Therefore the tumor of eye black often occurs at the corneal limbus. According to the property and shape of the tumor, it can be diagnosed as the dermoid tumor or the cancer.

(5) 黑睛肿物:由于黑睛本身无血管,而黑睛与白睛交界处(角膜缘)有丰富的血管,因而黑睛肿物好发于角膜缘,根据肿物的性状分辨为皮样瘤或癌。

2.13 Anterior chamber

2.13 前房

The space formed by the eye black, iris and pupil is called the anterior chamber. In the intraocular diseases, such as acute angle-closure glaucoma, bluish glaucoma, malignant glaucoma, senile cataract in intumescent stage, localized dislocation of crystalline lens, suprachorodal hemorrhage, diastasis or intraocular occupying lesions, postoperation of eye, etc., it is helpful to judge the progression of the disease by observing the depth change of the anterior chamber.

黑睛与黄仁、瞳神形成的空间为前房。在绿风内障、青风内障、恶性青光眼、圆翳内障膨胀期、晶珠局限性脱位、脉络膜上腔出血、脱离或眼内占位、内眼术后等内障眼病时,前房深度的改变有助于判断疾病的进展。

(1) The shallow anterior chamber is divided into three degrees according to the Spaech Classifica-

(1) 浅前房按 Spaech 分类法分为三级:

tion:

Degree Ⅰ: The central anterior chamber is formed, and the peripheral iris contacts with the corneal endothelium.

Ⅰ级:中央区前房形成,周边部虹膜与角膜内皮接触;

Degree Ⅱ: The whole iris contacts with the corneal endothelium, but there is a certain gap between the surface of crystalline lens and the corneal endothelium.

Ⅱ级:全虹膜与角膜内皮接触,但晶状体表面与角膜内皮之间仍有一定的间隙;

Degree Ⅲ: The anterior chamber disappears, and the iris and crystalline lens completely adhere to the corneal endothelium.

Ⅲ级:前房消失或无前房,虹膜面、晶状体前表面与角膜内皮完全相粘。

(2) Aqueous humor: In normal condition, the aqueous humor is transparent. In the inflammation of iris, the protein and inflammatory cells permeate into the anterior chamber from the blood vessels of iris and ciliary body. The wondering cells in the aqueous humor can be found under the slit lamp, the so-called Tyndall Phenomenon in western medicine. A large amount of cells permeates into the anterior chamber to cause hypopyon which can be seen by naked eyes. In anterior chamber bleeding accompanied by eye operation, rubeosis of iris, diabetic retinopathy, etc., there are the hemacytes in the aqueous humor to make aqueous humor reddish in color, even hyphema and vitreous hemorrhagia observed by naked eyes in severe condition. In the sitting or standing position, the hemacytes sink, and the condition of transparent aqueous humor in the upper and hematocele in the lower occurs. In traditional Chinese medicine, it is diagnosed as the pattern of heat or stasis.

(2) 神水(即房水):正常情况下房水是透明的,在黄仁炎症时,蛋白质和炎性细胞由虹膜和睫状体上的血管渗入前房,房水中的游浮细胞可以在裂隙灯显微镜下被发现,即西医丁道尔(Tyndall)现象。大量的细胞渗出到前房可形成肉眼可观的“黄液上冲”。外伤或内眼手术、虹膜红变、糖尿病视网膜病变等伴发前房出血时,可导致神水中会有血细胞,致使神水呈现红色,甚则出现肉眼可观的“血灌瞳神”,坐立后,血细胞下沉,可见上方透明神水,下方积血。中医辨证审因皆为热、瘀之变证。

(3) Chamber angle: The judgement of the width of the anterior chamber angle is importantly significant to the diagnosis, classification, preven-

(3) 房角:判断前房角的宽窄对青风内障、绿风内障的诊断、分类和防治具有重

tion and treatment of bluish glaucoma and acute angle-closure glaucoma.

要意义。

(4) Pupil: In traditional Chinese medicine, it refers to the pupil in narrow sense, and to the invisible part posterior to the pupil in broad sense. With the advent of modern times, the clinic oculists need to apply various instruments to confirm the diagnosis and achieve the various patterns and causes.

(4) 瞳神:中医学中狭义仅指瞳孔(黄仁),广义之瞳神则泛指瞳孔后所有肉眼不可观之变。因而随着时代的进步,临床眼科医师必须借助多种仪器丰富望诊获得的各种证候并辨证审因。

(5) Iris: In the observation of the iris, it is firstly necessary to observe the color. If the iris of the single eye becomes lighter, it indicates the heterochromia. If the local white patches occur, it indicates the atrophy of iris. If the black patches occur, it indicates the iris moles or malignant melanoma. If the red spots or red strips occur, it indicates the iris neovasularization or hemorrhage. Secondly, it is necessary to observe the iris texture. If the sludge-like texture occurs, it indicates the swelling and distension of iris due to infection. If the texture is loose like a loofah sponge, it indicates the atrophy of iris. Thirdly, it is necessary to observe the synechia of iris. The posterior synechia of iris involves the crystalline lens, and it needs to identify the local synechia from the complete synechia. The anterior synechia of iris involves the eye black. In the traumatic injury, it is necessary to observe if the iris occurs or not, and if the iris root detachment occurs or not. When the eyeball rotates, it is necessary to observe if the tremor phenomenon of iris occurs or not.

(5) 黄仁(即虹膜):观察黄仁,需要一看颜色:单眼变淡,可能患有虹膜异色症;局部白斑,提示黄仁萎缩;有黑斑,可能患有虹膜黑痣或恶性黑色素瘤;红点或红条,说明有黄仁新生血管或出血。二看黄仁纹理:如黄仁污泥状纹理不清,说明黄仁有炎症肿胀;如呈丝瓜络状疏松,提示黄仁萎缩。三看黄仁粘连:后粘连晶珠,呈部分还是全部;前粘连黑睛。如有外伤,要注意黄仁是否存在,根部是否断离;当眼球转动时,黄仁有无震颤现象。

2.14 Crystalline lens

As the most important ocular media, it is the effect organ to adjust the ocular refraction in virtue

2.14 晶珠

作为眼内最重要的屈光介质,晶珠凭借附着的悬韧

of the contraction and release actions of the attached suspensory ligament of lens and ciliary body. With the help of the narrow band of the slit lamp, it can be seen a rich-layer broad band inside the pupil area, i. e. the structure of different layers, as the anterior lenticular capsule, the anterior lenticular cortex, the lenticular nucleus, the posterior lenticular cortex and the posterior lenticular capsule in sequence. The density of the normal crystalline lens is gradually increasing along with the age. It is necessary to observe if there is the pigmentation at the lenticular antetheca. The density change and the various types of turbidity of the crystalline lens can help to judge the degrees of senile cataract and the possible causative factors. In the mydriasis test, it is possible to observe the mutual relation between the lenticular location and iris, and to observe if the latent lens dislocation, so as to possess the indicating action to the intraocular surgery.

带和睫状体的收放作用而成为眼部屈光调节的效应器官。借助裂隙灯的窄光带，可以看到瞳神区域内一个层次丰富的宽光带，依次显示的是：晶珠前囊、晶珠前皮质、晶珠核、晶珠后皮质、晶珠后囊的各层结构。正常晶珠随年龄增长密度逐步增加，注意晶珠前壁是否有色素沉着；晶珠的密度变化、形态各异的混浊以更好地判断圆翳内障程度和可能的致病原因，在散瞳条件下还可以观察到晶珠的位置与黄仁间的相互关系，是否存在隐匿的晶珠脱位，对内眼手术具有很好的提示作用。

2.15 Vitreous body

It fills the retrobulbar cavity and the space between the posterior surface of crystalline lens and retina, attaching to the retina. It is a transparent gelatinous structure in normal condition. Vitreous opacity may be caused by infection, hemorrhage, degeneration or character change. Clinically, the examination result is taken as the evidence of pattern identification.

(1) Vitreous opacity: The dusty, flocculent or stripe opacity occurs inside the vitreous body, accompanied by decrease of vision. There is the possibility of inflammatory diseases inside the eye. In traditional Chinese medicine, it is mostly caused by the damp-heat fumigation or by heat-toxin in liver

2.15 神膏(玻璃体)

充满于眼球后腔内，充填于晶珠的后表面与视衣(视网膜)间，与视衣相贴。正常是全透明凝胶状结构。神膏的混浊可因炎症、出血、变性或性状改变所致，临证依据检查所得作为辨证审因的佐证。

(1) 神膏混浊：瞳神内出现尘埃状、絮状、条状混浊，合并视力下降；眼内有炎性病变可能，多为湿热蕴蒸或为肝胆热毒煎灼；临证需结合其他检查以协诊。

and gallbladder. It is necessary to combine the other examinations to assist the diagnosis.

(2) The red-colored flaky or stripe opacity occurs inside the vitreous body, indicating the intraocular bleeding diseases or traumatic injury. In traditional Chinese medicine, it is mostly caused by upward attack of fire-heat, bleeding in collaterals or qi stagnation and blood stasis.

（2）神膏内出现红色片状或条状混浊，眼内有出血性病变或有外伤史，多为火热上攻，脉络出血，或为气滞血瘀。

(3) The filiform, flocculent or reticular opacity occurs inside the vitreous body, indicating the possibility of degeneration diseases, such as high myopia. With the combination of B-ultrasonic examination, it is possible to judge the character of vitreous opacity. In traditional Chinese medicine, it is mostly caused by insufficiency of liver and kidney or by qi and blood deficiency.

（3）神膏内出现丝状或棉絮状或网状混浊，有高度近视等退行性病变可能，结合 B 超检查，判断神膏性状。多为肝肾不足，或气血虚弱。

(4) A large amount of crystalline reflective material can be seen inside the vitreous opacity. It does not influence the vision, mostly caused by cholesterol crystal.

（4）神膏内见大量结晶样反光物，不影响视物，多为胆固醇结晶。

2.16 Retina-choroids and blood vessels

2.16 视衣与血管

The normal retina is diffuse-tangerine in color. The clinical abnormality is nothing but pigmentation degeneration of retina, retinal microvascular abnormalities, retinal edema, exudation or thickening, with the symptoms of strange feeling, retinal bleeding, etc.

正常视网膜呈弥漫性橘红色，临证的异像不外乎视网膜变性，视网膜血管异常，视网膜水肿、渗出、增厚所表现出的异样感以及视网膜出血等。

(1) Abnormalities of macula region: The macular cherry-red spot, the macular hole, the macular epiretinal membrane, the macular edema, the macular reflex halo, etc. indicate respectively the obstruction of central retinal artery or obstruction of macular branches of retinal artery, the macular hole or idiopathic macular hole, the vitreous macular

（1）黄斑区异常有：樱桃红、裂孔、前膜、水肿轮状反光晕等分别提示：视网膜中央动脉阻塞或者视网膜黄斑分支动脉阻塞；黄斑裂孔或特发性黄斑孔；玻璃体黄斑牵引综合征、中心性浆液性

traction syndrome, the central serous chorioretinitis, etc.

脉络膜视网膜炎等。

(2) Ratio imbalance of retinal vessel and vascular abnormality: It indicates hypertensive retinopathy, retinal arteriosclerosis, retinal angioma, etc.

(2) 视网膜血管比例失调与血管异常提示:高血压性视网膜病变;视网膜动脉硬化;视网膜血管瘤等。

(3) Retinal edema or retinal exudation: It indicates various types of retinal inflammation and retinal vascular diseases. The retinal yellow exudation is a hard lipid exudation of retina, often seen in the chronic vascular diseases. The retinal white exudation in flocculence indicates local retinal ischemia and anoxia.

(3) 视网膜水肿、渗出提示:见于各种视网膜炎性、血管性疾病。视网膜上黄色渗出,为视网膜的硬性脂质样渗出,常见于慢性血管性疾病。视网膜上类似棉绒样白色渗出提示局部视网膜缺血缺氧。

(4) Retinal hypertrophy: It indicates all types of retinal exudation or hemorrhage.

(4) 视网膜肥厚提示:所有视网膜渗出或出血性疾病。

(5) Retinal pigment abnormalities: It is mainly caused by abnormal melanin performance and distribution of fundus oculi, such as retinal pigmentation degeneration, retinal laser surgery, choroidal melanoma, choroidal melanocytoma, retinal pigmented nevus, etc.

(5) 视网膜色素异常:主要是指眼底的黑色素异常表现和分布,如:视网膜色素变性;视网膜激光术后;脉络膜黑色素瘤;脉络膜黑色素细胞瘤;视网膜色素痣等。

(6) Retinal degeneration area: It is often seen in the peripheral retina, including lattice degeneration of retina, paving stone degeneration of retina, snail track degeneration of retina, and oppressive or non-oppressive white degeneration of retina. In lattice degeneration, retinal hole often occurs.

(6) 视网膜变性区:多见于视网膜中周边。有状似格子样变性、形似铺路石样变性、蜗牛迹样变性以及压迫或不压迫变白样变性等。其中格子样变性易发生视网膜裂孔。

(7) Retinal hemorrhage: It is the most complicated. The different symptoms indicate different diseases, which need to be identified in virtue of other examination instruments. The common causes

(7) 视网膜出血:视网膜出血最为复杂,不同症状提示不同疾病,需要辅助其他检测设备加以鉴别。常见原

are as follows: ① Obstruction of central retinal vein or of its branches causes flame-shaped hemorrhage; ② Diabetic retinopathy is manifested by punctuate or splinter hemorrhage in different layers of retina or vitreous hemorrhage; ③ Retinal periphlebitis is manifested by peripheral retinal hemorrhage and exudation; ④ Retinal macroaneurysm is manifested by massive bleeding on the retinal surface, accompanied by visible aneurysm.

因有：①中央或者分支视网膜静脉阻塞：相应区域火焰状出血；②糖尿病性视网膜病变：可见视网膜不同层次的点、片状出血甚至玻璃体出血；③视网膜静脉周围炎：视网膜中周部出血和渗出；④视网膜大动脉瘤：视网膜表面大片出血，伴见动脉瘤体。

Section 2　Pattern identification in ophthalmology

第2节　眼病辨证法

1　Traditional pattern identification of circumocular and intraocular diseases

It is said in Important Secrets of Experiential Therapy of Ophthalmology, *The Golden Mirror of Medicine* (Yi Zong Jin Jian): "Screen means shielding. The intraocular diseases are caused by shielding from the inner part, while the circumocular diseases are caused by shielding from the outer part."

1　传统辨证之内外障辨证

《医宗金鉴·眼科心法要诀》："障，遮蔽也。内障者从内而蔽也；外障者从外而蔽也。"

1.1　Circumocular disease

It refers to the disease locating at the eyelid, outer or inner canthus, eye white and eye black. The disease is often caused by the invasion of the six exogenous factors, or caused by damp-heat, pathogenic fire of liver and lung, etc. Usually the manifestations are more obvious, and the symptoms are redness, swelling and distension, pain, lacrimation, photophobia, eyelid twitching, etc.

1.1　外障

外障是指病位在胞睑、两眦、白睛、黑睛的疾病。多由六淫之邪外袭或湿热、肝肺火邪等所致。一般症状表现比较明显，多有红赤、肿胀、疼痛、流泪、羞明、胞睑痉挛等症状。

1.2 Intraocular disease

It refers to the diseases of the intraocular tissues of pupil, crystalline lens, vitreous body, retina-choroid, eye system, etc. The disease is often caused by seven emotional factors, internal injury of zang-fu organs, disharmony of qi and blood, qi stagnation and blood stasis, invasion of the exogenous factors, or traumatic injury. Usually the appearance is quite good, but there are the symptoms of visual functional changes, such as visual disturbance, diminution of vision, or blurred or cloudy vision.

1.2 内障

内障是指发生在瞳神、晶珠、神膏、视衣、目系等眼内组织的眼病。多由七情内伤、脏腑内损、气血失调、气滞血瘀,或外邪入里、眼部外伤引起。一般外观端好,以视物障碍、视力下降、云雾移睛等视功能的改变为主要表现。

2 Pattern identification of zang-fu organs according to unity of wheels and organs

2 轮脏合一之脏腑辨证

2.1 Muscle wheel

It refers to the upper and lower eyelids, attributive to the spleen. The spleen is attributive to the earth and yellow colour in five elements, and dominates transportation and transformation. The muscle wheel is normal when it is yellow-colored and lustrous, and normal in opening and closing. The spleen and stomach are exteriorly-interiorly related, so the muscle wheel diseases are related to the spleen and stomach.

(1) Swelling and distension of eyelid: If it is soft by palpation without redness or pain, it is caused by the deficiency of the spleen which fails to dominate transportation.

(2) Erosion of eyelid skin with blister or pustule is caused by upward-flow of damp-heat in spleen and stomach.

(3) Ptosis of eyelid: If it is weak and fails to uplift, it is caused by sinking of the Zhong (Central) Qi in spleen and stomach.

2.1 肉轮

肉轮指上下胞睑,在脏属脾,脾于五行属土,其色黄,主运化。肉轮以色黄润泽,开合为顺。脾与胃相表里,肉轮之疾责于脾胃。

(1) 胞睑肿胀,按之虚软不赤无痛为脾虚失运。

(2) 睑肤糜烂,水或脓疱为脾胃湿热上泛。

(3) 胞睑垂下,无力提举为脾胃中气下陷。

(4) Twitching of eyelid is caused by the decrease of transportation and transformation of spleen and stomach, and deficiency of the Ying (Nutrient) Qi and blood.

(4) 胞睑瞤动为脾胃运化不足,营血虚少。

2.2 Blood wheel

2.2 血轮

It refers to the outer canthus, inner canthus, lacrimal punctum and blood vessels of lacrimal caruncle, attributive to the heart. The heart is attributive to the fire and red colour in five elements, and dominates the blood and vessels. The blood wheel is normal when it is red, energetic and lustrous. The heart and small intestines exteriorly-interiorly related, so the blood wheel diseases are related to the heat and small intestine.

指内外两眦、泪小点、泪阜之血络,在脏属心,心于五行属火,其色赤,主血脉血轮以红活润泽为顺。心与小肠相表里,血轮之疾责于心及小肠。

(1) Redness, swelling, hard mass or pain which is worsened by press at the inner canthus is caused by upward-flaming of heart fire.

(1) 内眦红肿硬结拒按疼痛为心火上炎。

(2) Pus exuded by palpation from the inner canthus without redness or pain is caused by the stagnant heat in the Heart Meridian.

(2) 内眦不红无痛,按之出脓为心经郁热。

(3) The visible red vessels which are thick at the outer or inner canthus are caused by the fire of excess type in the Heart Meridian. The visible red vessels which are thin are caused by the fire of deficiency type of the Heart Meridian.

(3) 两眦赤脉为心经实火,赤脉细小为心经虚火。

(4) Red and swollen pteryglum which involves the eye white is caused by wind-heat in heart and lung.

(4) 胬肉红赤臃肿攀及白睛为心肺风热。

2.3 Qi wheel

2.3 气轮

It refers to the eye white (conjunctiva and sclera), attributive to the lung. The lung is attributive to the metal and white colour in five elements, and dominates the protection of the body surface. The qi wheel is normal when it is white-colored and

气轮指白睛(结膜、巩膜),在脏属肺,肺于五行属金,其色白,主卫外。气轮以白而坚固为顺,肺与大肠相表里,气轮之疾责于肺和大

firm. The lung and large intestine are exteriorly-interiorly related, so the qi wheel diseases are related to the lung and large intestine.

肠。

(1) The red vessels occurring at the superficial layer of eye white are caused by wind-heat in the Lung Meridian. The red vessels which are thick occurring at the eye white are caused by the heat stagnation in lung.

(1) 白睛浅层赤脉为肺经风热,白睛赤脉粗大为肺热郁滞。

(2) Herpetiflorm nodule occurring at the superficial layer of eye white is caused by dryness-heat in the Lung Meridian. Nodule which is purple-colored and painful occurring at the deep layer of eye white is caused by hyperactivity and excess of lung fire.

(2) 白睛浅层疱性结节为肺经燥热,白睛深层结节,色紫拒按为肺火亢盛。

(3) If the eye white becomes bluish accompanied by unclear iris, it is caused by heat-toxin in lung and liver.

(3) 白睛变青,兼见黄仁不清,为肺肝热毒。

(4) **Turbidity of eye white:** If intolerable itching at eyelid is accompanied, it is caused by damp-heat in lung and spleen.

(4) 白睛污浊,兼见胞睑痒极难忍,为肺脾湿热。

2.4 Wind wheel

It refers to the eye black (cornea, aqueous humor and iris), attributive to the liver. The liver is attributive to the wood and green colour in five elements, and dominates draining-dispersing and free growing. The wind wheel is normal when it is sparkling clear. The liver and gallbladder are exteriorly-interiorly related, so the wind wheel diseases are related to the liver and gallbladder.

2.4 风轮

风轮指黑睛(角膜、神水、黄仁),在脏属肝,肝于五行属木,其色青,主疏泄条达,风轮以青莹明润为顺,肝与胆相表里,风轮之疾责于肝胆。

(1) The early nebula of eye black is caused by the wind-heat in the Liver Meridian. The big nebula with ulceration is caused by liver fire burning and flaming.

(1) 黑睛初生星翳为肝经风热;翳大溃陷为肝火灼盛。

(2) The verall nebula of eye black with red thread-like vessels is caused by damp-heat in liver

(2) 翳漫黑睛,赤脉渐入为肝胆湿热,翳久不敛为肝

and gallbladder. The chronic and unhealed nebula is caused by liver yin insufficiency.

阴不足。

(3) The hemorrhagic eye white, petal nebula and vascular nebula are caused by heat excess in lung and liver.

(3) 白睛赤脉、黑睛翳漫包睛为肺肝热盛。

(4) The peripheral prominence of eye black is caused by liver qi hyperactivity.

(4) 黑睛周边突起为肝气过旺。

2.5 Water wheel

2.5 水轮

It refers to the crystalline lens, vitreous body, retina, choroids and optic nerve, attributive to the kidney. The kidney is attributive to the water and black colour in five elements, and dominates the storage of essence. The water wheel is normal when it is black and clear. The kidney and bladder are exteriorly-interiorly related, so the water wheel diseases are related to the kidney and bladder. Furthermore, the liver and kidney share a same source, so the water wheel diseases are also related to the liver and kidney.

水轮指瞳神内含晶珠、神膏、视衣及目系(晶状体、玻璃体、视网膜、脉络膜、视神经)在脏属肾。肾于五行属水,其色黑,主藏精。水轮以黑莹清澈为顺,肾与膀胱相表里,水轮之疾责于肾、膀胱。由于肝肾同源,故水轮病变常与肝肾两脏相关。

(1) Corediastasis or iridocyclitis, accompanied by distending pain at eyes, it is caused by upward disturbance of wind-fire in liver and gallbladder. Afterwards, the pupil becomes dry and out of round, it is caused by yin deficiency of liver and kidney, leading to up-flaming of the false fire.

(1) 瞳神散大或紧小,伴眼胀痛,为肝胆风火上扰,久而瞳神干缺不圆,为肝肾阴亏,虚火上炎。

(2) Lens opacity and white-colored pupil is mostly caused by liver and kidney deficiency and by essence and blood insufficiency.

(2) 晶珠混浊,瞳神色白,多为肝肾亏虚,精血不足。

(3) Vitreous opacity accompanied by black shadow before eyes: If it is chronic, it is mostly caused by insufficiency of liver and kidney which fail to nourish the eyes. If it is acute, it is mostly caused by kidney yin deficiency, leading to the flaming of the false fire.

(3) 神膏混浊,眼前黑影,日久者多为肝肾不足,目失所养;骤然发生者可因肾阴亏虚,阴虚火旺而致。

(4) Retina-choroid edema is mostly caused by

(4) 视衣水肿者多为脾

yang deficiency of spleen and kidney, leading to upward attack of water-damp. Retina-choroid atrophy accompanied by pigmentation is mostly caused by liver and kidney insufficiency or fire failure in the Vital Gate (Ming Men).

肾阳虚,水湿上犯所致;视衣萎缩或伴色素沉着,多为肝肾不足或命门火衰。

The pattern identification according to five wheels has the guiding significance in the clinic. But in the clinic diagnosis, it is not advisable to stand on five wheels. For example, lacrimation is a disease locating at the canthi, but its pathogenesis is related to the draining and dispersing function of the liver and to the controlling and checking function of the spleen qi. Therefore, in the clinic pattern identification, it is necessary to consider the concept of wholism, to combine the four diagnostic methods and to integrate with the theory of five wheels, so as to achieve the therapeutic effects.

五轮辨证对临床有重要的指导意义,但临证切不可拘泥于五轮,如流泪症,病位虽在两眦,但其病机多与肝之疏泄功能及脾气之收摄功能有关。因而临证辨证需从整体观念出发,四诊合参,结合五轮学说,方可取得疗效。

3 Pattern identification of pathogenesis according to unity of heaven and human

3 天人合一之病因辨证

The normal climatic phenomena of wind, cold, summer-heat, damp, dryness and fire are regarded as the qi of the nature, but the excess of them is regarded as the six exogenous pathogens. The circumocular diseases are mostly caused by the six exogenous pathogens, manifested by redness, swelling, hotness, pain, itching, dryness, erosion, lacrimation and nebula in observationof appearance. It is to describe the properties of the diseases according to the attribution of the natural phenomena, while to determine the causative factors of diseases according to the manifestations of the diseases. It is actually the simple culture to observe the human beings and nature in traditional Chinese medicine. It is to apply

风、寒、暑、湿、燥、火顺条则为自然之气,过而致病则为六淫之邪。眼之外障病,多六淫为患,观其外候,无非红、肿、热、痛、痒、涩、湿烂、眦泪、翳障而概之。以自然属性来归纳描述疾病特性,以疾病表现形式来审别病因,是中医学观察人与自然的朴素文化。中医学采用取类比象之思维,提炼其自然属性,用以分析临证,获取表象以判其源。《银海指南·六气总论》有"寒暑燥湿

the analogy, a traditional pattern of thinking in traditional Chinese medicine, to refine the natural phenomena into their natural attribution, so as to analyze the clinic patterns and determine the source from the superficial phenomena. It is said in General Introduction to Six Climatic Phenomena, *A Guide to Silver Sea* (Yin Hai Zhi Nan): "Cold, summer-heat, dryness, damp, wind and fire are the six climatic phenomena. When they are proper, it is normal. When they are excessive, it is sick. If the human body is attacked, his eyes are sick. The wind causes lacrimation, redness and swelling, the cold causes purple colour and distension due to blood stasis, the summer-heat causes redness and blurred vision. The damp causes erosion tinea, the dryness causes dry and binding sensation at the canthus, and the fire causes redness, swelling and pain." The therapeutic methods are thus decided as to eliminate wind, to warm cold condition, to disperse summer-heat, to dissolve damp, to moisturize dry condition, to reduce fire and to relieve pain. The six exogenous pathogens attack the body one with the other, so that the clinical manifestations are more complicated and multifarious.

风火，是为六气，当其位则正，过则淫。人有犯其邪者，皆能为目患。风则流泪赤肿，寒则血凝紫胀，暑则红赤昏花，湿则沿烂成癣，燥则紧涩眦结，火则红肿壅痛。"从而衍生出疏风、温寒、祛暑、化湿、润燥、泻火、解痛之治法。且六淫常相伴为患，使临证表现更为复杂多样。

(1) The condition with eye itching and photophobia is often caused by the pathogenic wind, which may cause redness, swelling and warm tears if the pathogenic heat is accompanied, or cause frequent lacrimation with cold tears, spasm and purple colour of eyelid if the pathogenic cold is accompanied.

(1) 目痒、羞明者，常因风邪为患；合并热邪者可伴红肿而赤，热泪如汤；合并寒邪者常伴冷泪频流，胞睑拘挛或紫暗。

(2) The condition with twitching of eyelid, squinting eye and deviation of mouth and eye is caused by the invasion of the pathogenic wind which

(2) 胞轮振跳、目偏视、口眼㖞斜者为风邪乘虚侵入，阻滞经络而致病。

blocks the meridians and collaterals.

(3) The condition with erosion of eyelid, excessive eye discharge, turbidity of eye black and edema of eye white is caused by the pathogenic damp, and the symptoms and signs of damp-heat may occur if it is combined with the pathogenic heat or with the pathogenic summer heat.

（3）胞睑湿烂、眵多泪黏、黑睛混浊生翳、白睛水肿常因湿邪为患，且常与热邪、暑邪相合致病而表现为湿热征象。

(4) The condition with redness and pain of eyelid, excessive and yellow-colored eye discharge, jugular vessels, redness and swelling of eye white, hyphema and vitreous hemorrhagia, and hypopyon is mostly caused by the pathogenic fire, which is featured by the symptoms of yang-heat, such as quick and fierce onset, severe condition, rapid progression, etc.

（4）胞睑红赤焮痛，眵多黄稠，血脉怒张、白睛红赤浮肿、血灌瞳神、黄液上冲者多为火邪之来势猛、病情重、发展快的阳热证表现。

(5) The condition with dry skin of eyelid, dry and uncomfortable sensation, dryness and lusterless of eye white and eye black is caused by the pathogenic dryness which consumes yin and causes loss of nourishment of eyes.

（5）胞睑皮肤干燥、干涩不舒，白睛、黑睛干燥无光泽者则因燥邪伤阴，目失濡养所致。

(6) The condition with redness of eye, blurred vision, excessive eye discharge and tears, swelling and distension of eye is caused by the pathogenic summer-heat. This type of condition is rarely seen in the clinic and its symptoms and signs are similar to those of the damp-heat pattern. Therefore, it is often diagnosed as damp-heat pattern in the clinic.

（6）目赤视昏、眵泪多、目肿胀为暑邪致病表现，但临床上较为少见，且症状与湿热证候相似，故临证多以湿热为辨。

In western medicine, based upon the investigation of etiology, it is to identify the common basic pathology caused by the bacteria, virus, allergy and traumatic injury in the process of the inflammatory diseases. The congestion, exudation and edema are used to illustrate the origin the features of the clinical manifestations and to confirm some pathogenic

西医基于对病因病源学的探究，分辨细菌、病毒、过敏、外伤在炎性病变过程中导致的共同的基本病理。充血、渗出、水肿，很好地解释了临证外候的特征由来，明确了某些具有传染特性的病

microorganisms which possess the infectivity. The eye diseases caused by the viral infection are mostly related to the pathogenic wind-heat. The eye diseases caused by the bacterial infection are mostly related to the pathogenic heat-toxin. The eye diseases caused by the fungus infection are mostly related to the pathogenic damp-heat.

原微生物：病毒感染所致的眼病多于风热有关，细菌感染所致的眼病多与热毒有关，真菌感染所致的眼病多与湿热有关。

4 Pattern identification of zang-fu organs according to relationships between eyes and zang-fu organs

4 眼与脏腑关联之脏腑辨证

The dysfunction of five zang organs and six fu organs can cause various eye diseases. In traditional Chinese medicine, it is to presume the inner pathogenesis according to the superficial features and progression regulation of the eye diseases, and then to search for the healing methods. As for the pathogenesis of the zang-fu organs, it is nothing but two categories of deficiency and excess.

五脏六腑功能失调，在目表现为各种病征，中医学根据眼部的外显特征及其病程规律，推测内在病机，寻求治疗方法。而脏腑病机不外乎虚实两类。

4.1 Heart and small intestine

4.1 心与小肠

The heart dominates the spirit and mind, while the eyes are the messenger of the heart and pertain to the heart internally. If the heart is sick and affects the eyes, the diseases are of the visual changes, blood vessels in eyes and both canthi.

心主神明，目为心之使，内属于心，故心有病影响到眼，主要反映在视觉的变化和眼中血脉及两眦的病变。

(1) **Internal excess of heart fire:** Redness of both canthi, pterygium and dacryocystitis.

(1) **心火内盛：**两眦红赤，胬肉增生，漏睛生疮。

(2) **Heart fire disturbing spirit:** Derangement and seeing but failing to recognize somebody.

(2) **心火扰神：**神乱发狂，目不识人。

(3) **Heart blood deficiency or heart qi insufficiency:** Staring blankly, failure to watch for long time and blurring of vision after watching for long time.

(3) **心血亏耗或心气不足：**神光涣散，不耐久视，久视目昏。

4.2 Liver and gallbladder

4.2 肝和胆

The liver opens into the eyes. The Liver Merid-

肝开窍于目，肝脉连于

ian connects with the eyes. The liver qi flows to the eyes. The liver and gallbladder are the most related to the eyes.

目,肝气通于目,肝胆与目关系最为密切。

(1) Wind-heat in Liver Meridian: Redness of eyes, lacrimation, nebula of eye black and papillary seclusion.

(1) 肝经风热:目赤流泪,黑睛生翳,瞳神紧小。

(2) Liver qi stagnation: Distension and pain at eyeball and bluish glaucoma.

(2) 肝气郁结:目珠胀痛,青风内障。

(3) Liver yang hyperactivity or liver fire flaming upwards: Acute angle-closure glaucoma, subconjunctival ecchymosis and sudden visual loss.

(3) 肝阳上亢或肝火上炎:绿风内障,白睛溢血,暴盲。

(4) Internal movement of liver wind: Strabismus and deviation of mouth and eye.

(4) 肝风内动:目偏视,口眼㖞斜。

(5) Damp-heat in liver and gallbladder: Keratitis due to herpes simplex, purulent keratitis, interstitial keratitis and papillary seclusion.

(5) 肝胆湿热:聚星翳障,凝脂溃翳,混睛赤障,瞳神紧小。

(6) Liver blood insufficiency: Dryness of eyes, failure to watch for long time, blurring of vision, night blindness and kerotomalacia due to vitamin A deficiency.

(6) 肝血不足:眼干涩,不耐久视,视物昏花,夜盲,疳积上目。

4.3 Spleen and stomach

4.3 脾和胃

The spleen and stomach are the acquired basis and the source to produce qi and blood. If the stomach functions to accept food and the spleen functions to transport food essence normally, the eyes are nourished to maintain the normal physiological functions.

脾胃为后天之本,气血生化之源,胃纳脾输正常,目得濡养,维持正常生理功能。

(1) Spleen qi deficiency: Ptosis of upper eyelid, dryness of eyeballs, failure to watch for long time, blurring of vision, vitreous opacity and kerotomalacia due to vitamin A deficiency.

(1) 脾气虚弱:上胞下垂、目珠干涩、不耐久视、视物昏矇、云雾移睛、疳积上目。

(2) Spleen failing to control blood: Subconjunctival ecchymosis, hyphema and vitreous hemorrhagia.

(2) 脾不统血:白睛溢血、血灌瞳神。

(3) Stomach fire flaming and excess: Blephari-

(3) 胃火炽盛:睑弦赤

tis marginalis and hordeolum.

(4) Damp-heat in spleen and stomach: Blepharitis marginalis, vitreous opacity, retinal edema and exudation.

4.4 Lung and large intestine

The lung dominates qi and governs dispersing and descending. If the lung qi is harmonious, the eyes are bright.

(1) Lung qi deficiency or Wei (Defensive) Qi weakness may lead to attack of pathogens: Allergic conjunctivitis and epidemic keratoconjunctivitis.

(2) Lung yin insufficiency: Dryness of eyes and visible red vessels in eye white.

(3) Excessive heat in lung or heat accumulating in intestines: Dark-red colour in eye white and nodular prominence in eye white.

4.5 Kidney and bladder

The kidney stores the essence. If the kidney essence is sufficient, the eyes are nourished by the Jing (Essence) Qi and bright in watching things. The kidney dominates the body fluid. The aqueous humor and vitreous body rely on the body fluid of five zang organs and six fu organs, flowing upwards to the eyes and becoming the fluid to moisturize and nourish the eyes. The bladder dominates qi transformation.

(1) Kidney yang insufficiency leading to upward invasion by water-damp: Blurring of vision, vitreous opacity, retinal edema or detachment.

(2) Vital Gate fire deficiency or kidney yang insufficiency: Myopia, night blindness and primary pigmentary degeneration of retina.

(3) Kidney yin deficiency and false fire burning collaterals: Papillary metamorphosis, fundus hem-

烂、针眼。

（4）脾胃湿热：胞睑湿烂、神膏混浊、视衣水肿渗出。

4.4 肺和大肠

肺主气，主宣发肃降，肺气调则气和目明。

（1）肺气虚弱，卫气不固易受邪：暴风客热、天行赤眼。

（2）肺阴不足：眼干涩、白睛赤脉隐隐。

（3）肺热壅盛或热结肠腑：白睛暗红，呈结节状隆起。

4.5 肾和膀胱

肾藏精，肾精充足则目得精气充养，视物精明；肾主津液，目之神水、神膏依赖五脏六腑津液在肾的调节下上输于目，为目外润泽之水及目内充养之液。膀胱司气化。

（1）肾阳不足，水湿上犯：视瞻昏渺、云雾移睛、视衣水肿或脱离。

（2）命门火衰，肾阳不足：近视、夜盲、高风内障。

（3）肾阴亏虚，虚火灼络：瞳神干缺、眼底络脉出

orrhage and vitreous opacity.

(4) Heat accumulating in bladder which fails to dominate qi transformation: retinal edema.

The pattern identification according to zang-fu organs is the most important component part of the pattern identification system in traditional Chinese medicine. It is necessary in the clinic to consider the symptoms of both eyes and whole body, and to combine with the pattern identification according to five wheels, so as to guide the correct treatment.

血、云雾飘移。

（4）热结膀胱、气化失司：视衣水肿。

脏腑辨证是中医学辨证体系的重要组成部分，临证仍需考量眼部及全身症状，同时可与五轮辨证相结合，方可指导正确治疗。

5 Pattern identification of meridians and collaterals according to relationship between eyes and zang-fu organs

The twelve meridians connect head-to-tail in sequence and run in full circle. It is said in Chapter 47, Internal Organs as Roots and Causes, *Spiritual Pivot* (Ling Shu): "The meridians function to circulate qi and blood and to construct yin and yang." The meridians and collaterals run over the whole body, move qi and blood, communicate the Ying (Nutrient) and Wei (Defense) Phases and regulate zang-fu organs. The essence, blood and body fluid flow and infuse to the whole body through the qi activity and movement of the zang-fu organs, upwards to the head and eyes to moisturize and nourish the head. Therefore it is said in Chapter 10, Birth and Growth of Five Viscera, *Essential Questions* (Su Wen): "All meridians pertain to the eyes." The meridians and collaterals are the pathway to transport the nutrient substances, and also the transmitting routes of the exogenous pathogens. All the pathogens may attack the eyes along with the meridians to decrease the vision. For example, keratitis due to

5 眼与脏腑关联之经络辨证

十二经脉，首尾相贯，周而复始。《灵枢·本脏》曰："经脉者，所以行气血而营阴阳。"经络循环周身，行气运血，沟通营卫，调节脏腑，精血津液因脏腑气机运行推注于周身，上乘头目，濡养神明之府。故有《素问·五脏生成》之"诸脉者，皆属于目"之说。经络既是营养物质上传的通道，也是疾病外邪传输的途径，病邪皆可循经而上犯目折明，如典型眼疾聚星翳障，卫阳不固，初受风邪，循肝经侵扰黑睛，入里久伏，客于其间。

herpes simplex, a typical eye disease, is caused by the Wei (Defensive) Qi weakness and invasion of the pathogenic wind, which attack the eyes along with the Liver Meridian.

All the three yang meridians of foot start at the eye or periocular region. The branches of the three yang meridians of hand end at the eye or periocular region. The Liver Meridian of Foot-Jueyin, the Heart Meridian of Hand-Shaoyin and the Bladder Meridian of Foot-Taiyang directly connect with the eye system. It is common to see that the pathogenic wind-heat attacks the Liver Meridian and goes upward along the meridian to cause various eye diseases, from eye black to pupil, such asserpent corneal ulcer and corneal ulcer, papillary seclusion, etc. The stagnant heat in the Liver Meridian or the liver fire flaming upward may cause corediastasis and acute angle-closure glaucoma, manifested by headache radiating along meridians to the vertex of head. The Bladder Meridian of Foot-Taiyang and the Kidney Meridian of Foot-Shaoyin are exteriorly-interiorly related. If the kidney and bladder are abnormal in their qi transforming function, there can be various diseases caused by the retained water attacking the eyes, such as swelling and distension of eyelids, retinal edema, macular effusion, retinal detachment, etc. Therefore it is said in Diseases of Bladder, *Silver Sea's Essentials* (Yin Hai Jing Wei): "Whenever the eyes are treated, it must consider the bladder carefully."

足三阳经均起于眼或眼周；手三阳经亦有支脉止于眼或眼周；足厥阴肝经、手少阴心经、足太阳膀胱经则直接与目系相连。风热之邪客于肝经较为多见，循经而上，可致从黑睛到瞳神的各种眼疾，如黑睛生翳、瞳神紧小等。如肝经郁热，肝火上炎致瞳神散大，绿风内障者，头痛循经，痛连巅顶。足太阳膀胱经与足少阴肾经相互络属而互为表里，肾与膀胱气化功能失常，常可致水液潴留上犯目窍的各种病证，如胞睑肿胀、视衣水肿、黄斑积液、视衣脱离等，故《银海精微·膀胱主病》中有"故凡治目，不可不细究膀胱"一说。

The twelve muscle regions are the connective and adjunctive parts of the twelve meridians, making qi to accumulate at the tendons, muscles, joints and body surface, and acting to restrain the bones

十二经筋是十二经脉之气结聚于筋肉关节体表，约束骨骼，保持关节活动的连属部分。手足三阳之筋网结

and maintain the joint movements. The yang muscle regions of hand and foot spin the web at the eyes and periocular region and act to dominate the opening and closing of the eyelids and the eye movement. If the pathogens attack the muscle regions, their functions are lost, leading to the symptoms of ptosis of upper eyelid, twitching of eyelid, strabismus, deviation of mouth and eye, etc.

聚于眼及其周围，共同作用支配胞睑的开合、目珠的转动，而邪客于经络使经筋运动功能失司，出现上胞下垂、胞轮振跳、目偏视、口眼喎斜等症。

6 Pattern identification of function according to qi, blood and body fluid

6 气血津液之机能辨证

6.1 Qi

6.1 气

The Wei (Defensive) Qi, the Ying (Nutrient) Qi, the Yuan (Primary) Qi and the Zong (Pectoral) Qi are closely related to the eyes. The Ying (Nutrient) Qi flows inside the vessels, while the Wei (Defensive) Qi flows outside the vessel. The Ying (Nutrient) Qi and the Wei (Defensive) Qi mutually coordinate to connect the internal with the external and to protect the body surface. If the Ying (Nutrient) Qi is strong while the Wei (Defensive) Qi is weak, there can be the circumocular diseases. If the Ying (Nutrient) Qi is weak while the Wei (Defensive) Qi is strong, there can be the intraocular diseases.

卫气、营气、元气、宗气皆与目关系密切。营气行于脉中，卫气护于脉外，营卫之间，沟通里外，相互协调，护卫周全。营强卫弱则有外障之侵；营弱卫强则有内障之忧。

(1) Qi deficiency: Mostly the chronic and deficient diseases, such as senile cataract, frequent lacrimation with cold tears, failure to watch for long time, recurrent and unhealed attacks of eye diseases, etc. Qi deficiency may also cause ocular hemorrhage.

(1) 气虚：可见较多慢性虚衰病证，如圆翳内障、冷泪频流，不耐久视，眼病后期反复不愈等。气虚也可出现眼内出血性疾病。

(2) Qi sinking: Ptosis of upper eyelid and visual fatigue.

(2) 气陷：眼睑下垂，视力疲劳。

(3) Qi stagnation: Distension and pain of eye-

(3) 气滞：目珠胀痛，青

ball and bluish glaucoma.

(4) Up-reverse flow of qi: Distension and pain in head and eyes, acute angle-closure glaucoma, subconjunctival ecchymosis, sudden blindness.

风内障。

(4) 气逆:头目胀痛,绿风内障,白睛溢血,暴盲等。

6.2 Blood

The essence and blood share a same source which given by the essentials of the five zang organs and six fu organs. If the body is healthy, the eyes are bright and visualize. Qi is the commander of the blood, while the blood is the mother of qi, so they are mutually dependent and transformed. If qi is flouring and the blood is sufficient, the body is healthy. If qi is deficient and blood is weak, the diseases, such as blurring of vision, senile cataract, diabetic ophthalmopathy, etc., may occur.

(1) Blood deficiency: Blurring of vision and dryness of eyes.

(2) Heat in blood: Various types of hemorrhage in circumocular diseases due to heat forcing blood to flow recklessly.

(3) Blood stasis: It refers to the unsmooth flow of blood or accumulation of blood out of meridians, such as blue or purple colour of eyelid, trachomatous pannus, subconjunctival ecchymosis, hyphema and vitreous hemorrhagia, old fundus hemorrhage, fundus proliferation, or retinal scarring.

6.2 血

精血之源由五脏六腑之精华所赋,故身不病乃有目明视。气为血之帅,血为气之母,相互依存,相互生化。气旺血润(盛)则机体强健,气虚血枯(弱)则病影随行,视瞻昏渺、圆翳内障、消渴目病皆可不期而至。

(1) 血虚:视物昏花,目珠干涩不润;

(2) 血热:迫血妄行致内外障各种出血性眼病;

(3) 血瘀:各种原因致血行不畅或离经之血不散:胞睑青紫,赤膜下垂,黑睛赤脉,血灌瞳神,眼底陈旧性出血、增殖,瘢痕形成。

6.3 Body fluid

The bright vision relies on qi transformation of the lung, spleen, kidney and triple energizer. The lung in the upper energizer dominates spreading and transformation, the spleen in the middle energizer dominates transportation and transformation, and the kidney in the lower energizer dominates qi transformation. The triple energizer spreads the

6.3 津液

眼之明视,依赖肺、脾、肾、三焦气化,上焦肺主宣化,中焦脾主运化,下焦肾主气化,三焦为用则津液匀布濡养周身。津液在目外为润泽之水,如泪液;在内为充养之液,如神水、神膏。津液不

body fluid evenly all over the body to moisturize and nourish the body. The body fluid is transformed to the moisturizing fluid, as the tear at the circumocular area, and to the nourishing fluid, as aqueous humor or vitreous body at the intraocular area. Insufficiency of body fluid is manifested at the circumocular area by dryness of eyeball, dryness of eye white and lusterless eye black, and at the intraocular area by blurring of vision due to insufficiency of aqueous humor and malnutrition of vitreous body. Water retention, damp accumulation and phlegm blockage are the abnormal conditions of the body fluid and essence, leading to swelling and distension of eyelid, edema of eye white, lusterless eye black, iris opacity, choroids-retina exudation, macular effusion, retinal detachment and vitreous degeneration. The causative factors can be exogenous or endogenous, and can be the six pathogens or the seven emotional factors. When water retention, damp accumulation or phlegm blockage causes the disease, such as obstruction of central retinal vein, the diffuse edema of choroids-retina leads to blood stasis and collateral obstruction. In the end, both the essence and spirit of the eyes are damaged, and the eyes fail to see.

足则目外表现为目珠干涩、白睛不润、黑睛失泽；目内表现为神水不足，神膏失养所致视物昏花。水停、湿聚、痰阻反应的是津、精、液之失常，胞睑肿胀、白睛水肿、黑睛失泽、黄仁污秽、视衣渗出、黄斑聚液、网膜脱离、玻璃体机化皆由此生。其因或外或内，六因七情皆可为患。但水停、湿聚、痰阻继而为害如视网膜静脉阻塞，其视衣漫肿碍阻营血，脉络瘀而为患，眼之精、神俱损，不得而视。

Section 3 Diagnostic methods in ophthalmology

第3节 眼科诊法

1 Vision examination

Vision examination includes the distant vision examination and near vision examination. In the ex-

1 视力检查方法

视力检查方法包括远视力和近视力，检查时需要两

amination, it is necessary to examine the two eyes separately, usually the right eye first and then the left one. In the examination of one eye, apply a palm or other object to cover the other eye without compressing the eyeball.

眼分别进行，一般先右后左，检查一眼时，可用手掌或其他物遮挡另一眼，盖时不可压迫眼球。

1.1 Distant vision examination

The International Standard Visual Chart or the Logarithmic Visual Acuity Chart is often applied in the examination. The subject to be examined must be 5 meters away from the test chart, or a reflecting mirror can be used if the distance is not far enough. Take the International Standard Visual Chart as an illustrating example. The 1.0 line of the test chart and the subject's eyes must be at the same high level. The examiner then points to the chart letters line by line with an indicating bar and asks the subject to tell or gesticulate the opening side of the pointed letter in order to find out the utmost line of the letters that the subject can completely identify without any mistakes. The marked figure on the line will be the visual acuity of the subject. The standard of normal vision is 1.0. If he cannot identify the biggest letter (0.1 line) on the test chart, the subject is permitted to come near the chart step by step till he can identify the biggest letter. The distance between the patient and the test chart is measured and his vision is calculated according to the following formula:

Vision = (distance between subject and chart/5 m)×0.1

If the subject can identify the 0.1 line of the test chart in a distance of 4 meters, his vision should be 4/5 * 0.1 = 0.08, vision of 0.06 in a distance of 3 meters, vision of 0.04 in a distance of 2 meters, and

1.1 远视力检测法

常用国际标准视力表或对数视力表。被检查者距离视力表 5 米，如距离不足，可采用反光镜法。现以国际标准视力表举例加以说明，视力表的 1.0 行应与被检查者眼同高，检查者用杆指着视力表上的字符，嘱被检查者说出或用手势表示该字符缺口方向，逐行检查，找出被检查者最多能将哪一行的字符完全正确认识，该行标志的数字即表示被检查者的视力。正常视力 1.0.如果患者在 5 米处连最大的字符(0.1 一行)也不能认出，则嘱患者逐步向视力表走近，直到认出为止，测量与视力表的距离，然后按照下列公式计算：

视力 =（被检查者与视力表距离/5 米）×0.1。

如检查者在 4 米处才能辨别 0.1，则该眼视力为 4/5 ×0.1 = 0.08，3 米为 0.06，2 米为 0.04，1 米为 0.02。

vision of 0.02 in a distance of 1 meter.

If the subject cannot identify the visual target in a distance of 1 meter, he is asked to move forwards a distance of some centimeters to identify the fingers or moving hand of the examiner, and the result is recorded. If he even cannot identify the fingers or the hand, the light perception of the subject is examined in a dark room. If he can tell the on and off of the light with the sick eye, the distance of the light sense or ocular sensation of light is recorded. If he cannot identify the light in the dark room, he can be diagnosed as the absence of light perception.

如被检查者已经前至视力表 1 米，仍不能辨别视标时，则嘱其辨别距离眼前若干厘米的指数或手动，并加以记录。若被检查者手动都无法辨别，则应进入暗室，测其光感。患眼如能辨别灯光明灭，亦应记录距离，写出几米光感或眼前光感。如在暗室内完全不能辨别灯光，则该眼视力为无光感。

1.2 Near vision examination

The International Standard Visual Chart or the Logarithmic Visual Acuity Chart is applied in the examination. The examination should be done in the natural sunlight or lamplight. With the visual test chart placed 30 cm far away from the subject, both eyes must be examined respectively from the biggest visual target 0.1 downwards in order. If the visual targets above 1.0 can be identified, the near vision of the eye is normal. If the 1.0 visual target cannot be identified in 30 cm distance, the visual test chart is moved forwards or backwards before the subject till he can identify the smallest visual target, and the result is recorded, such as 1.0 / 20 cm or 0.5 / 30 cm. The normal reading is 1.0 / 30 cm.

1.2 近视力检查法

近视力检查法用标准近视力表或对数近视力表。检查须在充足自然光线或灯光下进行，把近视力表置于眼前 30 厘米处，分别检查两眼，由最大视标 0.1 开始，顺序向下。凡能辨认出 1.0 以上视标字向者，该眼近视力正常。如不能在 30 厘米处辨认出 1.0，则将视力表向眼前或后移动，直至能辨认出最小视标字向的距离为止，然后分别记录，如 1.0/20 厘米，或 0.5/30 厘米等，正常为 1.0/30 厘米。

2 Visual field examination

The visual field is the portion of space which the fixed eye can see. Compared with the central vision, it is the extent of the peripheral field of vi-

2 视野检查方法

视野是当眼球向正前方固视不动时所见的空间范围。与中央视力相对应，它

sion. The central visual field is termed as the 30° extent around the fixed visual point. The field beyond that extent is called the peripheral visual field. When the visual field is less than 10° extent, according to WHO's standard, the case can still be determined as a kind of visual field defect even if the vision is normal.

是周围视力。距注视点 30°以内的范围称为中央视野。30°以外者称周边视野。现世界卫生组织规定视野小于10°者即使视力正常也属于盲。

Visual field defect can be caused by many intraocular diseases, so the visual field examination plays an important role in the diagnosis of different of fundus diseases, especially the pathogenic changes concerning the central nervous system.

许多内障眼病都可引起视野缺损，所以视野检查对许多眼底疾病，特别是有关中枢系统病变，具有十分重要意义。

2.1 Contrast examination

2.1 对比法

With no need of any facilities, this is a simple and convenient method. In the examination, the examiner and the subject are sitting face to face in a distance of 0.5 meter and at the same height of eyesight. If, for instance, the right eye of the subject is to be examined, the left eye of the subject and the right one of the examiner are covered to have the subject's right fixed on the examiner's left eye. The examiner then places his fingers in the space between himself and the subject and moves his fingers from the outside to the center in every direction. If the subject can see the examiner's fingers in any direction at the same time as the examiner see them, his visual field can be determined as normal. The visual field of the other eye can examined with the same method which, thought simple, convenient and reliable, is not accurate enough and the result is hard to be recorded for the later references.

这是一种简单易行不需要任何设备的方法。检查时医生与被检查者距 0.5 米相对而坐，眼位等高。如检查右眼，则遮盖被检查者的左眼和医生的右眼，让被检查者的右眼与医生的左眼相互注视，医生将手指置于与两人等距离之处，在各个方向从外向中央移动，如被检查者能在各个方向与医生同时看到手指，即可认为视野大致正常。同法检查另一眼。此法简单，有一定可靠性，但不够精确，并且无法作记录，以供参考。

2.2 Arc perimeter examination

2.2 弧形视野计检查法

The arc perimeter is a quite simple instrument for the dynamic examination of the peripheral vi-

弧形视野计是比较简单的动态检查周边视野的器

sion. In the examination, the subject is asked to put his mandible on the support, with one eye covered and the other eye to be examined placed at the same high level of the 0° position and concentrating on the fixed central point. Then the examiner slowly moves the light visual target from the periphery to the center till the subject can see the light target and the angulation marked on the arc perimeter is recorded. With the arc plate rotated, the examination is continued on the twelve radial lines successively in the same way and the angles of light target of all the twelve radial lines, which are first seen by the patient, are linked to form a line on the visual field form, so that the extent of the visual field of the examined eye can be determined.

械。检查时，令被检查者的下颌放在支架上，遮盖一眼，使受检眼与0°在同一水平线上，并注视中央固定点不动，然后医生将光标由周边向中央缓缓移动，直到被检查者看见为止，记下弧上所标的角度，旋转弧板，依次查12个径线，将各径线开始看见光标的角度在视野表上连线画线，即为被检眼的视野范围。

The extent of visual field may vary with the sizes and colors of the light targets, examining distances, light intensity, height of the subject's nose bridge, sizes of the pupil and palpebral fissure as well as the spiritual and healthy conditions of the subject. The usual visual target is white and 3 mm in diameter and, if the subject's vision is too poor, the visual target of 5 mm or 10 mm in diameter can be used. The colors can be chosen on the basis of diseases, for example, blue or yellow colour for retinal diseases and red or green colour for optic nerve diseases.

视野的大小可因视标的大小颜色、检查距离、光线的强弱以及被检查者的鼻梁高低、瞳孔和睑裂的大小及其精神与健康状况而有所变化。通常3毫米直径的白色视标。若是你很差，则可改为5毫米或10毫米的视标，并可根据疾病选用不同颜色的视标，如视网膜疾病用蓝色或黄色，视神经疾病用红色或绿色的视标。

The normal plane extent of visual field (white color) include the temporal 90°, the paranasal 60°, the lower 70° and the upper 55°. About 10° is successively reduced when the colour is blue, red and green.

正常视野(白色)的平面范围，颞侧90°、鼻侧60°、下方70°、上方55°，蓝、红、绿色视野依次递减10°左右。

2.3 Campimetry

2.3 平面视野计检查法

The method is mainly used to examine scotoma

此法主要检查围绕固视

of the visual field within 30° extent around the visual point. In the examination, the subject is sitting in front of the campimeter in a distance of 1 meter, with one eye covered and the other one to be examined fixed on the visual point on the front central screen. Then the examiner holds the visual target and moves it slowly along each radial line from the periphery to the center to find out the scale of the scotomata which are marked out first in black dots with a pin and then recorded in the table. All the scotomata in the extent of such visual field are pathogenic except those physiological ones.

点30°以内视野范围的暗点。检查时，被检查者坐在平面视野计的1米处，遮盖一眼，受检眼在屏幕中央的注视点正前方，并注视不动。然后检查者持视标由周边向中央在各子午线上缓慢移动，检查出来的暗点范围先用小黑点大头针作标记，最后描记在记录表上。在此视野范围内，除了生理盲点外所出现的任何暗点，皆为病理性暗点。

2.4 Automatic perimeter examination

It is a kind of up-to-date perimeter which, on the basis of the improvement of the above methods, is equipped with a computer and can automatically show the photostimuli from the weak to the strong on each visual field position in accordance with the program. It can print a report according to the subject's positive and negative responses (by means of touching the buttons) when the examination is finished. In the report, the light threshold value of the subject on every position and the difference compared with the normal value of the same age group are recorded in the forms of figure, make and number, so that the extent and depth of total loss of vision and local visual defects are signified.

2.4 自动化视野计

此为最新的视野计，在上述改进的基础上配备微机，自动按照程序在视野的各个位点显示由弱到强的光刺激，并根据被检查者的应答（以按钮的方式表示看见与否），在检查完毕后答应报告，以图形、记号及数字记录被检查者视野中各个位点的光阈值及其同年龄组正常眼差别，从而给出视野总丢失量和局限性缺损的范围与深度。

3 Chromometry examination

Color sense is the faculty of the retina by which various colors are perceived and distinguished. The pseudoisochromatic table (plate), also called colour blindness test cards, is the most commonly used in

3 色觉检查法

视网膜辨别各种颜色的感觉，称为色觉。检查色觉最常用的是假同色表。假同色表常称为色盲本。检查应

the chromoscopy. The examination should be carried out on a fine day, and both eyes must be examined at the same time. The pseudoisochromatic table is placed 0.5 m away from the subject, and the subject is asked to identify the number or figure in the table in five seconds. If it is difficult for him to identify or if he makes mistakes or cannot recognize, the condition can be determined as a certain kind of colour blindness or weakness according to the attached instruction in the table.

在晴天自然充足的光线下进行，两眼同时进行，方法是将假同色表放在距离被检查者眼前 0.5 米处，让其在 5 秒内读出表内数字和图案。如果辨认有困难，读错或不能读出，可按假同色表内所附说明判定为何种色盲或色弱。

4 Slit-lamp microscopy

Slit-lamp microscope consists of a slit-lamp system and a microscope system. It can amplify the pathogenic changes of the eye to 10 to 16 times under strong light beams. Of its various operating procedures, six methods are often used in clinic because of different ways of illumination and different tissues to be illuminated. They are the diffuse illumination, the corneosclearal scatter illumination, the direct focal illumination, retro illumination, specular reflection and indirect illumination. The direct focal illumination, which is more often applied in clinical practice, throws light onto the conjunctiva, sclera and iris to produce a clear illuminated area by the joint of the light focus and the microscope focus. So lesions in the part can be observed thoroughly. When the light of the slit-lamp is thrown onto the transparent cornea or lens, a cream white optical section will show up. At this time, the examiner can observe the curvature and thickness of the section, find if there is any foreign body or corneal deposit, and determine the layers and forms of such pathogenic changes as infiltration, ulcer and

4 裂隙灯显微镜检查法

裂隙灯显微镜是由裂隙灯和显微镜两个系统组成。可在强光下放大 10～16 倍检查眼部病变。其操作方法很多，因光线照射的方式及被照射组织的不同，临床常用六种照射方法，即弥散光线照射法、角巩膜缘分光照射法、直接焦点照射法、后方反光照射法、镜面反光带照射法、间接照射法等。临床常用的是直接焦点照射法，此法是将灯光焦点与显微镜焦点联合在一起，将光线投射在结膜、巩膜和虹膜上，可见一境界清楚的射亮区，以便细致地观察该区的病变。将裂隙灯照在透明的角膜或晶状体上，则呈一种乳白色的光线切面，借此可以观察其弯曲度、厚度、有无异物或角膜后沉着物，以及浸润、溃

necrosis. Then the light is, by regulation, turned into a beam which is thrown onto the anterior chamber to see if there is aqueous flare (also called Tyndall phenomenon), i.e. when the optical density is raised, a cream white band of light will appear between the cornea and the lens if protein in the aqueous humor increases or cellular endosmosis exists. Again the focus point is moved backward in order that the lesions in the lens and one-third vitreous body can be observed.

疡、坏死等病变的层次和形态。将光线调成细小光柱射入前房，可检查有无房水闪辉（又称 Tyndall 现象），即在房水中蛋白质增加或有细胞渗入，因而使其光密度增加时，可见角膜与晶状体之间有一乳白色的光带。再将焦点向后移，还可以观察晶状体及前 1/3 玻璃体的病变。

5 Intraocular pressure examination

5 眼压检查法

5.1 Digital compression

This is a very simple and easy examining method of intraocular pressure through which the softness or hardness of the eyeball can be estimated. In the examination, the subject is asked to look downwards as possible as he can, and the examiner places the tips of his two index fingers on the upper margin skin of the subject's superior tarsus and slightly presses his eyeball alternately to estimate the subject's intraocular pressure through the resistance that the finger tips can feel. The symbols used in the method are: Tn indicating normal, T+1 slightly high, T+2 very high, and T+3 extremely high or as hard as a stone. On the other hand, symbols T-1, T-2 and T-3 represent slight low, very low and extremely low respectively.

5.1 指测法

简单容易操作，能估计眼球的软硬度。检查时，嘱患者两眼尽量向下注视，检查者用两手食指尖放在睑板上缘的皮肤上，两指尖交替轻压眼球，凭借指尖触知的抵抗力估计眼压的高低。记录时，以 Tn 表示眼压正常，T+1 表示眼压轻度增高，T+2 表示眼压很高，T+3 表示眼压极高，眼球坚硬如石。反之，则以 T-1、T-2、T-3 分别表示眼压稍低、很低、极低。

5.2 Ophthalmotonometry

(1) Schiotz Tonometer: The subject takes a supine position with a low headrest and the eye to be examined is dropped 2 or 3 times with 0.5% dicaine. Before the examination, the tonometer is examined on the standard plate, so that the needle can

5.2 眼压计量测量法

(1) Schiotz 眼压计：患者仰卧低枕，被检查眼滴入 0.5%地卡因 2～3 次。测前，眼压计先在标准试板上测试，指针指在零度时为正常。

point to zero, and then the plate is cleaned with 75% alcohol cotton and dried. The subject is asked to lift his left hand with the index finger as the fixed point, and the cornea right on the middle horizontal position. The examiner, holding the tonometer in his right hand, slightly opens the subject's eyelids with his left thumb and index finger, and fixes them on the orbital margin without compressing the subject's eyeball. Then the tonometer plate is vertically placed in the center of the cornea. With a 5.5 weight added, the examiner immediately reads the graduation pointed by the needle, and then instantly takes up the tonometer in case the corneal epithelium might be abraded. If the reading is less than 3, a heavier wight is used and another examination is performed. The actual number should be calculated by the conversion of the reading according to the conversion table. When the examination is finished, antibiotic eye drops should be applied to the conjunctival sac. Since the tonometer is of depression type, the reading number is determined by the depression of the cornea under the compression of the tonometer needle, and as the ocular volume may change greatly during the procedure, the reading number is often influenced by the hardness of the eyeball wall. In the case of abnormal hardness of eyeball wall, some slightly high or low incorrect readings ma by obtained. Although such errors can be avoided through the examination with two weights and the correct table, the final result is no as accurate as that with an applanation tonometer.

用75%酒精棉球擦拭底板待干。测量时嘱患者举起左手伸出食指作为注视点,使角膜恰在水平正中位,检查者右手持眼压计,左手拇指及食指轻轻分开上下睑,固定在眶缘上,不得给眼球施加任何压力。将眼压计底板垂直放在角膜中央,先用5.5砝码,迅速读指针刻度,立即提起眼压计,以免擦伤角膜上皮。如读数小于3,则需要更换较重砝码,再测量。测出的读数查换算表,得出眼压的实际数字。测毕,结膜囊内滴抗生素眼药水。此眼压计为压陷式,其刻度的多少取决于在眼压计压针的压迫下角膜向下凹陷的程度。如果测量时引起眼球容积的变化较大,则测出的数值会受到球壁硬度的影响。在球壁硬度显著异常者会给出偏高或偏低的数据,用两个砝码测量后查表校正可消除球壁硬度造成的误差,但仍不如压平眼压计准确。

(2) Goldmann Applanation Tonometer: This is the most accurate international tonometer. It is attached to a slit-lamp microscope to measure the in-

(2) Goldmann压平眼压计:这是目前国际通用的最准确的眼压计,它是附装

traocular pressure through the microscope in a sitting position. Since it is a kind of applanation tonometer, the cornea in the examining process becomes slightly applanated, but the eyeball volume does not change greatly without depression, avoiding the affection of the hardness of the eyeball wall. The Perkin applanation tonometer which, in principle, is the same as the Goldmann tonometer, is a hard tonometer and has the advantage of operating with the subject either in a sitting position or in a lying position without the need of slit-lamp microscope.

(3) Non-contact applanation tonometer: The principle of the applanation tonometer is to make use of a sort of controlled air pulse, the pressure of which is indicated by the characteristics of the linear increase. When the cornea is applanated within a certain area, the monitoring system is applied to receive the light reflected from the corneal surface, and the time to applanate the cornea to a certain extent is recorded and calculated in the unit of kPa. The biggest advantage of the applanation tonometer is that the cross infection sometimes caused by using the ophthalmonometry is thoroughly prevented, and the method is applicable to those who are allergic to surface anesthesia, while its disadvantage is that the obtained values may be a little lower.

在裂隙灯显微镜上，用显微镜观察，坐位测量。它是一种压平眼压计，在测量时仅仅使角膜凸面稍稍变平而不下陷，眼球容积改变很小，所以基本上不受球壁硬度的影响。还有 Perkin 压平眼压计，原理与 Goldmann 眼压计相同，其优点是可以手持使用，不需要裂隙灯显微镜，被检查者取坐位卧位都可以测量。

(3) 非接触压平眼压计：其原理是利用一种可控的空气脉冲，其压力具有线性增加特性，将角膜压平一定面积，再利用监测系统感受角膜表面反射的光线，并将角膜压平到一定程度所需的时间记录下来，换算成眼压的 kPa 数。它的最大优点是彻底避免了通过眼压计引起的交叉感染，并能应用于对表面麻醉药过敏的患者。其缺点是所得数值可能偏低。

6 Fundus examination

The fundus examination is always done in a dark room. If it is hard for the speculum examination in the case of stenocoriasis, the subject's pupil is treated with mydriatic agents. Before the mydriatic agentsare applied, the depth of the anterior

6 眼底检查方法

眼底检查一般在暗室进行，如患者瞳孔小，不容易窥入，需用药物散大瞳孔，详查眼底，在点散瞳药之前，必须先了解前房深浅、房角的宽

chamber and the width of its angle must be found out, for mydriasis, in a narrow anterior chamber condition, has the potential risk to start angle-closure glaucoma.

窄，注意窄房角眼散瞳有激发闭角型青光眼发作的潜在危险。

In the fundus examination, two kinds of ophthalmoscopes, indirect and direct, are used. With an indirect ophthalmoscope, the examiner can see an inverted image of a larger area amplified four times, while what he sees is an ortho-image of a smaller part amplified about 10 times with a direct one.

检查眼底用的检眼镜有间接检眼镜和直接检眼镜两种。间接检眼镜所见眼底范围为倒像，放大 4 倍，可见方位大；直接检眼镜所见眼底为正像，放大 10 倍，可见范围小。

6.1 Direct ophthalmoscopy

6.1 直接检眼镜检查方法

With his index finger putting on the ophthalmoscope plate for the convenient regulation of the diopter, the examiner holds the ophthalmoscope handle with the other fingers. When examining the right eye, the examiner should stand on the subject's right side with the ophthalmoscope in the right hand to check with the right eye. Likewise, when the left eye is examined, the examiner has to stand on the left side of the subject, with the ophthalmoscope in the left hand to check with left eye. In the examination, the transillumination is used first to find out if there is any cloudiness in the refracting media, then the ophthalmoscope turntable is set at the +8～+10D, and the light is right thrown into the pupil 10～20 cm awayfrom the examined eye. In a normal condition, the pupil area shows the orange-colored reflection. If the cloudiness exists in the cornea, lens or vitreous body, there may appear a dark shadow in the red reflection. At this moment, the subject is asked to move his eyeball around, and if the dark shadow turns together with his eyeball, it indicates that the cloudiness is in front of the

将食指放在检眼镜的盘上，以便随时调整屈光度数，拇指及其余手指握住镜柄。检查右眼时，检查者站在被检者右侧，用右手持检眼镜，用右眼检查。检查左眼时，检查者站在被检者左侧，用左手持检眼镜，用左眼检查。检查时，应先用彻照法检查眼的屈光间质有无混浊，用食指将检眼镜转盘拨到 +8～+10D，距受检眼 10～20 厘米，将检眼镜灯光射入瞳孔，正常者瞳孔区呈橘红色反光，如角膜、晶状体或玻璃体有混浊，则在红色反光中出现黑影。此时嘱患者转动眼球，如黑影转动的方向与眼球一致，则表明混浊位于晶状体前方，反之则位于晶状体后方，如不动，则在晶状体。

lens, conversely in the back of the lens, or inside the lens if immovable.

After the transillumination, the turntable is turned back to the "0 to −3" position and the ophthalmoscope is moved near the eye about 2 cm away to examine the fundus. If both the examiner and the subject are of emmetropia, the fundus can clearly be seen. If it cannot clearly be seen, the turntable is turned till the fundus can clearly be seen. The subject is asked to look straightly ahead, and the ophthalmoscope light is thrown at a 15° angle from the temporal to examine the optic disc. Then the subject is asked to take a round look for the examination of the periphery of the optic disc, and finally the macular retina is examined with the subject's eye fixed on the light of the ophthalmoscope.

彻照完毕后，将转盘拨回到 0～−3 处，同时将检眼镜移近受检眼约 2 厘米处，检查眼底，如检查者与被检者都是正视眼，则可看清眼底，如不能看清，可拨动转盘直至看清为止，嘱患者向正前方注视，检眼镜从颞侧约 15°处投入光线，以检查视盘，再嘱患者向上下左右方向注视，以检查周边部。最后嘱患者注视检眼镜灯光，以检查黄斑部。

The normal optic disc takes an ellipsoid-like shape in a light red-colored light, clearly bounded, and with the excavation in the center, which is also called the physiological excavation or cup. At the bottom of this physiological excavation, where some gry dots can be dimly seen, is the cribriform plate.

正常眼底可见视盘略呈椭圆形，浅红色，境界清楚，中央有凹陷，色泽稍淡，称为生理凹陷，亦称为杯。生理凹陷底部隐约可见一些暗灰色小点，该处为筛板。

Normally, the central retinal artery is bright red in color, its vein is dark red in color, and the diametric proportion of the retinal artery and vein is 2: 3. If the artery becomes thinned and the cross points of the artery and vein are broken of blunt, it indicates retinal angiospasm or arteriosclerosis.

视网膜中央动脉呈亮红色，静脉呈暗红色，动静脉管径之比为 2∶3，如动脉变细，或动脉交叉处静脉中断或尖削，则表明有视网膜动脉痉挛或硬化。

The normal retina is transparent with the pigmented epithelium and choroids seen, thus showing an even orange colour or leopard retina. A lot of fundus disorders and general diseases can cause edema, hemorrhage, exudation, necrosis or pigmental abnormality in the retina.

视网膜正常时透明，可见下方之色素上皮及脉络膜，故呈均匀橘红色或豹纹状，许多眼底病或全身疾病都可使视网膜出现水肿、出血、渗出、坏死或色素异常。

The macular retina which lies lightly below the temporal optic disc 2 PD (disc diameter) away is dark red in colour and has no blood vessels but a reflection point in the center called the central fovea reflection. A reflection areola can be seen around the macula of the young people and children.

黄斑部位于视盘颞侧2PD(视盘直径)稍偏下方,呈暗红色,无血管,其中央有一反光点,称中心凹光反射,青少年黄斑周围可见一反光晕。

6.2 Indirect ophthalmoscopy

6.2 间接检眼镜检查法

What can be seen in the examination is an inverted image of the larger scale of the fundus amplified 4 times, but the pupil must be treated with the mydriatic agents. At present, the binocular indirect ophthalmoscope is usually applied. The frontal mirror is fixed on the examiner's head with the illuminator installed in the headband and the convex lens held in the examiner's left hand. The visual field in the fundus examination by the indirect ophthalmoscope is larger than that by the direct one, so more general conditions of the fundus can be found without missing any pathological changes, particularly in the examination of the retinal hole. Besides, since the examination is performed in a quite far distance, the operations of blocking and padding the retinal hole and so on can be carried out in an audiovisual way. The indirect ophthalmoscope, therefore, is now the necessary instrument in the examination and treatment of the retinal detachment.

此镜所见的眼底为倒像、放大4倍,可见范围较大,但必须散大瞳孔,现多用双目间接眼底镜,用额头套固定于头部,光源也装在额带上,左手持一凸透镜,用间接检眼镜检查眼底,所见视野比直接检眼镜大,能比较全面了解眼底情况,不易遗漏眼底的病变,尤其有利于寻找视网膜裂孔,又因其可在较远距离检查眼底,从而使视网膜裂孔的封闭及垫压等操作可以在直观下进行,因此它已成为检查和治疗视网膜脱离的必备仪器。

7 Optical coherence tomography (OCT) scanning

7 光学相干断层扫描

Optical coherence tomography (OCT) scanning is a kind of non-contact and non-invasive image examination method by CT scanning theintraocular tissues, rapidly developed in the recent 10 years. In the examination, it clearly shows the 10-layer struc-

光学相干断层扫描(OCT)是近十年来迅速发展起来的非接触性、非损伤性对眼内组织结构进行断层扫描的影像学检查方法,可以

ture of the retinal section, the interface between the vitreous body and retina, and the relationship between the integrity of the retinal pigment epithelium and the choroid membrane, similar to the biopsy. It is a clinic diagnostic method to supply a clearer retinal structure at moment, so as to provide the diagnostic information for the common diseases, such as macular hole, macular epiretinal membrane, cystoid macular edema, choroidal neovascularization at macular region, central serous lesions of retina and choroids, retinoschisis, etc. The visual field analysis mentioned above is the reference standard in the diagnosis and progression of glaucoma, but it is impossible to find out the damage manifestations in suspected glaucoma in early stage in the visual field examination. Only in the massive loss (>40%) of the neural fibers, can the visual field defects be manifested in the visual field examination, so as to find out the optic neuropathy. Therefore, OCT becomes a kind of new, objective and quantitative index for the evaluation of glaucoma. Furthermore, in the selection of treatment and observation of therapeutic effect for the fundus diseases, OCT is more valuable than the other image examinations.

清晰地显示视网膜切面的10层结构、玻璃体与视网膜交界面、视网膜色素上皮的完整性及视网膜与脉络膜之间的关系，类似在活体组织进行病理检查。这是现阶段可以提供较清晰的视网膜结构的临床诊断方法，可为黄斑裂孔、黄斑视网膜前膜、黄斑囊样水肿、黄斑脉络膜新生血管、中心性浆液性脉络膜视网膜病变、视网膜劈裂等常见视网膜疾病提供量化的诊断信息，前面谈到的视野分析是青光眼的诊断和疾病进展评估的参考标准，但是通过视野检查却不能发现可疑青光眼早期的视功能损害表现。只有在大量神经纤维丢失时（>40%），视野检查才表现出视野缺损，从而发现视神经损害。因此，OCT为青光眼的评估提供了一种新的客观、定量指标。并且对眼底疾病的治疗选择与疗效观察，OCT的应用价值也是其他影像检查无法比拟的。

8 Fundus fluorescence angiography

The fundus fluorescence angiography (FFA) is a kind of technique to truly record the dynamic changes of the fundus, through the fluorescence occurring in the intraocular blood circulation after the

8 荧光眼底血管造影术

荧光眼底血管造影术（FFA），是通过静脉注射荧光素在眼内血液循环时所发出的荧光，利用装有特殊滤

intravenous injection of fluorescein and by using the fundus camera with specific filtering combination. In the process of the fundus fluorescence angiography, it is possible to clearly observe the fine structure of microcirculation, even the capillary vessels. The photos are taken for permanent preservation, to illustrate comprehensively, systematically and dynamically the normal or abnormal state of human body circulation, so as to provide the objective basis for the diagnosis, treatment or research of the fundus diseases. It is a necessary new technology of examination in the clinic.

光片组合的眼底照相机，真实地记录下眼底情况动态变化的技术。在眼底荧光血管造影过程中，能够清楚地观察到微循环的细微结构，直到毛细血管水平，并且可以拍照下来永久保存，它可以完整地系统地以动态说明人体循环的正常或异常状态，从而为诊断、治疗或研究眼底病提供客观依据，是一项临床上不可缺少的检查新技术。

In the process of FFA, it is possible to observe the conditions of the fundus and choroid circulation and the retinal blood vessel circulation with different manifestations. The choroid circulation in FFA can be seen as the rough, hazy and geographicchoroid fluorescence. It is difficult to see the details of the choroid circulation, because the yellow-green spectrum from the fluorescein in blood is almost absorbed by the retinal pigment epithelium. Besides, the fluorescein may leak out from the choroid capillary vessels, while the choroid contains a large amount of fluorescein, which may enter the subretinal area through the break of the retinal pigment epithelium, to cause the abnormal fluorescence phenomena (such as central serous retinopathy, retinal pigment epithelitis, macular degeneration, choroid neoplasms and choroid neovascularization).

眼底荧光血管造影过程中可以观察到眼底脉络膜循环及视网膜血管循环情况，其各有不同的表现，脉络膜循环在荧光造影过程中，只能粗略地朦胧地见到地图状脉络膜荧光，很难见到脉络膜循环的细节，因为血液中荧光素所发出的黄绿色光谱几乎大部分被视网膜色素上皮所吸收。同时荧光素可以从脉络膜毛细血管内向外渗漏，致使在造影过程中，脉络膜内含有多量的荧光素，当脉络膜毛细血管产生病变而使视网膜色素上皮出现病变时，含有高浓度荧光素的脉络膜液就会通过视网膜色素上皮损害处进入视网膜下而出现异常荧光现象（如中浆病、视网膜色素上皮炎、黄斑变性、脉络膜肿瘤、脉络膜新生血管）。

In the diabetic patients, it is possible through FFA the diabetic retinopathy in early stage. The staging criteria of the diabetic retinopathy are as follows:

Stage I: Microaneurysms accompanied by small hemorrhagic spots.

Stage II: Yellow-white colored "hard exudates" accompanied by hemorrhagic blotches.

Stage III: Grey-white colored "soft exudates" accompanied by Stage II.

Stage IV: Neovascularization accompanied by vitreous hemorrhage.

Stage V: Neovascularization and fibrous proliferation.

Stage VI: Neovascularization and fibrous proliferation leading to retinal detachment.

尤其在糖尿病患者，FFA能够比较好地发现早期糖尿病性视网膜病变，糖尿病视网膜病变分期标准如下：

Ⅰ期：微血管瘤合并小出血点；

Ⅱ期：黄白色"硬性渗出"合并出血斑；

Ⅲ期：灰白色"软性渗出"合并Ⅱ期；

Ⅳ期：新生血管合并玻璃体出血；

Ⅴ期：新生血管和纤维增殖；

Ⅵ期：新生血管和纤维增殖，引起视网膜脱离。上述微血管瘤、出血、渗出、新生血管及纤维增殖均为检眼镜下观察结果。

All the above-mentioned conditions of microaneurysms, hemorrhage, exudes, neovascularization and fibrous proliferation are the results observed under the optic microscope. In FFA, it is possible to observe instantly the fluorescein in the fundus along with the blood circulation, and to dynamically reflect the retinal blood circulation state and the blood shape, so as to find out the organic changes of the retinal micro-vessels before the above-mentioned lesions found by the optic microscope, manifested by fluorescein leakage, localized dilation of capillary vessels, filling defects of capillary vessels and tumor-like dotted fluorescein. Therefore, it is nec-

FFA可通过即时观察荧光素在眼底随血液循环状况，动态反映视网膜血液循环状态和血管形态，可以在眼底镜发现上述病变之前更早发现视网膜微血管的器质性改变，其表现为：荧光渗漏、毛细血管局限性扩张、毛细血管充盈缺损、瘤样点状荧光。因此，糖尿病患者尽早行FFA检查，及早发现黄斑病变，有利于尽早采取合理的治疗措施，减缓视网膜

essary to take FFA for the diabetic patients as early as possible, so as to find the macular lesions early, and then to apply the reasonable and proper therapeutic measures, for the purpose to slow down the development of retinopathy and decrease the damage to the visual function.

病变的发展速度,减少对视功能造成的损害。

Chapter 4 Essentials of Therapeutics in Ophthalmology

第4章 治疗概要

Section 1 Internal therapies

第1节 内治法

1 Wind-eliminating and heat-clearing method

This method is to apply the prescription formed by the pungent-cool and exterior-relieving drugs, to eliminate wind and reduce heat, so as to treat the eye diseases caused by pathogenic wind-heat. It is applied to treat the eye diseases due to exogenous wind-heat, manifested by sudden onset of disease, eye itching and pain, swelling of eyelids, redness of eye white, nebula of eye black, etc., accompanied by the general symptoms of headache, aversion to cold, fever, superficial-rapid pulse, etc.

1 疏风清热法

本法是用具有辛凉解表作用的药物组成方剂，通过疏风散热、解除风热所致眼病的治法。适用于外感风热所致眼病的治法，适用于外感风热眼病。常见症状如：病起突然，目痒目痛，胞睑浮肿，白睛红赤，黑睛星翳等，常伴有头痛，恶寒发热，脉浮数等全身症状。

2 Fire-reducing and toxin-relieving method

This method is to apply the prescription formed by the fire-reducing and toxin-relieving drugs, to remove the heat-toxin in eye diseases, so as to treat the eye diseases caused by the six exogenous pathogens transforming to heat and entering the interior, or the eye diseases caused by the upward attack of heat-toxin, manifested by quick and severe onset of

2 泻火解毒法

本法是用性质寒凉的药物组成方剂，通过泻火解毒以清除眼病热毒的方法，适用于外感六淫化热入里，或热毒上攻的眼病。常见症状：发病急重、眼病疼痛拒按、羞明灼痛、热泪如汤、眵

disease, eye pain which is worsened by pressure, photophobia, burning pain, hot and excessive tears, excessive and sticky eye discharge, swelling of eyelids, turbidity and redness of eye white, necrosis of eye black, hypopyon, papillary seclusion, etc., accompanied by the general symptoms of thirst, constipation, red tongue body, yellow tongue coating, etc.

多粘结，胞肿如桃、白睛混赤、黑睛溃陷、黄液上冲、瞳神紧小等，常伴有口渴、便秘、舌红、苔黄等全身症状。

It is a cooling and attacking method, which may damage the yang qi of spleen and stomach, so it is not advisable to apply it for long time. Clinically, it is necessary to select the drugs carefully according to the seriousness of the disease and the body constitution of the patient. Furthermore, the cooling drugs applied for long time may cause qi stagnation and blood stasis, so it is difficult to dissolve the nebula. Therefore, it is necessary to grasp the scale of the method in the treatment of cornea diseases and fundus hemorrhage. It is prohibited to apply this method for the patient of false fire pattern.

本法为寒凉直折之法，容易损伤脾胃阳气，故不宜久用，临床上根据患者病情轻重和体质强弱慎重选择，又因寒凉药久用可导致气血凝滞，翳障难消，故对黑睛疾患，眼底出血，用本法必须掌握尺度。虚火者，禁用此法。

3 Yin-nourishing and fire-subduing method

3 滋阴降火法

This method is to apply the prescription formed by the cooling and nourishing drugs, to nourish the yin fluid, clear and reduce the false fire, relieve the symptoms of yin deficiency and fire hyperactivity, so as to brighten the eyes, applied to treat the eye diseases caused by yin deficiency and fire hyperactivity, manifested by dryness of eyes, slight red-color of eye white, appearing and disappearing nebular of eye black, papillary metamorphosis, corediastasis, increase of intraocular hypertension, blurring of vision, etc., accompanied by the general symp-

本法是用具有寒凉滋润作用的药物组成方剂，通过滋阴液，清降虚火，解除阴虚火旺的证候而达到明目效果的治法，适用于阴虚火旺的眼病。常见症状：眼球干涩、白睛微赤、黑睛星翳乍隐乍现，瞳神干缺，或瞳神散大，眼压增高，视物昏矇等。常伴有潮热颧红，手足心热，头晕心烦，口苦口干，舌红少

toms of tidal fever, flushed cheeks, feverish sensation in palms and soles, dizziness, irritability, bitter taste in mouth, dry mouth, red tongue body with scanty coating, thready-rapid pulse, etc.

苔，脉细数等全身症状。

Clinically, the eye diseases due to yin deficiency and fire hyperactivity are rather common, but it is necessary to further identify the patterns in the application of this method. For example, red colour of canthi, irritability and insomnia are of the false fire in the Heart Meridian. Slightly red colour of eye white, dry nose and dry throat are of the false fire in the Lung Meridian. Nebula of eye black, ciliary hyperemia, restlessness and anger are of the false fire in the Liver Meridian. It is advisable to select the proper formulas and herbal drugs by integrating the pertained zang-fu organs.

临床上阴虚火旺的眼病较多，但在具体应用本法时，尚须进一步辨证。如两眦红赤，心烦失眠，属心经虚火；白睛淡红，鼻干咽燥，属肺经虚火；黑睛生翳，抱轮红赤，烦躁易怒，属肝经虚火等；可结合脏腑所属，选方用药。

The yin-nourishing and fire-reducing drugs are mostly sticky, so it is prohibited to apply this method for the eye diseases caused by the exogenous pathogens, by deficiency and weakness of spleen and stomach, or by the existence of damp.

滋阴降火药物性多滋腻，故外感眼病、脾胃虚弱或湿邪未化者忌用本法。

4 Damp-removing method

4 祛湿法

This method is to apply the prescription formed by the damp-removing drugs, to remove the pathogenic damp, applied to treat the eye diseases caused by invasion of exogenous damp or internal accumulation of damp, manifested by erosion of eyelids, swelling of eyelids leading to failure to open eyes, millet-like boils inside eyelid, turbidity and yellow colour of eye white, excessive and sticky eye discharge, nebula of eye black, vitreous opacity, blurring of vision, etc., accompanied by the general symptoms of heavy sensation in head with a banding

本法是用祛湿药物组成方剂，通过祛除湿邪而治疗眼病的方法，适用于湿邪外侵或湿浊内蕴所引起的一切眼病，常见症状：睑弦湿烂，胞肿难睁，睑内粟疮或有膜形成，白睛污黄，眵多胶黏，黑睛有翳如虫蚀，神水混浊，视瞻昏渺等。常伴有头重如裹，口干不渴或口渴不欲饮，四肢乏力，胸闷少食，腹胀便

sensation, dry mouth without thirst, or thirst without desire to drinking water, fatigue of four limbs, stuffy chest, poor appetite, abdominal distension, loose feces, sticky tongue coating, etc.

溏,舌苔腻等全身症状。

The eye diseases due to damp are rather intractable, while the damp-removing drugs applied for long time may exhaust the body fluid, so that it is necessary to select the herbal drugs carefully according to the seriousness of the disease and the general condition of the patient. It is especially cautious to apply the herbal drugs for those with yin deficiency, blood insufficiency or body fluid defects.

湿症眼病比较顽固,祛湿药物久用易耗液伤津,故要根据病情轻重及患者全身情况慎重选药。阴虚血少与津液亏损者,尤宜注意。

5 Blood-stanching method

5 止血法

This method is to apply the prescription formed by the blood-stanching drugs, to stop bleeding in eyes, applied to treat the eye diseases with bleeding as the major symptom due to various causes, manifested by subconjunctival ecchymosis, hyphema and vitreous hemorrhage, retinal hemorrhage, macular hemorrhage, choroid hemorrhage, etc.

本法是用具有止血作用的药物组成方剂来终止眼病出血的方法,适用于各种原因引起的以出血症状为主的眼病。常见症状:白睛溢血,血灌瞳神,视网膜出血,黄斑出血,脉络膜出血等。

Bleeding is a common symptom in the eye diseases. This is a method applied in "the treatment of branch for emergent condition", suitable for bleeding in early stage. If bleeding stops, it is necessary to stop the method. In case when there is no bleeding tendency, it is advisable to change the method to the blood-activating and stasis-dissolving method, for the purpose to absorb the bled blood, so as to prevent the occurrence of stasis.

眼科出血症状较多常见,本法属急则治标之法,仅适用于出血早期,若出血停止,已无再出血的倾向,应逐渐转向活血化瘀治法,以促进出血的吸收,以免导致留瘀之弊。

6 Blood-activating and stasis-dissolving method

6 活血化瘀法

This method is to apply the prescription formed by the blood-activating and stasis-dissolving drugs, to improve the blood circulation, dissolve the stasis

本法是用具有活血化瘀作用的药物组成方剂,以改善血行,消散瘀滞,促进眼部

and promote the absorption of stasis, applied to treat the eye diseases and eye trauma caused by various types of blood vessel blockage, unsmooth blood flow or blood stasis, manifested by blue-purple colour and hard swelling of eyelid, thickening and red vessels of eye white, hemorrhage, blood stasis in all intraocular and circumocular areas, retinal vessel obstruction, fixed pain worsened by pressure in eye, purple spots on the tongue, etc.

瘀血吸收的方法，适用于各种血脉阻滞，血流不畅，或瘀血停聚的眼病及眼外伤。常见症状：胞睑青紫肿硬，白睛赤脉粗大，溢血，眼内外各个部位的瘀血，视网膜血管阻塞，眼部固定性疼痛拒按，以及舌有瘀斑等。

Besides, if the relevant symptoms occur in the disease progression due to other causative factors, it is advisable to apply the blood-activating and stasis dissolving drugs in the treatment.

此外，其他原因引起的眼病在病变的发展过程中若出现证候，在治疗时宜适当应用活血化瘀。

Qi is the commander of the blood, and the blood can flow smoothly if qi flows smoothly. Therefore, in the clinic application, it is necessary to combine the qi-moving drugs, so as to increase the therapeutic effects.

气为血之帅，气行则血行，故临床运用时，常配伍行气导滞药物，以提高疗效。

It is not advisable to apply the method for long time, so as to prevent the damage of the Zheng (Anti-Pathogenic) Qi. For those with blood stasis in eye and qi deficiency, it is necessary, on the basis of the method, to combine the qi-reinforcing drugs. It is prohibited to apply the method for those with qi and blood deficiency and pregnant women.

本法不宜久用，以免耗伤正气，对眼部既有瘀滞又见气虚症状者，应用本法需适当配伍补气药物。气血虚弱者及孕妇忌用本法。

7 Liver-soothing and qi-regulating method

7 疏肝理气法

This method is to apply the prescription formed by the liver-soothing, qi-regulating and depression-relieving drugs, to improve or removethe symptoms of liver qi stagnation, so as to brighten the eyes, applied to treat all types of intraocular and circumocular diseases due to liver qi stagnation, qi activity stoppage or eye orifice obstruction. It is advisable to

本法是用具有疏肝解郁、调理气机作用的药物组成方剂，以改善或清除肝郁气滞证候而达到明目作用的治法，适用于肝气郁滞，气机不畅，目窍不利的一切内外障眼病。临床无论内外障眼

apply the liver-soothing and qi-regulating method to treat all types of intraocular and circumocular diseases, accompanied by the symptoms of hypochondriac distension, belching, stuffy chest, restlessness, anger, foreign-body sensation in throat, irregular menstruation in females, wiry pulse, etc. For those with liver qi stagnation transforming to fire, it is advisable to add some fire-reducing drugs, for the purpose to clear the liver and relieve depression. For those with liver qi stagnation and qi and blood deficiency, it is advisable to add the blood-nourishing and spleen-strengthening drugs.

病，只要兼有胁胀，嗳气，胸闷，急躁易怒，咽部似有物阻，妇女月经不调，脉弦等症者，皆可用疏肝理气法治之。肝郁化火者，宜酌加清火之品，以清肝解郁；肝郁兼有气血虚弱者，宜与养血健脾药同用。理气药物多辛燥，故对阴亏之人须慎用，并注意配伍。

8 Qi-benefiting and blood-nourishing method

This method is to apply the prescription formed by the qi-benefiting and blood-nourishing drugs, to treat qi and blood deficiency pattern, so as to brighten the eyes, applied to treat eye diseases of qi and blood insufficiency pattern due to various causes. Clinically, it is applied to treat chronic intraocular and circumocular diseases, accompanied by the general symptoms of weakness in opening eyes, eye distension after using eyes for long time, unhealed nebula of eye black, blurring of vision, etc.

The spleen and stomach are the acquired basis and the source to produce qi and blood. Only when the spleen qi is strong and the spleen is normal in transporting and transforming function, can qi and blood be sent constantly upwards to the eyes. Therefore, at the same time when reinforcing qi and nourishing blood, it is advisable to regulate the spleen and stomach as well. For the condition with both deficiency and excess, it is advisable to apply both the attacking method and reinforcing method,

8 益气养血法

本法是用具有补益气血作用的药物组成方剂，以消除气血虚弱证候而达到明目作用的治法，适用于各种原因引起的气血不足的眼病。临床上多见于慢性内外障眼病，全身兼有气血不足的证候。常见症状：眼睁乏力，久视眼胀，黑睛翳陷日久不愈，视物渐昏等。

脾胃为后天之本，气血生化之源，脾气健运，气血才能不断上注于目，故补气养血时，还要注意调理脾胃，如属虚实夹杂，则可攻补兼施，或先攻后补，或先补后攻。因气血相依，故益气与养血往往同用，但根据气血偏虚程度的不同，治疗时又有所侧重，偏于气虚者，见眼睁乏

or the attacking method first and then the reinforcing method, or the reinforcing method first and then the attacking method. Since qi and blood are closely related, the qi-benefiting method and blood-nourishing method are applied simultaneously. According to the different degrees of qi deficiency and blood deficiency, it is necessary to stress on that is more serious in the treatment. For that qi deficiency is more serious, manifested by tiredness in opening eyes, preference for closing eyes, pale tongue body and weak pulse, it is advisable to take the qi-benefiting method as the major one. For that the blood deficiency is more serious, manifested by dizziness, blurring of vision, failure to watch for long time, dream-disturbed sleep, irritability, poor sleep, pale tongue body and thready pulse, it is advisable to take the blood-nourishing method as the major one.

力，常欲闭垂，舌淡脉弱，应以益气为主；偏于血虚者，见头昏眼花，不耐久视，多梦易醒，心烦失眠，舌淡脉细，应以养血为主。

It is prohibited to apply the method for those with excess of Xie (Pathogenic) Qi without symptoms of deficiency.

本法忌用于邪气亢盛而无虚候者。

9 Liver-reinforcing and kidney-benefiting method

This method is to apply the prescription formed by the liver-reinforcing and kidney-benefiting drugs, to treat the eye diseases due to liver and kidney insufficiency, manifested by milder condition with longer diseased course, repeated attacks of chronic circumocular diseases, fundus diseases in late stage, degenerative changes in intraocular diseases, etc., accompanied by the general symptoms ofaching and weakness of low back and knees, insomnia, poor memory, seminal emission in males, irregular menstruation in females, red tongue with scanty tongue coating, thready-weak pulse, etc.

9 补益肝肾法

本法是用具有补益肝肾作用的药物组成方剂，以消除肝肾亏虚证候而达到明目作用的治法，适用于肝肾不足的眼病。常见症状：症状较轻，病程较长，易反复发作的慢性外障眼病及眼底病后期，有退行性变化的内障眼病，全身兼有腰膝酸软，失眠健忘，男子遗精，女子月经不调，舌红少苔，脉细无力等，皆可用本法治疗。

It is prohibited to apply the method for those with excess patterns, and cautious to apply for those with existence of damp.

本法忌用于实证，湿邪未尽者慎用。

10 Hard-softening and stasis-dissolving method

10 软坚散结法

This method is to apply the prescription formed by the hard-softening and stasis-dissolving drugs, to treat various types of intraocular and circumocular diseases with the tangible pathological products as accumulation of phlegm and damp and qi and blood stasis, manifested chalazion, vitreous machine cords, old vitreous exudation, nebular prominence of eye white, etc.

本法是用具有化痰软坚散结作用的方药来治疗眼病的方法。适用于各种内外障眼病中出现痰湿互结，气血凝滞而成为有形之物者。常见症状：胞睑肿核，眼内机化条索及陈旧性渗出，白睛结节隆起等，可用本法消散之。

For qi and blood stasis, it is advisable to combine with the qi-regulating and blood-activating drugs. For accumulation of phlegm and damp, it is advisable to combine with the damp-removing and phlegm-dissolving drugs.

属气血凝滞者须配伍理气活血药物；属痰湿互结者，须配伍祛湿化痰药。

11 Nebula-removing and eye-brightening method

11 退翳明目法

This method is to apply the prescription formed by the nebula-removing and eye-brightening drugs to treat nebula of eye black, for the purpose to brighten the eyes.

本法是用具有退翳明目作用的方药以消退黑睛翳障，而达到明目作用的眼科独特治法。适用于黑睛生翳者。

The application of the method is layered. For the eye black diseases in early stage, manifested by scattered nebular spots, redness of eyes and lacrimation, it is advisable to apply the wind-eliminating and heat-clearing method, by combining with a small amount of nebula-removing drugs. If the pathogenic wind-heat is gradually decreasing, it is advisable to transit to the nebula-removing method as the major one. For the eye black diseases in late

运用本法须有层次。黑睛病初起，属外感风热，表现为星翳散在，红赤流泪，治以疏风清热为主，配伍少量退翳药；若风热渐减，则应逐渐过渡至退翳明目为主，病后期，邪气已退，而正气已虚，黑睛遗留翳障，则需兼顾扶正，结合全身病情，酌加益气

stage, when the Xie (Pathogenic) Qi is removed and the Zheng (Anti-pathogenic) Qi is deficient, manifested by the existence of nebula in eye black, it is advisable to give consideration to strengthening the Zheng (Anti-pathogenic) Qi, and to add the qi-benefiting and blood-nourishing drugs or the liver-reinforcing and kidney-benefiting drugs according to the general condition.

养血或补益肝肾之品。

The eye black pertains to the liver, and a certain amount of liver-purifying, liver-calming and liver-soothing drugs function to treat nebula and can be added in the treatment.

黑睛属肝,不少清肝、平肝、疏肝药物多有退翳作用,故可配伍应用。

For the nebula of eye black in late stage, it is advisable to apply thenebula-removing method as the major one, in which the herbal drugs too cold in property are not advisable, so as to prevent qi and blood stasis, congealing of Xie (Pathogenic) Qi and difficulty in removing nebula. If the nebula of eye black exists for long time and becomes smooth as porcelain, it indicates the formed stasis of qi and blood and it is difficult to remove the nebula with the herbal drugs. Therefore, it is necessary to treat nebula as early as possible.

黑睛生翳后期,以退翳为主,用药不可过于寒凉,以免气血凝滞,邪气冰伏,翳不易退,若宿翳已久,光滑如瓷,为气血已定,用药则难以消散;故退翳必须抓紧时机,及时辨证用药。

Section 2 External therapies

第2节 外治法

1 Eye-dropping method

This is a therapeutic method by applying the drugs directly into the eyes to relieve redness, swelling, itching and nebula, or for the mydriasis or miosis purposes. It is applied to treat the circumocular diseases at the eyelid, eye white, eye black and can-

1 点眼药法

本法是将药物直接点入眼部,用来消红肿,止痛痒,除翳膜,散大或缩小瞳孔,适用于胞睑、白睛、黑睛、两眦部位的外障眼病及部分内障

thi and some of the intraocular diseases. The commonly-used agents are the eye drops, eye powders and eye ointments.

眼病，常用的有眼药水，眼药粉及眼药膏三种。

1.1 Eye drops

The prescribed drugs are made into a kind of liquid agent. In the application, the patient is advised to look upwards and the doctor, with the dropper or dropping bottle in his right hand, opens the patient's lower eyelid with his left hand, applies 1 to 2 drops of the liquid into the inner canthus or below the cornea, and then, with the lower eyelid free, lift the upper eyelid at the same time, so that the liquid can be well-distributed in the eye. Finally, the patient closes his eye for several minutes. The method is applied 3 to 4 times a day, or more times in a very severe case.

1.1 点眼药水

将药物配成水剂应用。滴时令患者双目上视，医生用左手向下拉开下睑，右手持滴管或滴瓶，将药水滴入大眦角或白睛下方 1～2 滴，然后轻轻将上睑提起，并同时放松下睑，使药液充分均匀地分布于眼内，轻轻闭目数分钟，一般每日 3～4 次。对于病情急重者，次数可以增加。

1.2 Eye powders

The prescribed drugs are made into a kind of very fine powder. In the process, the doctor gently opens the patient's eyelids with his fingers and applies into the patient's inner canthus a small amount of the powder (half or one sesame-seed size) which is dipped with the smooth end of a sterilized glass rod soaked in the normal saline. Then the patient is asked to close his eyes with a cool but no irritant sensation as the limit. Finally, Point Yuwei (EX-HN) is pressed several times by the patient himself, so the circulation of qi and blood is effectively improved. After a few minutes, the patient gently opens his eyes. The method is applied 2 to 3 times a day.

1.2 点眼药粉

将药物制成极为细腻的粉末后应用。用时用消毒的小玻璃棒光滑头部粘生理盐水后，再蘸药粉约半粒到一粒芝麻大小，医生用手指轻轻分开患者胞睑，将药物轻轻放置于大眦角处，令患者闭目，以有清凉而无刺激感为度。点闭，患者用手按鱼尾穴数次，以助气血流行。闭目数分钟后，渐渐睁眼即可。一般每日 2～3 次。

1.3 Eye ointments

The prescribed drugs are made into a kind of ointment and a small amount of it is squeezed out and applied to the affected part of the eyelid or be-

1.3 涂眼药膏

将药物配成膏剂应用，用时将药膏挤出少许，置于胞睑皮肤患处或眼内白睛下

low the eye white and inside the lower eyelid. Then with the lower eyelid gently raised by the doctor, the patient is asked to close his eye slowly and the eyelid is gently pressed and kneaded with a cotton ball for 2 to 3 minutes (no pressing-kneading in the case of corneal nebula). And the ointment can also be applied with a glass rod, i.e. when the patient is closing his eye, the glass rod with the ointment is slowly drawn out in the canthus direction without touching the surface of the eye black in case the cornea might be injured.

方,下睑内面,轻轻提拉下睑后,令患者轻轻闭眼,用棉球轻轻按揉胞睑 2～3 分钟即可(黑晶生翳者,不用按揉)。也可用玻璃棒点药,在患者闭目时,将玻璃棒徐徐自眦角方向抽出,每日 3 次或临睡前用 1 次,抽玻璃棒时,切勿在黑睛表面擦过,以防擦伤黑睛。

2 Fumigating-washing method

The fumigating method is a therapeutic method to fumigate the affected part of the eye with the steam of the hot boiled decoction, while the washing method as to shower the sick eye with the filtrated liquid of a decoction. Usually the fumigating method is applied first, and then the washing method. As a whole, the both methods are called the fumigating-washing method. It is applied to treat the circumocular diseases of redness and swelling of eyelids, photophobia, dryness and pain, redness of eye white, excessive eye discharge. By using the warming action of the decoction, the method has the function to improve the qi and blood circulation in the eye, so as to remove the Xie (Pathogenic) Qi. Besides, because of the direct effect of different drugs on the affected part of the eye, it can dredge the meridians, relieve redness and swelling, arrest tears and relieve itching.

2 熏洗法

熏法是用药液煮沸后的热气蒸腾上熏眼部;洗法是将煎剂滤清后淋洗患眼。一般多是先熏后洗,合称熏洗法,适用于胞睑红肿,羞明涩痛,白睛红赤,眵泪较多的外障眼病。本法除利用药液的温热作用,使眼部气血流畅,能疏邪导滞外,还可通过不同的药物,直接作用于眼部,达到疏通经络,退赤消肿,敛泪止痒等效果。

Clinically, the decoction for the fumigating-washing method is prepared, according to the different eye diseases, by decocting the properly pre-

临床上根据不同病情,选择适当的药物煎成药汁,也可将内服药渣再煎水作成

scribed herbal drugs, or by boiling again the herbal dregs as an oral decoction. Before the treatment, a cover is made for the medicinal earth-ware pot or the container of the decoction with a hole as big as the patient's orbit. And two holes are made if both eyes are to be treated. When the decoction is ready, the pot or the container is covered with the cover, and then the sick eye is fumigated on the hole in the cover. In the cases of eyeball diseases, a frequent nictation is needed. In case of the eyelid diseases, the eye can be closed during the fumigation.

熏洗剂。使用前，在煎药锅或盛药液的器皿上作一盖板，盖上开一洞，洞口大小与眼眶范围大小一致，双眼患病可开两个相同的小洞，药物煎毕，用盖板覆盖在药锅或器皿口上，将患眼置于洞口熏之。如属眼珠病患，熏时要频频瞬目，使药力达到病所；如胞睑疾患，熏时闭目即可。

During the washing treatment, the eye can be showered or washed with the antiseptic gauze or sterilized cotton ball soaked with normal saline. Or with his head bowing, the patient first puts his eye closely on a sterilized eye-cup which contains the washing solution, and then raises his head, frequently nictitates and moves the eyeball, so that the eyeball may be thoroughly washed. Such a washing method continued for 20 minutes each time, and 2 to 3 times a day.

洗眼时，可用消毒纱布或消毒棉球渍水，不断淋洗眼部；亦可用消毒眼杯与眼窝紧紧贴靠，然后仰后，并频频瞬目，转动眼珠，进行眼浴，每日 2～3 次，每次 20 分钟。

The temperature for the fumigation should neither be too high in order to avoid eye from scalding, nor too low in order to prevent losing its therapeutic effect. The washing solution must be filtrated in case the fine drugs enter the eye to cause uncomfortable sensation. At the same time, all the containers, cotton balls, gauze and fingers must be sterilized and, in particular, special attention must be paid to the treatment of ulcerative nebula of cornea. It is prohibited to apply this method for those with new bleeding and malignant boils in the eye.

熏眼温度不宜过高，以免烫伤，但也不宜过冷以免失去治疗作用；洗剂必须过滤，以免药渣入眼，引起不适。同时，一切器皿、棉球、纱布及手指必须消毒，尤其是黑睛有陷翳者，用洗法时更须慎重，眼部有新生出血或患有恶疮者，忌用本法。

3 Irrigating method

3.1 Irrigating method for conjunctival sac

This is a method directly to irrigate the conjunctival sac with the clean water or the liquid of a decoction in order to remove the eye discharge, foreign bodies and chemical substances in the conjunctival sac. It is applied to treat the diseases of bulbar conjunctiva with foreign bodies and excessive discharge, and to act for the preoperative preparation and emergency treatment of chemical injury of the eye.

Procedure: The irrigation is done with an undine or a piece of rubber tube attached to a pendent bottle loaded with normal saline or medicinal liquid. If the patient takes a sitting position, he is asked to hold his head a little backward and the water or drug container closely touches his cheek. If he takes a lying position, he is ordered to divert his head a little to the sick eye side and the container closely touches the front part of his ear. Then the eyelids are gently opened and the irrigation starts slowly from the lower eyelid to the intraocular part. At the same time, the patient is asked to open his eye and moves the eyeball, so as to enlarge the irrigation area. In the cases of excessive eye discharge or those with a foreign body on the conjunctiva, the eyelids are turned up to expose the inner part of the upper eyelid and the conjunctival part of the superior fornix for a thorough irrigation. When the irrigation is finished, the eye is dried with the antiseptic gauze and the container is taken away.

3.2 Irrigating method for lacrimal passage

This is a method to irrigate the lacrimal passage with the normal saline or medicinal lotion. It is of-

3 冲洗法

3.1 结膜囊冲洗法

用水或中药药液直接冲洗结膜囊，其目的是除去结膜囊内的眼眵、异物和化学物质等。适用于结膜囊异物、眵泪较多的白睛疾患，术前准备及眼化学伤的急救措施。

方法：用盛有生理盐水或药液的洗眼壶或吊瓶的胶管来冲洗，冲洗时，患者如是坐位，头稍后仰，将受水器紧贴颊部；如患者取卧位，令头稍偏向患眼侧，将受水器紧贴耳前皮肤，轻轻拉开胞睑，冲洗液渐渐由下睑皮肤移到眼内，嘱患者睁眼及转动眼球，以扩大冲洗范围。眼分泌物较多者或结膜有异物者，应翻转上下胞睑，暴露上睑内面及上穹窿部结膜，彻底冲洗。冲洗完毕，用消毒纱布揩干眼周围，然后除去受水器。

3.2 泪道冲洗法

这是用生理盐水或药液冲洗泪道的方法。它多用来

ten applied to detect the lacrimal condition and remove the accumulated discharge in the lacrimal sac. It is applied to treat epiphora and chronic dacryocystitis, and to act as the routine preparation of intraocular operation.

探测泪道是否通畅及清除泪囊中积存的分泌物，适用于泪溢症、慢性泪囊炎及内眼手术前的常规准备。

Procedure: A short cotton stick dipped with the 0.5% to 1% decaine is inserted between the inner canthi, or the eye is dropped with the 0.5% to 1% decaine twice. After 2 to 3 minutes, the patient is asked to hold his head backwards, and the doctor pulls the patient's lower eyelid downwards with his index finger and fixes it on the orbital margin to expose the lower lacrimal punctum. If it is too small, the lacrimal punctum is dilated with a canaliculus dilator. Then the doctor holds in his right hand a syringe which contains 5 to 10 ml normal saline and as a syringe needle of gauge 5 to 6, curved nearly to a right angle and vertically inserts the needle into the lacrimal punctum 1.5 mm deep, then the needle is turned inwards 90° to a horizontal level and pushed towards the nasal side 3 to 5 mm, the irrigating lotion is slowly injected. If there is a resistance, the needle should not be inserted with a great force.

方法：用蘸有0.5%～1%的地卡因溶液的短棉签，夹在大眦头，或用0.5%～1%的地卡因液点眼2次，约2～3分钟后，嘱患者头向后仰，医生左手食指将下睑往下拉，固定于下眶缘部，暴露下泪点。若泪点较小，可先用泪点扩张器扩张之。右手持装有5～10毫升生理盐水的注射器，将磨成钝头并弯成近直角的5～6号注射针头，垂直插入下泪点约1.5毫米深，然后向内转90°成水平，沿泪小点缓慢向鼻侧推进，再进针3～5毫米时，缓缓注入冲洗液，若有阻力，不可用力强行通过。

If the lacrimal passage is unblocked, the irrigating lotion may flow from the passage into the nose and out of the nostrils. If the passage is obstructed, the lotion may be totally refluent in the upper and lower lacrimal puncturms. If the mucopurulent discharge is refluent out from the small lacrimal punctum, it is diagnosed as chronic lacryocystitis. If the lacrimal duct is obstructed, the lotion may flow out from the upper lacrimal punctum. If it is of stenosis of the nasolacrimal duct, there may be some resistance during the irrigation, and most lotion may be

如泪道通畅，冲洗液从泪道流入鼻内，从两侧鼻孔流出；如鼻泪管阻塞，冲洗液全部从上、下泪点返流；若从泪小点返流出黏液脓性分泌物，则为慢性泪囊炎；如泪总管阻塞，冲洗液从上泪点返流；如鼻泪管狭窄，冲洗时有一定阻力，大部分冲洗液从上泪点返流，仅少量冲洗液通过，鼻孔流出水液呈滴状。

refluent from the upper punctum with a little through and drops out of the nostrils.

4 Sickling-washing method

This is a therapeutic method gently to prick or scale the affected part with asword-like needle or materials with the course surface, and then to irrigate the wound with normal saline. It acts to directly remove the blood stasis of the sick area by relieving toxin and promote qi and blood flow. The method is applied to treat ocular granular diseases due to blood stasis in the eyelids, such as granular trachoma, conjunctival folliculosis, follicular conjunctivitis, etc.

Procedure: After the local surface anesthesia by dropping 0. 5% to 1% dicaine, the eyelids are turned up and blood stasis or the big rough granule is pricked or scaled with the sterilized sword-like needle or the materials like cuttlebone rod specially prepared till the mild bleeding occurs. Then the eye is dropped with normal saline or anti-inflammatory eye drops to irrigate the stagnant blood. The method can be performed again in 2 to 3 days. Attention is paid to that the method should not applied for the conditions of hyperemia of bulbar conjunctiva, excessive mucupurulent eye discharge, new nebula of eye black.

4 劆洗法

本法是用锋针或表面粗糙之器物轻刺或轻刮患部然后用水冲洗的治法，具有直接对病患处祛瘀消滞，散邪泻毒，疏通气血的作用。适用于胞睑内面的疾患，如沙眼、结膜滤泡症、滤泡性结膜等。

方法：局部滴 0.5%～1%的地卡因溶液表面麻醉后，翻转胞睑，以消毒后的锋针或特制的海螵蛸棒之类器物轻刺或轻刮睑内的瘀积或粗大颗粒，以微出血为度，劆毕用生理盐水或消炎眼药水点眼冲洗瘀血，隔 2～3 日可再施行 1 次。但要注意，如为白睛暴赤，眵多稠结，黑睛新翳者，不用此法。

Section 3 Common drugs for oral administration in ophthalmology

第 3 节 眼科常用内服药

1 Wind-eliminating drugs

The wind-eliminating drugs act to eliminate

1 祛风药

祛风药具有祛风解表，

wind, reliever the exterior, subside swell, stop pain, stop itching, astringe tears and treat nebula, so they are applied extensively in the ophthalmology, especially for the circumocular diseases of early stage.

消肿止痛,止痒敛泪及退翳作用,故在眼科运用较为广泛,尤其是外障眼病初期。

The wind-eliminating drugs applied in ophthalmology are divided into two categories of pungent-cool and exterior-relieving drugs and pungent-warm and exterior-relieving drugs.

眼科常用祛风药有辛凉解表药和辛温解表药两类。

1.1 Pungent-cool and exterior-relieving drugs

This type of herbal drugs are mainly to treat the eye diseases due to wind-heat, such as *Folium Mori* (Sang Ye), *Flos Chrysanthemi* (Ju Hua), *Herba Menthae* (Bo He), *Radix Puerariae* (Ge Gen), *Periostracum Cicadae* (Chan Tui), *Fructus Viticis* (Man Jing Zi), etc. This type of herbal drugs act to eliminate wind-heat, stop itching and pain, benefit head and eyes and relieve swelling and redness. *Folium Mori* (Sang Ye) and *Flos Chrysanthemi* (Ju Hua) act to eliminate wind-heat, purify liver and brighten eyes, applied to treat the eye diseases due to wind-heat in the Liver Meridian. *Herba Menthae* (Bo He) acts to treat the eye diseases due to wind-heat. *Radix Puerariae* (Ge Gen), attributive to the Yangming Meridians, acts to eliminate wind-heat in the Yangming Meridians, applied to treat the eye diseases due to wind-heat, accompanied by frontal headache. *Periostracum Cicadae* (Chan Tui) acts to eliminate wind-heat, treat nebula and stop itching, applied to treat the eye diseases with obvious itching eyes, such as nebula of eye black, blepharitis marginalis, etc. *Radix Bupleuri* (Chai Hu) acts to reduce heat, soothe liver, uplift the Zhong (Central) Qi and remove nebula, so it is widely applied to treat

1.1 辛凉解表药

该类药主要治风热眼病,常用药有桑叶、菊花、薄荷、葛根、蝉蜕、蔓荆子等。此类药具有疏散风热、止痒止痛、清利头目、消肿退赤的作用。桑叶、菊花能疏散风热,清肝明目,二者配伍常应用于肝经风热眼病;薄荷为治疗风热眼病的常用药,葛根入阳明经,能清阳明经风热,常用于风热眼病兼有前额头痛者;蝉蜕散风热,退翳止痒,故常用于黑睛翳障,睑弦赤烂等目痒症状较明显者;柴胡有解热、疏肝、升提与退翳作用,故可以通过不同配伍,广泛应用于风热或肝热所致的黑睛翳障,或中气不足所致的上睑下垂及肝气郁结所致的多种内外障眼病。

nebula of eye black due to wind-heat or heat in liver, or to treat ptosis of upper eyelid due to insufficiency of Zhong (Central) Qi, or to treat various types of intraocular and circumocular diseases due to liver qi stagnation.

1.2 Pungent-warm and exterior-relieving drugs

This type of herbal drugs are mainly to treat the eye diseases due to wind-cold, such as *Herba Schizonepetae* (Jing Jie), *Radix Ledebouriellae* (Fang Feng), *Rhizoma seu Radix Notopterygii* (Qiang Huo), *Rhizoma Ligustici* (Gao Ben), *Herba Asari* (Xi Xin), *Radix Angelicae Dahuricae* (Bai Zhi), etc. This type of herbal drugs act to eliminate wind-cold, subside swell, stop pain, relieve itching and remove nebula. *Herba Schizonepetae* (Jing Jie), *Radix Ledebouriellae* (Fang Feng) and *Rhizoma seu Radix Notopterygii* (Qiang Huo) act to treat eye pain, headache, intolerable itch of eye, redness of eye and nebula due to exogenous wind-heat. *Rhizoma seu Radix Notopterygii* (Qiang Huo) also acts to treat eye pain due to wind-damp. *Rhizoma Ligustici* (Gao Ben), attributive to the vertex of head, acts to eliminate wind-cold, applied to treat the eye diseases due to exogenous wind-cold accompanied by vertex headache. It is more effective by combining with other wind-eliminating drugs. *Herba Asari* (Xi Xin) acts to eliminate wind and relieve pain, applied to treat the eye diseases due to wind-cold accompanied by severe headache and eye pain. But it is not advisable to apply for long time. *Radix Angelicae Dahuricae* (Bai Zhi), attributive to the Yangming Meridians, acts to relieve pain and stop lacrimation, applied to treat the eye diseases due to exogenous wind-cold manifested by headache and

1.2 辛温解表药

该类药物主治风寒眼病。常用药有荆芥、防风、羌活、藁本、细辛、白芷等。此类药物有发散风寒，消肿止痛，止痒退翳的作用。荆芥、防风、羌活的祛风止痛和止痒退翳作用强，三药配伍应用于外感风寒所致的目痛头痛、目痒难忍、目赤生翳，羌活更擅长于风湿眼痛；藁本发散风寒，善达头顶，故对外感风寒眼病兼有头顶痛者，常以之与其他祛风药配伍同用效果更好；细辛止痛作用尤强，故风寒眼病，头目疼痛剧烈者，常用本药祛风止痛，但不宜久用；白芷入阳明经，有镇痛止泪作用，多用于外感风寒而头痛多眵者。

excessive eye discharge.

2 Heat-clearing drugs

2.1 Heat-clearing and toxin-relieving drugs

This type of herbal drugs are mainly to treat all types of eye diseases of excess heat pattern due to heat-toxin, such as *Flos Lonicerae* (Jin Yin Hua), *Fructus Forsythiae* (Lian Qiao), *Folium Isatidis* (Da Qing Ye), *Radix Isatidis* (Ban Lan Gen), *Herba Violae* (Zi Hua Di Ding), *Herba Taraxaci* (Pu Gong Ying), etc.

2.2 Heat-clearing and fire-reducing drugs

This type of herbal drugs are mainly to treat the eye diseases due to excess of pathogenic heat, such as *Radix Gentianae* (Long Dan), *Rhizoma Coptidis* (Huang Lian), *Radix Scutellariae* (Huang Qin), *Cortex Phellodendri* (Huang Bo), *Fructus Gardeniae* (Zhi Zi), *Gypsum Fibrosum* (Shi Gao), *Rhizoma Anemarrhenae* (Zhi Mu), *Cortex Mori Radicis* (Sang Bai Pi), *Herba Lophatheri* (Dan Zhu Ye), etc. *Radix Gentianae* (Long Dan) acts to treat the eye black diseases due to liver fire upward-flaming. *Rhizoma Coptidis* (Huang Lian) acts to reduce the heart fire, purify the heat and relieve restlessness, applied to treat redness, swelling and pain of eye or redness of canthi. *Radix Scutellariae* (Huang Qin) and *Cortex Mori Radicis* (Sang Bai Pi) act to reduce the lung fire, applied to treat redness of eye white. *Cortex Phellodendri* (Huang Bo) acts to reduce the kidney fire, clear the false fire and astringe the Xiang (Premiere) Fire. It acts to clear the false heat and nourish the kidney yin by combining with *Rhizoma Anemarrhenae* (Zhi Mu), applied to the eye diseases due to yin deficiency and

2 清热药

2.1 清热解毒药

该类药物主治一切热毒引起的实热证眼病。常用药有金银花、连翘、大青叶、板蓝根、紫花地丁、蒲公英等。

2.2 清热泻火药

该类药主治邪热炽盛的眼病。常用药有龙胆草、黄连、黄芩、黄柏、栀子、石膏、知母、桑白皮、淡竹叶等。其中龙胆草清肝胆实热，常用于肝火上炎所指的黑睛疾患；黄连泻心火，清心除烦，可用于眦帷赤肿痛或两眦红赤；黄芩、桑白皮泻肺火，多用于白睛红赤；黄柏泻肾火，可用于清虚火，制相火，临床常用黄柏和知母配伍以清虚热、滋肾阴，治疗阴虚火旺之眼病，与黄连、黄芩配伍治疗湿热眼病；栀子泻三焦之火，与其他清热药配伍，可用于各种实热眼病；石膏、知母泻胃火，可用于胞睑红肿与黄液上冲；淡竹叶清心火，利小便，用于胬肉红赤，两眦红赤等。

fire hyperactivity. It acts to treat the eye diseases due to damp-heat by combining with *Rhizoma Coptidis* (Huang Lian) and *Radix Scutellariae* (Huang Qin). *Fructus Gardeniae* (Zhi Zi) acts to reduce the fire of triple energizer, applied to treat various types of eye diseases due to excess heat by combining with other heat-reducing drugs. *Gypsum Fibrosum* (Shi Gao) and *Rhizoma Anemarrhenae* (Zhi Mu) act to reduce the stomach fire, applied to treat redness and swelling of eyelids and hypopyon. *Herba Lophatheri* (Dan Zhu Ye) acts to reduce the heart fire and promote urination, applied to treat pterygium, redness of canthi, etc.

2.3 Bowel-dredging and heat-reducing drugs

This type of herbal drugs are mainly toredness, swelling and pain of eyes and sticky eye discharge due to excess patterns of Yangming-fu organs or upward attack of interior heat, such as *Radix et Rhizoma Rhei* (Da Huang), *Natrii Sulfas* (Mang Xiao), etc.

2.3 通腑泻热药

该类药主治阳明腑实，里热上攻引起的目赤肿痛，眵泪胶黏。常用药有大黄、芒硝等。

2.4 Heat-clearing and eye-brightening drugs

This type of herbal drugs include *Spica Prunellae* (Xia Ku Cao), *Semen Cassiae* (Jue Ming Zi), *Semen Celosiae* (Qing Xiang Zi), *Flos Buddlejae* (Mi Meng Hua), *Herba Equiseti Hiemalis* (Mu Zei), etc. *Spica Prunellae* (Xia Ku Cao) acts to reduce the stagnant fire in liver and gallbladder, applied to treat redness, swelling and pain of eyes and fundus hemorrhage due to liver fire. It acts to treat eye pain due to liver qi stagnation by combining with *Rhizoma Cyperi* (Xiang Fu). *Semen Cassiae* (Jue Ming Zi) and *Semen Celosiae* (Qing Xiang Zi) act to purify the liver and brighten the eyes. *Flos Buddlejae* (Mi Meng Hua) acts to eliminate wind-

2.4 清热明目药

常用药有夏枯草、决明子、青葙子、密蒙花、木贼等。夏枯草泻肝胆郁火，用于肝火所致目赤肿痛，眼底出血，配伍香附还可治肝郁目痛；决明子、青葙子清肝明目；密蒙花祛风热，养肝润燥，不论虚实眼病皆可用，肝肾阴亏有热者更为适宜；木贼能疏风热，退翳明目。

heat, nourish the liver and moisturize the dry condition, applied to the eye diseases of both deficiency and excess patterns, more effective for yin deficiency of liver and kidney with symptoms of heat. *Herba Equiseti Hiemalis* (Mu Zei) acts to eliminate wind-heat, remove nebula and brighten the eyes.

2.5 Heat-clearing and blood-cooling drugs

This type of herbal drugs act to treat the eye diseases caused by heat entering the Ying (Nutrient) and Xue (Blood) Phases, especially by heat forcing blood to flow recklessly and sudden decrease of vision, such as *Radix Rehmanniae Cruda* (Sheng Di Huang), *Cortex Moutan Radicis* (Mu Dan Pi), *Radix Scrophulariae* (Xuan Shen), *Radix Paeoniae Rubra* (Chi Shao), *Radix Arnebiae seu Lithospermi* (Zi Cao), etc. *Cortex Moutan Radicis* (Mu Dan Pi) and *Radix Paeoniae Rubra* (Chi Shao) act to reduce heat, cool blood, activate blood and dissolve stasis. *Radix Rehmanniae Cruda* (Sheng Di Huang) and *Radix Scrophulariae* (Xuan Shen) act to reduce heat, cool blood, nourish yin and produce fluid. *Radix Arnebiae seu Lithospermi* (Zi Cao) acts to cool blood and relieve toxin.

2.5 清热凉血药

该类药主治热入营血所致的眼病，尤其是血热妄行、视力骤降者。常用药有生地黄、牡丹皮、玄参、赤芍、紫草等。牡丹皮、赤芍清热凉血，活血化瘀；生地黄、玄参清热凉血，养阴生津；紫草偏于凉血解毒。

3 Reinforcing drugs

The deficient patterns in the eye diseases are mostly caused by the insufficiency of qi and blood or by the insufficiency of liver and kidney, so that the reinforcing drugs for the eye diseases are qi-benefiting drugs, blood-nourishing drugs and liver-kidney reinforcing drugs.

3 补益药

眼病之虚证，多属气血不足或肝肾不足，眼科补益药以益气养血及补益肝肾药物为常用。

3.1 Qi-benefiting and blood-nourishing drugs

(1) Qi-benefiting drugs: This type of herbal drugs are applied to treat qi deficiency manifested

3.1 益气养血药

(1) 益气药：该类药适用于气虚所致的胞睑乏力，常

by fatigue of eyelids, preference for closing eyes and unhealed nebula, such as *Radix Astragali* (Huang Qi), *Rhizoma Atractylodis Macrocephalae* (Bai Zhu), *Radix Codonopsis Pilosulae* (Dang Shen), *Rhizoma Dioscoreae* (Shan Yao), etc.

欲闭垂及陷翳不愈等症。常用药有黄芪、白术、党参、山药等。

(2) Blood-nourishing drugs: This type of herbal drugs are applied to treat blood deficiency manifested by dryness of eyes, blurring of vision and night blindness, such as *Radix Rehmanniae Praeparata* (Shu Di Huang), *Radix Paeoniae Alba* (Bai Shao), *Radix Angelicae Sinensis* (Dang Gui), *Radix Polygoni Multiflori* (He Shou Wu), *Fructus Mori* (Sang Shen Zi), *Colla Corii Asini* (E Jiao), *Arillus Longan* (Long Yan Rou), etc.

(2) 养血药:该类药适用于血虚所致的眼干涩昏花,夜盲等。常用药有熟地黄、白芍、当归、何首乌、桑葚子、阿胶、龙眼肉等。

3.2 Liver-reinforcing and kidney-benefiting drugs

3.2 补益肝肾药

This type of herbal drugs are applied to treat the intraocular and circumocular diseases caused by insufficiency of liver and kidney, such as *Fructus Lycii* (Gou Qi Zi), *Fructus Ligustri Lucidi* (Nü Zhen Zi), *Semen Cuscutae* (Tu Si Zi), *Fructus Broussonetiae* (Chu Shi Zi), *Cortex Eucommiae* (Du Zhong), *Herba Ecliptae* (Mo Han Lian), *Fructus Rubi* (Fu Pen Zi), *Radix Rehmanniae Praeparata* (Shu Di Huang), etc. *Fructus Lycii* (Gou Qi Zi) acts to nourish and reinforce liver and kidney, benefit essence and brighten eyes, applied to treat intraocular and circumocular diseases due to liver and kidney insufficiency. *Fructus Ligustri Lucidi* (Nü Zhen Zi) acts to nourish yin of liver and kidney, applied to treat yin deficiency with internal heat. By combining with *Herba Ecliptae* (Mo Han Lian), it acts to nourish yin, cool blood and stanch blood, applied to treat intraocular hemorrhage in the early

该类药适用于肝肾不足之内外障眼病。常用药有枸杞子、女贞子、菟丝子、楮实子、杜仲、墨旱莲、覆盆子、熟地黄等。枸杞子滋补肝肾,益精明目,广泛用于肝肾不足引起的内外障眼病;女贞子滋养肝肾之阴,善治阴虚内热,与墨旱莲配伍,滋阴凉血止血,常用于眼内出血的早期;菟丝子补益肝肾,明目;楮实子平补肝肾,养肝明目;覆盆子补肝肾,固精明目;杜仲补肝肾,强筋骨,通过配伍可以广泛用于肝肾不足内障眼病兼有腰膝酸软或萎软无力者;熟地黄滋阴力较强,故阴虚内障眼病常用

stage. *Semen Cuscutae* (Tu Si Zi) acts to reinforce and benefit liver and kidney, and brighten eyes. *Fructus Broussonetiae* (Chu Shi Zi) balance and reinforce liver and kidney, nourish liver and brighten eyes. *Fructus Rubi* (Fu Pen Zi) acts to reinforce liver and kidney, astringe essence and brighten eyes. *Cortex Eucommiae* (Du Zhong) acts to reinforce liver and kidney, and strengthen tendons and bones, applied to treat intraocular diseases due to liver and kidney insufficiency accompanied by aching and weakness in low back and knees, by combining with other herbal drugs. *Radix Rehmanniae Praeparata* (Shu Di Huang) acts to nourish yin, applied to treat intraocular diseases due to yin deficiency.

之。

4 Damp-removing drugs

The eye diseases caused by pathogenic damp are quite common. The damp-dissolving drugs act to dissolve damp, astringe sores, subside swell, remove nebula and brighten eyes, so widely applied in the ophthalmology. But it is cautious to apply them for yin deficiency, blood scantiness or body fluid loss. The commonly-used damp-removing drugs include two types of fragrant and damp-dissolving drugs and water-promoting and damp-removing drugs.

4 祛湿药

湿邪所致眼病较为多见，祛湿药能收湿敛疮，退肿去翳明目，故眼科应用也很广泛，但阴虚血少或津液已伤当慎用。常用的祛湿药有芳香化湿药与利水渗湿药两类。

4.1 Fragrant and damp-dissolving drugs

This type of herbal drugs are applied to treat the eye diseases caused by internal accumulation of damp-turbidity, such as *Herba Agastachis* (Huo Xiang), *Herba Eupatorii* (Pei Lan), *Rhizoma Atractylodis* (Cang Zhu), *Rhizoma Acori Graminei* (Shi Chang Pu), *Semen Amomi Cardamomi* (bai dou kou), *Fructus Amomi* (Sha Ren), etc. *Herba*

4.1 芳香化湿药

该类药适用于湿浊内阻所致的眼病。常用药有藿香、佩兰、苍术、石菖蒲、白豆蔻、砂仁等。藿香、佩兰发表祛湿以和中化浊，往往同用，治疗外感湿邪或湿困脾胃所致的内外障眼病。苍术燥湿

Agastachis (Huo Xiang) and *Herba Eupatorii* (Pei Lan) act to remove damp, harmonize middle energizer and dissolve turbidity, applied to treat intraocular and circumocular diseases caused by invasion of exogenous damp or damp blocking spleen and stomach. *Rhizoma Atractylodis* (Cang Zhu) acts to dry the damp and strengthen spleen, applied to treat blepharitis marginalis, keratitis due to herpes simplex, retinal edema, etc. It is also applied to treat primary pigmentary degeneration of retina by combining with the pork liver. *Rhizoma Acori Graminei* (Shi Chang Pu) is fragrant, and acts to dissolve turbidity, open aperture and brighten eyes. *Semen Amomi Cardamomi* (bai dou kou) and *Fructus Amomi* (Sha Ren) act to dry the damp and warm middle energizer, applied to treat the eye diseases accompanied by the symptoms of pathogenic damp blocking spleen and stomach.

健脾，用于胞睑赤烂，翳膜遮睛，视网膜水肿等，与猪肝同煮，可治肝虚雀目；石菖蒲芳香化浊，开窍明目；白豆蔻、砂仁有燥湿温中作用，常用于眼病兼有湿邪阻滞脾胃证候者。

4.2 Water-promoting and damp-removing drugs

This type of herbal drugs are applied to treat the eye diseases caused by overflow of water-damp or upward-steaming of damp-heat, such as *Sclerotium Poriae* (Fu Ling), *Polyporus Umbellatus* (Zhu Ling), *Rhizoma Alismatis* (Ze Xie), *Talcum* (Hua Shi), *Semen Plantaginis* (Che Qian Zi), *Semen Coicis* (Yi Yi Ren), *Semen Phaseoli* (Chi Xiao Dou), *Caulis Akebiae* (Mu Tong), etc. *Sclerotium Poriae* (Fu Ling) and *Semen Coicis* (Yi Yi Ren) act to strengthen spleen, remove damp and promote water flow, applied to treat the eye diseases caused by spleen deficiency with water overflow. *Polyporus Umbellatus* (Zhu Ling) acts to remove damp, applied to treat tissue edema in eye diseases, especially severe retinal edema, by combining with *Sclerotium*

4.2 利水渗湿药

该类药适用于水湿上泛或湿热熏蒸所致的眼病。常用药有茯苓、猪苓、泽泻、滑石、车前子、薏苡仁、赤小豆、木通等。茯苓、薏苡仁健脾渗湿利水，用于脾虚湿泛眼病；猪苓淡渗利湿作用较强，可于茯苓配伍应用，用于眼病组织水肿，尤其是视网膜水肿严重者；泽泻利水渗湿，且能泄肾与膀胱之湿热，与车前子、猪苓配伍，可用于水湿滞留或湿热眼病；车前子还能清肝明目，故凡肝热所致红肿翳膜，也可用车前子

Poriae (Fu Ling). *Rhizoma Alismatis* (Ze Xie) acts to promote water flow, remove damp, and reduce damp-heat in kidney and bladder, applied to treat the eye diseases caused by water-damp retention or damp-heat, by combining with *Semen Plantaginis* (Che Qian Zi) and *Polyporus Umbellatus* (Zhu Ling). *Semen Plantaginis* (Che Qian Zi) acts to purify liver and brighten eyes, applied singly or by combining with other liver-purifying drugs to treat conjunctivitis with nebula. *Talcum* (Hua Shi) acts to promote water flow, remove damp, reduce heat and relieve summer-heat, applied to treat the eye diseases caused by damp-heat. *Semen Phaseoli* (Chi Xiao Dou) acts to promote water flow, subside swell, relieve toxin and drain the pus, applied to treat retinal edema. It is also applied to treat eyelid sores and boils by combining with the heat-reducing and toxin-relieving drugs. *Caulis Akebiae* (Mu Tong) acts to reduce heat and remove damp, especially to reduce the pathogenic heat of heart and small intestine, applied by combining with *Herba Lophatheri* (Dan Zhu Ye), *Rhizoma Coptidis* (Huang Lian) and *Radix Rehmanniae Cruda* (Sheng Di Huang), to treat the eye diseases due to damp-heat, accompanied by redness of canthi, ulcers in mouth and tongue, yellow urine, red tongue tip, etc.

配伍其他清肝药同用；滑石利水渗湿，清热解暑，一般用于湿热眼病；赤小豆利水消肿，解毒排脓，既可用于视网膜水肿，也可配伍清热解毒药物治疗眼睑疮疖；木通清热利湿，擅长于清利心与小肠邪热，故湿热眼病，有两眦红赤、口舌生疮、尿黄、舌尖红等现象者，可用木通配伍淡竹叶、黄连、生地黄等药。

5 Blood-regulating drugs

This type of herbal drugs are applied to treat the eye diseases due to bleeding, blood stasis, heat in blood and blood deficiency. It is advisable to stanch blood for bleeding, to activate blood for blood stasis, to cool blood for heat in blood, and to

5 理血药

该类药适用于因血溢、血瘀、血热、血虚所致的眼病。血溢者宜止血，血瘀者宜活血，血热者宜凉血，血虚者宜补血。凉血药和补血药

reinforce blood for blood deficiency. The blood-cooling drugs and blood-reinforcing drugs are introduced in "heat-reducing drugs" and "reinforcing drugs", therefore the blood-stanching drugs and blood-activating drugs are introduced here below.

在清热药和补益药中已有介绍,这里仅介绍止血药和活血药化瘀药。

5.1 Blood-stanching drugs

This type herbal drugs are applied to treat hemorrhagic eye diseases. The blood-stanching drugs in ophthalmology include the blood-cooling and blood-stanching drugs, the astringent and blood-stanching drugs and the stasis-dissolving and blood-stanching drugs, which are selectively applied according to the different causes of bleeding.

5.1 止血药

该类药适用于出血性眼病。眼科常用的止血药,其作用有凉血止血,收敛止血和祛瘀止血的不同,故临证时当根据出血原因选择使用。

(1) Blood-cooling and blood-stanching drugs: The herbal drugs are applied to treat bleeding pattern due to heat in blood, such as *Herba seu Radix Cirsii Japonici* (Da Ji), *Herba Cephalanoploris* (Xiao Ji), *Caumen Biotae* (Ce Bai Ye), *Rhizoma Imperatae* (Bai Mao Gen), *Radix Sanguisorbae* (Di Yu), *Flos Sophorae* (Huai Hua), etc.

(1) 凉血止血药:适用于血热妄行的出血证。常用药有大蓟、小蓟、侧柏叶、白茅根、地榆、槐花等。

(2) Astringent and blood-stanching drugs: The herbal drugs are applied to treat new bleeding or traumatic bleeding in eye diseases, such as *Rhizoma Bletillae* (Bai Ji), *Crinis Carbonisatus* (Xue Yu Tan), *Herba Agrimoniae* (Xian He Cao), *Nodus Nelumbinis Rhizomatis* (Ou Jie), etc.

(2) 收敛止血药:适用于眼病的新出血及外伤出血。常用药有白及、血余炭、仙鹤草、藕节等。

(3) Stasis-dissolving and blood-stanching drugs: The herbal drugs are applied to treat bleeding due to blood stasis, such as *Radix Notoginseng* (San Qi), *Pollen Typhae* (Pu Huang), Radix Rubiae (Qian Cao), *Ophicalcitum* (Hua Rui Shi), etc.

(3) 化瘀止血药:适用于血瘀而致出血者。常用药有三七、蒲黄、茜草、花蕊石等。

5.2 Blood-activating and stasis-dissolving drugs

This type of herbal drugs are applied to treat

5.2 活血化瘀药

该类药适用于气滞血瘀

the eye diseases due to qi stagnation and blood stasis, by combining with the qi-moving drugs, such as *Semen Persicae* (Tao Ren), *Flos Carthami* (Hong Hua), *Radix Salviae Miltiorrhizae* (Dan Shen), *Rhizoma Ligustici Chuanxiong* (Chuan Xiong), *Herba Artemisiae Anomalae* (Liu Ji Nu), *Herba Lycopi* (Ze Lan), *Semen Vaccariae* (Wang Bu Liu Xing), *Resina Olibani* (Ru Xiang), *Myrrha* (Mo Yao), *Radix Paeoniae Rubra* (Chi Shao), *Cortex Moutan Radicis* (Mu Dan Pi), *Lignum Sappan* (Su Mu), *Caulis Spatholobi* (ji xue teng), etc.

所致的眼病，常与行气药同用。常用药有桃仁、红花、丹参、川芎、刘寄奴、泽兰、王不留行、乳香、没药、赤芍、牡丹皮、苏木、鸡血藤等。

6 Qi-regulating drugs

This type of herbal drugs are applied to treat the eye diseases caused by disharmony of qi activity. The qi-regulating drugs are mostly pungent, warm and dispersing in property, easy to consume qi and damage yin, therefore it is cautious to apply them for those with yin deficiency.

6 理气药

该类药适用于气机失调所致眼病。理气药多辛温发散，易耗气伤阴，故阴虚者慎用。常用的理气药有疏肝理气药与行气导滞药两种。

6.1 Liver-soothing and qi-regulating drugs

This type of herbal drugs are applied to treat the eye diseases caused by liver qi stagnation, such as *Radix Bupleuri* (Chai Hu), *Rhizoma Cyperi* (Xiang Fu), *Pericarpium Citri Reticulatae Viride* (Qing Pi), *Fructus Meliae Toosendan* (Chuan Lian Zi), *Radix Curcumae* (Yu Jin), *Fructus Citri Sarcodactylis* (Fo Shou), etc.

6.1 疏肝理气药

该类药适用于肝气郁结的眼病。常用药有柴胡、香附、青皮、川楝子、郁金、佛手等。

6.2 Qi-moving and digestion-promoting drugs

This type of herbal drugs are applied to treat the eye diseases caused by qi stagnation in spleen and stomach, such as *Pericarpium Citri Tangerinae* (Chen Pi), *Radix Aucklandiae* (Mu Xiang), *Fructus Aurantii Immaturus* (Zhi Shi), *Cortex Magnoliae Officinalis* (Hou Pu), *Semen Arecae* (Bing

6.2 行气导滞药

该类药适用于脾胃气滞的眼病。常用药有陈皮、木香、枳实、厚朴、槟榔、沉香等。

Lang), *Lignum Aquilariae Resinatum* (Chen Xiang), etc.

7 Hard-softening and stasis-dissolving drugs

This type of herbal drugs act to dissolve stasis and soften the hard, or to promote digestion and dissolve stasis, applied to treat the eye diseases manifested by masses, nodules or scars due to qi stagnation and blood stasis, or due to accumulation of phlegm and stasis, such as *Thallus Laminariae seu Eckloniae* (Kun Bu), *Sargassum* (Hai Zao), *Concha Arcae* (Wa Leng Zi), *Spica Prunellae* (Xia Ku Cao), *Bulbus Fritillariae Thumbergii* (Zhe Bei Mu), *Concha Ostreae* (Mu Li), *Rhizoma Sparganii Stoloniferi* (San Leng), *Rhizoma Zedoariae* (E Zhu), *Concha Meretricis seu Cyclinae* (Hai Ge Ke), *Pumex* (Hai Fu Shi), etc.

7 软坚散结药

该类药具有祛瘀软坚或消导积滞的作用，凡在眼病过程中，出现气血凝滞，痰瘀互结的肿块、结节及瘢痕等，均可配伍软坚散结药。常用药有昆布、海藻、瓦楞子、夏枯草、浙贝母、牡蛎、三棱、莪术、海蛤壳、海浮石等。

8 Nebula-removing and eye-brightening drugs

This type of herbal drugs act to eliminate wind-heat, purify and soothe liver, remove nebula and brighten eyes, such as *Periostracum Cicadae* (Chan Tui), *Cortex Fraxini* (Qin Pi), *Eriocaulon Buergerianum* (Gu Jing Cao), *Herba Equiseti Hiemalis* (Mu Zei), *Flos Buddlejae* (Mi Meng Hua), *Concha Haliotidis* (Shi Jue Ming), *Fructus Tribuli* (Bai Ji Li), *Semen Celosiae* (Qing Xiang Zi), *Concha Margaritifera Usta* (Zhen Zhu Mu), *Periostracum Serpentis* (she tui), *Os Sepiellae seu Sepiae* (Hai Piao Xiao), etc.

8 退明目药

该类药具有疏散风热，清肝平肝，退翳明目作用。常用药有蝉蜕、秦皮、谷精草、木贼、密蒙花、石决明、白蒺藜、青葙子、珍珠母、蛇蜕、海螵蛸等。

Specific Introduction

各　论

Chapter 1 Eyelid Diseases

第1章 胞睑疾病

Viral palpebral dermatitis

病毒性睑皮炎

Viral palpebral dermatitis is a kind of acute inflammatory reaction of the eyelid skin caused by herpes simplex virus or herpes zoster virus. It is divided into herpes simplex palpebral dermatitis and herpes zoster palpebral dermatitis according to the local signs, occuring in common cold, high fever or immunity decrease. The latter may involve the cornea, leading to severe corneal complications. Besides, the herpes zoster virus may damage the semilunar ganglion of the trigeminal nerve, so the pain occurred in the disease lasts for six months.

病毒性睑皮炎指由单纯疱疹病毒或带状疱疹病毒引起的眼睑皮肤急性炎性反应。临床依据局部体征分为单疱病毒性睑皮炎和带状疱疹病毒性睑皮炎。本病常发生于感冒、高热或抵抗力下降时，后者可侵犯角膜，出现严重的角膜并发症。由于带状病毒对三叉神经的半月神经的伤害，疼痛症状可延续半年之久。

In traditional Chinese medicine, the disease is called "vesiculated dermatitis of eyelid", manifested by redness of eyelid skin, burning pain, blisters or pustules, even ulcers and scars. The exogenous factor of the disease is the pathogenic damp-heat, while its endogenous factor is related to the spleen, stomach, liver and gallbladder. The exogenous and endogenous pathogens in combination attack the eyes upwards to cause the disease.

本病属于中医学"风赤疮痍"范畴，临床以胞睑皮肤红赤如朱，灼热疼痛，起水疱或脓疱，直至溃烂、收痂为主症。本病外因责之湿热之邪，内因责之于脾胃肝胆，内外合邪，上攻目系为患。

1 Etiology and pathogenesis

1.1 Damp-heat in Spleen Meridian and invasion of exogenous wind. The wind, damp and heat attack the body in combination and invade the eyelid along the meridian.

1.2 Damp-heat blocking spleen and stomach. When the earth is excessive, it counter-acts on the wood. When the spleen disease involves the liver, both the liver and spleen are sick. In such a situation, the pathogenic wind attacks the body, so that the wind, damp and heat attack the body in combination and invade the eyelid along the meridian.

1.3 Invasion of exogenous wind, heat and toxin which induce the endogenous fire. Both the liver and spleen are diseases, leading to the fire-toxin burning the muscle wheel and wind wheel.

2 Diagnostic essentials

2.1 Clinical manifestations

Itching, burning sensation and sharp-stabbing pain on eyelid skin, clusters of blisters, or burning pain at the areas of forehead, temple, cheeks, etc., then sporadic blisters, mucus exudation and scarring at the above-mentioned areas, or severe pain if the trigeminal nerve is involved.

2.2 Examination

(1) If it is caused by herpes simplex virus, the clusters of blisters occur at the skin of the eyelid, lip and nose, and the swollen nodules are palpable at the area anterior the ear on the same side. If the palpebral margin is attacked, the cornea, or lip and nasal vestibule can be involved.

1 病因病机

1.1 脾经湿热，外感风邪，风湿热裹挟，循经上犯胞睑。

1.2 脾胃湿热中阻，土盛侮木，脾病及肝，肝脾同病，复感风邪，风湿热邪循经上犯于目。

1.3 外感风热邪毒引动内火，肝脾共患，热毒灼盛于肉轮、风轮。

2 诊断要点

2.1 临床表现

眼睑皮肤瘙痒、灼热、刺痛，继之相对应的皮肤出现簇状水疱，或额、颞、腮等部位灼痛感，继之弥散于上述部位的散在疱疹、黏液渗出、结痂。三叉神经受累则疼痛剧烈。

2.2 眼部检查

（1）由单纯疱疹病毒所致者，胞睑或唇、鼻部皮肤出现团簇水泡，数日后水疱化脓，或可破溃糜烂、结痂；同侧耳前可扪及肿核。如发生于睑缘处，可蔓延至角膜，亦可见于在唇部、鼻前庭。

(2) If it is caused by herpes zoster virus, the clusters of blisters occur at the skin of eyelid, forehead and scalp on one side, without transcending the midline. If the cornea is involved, the nebula and visual decrease occur as well.

(2)由带状疱疹所致者,患侧眼睑、额部皮肤及头皮出现成簇的水疱,其分布不超过鼻中线;仅累及同侧颜面部及额部。病变累及角膜时,形成翳障,视力下降。

3 Therapeutic methods

3 治疗方法

3.1 Therapeutic principles

3.1 治疗原则

For the condition caused by herpes simplex virus, it is advisable to treat the local area only. For the condition caused by herpes zoster virus, it is advisable to apply the antiviral agents orally, even the glucocorticoids, besides the local treatment. It is necessary to observe if the cornea is involved or not and to prescribe reasonably.

由单纯疱疹病毒引起者局部治疗即可;带状疱疹病毒引起者除局部应用外,须口服抗病毒药,必要时使用糖皮质激素。合理辨证处方,观察角膜是否累及。

Principles of pattern identification: The eyelid is attributive to the muscle wheel and spleen, while the eye black to the wind wheel and liver. The exogenous factor is invasion of pathogenic wind, heat and damp, while the endogenous factor is related to the spleen or liver. It is advisable to treat the disease according to the manifestations and seriousness of the conditions respectively.

辨证原则:胞睑为肉轮在脏属脾,黑睛为风轮在脏属肝,辨证外因风热湿为邪,内因责之或脾或肝,临证应注意外显证候之孰轻孰重而分别处置。

3.2 Treatment based on syndrome differentiation

3.2 辨证论治

(1) **Wind-heat in Spleen Meridian**

(1) **脾经风热**

Main symptoms: Redness, itching, pain, burning sensation and blisters at the skin of eyelid, or accompanied by fever and aversion to cold, thin-yellow tongue coating and superficial-rapid pulse.

主症:胞睑皮肤红赤、痒痛、灼热,起水疱;或伴发热恶寒。舌苔薄黄,脉浮数。

Therapeutic methods: Purify spleen and remove damp.

治法:清脾除湿。

Herbal formulas and drugs: The major formula

方药:代表方为清脾除

is *Spleen-Purifying and Damp-Removing Drink* (Qing Pi Chu Shi Yin). The commonly-used herbal drugs are *Rhizoma Alismatis* (Ze Xie), *Rhizoma Atractylodis* (Cang Zhu), *Rhizoma Atractylodis Macrocephalae* (Bai Zhu), *Herba Artemisiae Scopariae* (Yin Chen), *Fructus Gardeniae* (Zhi Zi), *Radix Scutellariae* (Huang Qin), *Fructus Forsythiae* (Lian Qiao), *Natrii Sulfas Exsiccatus* (Xuan Ming Fen), *Radix Rehmanniae Cruda* (Sheng Di Huang), *Fructus Aurantii* (Zhi Ke), *Radix Glycyrrhizae Praeparata* (Zhi Gan Cao), etc.

湿饮，常用药如泽泻、苍术、白术、茵陈、栀子、黄芩、连翘、玄明粉、生地、枳壳、炙甘草等。

Modification according to symptoms: For those without constipation, subtract *Natrii Sulfas Exsiccatus* (Xuan Ming Fen) and add *Radix Paeoniae Rubra* (Chi Shao) and *Cortex Moutan Radicis* (Dan Pi), to clear heat, cool blood, relieve redness, dissolve stasis and stop pain. For those with severe itching of skin, add *Herba Menthae* (Bo He), *Periostracum Cicadae* (Chan Tui) and *Herba Equiseti Hiemalis* (Mu Zei), to eliminate wind, remove pathogens and relieve itching.

加减：无便秘者，去玄明粉，加赤芍、丹皮以清热凉血退赤；散瘀止痛，皮肤痒甚者，可加薄荷、蝉蜕、木贼以疏风散邪止痒。

(2) **Upward-attack of damp-heat**

(2) **湿热上攻**

Main symptoms: Redness, pain, blisters, clusters of pustules on eyelid, diabrosis, exudation and erosion, accompanied by stuffy chest, poor appetite, sticky sensation in mouth, unrelieved thirst after drinking water, etc., red tongue body with sticky tongue coating and rolling-rapid pulse.

主症：胞睑红赤疼痛，水疱、脓疱簇生，极痒，甚或破溃流水，糜烂；或伴胸闷纳呆，口中黏腻，饮不解渴等症。舌质红，苔腻，脉滑数。

Therapeutic methods: Reduce fire, relieve toxin and remove damp.

治法：泻火解毒除湿。

Herbal formulas and drugs: The major formula is *Universal Salvation Detoxifying Drink* (Pu Ji Xiao Du Yin) plus *Dampness-Dispersing Decoction* (Chu Shi Tang). The commonly-used herbal drugs are *Sclerotium*

方药：代表方为普济消毒饮合除湿汤，常用药如茯苓、滑石、车前子、黄芩、黄连、板蓝根、牛蒡子、连翘、薄

Poriae (Fu Ling), *Talcum* (Hua Shi), *Semen Plantaginis* (Che Qian Zi), *Radix Scutellariae* (Huang Qin), *Rhizoma Coptidis* (Huang Lian), *Radix Isatidis* (Ban Lan Gen), *Fructus Arctii* (Niu Bang Zi), *Fructus Forsythiae* (Lian Qiao), *Herba Menthae* (Bo He), *Herba Schizonepetae* (Jing Jie), *Radix Ledebouriellae* (Fang Feng), *Radix Platycodi* (Jie Geng), etc.

Modification according to symptoms: Add *Rhizoma Smilacis Glabrae* (Tu Fu Ling), *Semen Coicis* (Yi Yi Ren), *Flos Lonicerae* (Jin Yin Hua) and *Herba Taraxaci* (Pu Gong Ying) to assist the actions to remove damp, clear heat and relieve toxin. For blisters, pustules, diabrosis, erosion and extreme itch of eyelid skin, add *Fructus Kochiae* (Di Fu Zi) and *Cortex Dictamni* (Bai Xian Pi) to clear heat, remove damp and stop itching.

(3) **Heat-toxin in liver and spleen**

Main symptoms: Redness, itching, pain and clusters of blisters and pustules on eyelid, dry sensation, pain, photophobia and lacrimation of diseases eye, vesiculated dermatitis of eyelid, redness of eye white, nebula or erosion of eye black, accompanied by headache, fever, bitter taste in mouth, yellow urine and constipation, red tongue body with yellow tongue coating and wiry-rapid pulse.

Therapeutic methods: Clear heat, dissolve damp, eliminate pathogens and remove nebula.

Herbal formulas and drugs: The major formula is *Gentian Liver-Draining Decoction* (Long Dan Xie Gan Tang). The commonly-used herbal drugs are *Radix Gentianae* (Long Dan), *Fructus Gardeniae* (Zhi Zi), *Radix Scutellariae* (Huang Qin), *Rhizoma Alismatis* (Ze Xie), *Radix Angelicae Sinensis*

荷、荆芥、防风、桔梗等。

加减：①酌加土茯苓、薏苡仁、金银花、蒲公英等以助除湿清热解毒之功；②胞睑皮肤水疱、脓疱，破溃糜烂、极痒者，加地肤子、白鲜皮以清利湿热止痒。

（3）**肝脾热毒**

主症：胞睑红赤痒痛，水疱脓疱簇生，患眼碜涩疼痛，畏光流泪，抱轮红赤或白睛混赤，黑睛生星翳或黑睛生翳溃烂；全身可见头痛发热，口苦，溲黄便结。舌红苔黄，脉弦数。

治法：清热除湿，散邪退翳。

方药：代表方为龙胆泻肝汤，常用药如龙胆草、栀子、黄芩、泽泻、当归、生地、车前子、柴胡、炙甘草等。

(Dang Gui), *Radix Rehmanniae Cruda* (Sheng Di Huang), *Semen Plantaginis* (Che Qian Zi), *Radix Bupleuri* (Chai Hu), *Radix Glycyrrhizae Praeparata* (Zhi Gan Cao), etc.

Modification according to symptoms: Add *Radix Ledebouriellae* (Fang Feng), *Spica Schizonepetae Tenuifolia* (Jing Jie Sui) and *Rhizoma seu Radix Notopterygii* (Qiang Huo) to assist the actions to eliminate wind, remove pathogens and relieve photophobia and lacrimation. For severe pain, add *Resina Olibani* (Ru Xiang), *Myrrha* (Mo Yao) and *Radix Salviae Miltiorrhizae* (Dan Shen) to activate blood, regulate qi flow and stop pain.

加减：酌加防风、荆芥穗、羌活以助疏风散邪，解畏光流泪；疼痛剧烈，加乳香、没药、丹参活血理气止痛。

3.3 External therapies

(1) Eye drops: Apply 0.1% acyclovir eye drops 4 to 6 times a day, for the purpose to prevent or treat nebula of eye black (i.e. corneal infiltration).

(2) Eye ointment: Apply 3% acyclovir eye ointment inside the eye before sleep.

(3) Drug compress: For herpes zoster of eyelid, apply Six Spirits Pills (Liu Shen Wan) and *Yunnan's White Drug* (Yun Nan Bai Yao) in equal amounts and make into a paste for topical compress. Or apply *Indigo Naturalis Ointment* (Qing Dai Gao) for topical compress. For ulceration, apply 0.5% neomycin solution for wet compress, 3 to 4 times a day.

(4) If the cornea is involved, it is advisable to apply mydriatic to prevent complications.

3.3 外治法

（1）滴眼液：0.1%无环鸟苷滴眼液，每日4～6次，以预防或治疗黑睛生翳（即角膜侵润）。

（2）涂眼药膏：3%无环鸟苷眼膏，或睡前涂于眼内。

（3）药物敷：眼睑带状疱疹取六神丸和云南白药等份，调成糊状涂于患处；或用青黛膏外涂。若有溃烂者，可用0.5%新霉素溶液湿敷，每日3～4次。

（4）累及角膜需扩瞳以免出现并发症。

4 Speculative map

4 思辨导图

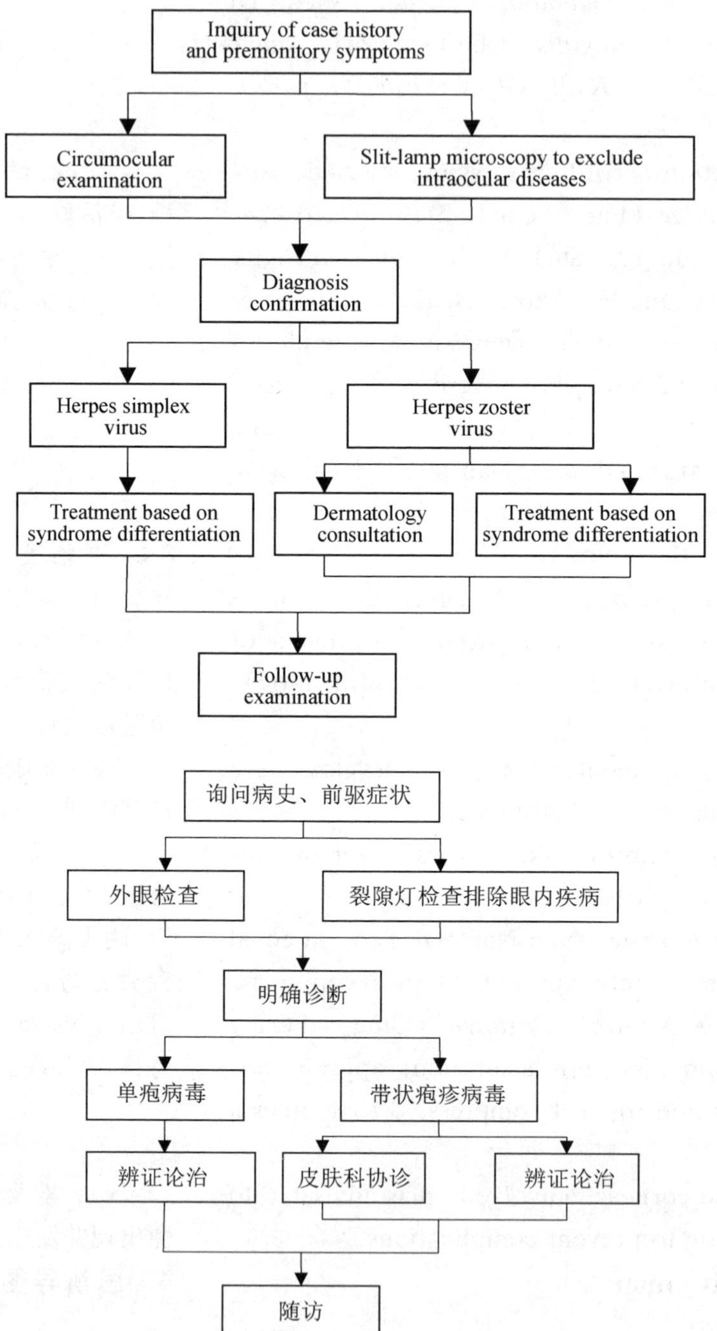
Inquiry of case history and premonitory symptoms
Circumocular examination
Slit-lamp microscopy to exclude intraocular diseases
Diagnosis confirmation
Herpes simplex virus
Herpes zoster virus
Treatment based on syndrome differentiation
Dermatology consultation
Treatment based on syndrome differentiation
Follow-up examination
询问病史、前驱症状
外眼检查
裂隙灯检查排除眼内疾病
明确诊断
单疱病毒
带状疱疹病毒
辨证论治
皮肤科协诊
辨证论治
随访

Hordeolum

麦粒肿

Hordeolum refers to acute and purulent infection of eyelid gland. The infection of eyelid sebaceous gland (Zeis gland) or eyelid sweat gland (Moll gland) is called external hordeolum, while the infection of meibomian gland is called internal hordeolum. It is mostly caused by staphy lococcus infection.

麦粒肿是眼睑腺体急性化脓性感染，眼睑皮脂腺(Zeis 腺)或汗腺(Moll 腺)感染为外麦粒肿，睑板腺(Meibomian 腺)受累时，称之为内麦粒肿。大多数由葡萄球菌感染所致。古籍中多有论述。

In traditional Chinese medicine, the disease is called "sty", "earth sore" or "earth ulcer", a kind of wheat-like furuncle occurring on the eyelid, becoming purulence and ulceration, manifested by redness, swelling, redness and pain. The exogenous factor of the disease is the pathogenic wind-heat, while its endogenous factor is the accumulated heat in spleen and stomach.

本病属于中医学"偷针眼""土疳""土疡"范畴，为眼睑发生形如麦粒的疖肿，易成脓、溃破；以红、肿、热、痛为特征性临床表现。其因中医外因责之风热之邪，内因为脾胃积热。

1 Etiology and pathogenesis

1 病因病机

1.1 The pathogenic wind-heat invades the eyelid and blocks the local meridians, leading to unsmooth flow of qi and blood.

1.1 风热之邪客于胞睑，滞留局部脉络，气血不畅。

1.2 Taking of pungent, spicy and fried food produces the accumulated heat in the spleen and stomach, and then the excessive heat-toxin leads to purulence and ulceration.

1.2 喜食辛辣炙煿，脾胃积热，热毒壅盛，酿脓溃破。

1.3 The residual pathogen or the weakened spleen qi makes the Wei (Defensive) Qi deficiency and causes repeated attacks of the exogenous wind-heat.

1.3 余邪未清或脾气虚弱，卫外不固，缕感风热外邪。

2 Diagnostic essentials

2 诊断要点

2.1 Clinical manifestations

2.1 临床表现

Redness, swelling, hotness and pain on eyelid, and rapid development of purulence and ulceration.

眼睑局部红、肿、热、痛，迅速成脓溃破。

2.2 Ocular examinations

In the early stage, there is a limited and tender nodule at the eyelid. After purulence, the swollen nodule becomes soft in property and fluctuant.

2.2 眼部检查

初期眼睑有局限性、压痛性结节。脓成肿块质软，可及波动感。

3 Therapeutic methods

3 治疗方法

3.1 Therapeutic principles

Before purulence, apply oral and external treatments, to promote disperse of nodule. After purulence, apply incision and drainage.

3.1 治疗原则

未成脓者内外兼治，促其消散；已成脓者，切开排脓。

3.2 Treatment based on syndrome differentiation

3.2 辨证论治

(1) **Wind-heat attacking eyelid**

Main symptoms: In the early stage, localized itching, distension, slight redness, unobvious nodule and sharp-stabbing pain on eyelid, thin-yellow tongue coating and superficial-rapid pulse.

Therapeutic methods: Eliminate wind and clear heat.

Herbal formulas and drugs: The major formula is *Lonicera and Forsythia Powder* (Yin Qiao San). The commonly-used herbal drugs are *Flos Lonicerae* (Jin Yin Hua), *Fructus Forsythiae* (Lian Qiao), *Radix Platycodi* (Jie Geng), *Fructus Arctii* (Niu Bang Zi), *Herba Schizonepetae* (Jing Jie), *Rhizoma Phragmitis* (Lu Gen), *Semen Armeniacae Amarum* (Ku Xing Ren), etc.

Modification according to symptoms: For severe itching, add *Folium Mori* (Sang Ye) and *Flos Chrysanthemi* (Ju Hua) to eliminate wind and relieve itching. For severe pain, add *Resina Olibani* (Ru Xiang) and *Myrrha* (Mo Yao) to activate blood and stop pain. For severe redness and swelling, add *Rhizoma Coptidis* (Huang Lian), *Fructus Gardeniae* (Zhi Zi) and *Herba Taraxaci* (Pu Gong

(1) **风热客睑**

主症：初起胞睑局限性痒胀，微红，硬结不显，刺痛。舌苔薄黄，脉浮数。

治法：疏风清热。

方药：代表方为银翘散。常用药如金银花、连翘、桔梗、牛蒡子、荆芥、芦根、杏仁等药。

加减：痒甚者，加桑叶、菊花以助祛风止痒；疼痛者，加乳香、没药活血止痛；若红肿较重者，加黄连、栀子、蒲公英清热解毒；便秘者，加大黄通腑泻热。

Ying) to clear heat and relieve toxin. For constipation, add *Radix et Rhizoma Rhei* (Da Huang) to dredge fu organs and clear heat.

(2) **Accumulation and excess of heat-toxin**

Main symptoms: Localized redness, swelling, hotness and pain on eyelid, growing hard nodule which is tender and worsened by pressure, or redness and swelling of eye white, accompanied by thirst with preference for drinking water, constipation and red urine, red tongue body with yellow tongue coating and rapid pulse.

Therapeutic methods: Clear heat, relieve toxin, subside swell and stop pain.

Herbal formulas and drugs: The major formula is *Fairy Formula Life-Saving Drink* (Xian Fang Huo Ming Yin). The commonly-used herbal drugs are *Flos Lonicerae* (Jin Yin Hua), *Radix Trichosanthis* (Tian Hua Fen), *Radix Angelicae Sinensis* (Dang Gui), *Radix Paeoniae Rubra* (Chi Shao), *Resina Olibani* (Ru Xiang), *Myrrha* (Mo Yao), *Squama Manitis* (Chuan Shan Jia), *Spina Gleditsiae* (Zao Jiao Ci), *Radix Angelicae Dahuricae* (Bai Zhi), *Bulbus Fritillariae Thumbergii* (Zhe Bei Mu), etc.

Modification according to symptoms: Combine with *Five Ingredients Detoxifying Drink* (Wu Wei Xiao Du Yin), to dissipate hard nodule and to increase the actions to clear heat and relieve toxin. For constipation, add *Radix et Rhizoma Rhei* (Da Huang) to reduce fire and dredge fu organs. For fever, aversion to cold and headache due to deep location of heat-toxin or due to heat entering the Ying (Nutrient) and Xue (Blood) Phases, combine with *Rhinoceros Horn and Rehmannia Decoction* (Xi Jiao Di Huang Tang), to clear heat, relieve toxin, cool

(2) **热毒壅盛**

主症：胞睑局部红肿热痛，硬结渐大成脓，压痛拒按，或白睛红赤肿，或伴口渴喜饮，便秘溲赤。舌红苔黄，脉数。

治法：清热解毒，消肿止痛。

方药：代表方为仙方活命饮，常用药如金银花、天花粉、当归、赤芍、乳香、没药、穿山甲、皂角刺、白芷、浙贝母等药。

加减：与五味消毒饮合用以消散硬结，增强清热解毒之功；便秘者，加大黄以泻火通腑；若发热、恶寒、头痛者，为热重毒深或热入营血，可与犀角地黄汤配合应用，以助清热解毒，并凉血散瘀滞。

blood and dissolve stasis.

(3) **Spleen deficiency complicated by pathogens**

Main symptoms: Repeated attacks of hordeolum, or unobvious redness and swelling in hordeolum, or chronic and unhealed hordeolum, accompanied by lusterless face, low spirit, lassitude, dietary bias, poor appetite and constipation, pale tongue body with thin-white tongue coating and thready-rapid pulse.

Therapeutic methods: Strengthen spleen, benefit qi, dissipate nodule and dissolve stasis.

Herbal formulas and drugs: The major formula is *Interior-Supporting and Detoxifying Powder* (Tuo Li Xiao Du San). The commonly-used herbal drugs are *Radix Ginseng* (Ren Shen), *Radix Astragali* (Huang Qi), *Rhizoma Atractylodis Macrocephalae* (Bai Zhu), *Sclerotium Poriae* (Fu Ling), *Radix Angelicae Sinensis* (Dang Gui), *Radix Paeoniae Alba* (Bai Shao), *Rhizoma Ligustici Chuanxiong* (Chuan Xiong), *Flos Lonicerae* (Jin Yin Hua), *Fructus Forsythiae* (Lian Qiao), *Radix Angelicae Dahuricae* (Bai Zhi), *Pericarpium Citri Tangerinae* (Chen Pi), etc.

Modification according to symptoms: For poor appetite and constipation, add *Fructus Hordei Germinatus* (Mai Ya), *Fructus Crataegi* (Shan Zha) and *Semen Raphani* (Lai Fu Zi) to strengthen spleen, digest food and dissolve stasis. For hard, small and ulcerative nodule, add *Semen Coicis* (Yi Yi Ren), *Radix Platycodi* (Jie Geng), *Radix Rhapontici seu Echinopsis* (Lou Lu) and *Herba Violae* (Zi Hua Di Ding), to clear heat and drain pus. For attack-free stage of hordeolum, select Ginseng, Poria and Atractylodes Powder (Shen Ling Bai Zhu San) to regulate spleen and stomach and to prevent recurrence.

(3) **脾虚挟邪**

主症：针眼屡发，或针眼红肿不甚，经久难消；或见面色无华，神倦乏力，小儿偏食，纳呆便结。舌淡，苔薄白，脉细数。

治法：健脾益气，散结消滞。

方药：代表方为托里消毒散，常用药如人参、黄芪、白术、茯苓、当归、白芍、川芎、金银花、连翘、白芷、陈皮等药。

加减：若纳呆便结者，加麦芽、山楂、莱菔子等以健脾消食行滞；若硬结小且将溃者，加薏苡仁、桔梗、漏芦、紫花地丁以清热排脓；在针眼未发之间歇期，可选用参苓白术散以调理脾胃防止复发。

3.3 External therapies

(1) Apply an herbal decoction, made of *Folium Isatidis* (Da Qing Ye), *Flos Lonicerae* (Jin Yin Hua), *Flos Chrysanthemi Indici* (Ye Ju Hua), etc. for fumigation or wet compress, in the early stage of the disease for the purpose to relieve the inflammation, and in the middle stage for the purpose to promote the maturity of nodule and diabrosis, 3 to 4 times a day and 15 minutes each time.

(2) Apply the incision and drainage for the purulence if it is maturated. It is necessary to have a neat incision. For external hordeolum, apply the incision on the skin surface with the incision parallel to the eyelid. For internal hordeolum, apply the incision on the palpebral conjunctiva surface with the incision perpendicular to the palpebral margin. For those whose drainage is not smooth, apply the medicated thread or lace for drainage, and change the medicated thread or lace till complete recovery.

3.3 外治法

（1）湿热或中药煎剂（大青叶、金银花、野菊花等）熏敷，发病初期可帮助炎症消散，中期可促使硬结成熟，以利溃破痊愈。每日 3～4 次，每次 15 分钟。

（2）脓肿成熟后，行切开引流。注意掌握切口齐整。外麦粒肿，选择皮肤面切开，切口与睑缘平行；内麦粒肿，选择睑结膜面切开，切口与睑缘垂直；脓液引流不畅者，放置药线或皮条引流，每日换药至愈。

4 Speculative map

4 思辨导图

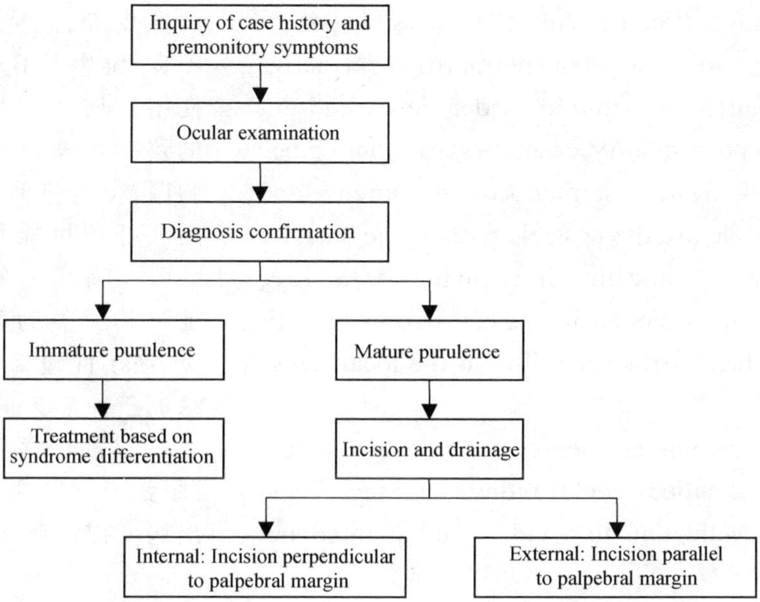

Inquiry of case history and premonitory symptoms
↓
Ocular examination
↓
Diagnosis confirmation
↓
- Immature purulence → Treatment based on syndrome differentiation
- Mature purulence → Incision and drainage
  - Internal: Incision perpendicular to palpebral margin
  - External: Incision parallel to palpebral margin

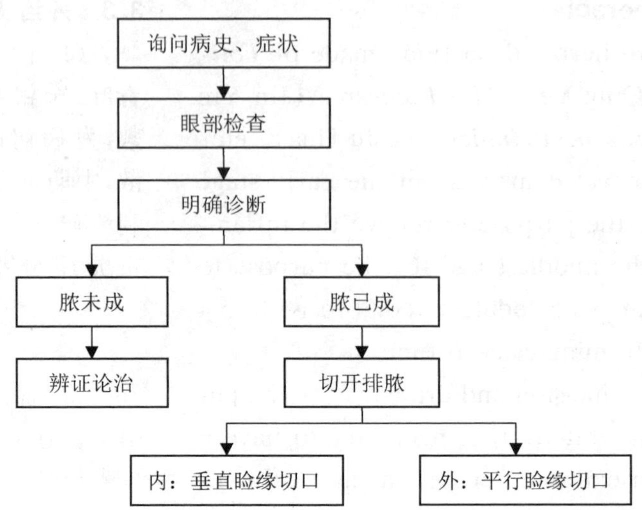

Blepharitis

Blepharitis refers to the sub-acute or chronic inflammation of palpebral margin surface, eyelash hair follicles and follicle gland tissue, with attack of both eyes, long course of disease and stubborn condition which is difficult to cure. The possible pathogenic factors are seborrheic dermatitis, refractive errors, malnutrition, vitamin B_2 deficiency and application of poor quality cosmetics for long time. Pityrosporum ovale, staphylococcus aureus and Morax-Axenfeld are the possible pathogenic bacteria of the disease. Clinically, it is divided into three types of squamous blepharitis, ulcerative blepharitis and angular blepharitis according to the local signs.

In the ancient classics of traditional Chinese medicine, it is called "eyelid redness and ulcer" and "ulcerative eyelid due to wind", and pointed out

睑缘炎

睑缘炎指睑缘表面、睫毛毛囊及其腺组织的亚急性、慢性炎症。双眼发病，病程长，病情顽固难愈。脂溢性皮炎、屈光不正、营养不良、维生素 B_2 缺乏及长期使用劣质化妆品均是可能的致病因素。卵圆皮屑芽胞菌，金黄色葡萄球菌，莫-阿双杆菌可能是该病的致病菌。临床上依据局部体征将其分类为鳞屑性睑缘炎、溃疡性睑缘炎和眦部睑缘炎三种。

早期中医古籍名之为"眼弦赤烂""烂弦风"，并指出病变以两眦为主；又有医

that the major affected areas are the canthi. It is also called "canthus redness and ulcer", or "redness and ulcer due to fetus wind" for the condition in children. Clinically, the distinctive manifestations are itching, redness and erosion of palpebral margin. In traditional Chinese medicine, the exogenous pathogens are wind, heat and damp, while the endogenous factors are related to the spleen and stomach. The both exogenous and endogenous factors attack the palpebral margin to cause the disease.

家名其为"眦帷赤烂";发于儿童者被称为"胎风赤烂"。临床以睑缘刺痒、红赤、糜烂为特征性表现。其因中医外责之风、热、湿三邪,内因责之于脾胃,内外合邪,相搏于睑缘而发病。

1 Etiology and pathogenesis

1 病因病机

1.1 Accumulated heat in spleen and stomach. Due to the invasion of pathogenic wind, the pathogenic wind and heat combine to attack the palpebral margin, to consume the body fluid and cause dryness.

1.1 脾胃蕴热,复受风邪,风热合邪触染睑缘,伤津化燥。

1.2 Damp-heat in spleen and stomach. Due to the invasion of pathogenic wind, the pathogenic wind, damp and heat combine to attack the palpebral margin to cause the disease.

1.2 脾胃湿热,外感风邪,风、湿、热邪相搏,循经攻于睑缘而发病。

1.3 Internal hyperactivity of heart fire. Due to the invasion of pathogenic wind which induces the heart fire, the pathogenic wind and fire combine and move upwards to burn the palpebral margin to cause the disease.

1.3 心火内盛,风邪犯眦,引动心火,风火上炎,灼伤睑眦。

2 Diagnostic essentials

2 诊断要点

2.1 Clinical manifestations

2.1 临床表现

Itching, burning sensation and pain at the palpebral margin of the affected eye, and redness at the canthus and palpebral margin, squama or erosion or ulcer at the root part of eyelash.

患眼睑弦刺痒灼痛。眦部、睑弦红赤,睫毛根部有鳞屑或糜烂溃疡。

2.2 Ocular examination

2.2 眼部检查

(1) Squamous blepharitis: Slight redness at the palpebral margin can be seen, with small and husk-

(1) 鳞屑性睑缘炎:仅见睑缘潮红,睫毛根部及睫毛

like squama attached to the root part of eyelash. After the squama is removed, redness at palpebral margin, easy loss of eyelash and regeneration of squama can be seen.

间附有细小糠皮样鳞屑,除去鳞屑后可见睑缘红赤,睫毛易脱落,但可再生为鳞屑性。

(2) Ulcerative blepharitis: Redness and erosion at the palpebral margin can be seen, with scars and sticky and fascicular eyelash. After the crust is removed, purulence and bleeding can be seen at the root part of eyelash. After dropping-off of eyelash, the eyelash cannot regenerate, becoming sparse eyelash or bald eyelash over long time.

(2) 溃疡性睑缘炎:如见睑缘红赤糜烂,结痂,睫毛胶黏成束,除去痂皮可见睫毛根部出脓、出血,乱生或脱落,睫毛脱落后不能再生,日久则睫毛稀疏或成秃睫者为溃疡性。

(3) Angular blepharitis: Symptoms of redness, erosion, etc. can be seen at the canthi.

(3) 眦部睑缘炎:或见红赤糜烂等症在两眦部为眦部性。

3 Therapeutic methods

3 治疗方法

3.1 Therapeutic principles

3.1 治疗原则

Eliminate the incentive cause, avoid the stimulation, pay attention to local cleaning, apply massage of meibomian glands, and apply local fumigation and compress at the local area. Besides, the method to eliminate wind, clear heat and dissolve damp is taken as the major one, while the method to regulate spleen and heart as the auxiliary one. It is advisable to combine both the external and internal therapy.

去除诱因,避免刺激,注意局部清洁,按摩睑板腺,局部药液熏敷。临证以驱风清热除湿为主,调理脾心为辅,内外合治。

3.2 Treatment based on syndrome differentiation

3.2 辨证论治

(1) **Hyperactivity of wind-heat**

(1) **风热偏盛**

Main symptoms: Redness, itching and burning sensation at palpebral margin, husk-like squama at the root part of eyelash, red tongue body with thin tongue coating, and superficial-rapid pulse.

主症:睑弦赤痒,灼热,睫毛根部有糠皮样鳞屑。舌红苔薄,脉浮数。

Therapeutic methods: Eliminate wind, stop

治法:祛风止痒,清热凉

itching, clear heat, and cool blood.

Herbal formulas and drugs: The major formula is *Lonicera and Forsythia Powder* (Yin Qiao San). The commonly-used herbal drugs are *Flos Lonicerae* (Jin Yin Hua), *Fructus Forsythiae* (Lian Qiao), *Radix Platycodi* (Jie Geng), *Fructus Arctii* (Niu Bang Zi), *Herba Schizonepetae* (Jing Jie), *Rhizoma Phragmitis* (Lu Gen), *Semen Armeniacae Amarum* (Ku Xing Ren), etc.

Modification according to symptoms: Add *Radix Paeoniae Rubra* (Chi Shao) to enhance the action to clear heat and cool blood. Add *Periostracum Cicadae* (Chan Tui) and *Zaocys* (Wu Shao She) to enhance the action to eliminate wind and stop itching. Add *Radix Trichosanthis* (Tian Hua Fen) to produce body fluid and moisturize the dry condition.

(2) **Hyperactivity of damp-heat**

Main symptoms: Itching and pain of the affected eye, redness, ulcer, purulence, bleeding, turbidity and scars at the palpebral margin, sticky eye discharge, sparse eyelash, or trichiasis, or bald eyelash, red tongue body with yellow-sticky tongue coating, and soft-rapid pulse.

Therapeutic methods: Clear heat, dissolve damp, eliminate wind and stop itching.

Herbal formulas and drugs: The major formula is *Dampness-Dispersing Decoction* (Chu Shi Tang). The commonly-used herbal drugs are *Sclerotium Poriae* (Fu Ling), *Talcum* (Hua Shi), *Semen Plantaginis* (Che Qian Zi), *Radix Scutellariae* (Huang Qin), *Rhizoma Coptidis* (Huang Lian), *Radix Ledebouriellae* (Fang Feng), *Herba Schizonepetae* (Jing Jie), *Fructus Aurantii* (Zhi Ke), *Pericarpium*

血。

方药：代表方为银翘散，常用药如金银花、连翘、桔梗、牛蒡子、荆芥、芦根、杏仁等。

加减：加赤芍以增清热凉血之功；加蝉蜕、乌梢蛇以助祛风止痒；加天花粉以增津润燥。

(2) **湿热偏盛**

主症：患眼痒痛并作，睑弦红赤溃烂，出脓出血，秽浊结痂，眵泪胶黏，睫毛稀疏，或倒睫，或秃睫。舌质红，苔黄腻，脉濡数。

治法：清热除湿，祛风止痒。

方药：代表方为除湿汤，常用药如茯苓、滑石、车前子、黄芩、黄连、防风、荆芥、枳壳、陈皮、炙甘草等。

Citri Tangerinae (Chen Pi), *Radix Glycyrrhizae Praeparata* (Zhi Gan Cao), etc.

Modification according to symptoms: Add *Flos Lonicerae* (Jin Yin Hua), *Herba Taraxaci* (Pu Gong Ying), *Cortex Phellodendri* (Huang Bo) and *Fructus Gardeniae* (Zhi Zi) to assist the action to clear heat and dissolve damp.

加减：加金银花、蒲公英、黄柏、栀子以助清热除湿之功。

(3) **Upward-flaming of heart fire**

(3) **心火上炎**

Main symptoms: Redness, burning sensation and itching at palpebral margin of canthus, or redness, erosion, purulence and bleeding at palpebral margin, red tongue tip with thin tongue coating, and rapid pulse.

主症：眦部睑弦红赤，灼热刺痒，甚或睑弦赤烂、出脓出血。舌尖红，苔薄，脉数。

Therapeutic methods: Purify heart and reduce fire.

治法：清心泻火。

Herbal formulas and drugs: The major formula is *Heat-Abducting Powder* (Dao Chi San) plus *Coptis Detoxifying Decoction* (Huang Lian Jie Du Tang). The commonly-used herbal drugs are *Radix Rehmanniae Cruda* (Sheng Di Huang), *Caulis Akebiae* (Mu Tong), *Herba Lophatheri* (Dan Zhu Ye), *Radix Glycyrrhizae* (Gan Cao), *Rhizoma Coptidis* (Huang Lian), *Radix Scutellariae* (Huang Qin), *Cortex Phellodendri* (Huang Bo), *Fructus Gardeniae* (Zhi Zi), etc.

方药：代表方为导赤散合黄连解毒汤，常用药如生地黄、木通、淡竹叶、生甘草、黄连、黄芩、黄柏、栀子等。

Modification according to symptoms: For severe redness at the sick area, add *Radix Paeoniae Rubra* (Chi Shao) and *Cortex Moutan Radicis* (Mu Dan Pi) to cool blood and relieve redness. For intolerable itching, add *Periostracum Cicadae* (Chan Tui), *Fructus Kochiae* (Di Fu Zi), *Cortex Dictamni* (Bai Xian Pi), *Flos Chrysanthemi* (Ju Hua), *Radix Ledebouriellae* (Fang Feng) and *Rhizoma Ligustici Chuanxiong* (Chuan Xiong) to eliminate wind and stop itching.

加减：若患处红赤较甚者，可加赤芍、牡丹皮以凉血退赤；痒极难忍者，酌加蝉蜕、地肤子、白鲜皮、菊花、防风、川芎以祛风止痒。

3.3 External therapies

(1) Fumigation and wash: In the fumigation and wash with herbal decoction, the moisturizing action of the wet steam acts to promote the dropping off of the squama, purulence and scars and to clear away the purulent fluid in the eyelash follicle, fully expose the sick area and improve the local blood circulation. The medication may reach the sick area. ① It is advisable to apply the soup decocted by the herbal dredge for oral administration, or the decoction composed of 30g *Herba Senecionis Scandentis* (Qian Li Guang), 15g *Cortex Dictamni* (Bai Xian Pi), 30g *Radix Sophorae Flavescentis* (Ku Shen), 15g *Flos Chrysanthemi Indici* (Ye Ju Hua), 30g *Herba Taraxaci* (Pu Gong Ying), 30g *Fructus Cnidii* (She Chuang Zi), etc., to fumigate and wash the local area, 2 to 3 times a day; ② Apply 0.9% sodium chloride injection or 3% boric acid solution to wash the palpebral margin; ③ Apply the decoction of *Two Sages Powder* (Er Sheng San) to wash the local area.

(2) Eye ointment: Apply antibiotic eye ointment, as Erythromycin Eye Ointment.

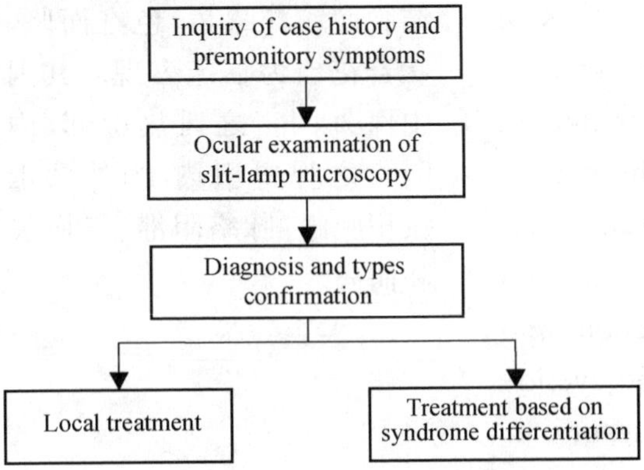

3.3 外治法

（1）熏洗：中药药液熏洗时，先通过蒸汽的湿润作用使鳞屑、脓痂松脱易于拭去并清除睫毛毛囊中的脓液，充分暴露病损处，改善局部血液循环，药力可达病处。①可用内服药渣煎液，或选用千里光30克，白鲜皮15克，苦参30克，野菊花15克，蒲公英30克，蛇床子30克等药煎水熏洗，每日2～3次；②用0.9%氯化钠注射液或3%硼酸溶液清洗睑缘，每日2～3次；③二圣散煎水外洗。

（2）涂眼药膏：涂抗生素眼膏，如红霉素眼膏等。

4 Speculative map

Inquiry of case history and premonitory symptoms
↓
Ocular examination of slit-lamp microscopy
↓
Diagnosis and types confirmation
↓
Local treatment | Treatment based on syndrome differentiation

4 思辨导图

询问病史、症状
↓
眼部裂隙灯检查
↓
明确诊断、类型
↓
局部治疗 | 辨证论治

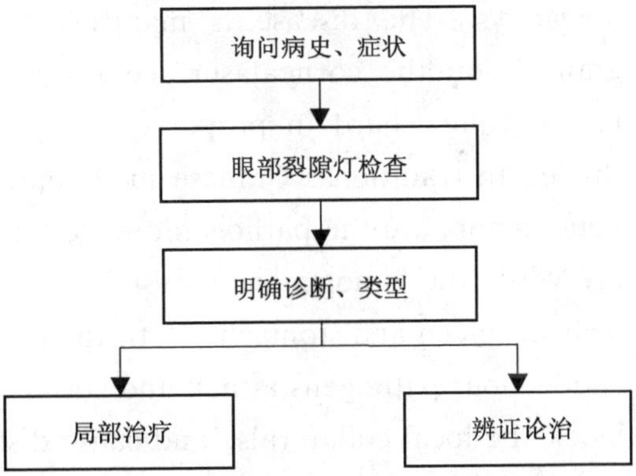

Trachoma

沙　眼

Trachoma is a kind of chronic inflammatory ocular disease of cornea and conjunctiva. The pathogenic factor is Chlamydia trachomatis. The infected conjunctival and corneal cells, as the host, produce the offspring of chlamydial in a binary fission. The protomer subunits are released in fragmentation of cytoplasm, and then the normal cells are reinfected in full circle. In the end, it is possible to cause conjunctival scarring, meibomian deformation and pannus which further lead to the complications as entropion, trichiasis, corneal opacity, etc., as a result, the blindness occurs. The disease affects the both eyes and lasts for a long period of time, easily becoming an epidemic disease in the areas with poor sanitary condition.

In traditional Chinese medicine, it is called "wind-swelling of eye", "redness of eye due to wind". "windy nodule inside eyelid", "red-colored nodule inside eyelid", etc. It is called "pepper-like eye sore" in *Standards of Diagnosis and Treatment* (Zheng Zhi Zhun Sheng) and has been in use till nowadays. The disease is manifested by massive granules on the corneal surface inside the eyelid, red in color, hard in property and pepper-like in shape. In traditional Chinese medicine, the exogenous factors are the pathogenic wind, heat and toxin, while the endogenous factor is the accumulated heat in spleen and stomach. Both the exogenous and endogenous pathogens attack and stay in the eyelid, block the local collaterals, and cause disharmony of qi and blood, leading to the disease as a result.

沙眼属于慢性传染性角结膜病变。病因为沙眼衣原体，感染后的结膜、角膜细胞作为宿主以二分裂方式形成子代原体，充满胞浆破裂释放出原体，再周而复始的感染正常细胞。最终导致结膜瘢痕、睑板变形、角膜血管翳等引发睑内翻、倒睫、角膜混浊等并发症而失明。双眼发病，病程迁延，通常在卫生条件差的地区易形成流行趋势。

本病属于中医学“目中风肿”“目风赤候”“睑生风粒”“眼睑皮里生赤肉入鸡冠”“椒疱”等范畴。自《证治准绳》名之“椒疮”后，中医眼科沿用至今。本病以眼睑内结膜面颗粒累累，色红而坚，状若花椒为临床表现。其因中医外因责之风热毒邪，内因责之脾胃积热，内外邪毒瘀积胞睑，脉络阻滞、气血失和而病。

1 Etiology and pathogenesis

The exogenous pathogens of wind, heat and toxin invade the body and combine with the endogenous accumulated heat in spleen and stomach. Both the exogenous and endogenous pathogens attack the eyelid to block the local collaterals and cause disharmony of qi and blood, leading to the disease as a result.

1 病因病机

外感风热毒邪，内有脾胃积热，内外邪毒上雍胞睑，以致脉络阻滞，气血失和，瘀积为疾。

2 Diagnostic essentials

2.1 Clinical manifestations

Slight itching inside eyelid, slight dry sensation and small amount of eye discharge, or absence of obvious abnormal sensation, redness, itching and burning sensation inside eyelid in severe condition, with photophobia, eye discharge, drop-weight sensation and blurring of vision.

2.2 Ocular examinations

(1) Diffuse conjunctival congestion of upper eyelid, papillary hyperplasia and follicular formation at the palpebral conjunctiva and upper formix.

(2) Corneal vessel nebula found in slit-lamp microscopy.

(3) Scars at the upper formix or palpebral conjunctiva.

(4) Trachoma inclusions found in conjunctiva scraping examination.

Clinically, the condition with above Item Ⅰ and one of any other items is diagnosed trachoma.

2 诊断要点

2.1 临床表现

睑内微痒，稍有干涩及少量眵泪，或无明显异常感觉；病情重者，睑内赤痒灼热，畏光流泪，伴分泌物，眼睑重坠感，视物模糊。

2.2 眼部检查

（1）弥漫性上睑结膜血管充血，上睑结膜及上穹窿部乳头增生、滤泡形成。

（2）裂隙灯显微镜检查见角膜血管翳。

（3）上穹窿部或上睑结膜瘢痕。

（4）结膜刮片找到沙眼包涵体。

临证时见到上述第一项兼有其他一项即可诊断为沙眼。

Appendix: Diagnosis and Staging of Trachoma

Stages	Bases	Grades	Affection areas
Stage I (Active stage)	Conjunctival follicles and papillary hyperplasia in upper formix or upper eyelid, obscure vessels of palpebral conjunctiva.	Mild (+) Moderate (++) Severe (+++)	<1/3 1/3~2/3 > 2/3
Stage II (Regression stage)	Above affections with scarring	Mild (+) Moderate (++) Severe (+++)	< 1/3 1/3~2/3 > 2/3
Stage III (Scarring stage)	Scarring		

附:沙眼的诊断与分期

分期	依据	分级	病变占上睑的面积
Ⅰ期(进行期)	上穹窿或上睑结膜滤泡、乳头增生,睑结膜血管模糊。	轻(+) 中(++) 重(+++)	<1/3 1/3~2/3 >2/3
Ⅱ期(退行期)	上述病变同时出现瘢痕	轻(+) 中(++) 重(+++)	<1/3 1/3~2/3 >2/3
Ⅲ期(瘢痕期)	仅见瘢痕		

2.3 Common complications

(1) Entropion and trichiasis: Contracture of conjunctival surface scar of eyelid causes entropion.

(2) Corneal vessel nebula: In mild condition, the nebula of angiogenesis forms trachomatous pannus. In severe condition, the complete angiogenesis of cornea affects the vision.

(3) Corneal opacity.

(4) Symblepharon: The repeated conjunctival infection causes adhesion of bulbar conjunctiva and palpebral conjunctiva, so as to affect the ocular movement.

(5) Chronic dacryocystitis: The Chlamydia trachomatis attacks the nasolacrimal canal to cause lacrimation disturbance.

2.3 常见并发症

(1) 睑内翻倒睫:眼睑结膜面瘢痕收缩形成眼睑内翻。

(2) 角膜血管翳:轻者新生血管翳自从上方呈垂帘状,重者角膜全部新生血管化从而影响视力。

(3) 角膜混浊。

(4) 睑球粘连:反复的结膜炎症致使球结膜与睑结膜发生粘连,影响眼球运动。

(5) 慢性泪囊炎:沙眼衣原体侵犯鼻泪管,造成泪液引流障碍。

(6) **Keratoconjunctivitis sicca:** The repeated inflammation destroys the discharge function of conjunctival goblet cells, to cause low Schirmer I score.

(6) **角结膜干燥症:**反复的炎症只是结膜杯状细胞分泌功能破坏,基础泪液分泌不足。

(7) **Ptosis.**

(7) **上睑下垂。**

3 Therapeutic methods

3 治疗方法

3.1 Therapeutic principles

3.1 治疗原则

For mild condition, apply local eye drop. For severe condition, it is necessary to combine with the internal treatment, and accompanied by surgery if it is necessary. For complication and sequela, treat it according to relevant symptoms. Most conditions are caused by accumulated heat in spleen and stomach, and pathogenic wind, heat and toxin attacking the qi wheel and muscle wheel.

本病轻症可以局部点药为主,重症则配以内治,必要时还须辅以手术。并发症和后遗症应对症治疗。临证多以脾胃积热,风热毒邪客于气、肉轮间论治。

3.2 Treatment based on syndrome differentiation

3.2 辨证论治

(1) **Wind-heat attacking eyelid**

(1) **风热客睑**

Main symptoms: Slight itching and discomfort at eye with eye discharge, obscure vessels and congestion of palpebral conjunctiva, with small amount of follicles, papillary or neovascular nebula, red tongue tip with thin tongue coating, and superficial-rapid pulse.

主症:眼微痒不适,伴分泌物,睑结膜面血管模糊、充血,有少量滤泡,乳头或有新生血管翳。舌尖红,苔薄,脉浮数。

Therapeutic methods: Eliminate wind, clear heat, reduce redness and dissolve stasis.

治法:疏风清热,退赤散结。

Herbal formulas and drugs: The major formula is *Lonicera and Forsythia Powder* (Yin Qiao San). The commonly-used herbal drugs are *Flos Lonicerae* (Jin Yin Hua), *Fructus Forsythiae* (Lian Qiao), *Radix Platycodi* (Jie Geng), *Fructus Arctii* (Niu Bang Zi), *Herba Schizonepetae* (Jing Jie), *Rhizoma Phragmitis* (Lu Gen), *Semen Armeniacae Amarum*

方药:代表方为银翘散,常用药如金银花、连翘、桔梗、牛蒡子、荆芥、芦根、苦杏仁等。

(Ku Xing Ren), etc.

Modification according to symptoms: Add *Radix Rehmanniae Cruda* (Sheng Di Huang), *Radix Paeoniae Rubra* (Chi Shao) and *Radix Angelicae Sinensis* (Dang Gui), to clear heat, cool blood and reduce redness.

加减：可于方中加生地黄、赤芍、当归以清热凉血退赤。

(2) **Heat and stasis in blood**

(2) **血热瘀滞**

Main symptoms: Sharp-stabbing pain, burning and foreign-body sensations inside eye, photophobia, lacrimation with eye discharge, drop-weight sensation of eyelid which is difficult to uplift, congestion of palpebral conjunctiva, alternate papillary follicles and scars, accompanied by neovascular nebula, visual decrease, dark-red tongue body with yellow tongue coating, and rapid pulse.

主症：眼内刺痛灼热，异物感，畏光，流泪伴分泌物，眼睑重坠难开，睑结膜充血，乳头滤泡与瘢痕相间，伴新生血管翳呈垂帘状，视力下降。舌质暗红、苔黄，脉数。

Therapeutic methods: Clear heat, cool blood, activate blood and dissolve stasis.

治法：清热凉血，活血散瘀。

Herbal formulas and drugs: The major formula is *Angelica, Peony and Safflow Powder* (Gui Shao Hong Hua San). The commonly-used herbal drugs are *Radix Angelicae Sinensis* (Dang Gui), *Radix Paeoniae Rubra* (Chi Shao), *Flos Carthami* (Hong Hua), *Fructus Gardeniae* (Zhi Zi), *Radix Scutellariae* (Huang Qin), *Radix et Rhizoma Rhei* (Da Huang), *Radix Angelicae Dahuricae* (Bai Zhi), *Fructus Forsythiae* (Lian Qiao), *Radix Ledebouriellae* (Fang Feng), *Radix Rehmanniae Cruda* (Sheng Di Huang), *Radix Glycyrrhizae Praeparata* (Zhi Gan Cao), etc.

方药：代表方为归芍红花散，常用药如当归、赤芍、红花、栀子、黄芩、大黄、白芷、连翘、防风、生地、炙甘草等。

Modification according to symptoms: ① For thickened and hard eyelid and patches of follicles, add *Radix Rehmanniae Cruda* (Sheng Di Huang), *Cortex Moutan Radicis* (Mu Dan Pi) and *Semen Persicae* (Tao Ren), to enhance the action to cool blood, dissolve stasis and reduce redness. ②For ex-

加减：①若眼睑厚硬，乳头滤泡成片者，加生地、牡丹皮、桃仁等，以助凉血化瘀退赤之功；②若分泌物多、沙涩羞明者，常加金银花、桑叶、菊花等以清热解毒；③若赤

cessive eye discharge, astringent sensation and photophobia, add *Flos Lonicerae* (Jin Yin Hua), *Folium Mori* (Sang Ye) and *Flos Chrysanthemi* (Ju Hua), to clear heat and relieve toxin. ③ For trachomatous pannus or corneal nebula, add *Concha Haliotidis* (Shi Jue Ming), *Flos Buddlejae* (Mi Meng Hua) and *Eriocaulon Buergerianum* (Gu Jing Cao) accordingly, to enhance the action to clear heat, brighten eyes and remove nebula.

膜下垂、黑睛生星翳者，酌加石决明、密蒙花、谷精草等以增清热明目退翳之功。

3.3 External therapies

(1) Eye drop: Apply the medications sensitive to Chlamydia, such as sulfonamide eye drop, rifampicin eye drop, etc.

(2) Eye ointment: Apply antibiotic eye ointment before sleep.

(3) Treatment for sequela: For dryness of eyeball, apply artificial tears to relieve the symptom. For severe entropion or trichiasis, apply correction of entropion or trichiasis, so as to avoid the damage to the cornea.

3.3 外治法

（1）滴眼药水：可选用对衣原体敏感药物如磺胺类、利福平眼药水滴眼。

（2）涂眼药膏：睡前涂抗生素眼药膏。

（3）后遗症的治疗：眼珠干燥者，可点滴人工泪液缓解症状；睑内翻倒睫严重者，可行睑内翻倒睫矫正术，以避免对角膜损伤。

4 Speculative map

4 思辨导图

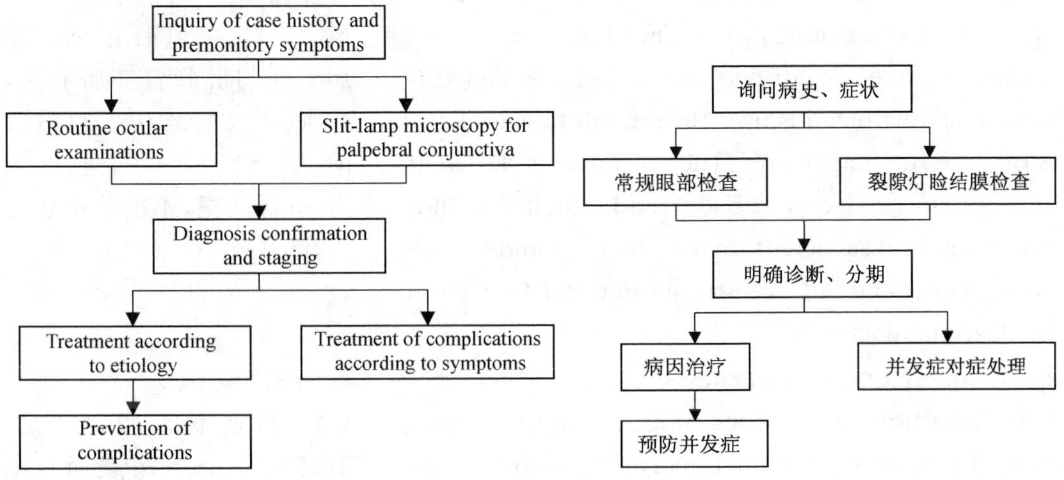

Chapter 2 Canthus Diseases

第 2 章 两眦疾病

Epiphora

溢 泪 症

It is a lacrimal duct disease caused by lacrimal punctum abnormality, stenosis or obstruction of lacrimal duct, or discharging dysfunction of lacrimal duct.

In traditional Chinese medicine, the disease is called "epiphora induced by wind" or "constant cold tear" according to its manifestations of lacrimation from extra duct or overflow of tears. In the ancient classics of traditional Chinese medicine, the symptoms are described as "lacrimation induce by wind", "constant lacrimation", etc. The disease is related mainly to three zang organs of liver, spleen and kidney. The liver blood is insufficient and fails to nourish the lacrimal aperture. The spleen qi is deficient and fails to produce the body fluid which does not transform into sufficient tears. The liver and kidney are deficient and fail to restrain the water flow from the lacrimal duct.

溢泪是指因泪小点位置异常、泪道狭窄或阻塞及泪道排泄功能障碍引起的泪道疾患。

中医依据泪液不寻常道,溢出睑弦而致经常流泪的临床表现归属为"迎风流泪""冷泪症"等范畴。中医古籍中常将其症状描述为"迎风洒泪""目泪不止","目风泪出","冲风泪出"等。本病主要与肝脾肾三脏有关,肝血不足,泪窍不密;脾气亏虚,生化乏源,失于收摄眼泪;肝肾两虚,不能约束皆可为其因。

1 Etiology and pathogenesis

1.1 Insufficiency of liver blood: The liver blood fails to nourish the lacrimal aperture, so the patho-

1 病因病机

1.1 肝血不足: 肝血不足,泪窍不密,风邪外袭而致泪

genic wind attacks to cause lacrimation.

1.2 Deficiency of spleen qi: The spleen fails to produce qi and blood which fail to restrain tears to cause lacrimation.

1.3 Deficiency of liver and kidney: The tear is the fluid of liver, while the liver and kidney share a same source, so the liver and kidney are deficient and fail to restrain tears to cause lacrimation.

2 Diagnostic essentials

2.1 Clinical manifestations

Frequent lacrimation or lacrimation induced by wind, more severe condition in winter and early spring when the cold wind stimulates the eyes.

2.2 Ocular examinations

If the inner canthus is wet, the lacrimal duct is oppressed without sticky fluid flowing out. The lacrimal punctum is not abnormal, or it is narrow, or evaginable, or obstructed. Or facial paralysis can be seen.

2.3 Special examinations

(1) Drop 2% fluorescein sodium solution into the conjunctival sac of the sick eye, then apply a cotton swab to wipe the nasal duct to observe if the cotton swab is stained by the fluorescein sodium. If it is, it indicates that the lacrimal duct is still unblocked; if it is not, it indicates that it is blocked.

(2) Apply the irrigation of lacrimal duct to determine if it is unblocked, semi-blocked or blocked.

3 Therapeutic methods

3.1 Therapeutic principles

For lacrimation with unblocked lacrimal duct or semi-blocked lacrimal, apply medication combined with acupuncture to treat. For lacrimation with

出。

1.2 脾气亏虚：生化乏源，气血不足，不能收摄眼泪而致泪出。

1.3 肝肾亏虚：泪为肝之液，肝肾同源，肝肾两虚，不能约束其液而流泪。

2 诊断要点

2.1 临床表现

患眼时有泪出或迎风泪出，在冬季、初春寒风刺激时更甚。

2.2 眼部检查

内眦部潮湿感；压迫泪囊无黏液溢出。泪小点无异样或偏小或外翻或闭塞，或面瘫。

2.3 特殊检查

（1）将2%荧光素钠溶液滴入患眼结膜囊内，将棉签擦下鼻道，观察棉签是否带荧光素钠之颜色，若有则说明泪道尚通畅；否则为不通。

（2）冲洗泪道判断其是通畅或通而不畅或不通。

3 治疗方法

3.1 治疗原则

流泪，但泪道通畅，或通而不畅者，可药物配合针灸等治疗，若泪道不通者，可行

blocked lacrimal duct, apply surgery to treat. Clinically, it is apply the treatment for the deficiency according to the pattern identification on zang-fu organs or the pattern identification on five wheels.

手术治疗。临证遵循脏腑辨证、五轮辨证原则，多以虚论治。

3.2 Treatment based on syndrome differentiation

3.2 辨证论治

(1) **Blood deficiency accompanied by wind**

(1) **血虚挟风**

Main symptoms: Lacrimation, more severe condition by irritation of wind, astringent sensation and discomfort, absence of redness, swelling and pain at the sick eye, accompanied by dizziness, blurring of vision, lusterless complexion, pale tongue body with thin tongue coating, and thready pulse.

主症：流泪，迎风更甚，隐涩不适，患眼无红赤肿痛；兼头晕目眩，面色少华。舌淡薄，脉细。

Therapeutic methods: Reinforce and nourish the liver blood, and eliminate the pathogenic wind.

治法：补养肝血，祛风散邪。

Herbal formulas and drugs: The major formula is *Tear-Restraining and Liver-Reinforcing Powder* (Zhi Lei Bu Gan San). The commonly-used herbal drugs are *Radix Rehmanniae Praeparata* (Shu Di Huang), *Radix Paeoniae Alba* (Bai Shao), *Radix Angelicae Sinensis* (Dang Gui), *Rhizoma Ligustici Chuanxiong* (Chuan Xiong), *Radix Ledebouriellae* (Fang Feng), *Spica Prunellae* (Xia Ku Cao), Herba Equiseti Hiemalis (Mu Zei), *Fructus Tribuli* (Bai Ji Li), etc.

方药：代表方为止泪补肝散，常用药如熟地黄、白芍、当归、川芎、防风、夏枯草、木贼、白蒺藜等。

Modification according to symptoms: For severe lacrimation induced by irritation of wind, add *Radix Cynanchi Atrati* (Bai Wei), *Flos Chrysanthemi* (Ju Hua) and *Pericarpium Granati* (Shi Liu Pi), to eliminate wind and stop lacrimation.

加减：若流泪迎风更甚者，可加白薇、菊花、石榴皮等以祛风止泪。

(2) **Insufficiency of qi and blood**

(2) **气血不足**

Main symptoms: Constant lacrimation with clear, cold and thin tears, failure to watch for long

主症：无时泪下，泪液清冷稀薄，不耐久视；面色无

time, lusterless complexion, low spirit, lassitude, palpitation, poor memory, pale tongue body with thin tongue coating, and thready-weak pulse.

华,神疲乏力,心悸健忘。舌淡,苔薄,脉细弱。

Therapeutic methods: Benefit qi, nourish blood and restrain tears.

治法:益气养血,收摄止泪。

Herbal formulas and drugs: The major formula is *Eight Jewel Decoction* (Ba Zhen Tang). The commonly-used herbal drugs are adix *Rehmanniae Praeparata* (Shu Di Huang), *Radix Paeoniae Alba* (Bai Shao), *Radix Angelicae Sinensis* (Dang Gui), *Rhizoma Ligustici Chuanxiong* (Chuan Xiong), *Radix Ginseng* (Ren Shen), *Rhizoma Atractylodis Macrocephalae* (Bai Zhu), *Sclerotium Poriae* (Fu Ling), *Radix Glycyrrhizae* (Gan Cao), etc.

方药:代表方为八珍汤,常用药如熟地黄、白芍、当归、川芎、人参、白术、茯苓、甘草等。

Modification according to symptoms: For severe lacrimation induced by irritation of wind, add *Radix Ledebouriellae* (Fang Feng), *Radix Angelicae Dahuricae* (Bai Zhi) and *Flos Chrysanthemi* (Ju Hua), to eliminate wind and stop lacrimation. For severe lacrimation induced by irritation of cold, accompanied by fear of cold and chills in limbs, add *Herba Asari* (Xi Xin), *Ramulus Cinnamomi* (Gui Zhi) and *Radix Morindae Officinalis* (Ba Ji Tian), to warm yang, eliminate cold and restrain tears.

加减:如迎风泪多者,加防风、白芷、菊花以祛风止泪;若遇寒泪多,畏寒肢冷者,酌加细辛、桂枝、巴戟天以温阳散寒摄泪。

(3) **Deficiency of liver and kidney**

(3) **肝肾两虚**

Main symptoms: Frequent lacrimation, occurrence of lacrimation just after wiping tears, accompanied by dizziness, tinnitus, aching and weakness at low back and knees, and thready-weak pulse.

主症:眼泪常流,拭之又生,或泪液清冷稀薄;兼头昏耳鸣,腰膝酸软。脉细弱。

Therapeutic methods: Reinforce and benefit liver and kidney, and restrain tears.

治法:补益肝肾,固摄止泪。

Herbal formulas and drugs: The major formula is *Kidney Yin-Reinforcing Drink* (Zuo Gui Yin). The commonly-used herbal drugs are *Radix Reh-*

方药:代表方为左归饮,常用药如熟地、山药、枸杞子、茯苓、山茱萸、炙甘草等。

manniae Praeparata (Shu Di Huang), *Rhizoma Dioscoreae* (Shan Yao), *Fructus Lycii* (Gou Qi Zi), *Sclerotium Poriae* (Fu Ling), *Fructus Corni* (Shan Zhu Yu), *Radix Glycyrrhizae Praeparata* (Zhi Gan Cao), etc.

Modification according to symptoms: ①For severe lacrimation, add *Fructus Schisandrae* (Wu Wei Zi) and *Radix Ledebouriellae* (Fang Feng), to eliminate wind and restrain tears. ② For lacrimation with clear and cold tears, add *Radix Morindae Officinalis* (Ba Ji Tian), *Herba Cistanchis* (Rou Cong Rong) and *Ootheca Mantidis* (Sang Piao Xiao), to warm and reinforce the kidney yang and enhance the action to restrain and stop tears.

加减:①若流泪较甚者,加五味子、防风以收敛祛风止泪;②若感泪液清冷者,加巴戟天、肉苁蓉、桑螵蛸以加强温补肾阳之利助固摄止泪之功。

3.3 Other therapies

(1) Diagnostic treatment: Apply the irrigation of lacrimal duct to confirm the causative factors.

(2) Surgical: For palpebral margin and lcrimal punctum abnormality, apply the corrective surgery. For lacrimal duct obstruction, try to apply laser therapy or silicon tube encumbrance in lacrimal duct.

(3) Acupuncture: For facial paralysis due to the liver blood insufficiency with re-affection of wind, apply the reinforcing method by puncturing the points of Ganshu (BL 18), Taichong (LR 3), Hegu (LI 4) and Fengchi (GB 20). For deficiency of liver and kidney which fail to restrain tears, apply the reinforcing method with both acupuncture and moxibustion, by puncturing the points of Ganshu (BL 18), Shenshu (BL 23), Yongquan (KI 1) and Taichong (LR 3). For lacrimation with clear and cold tears, apply the moxibustion on Shenque (CV 8) and warming-needle method on Jingming

3.3 其他疗法

(1) 诊断性治疗:冲洗泪道明确病因。

(2) 手术治疗:针对睑缘及泪点位置异常可行矫形手术;如泪道阻塞者,可试行激光治疗或使用泪道硅管留置治疗。

(3) 针灸治疗:针对面瘫肝血不足,复感风邪证,以补法为主,可针肝俞、太冲、合谷、风池;肝肾两虚,约束无权证,以补法为主,针灸并用,可针肝俞、肾俞、涌泉、太冲;若流泪清冷者,可加神阙艾灸及同侧睛明穴温针(将针用火烧热,待温后再针)治疗。

(BL 2) on the sick side.

(4) Patent herbal medicine: For deficiency of liver and kidney which fail to restrain tears, apply *Lycium, Chrysanthemun and Rehmannia Pills* (Qi Ju Di Huang Wan), 6g of bolus or 9g of pills each time, and twice a day.

(4) 中成药治疗：杞菊地黄丸适用于肝肾两虚，约束无权证，口服水蜜丸，每日2次，每次6克（小蜜丸每次9克）。

4 Speculative map

4 思辨导图

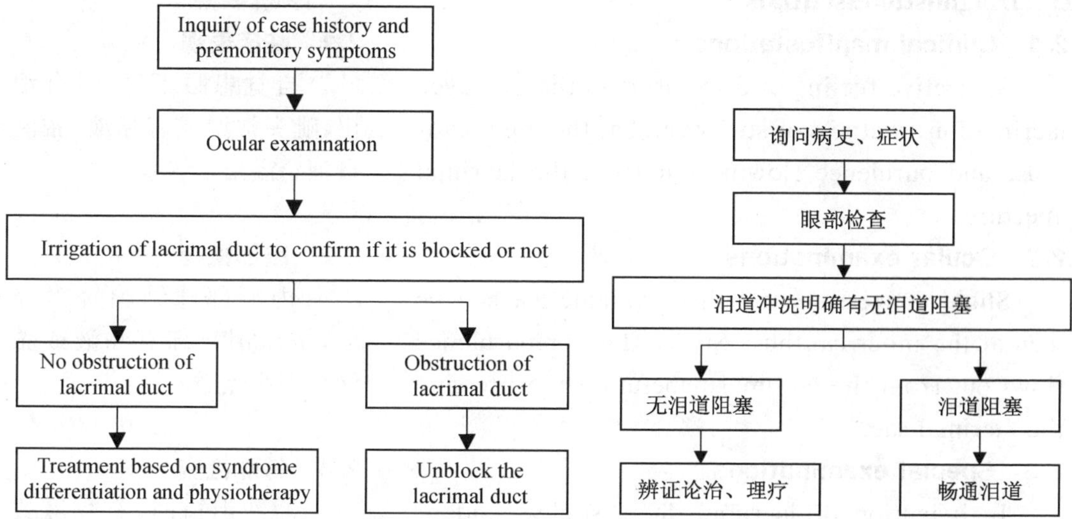

Chronic dacryocystitis

慢性泪囊炎

Chronic dacryocystitis is caused by stenosis or obstruction of the naso-lacrimal duct, to make the tears retain inside the lacrimal sac, leading to bacillary infection. Traumatic injury, rhinitis, nasal septal deviation, turbinate hypertrophy, etc. could be the possible incentive causes. The disease can be seen in newborn.

慢性泪囊炎是因鼻泪管狭窄或阻塞，致使泪液滞留于泪囊内而伴发细菌感染。外伤、鼻炎、鼻中隔弯曲或鼻甲肥大等是本病可能的诱因。亦有新生儿患本病者。

In traditional Chinese medicine, it is called “eye leakage” according to the feature of sticky flu-

中医因其内眦部常有黏液或脓液自泪窍漏出的临床

id or purulence leaking out from the lacrimal aperture at the inner canthus.

特征命名为"漏睛"。

1 Etiology and pathogenesis

The hidden fire in the heart, or the damp-heat in the spleen, goes to the meridians and attack upwards the lacrimal aperture along the meridians, corroding to form the purulence.

1 病因病机

心有伏火,脾蕴湿热,流注经络,上攻泪窍,腐而成脓。

2 Diagnostic essentials

2.1 Clinical manifestations

Subjective feeling of discomfort in the sick eye, lacrimation, wetness or sticky fluid at the inner canthus, and purulence flowing out from the lacrimal aperture.

2 诊断要点

2.1 临床表现

自觉患眼不舒,时有泪出,眦头常湿或有黏液、脓液自泪窍溢出。

2.2 Ocular examinations

Slight congestion of bulbar conjunctiva can be seen at the inner canthus. Sticky fluid or purulence flows out from the lacrimal punctum when pressing the lacrimal sac.

2.2 眼部检查

内眦部球结膜轻微充血,按压泪囊部有黏液或脓液自泪小点溢出。

2.3 Special examinations

In irrigation of lacrimal duct, sticky fluid or purulence flows out from the lacrimal punctum. In irrigation, there is prominence sensation at the lacrimal sac.

2.3 特殊检查

冲洗泪道时,有黏液或脓液自泪点反流,冲洗时泪囊部有隆起感。

3 Therapeutic methods

3.1 Therapeutic principles

The long-term retention of sticky fluid or purulence in the lacrimal sac, due to traumatic injury or surgery of the eye, may cause an inflammatory state, leading to the risk of endophthalmitis. Therefore, it is advisable to apply the preventive treatment to prevent the progression. In traditional Chinese medicine, the treatment is to focus on the accumulated heat in heart and spleen.

3 治疗方法

3.1 治疗原则

泪囊部长期滞留黏脓造成局部带菌状态,如眼部外伤或手术时,易致感染而酿成眼内炎风险,因此预先治疗防止生变。中医临证多以心脾积热论治。

3.2 Treatment based on syndrome differentiation

Main symptoms: Slight redness and wetness at the medial canthus, purulent fluid dipping, reoccurring fluid after wiping away, thick and excessive purulence, purulent fluid flowing out from lacrimal aperture by pressing the inferior part of Jingming (BL 1), yellow-red urine, red tongue body with yellow-sticky tongue coating, and soft-rapid pulse.

Therapeutic methods: Purify heart and dissolve damp.

Herbal formulas and drugs: The major formula is *Bamboo Leaf Heart-Reducing Decoction* (Zhu Ye Xie Jing Tang). The commonly-used herbal drugs are *Rhizoma Coptidis* (Huang Lian), *Fructus Gardeniae* (Zhi Zi), *Radix Scutellariae* (Huang Qin), *Radix et Rhizoma Rhei* (Da Huang), *Semen Cassiae* (Jue Ming Zi), *Rhizoma seu Radix Notopterygii* (Qiang Huo), *Radix Bupleuri* (Chai Hu), *Rhizoma Cimicifugae* (Sheng Ma), *Radix Paeoniae Rubra* (Chi Shao), *Rhizoma Alismatis* (Ze Xie), *Sclerotium Poriae* (Fu Ling), *Semen Plantaginis* (Che Qian Zi), *Herba Lophatheri* (Dan Zhu Ye), *Radix Glycyrrhizae Praeparata* (Zhi Gan Cao), etc.

Modification according to symptoms: For excessive, yellow and thick purulent fluid, subtract *Rhizoma seu Radix Notopterygii* (Qiang Huo) and add *Radix Trichosanthis* (Tian Hua Fen), *Radix Rhapontici seu Echinopsis* (Lou Lu), *Resina Olibani* (Ru Xiang) and *Myrrha* (Mo Yao), to enhance the action to clear heat, drain pus and dissolve stasis.

3.3 External therapies

(1) Eye drop: Before application of eye drop, press the lacrimal sac to make the sticky fluid or pu-

3.2 辨证论治

主症：内眦头微红潮湿，可见脓液浸渍，拭之又生，脓多且稠；按压睛明穴下方时，有脓液从泪窍沁出；小便黄赤。舌红，苔黄腻，脉濡数。

治法：清心利湿。

方药：代表方为竹叶泻经汤，常用药如黄连、栀子、黄芩、大黄、决明子、羌活、柴胡、升麻、赤芍、泽泻、茯苓、车前子、淡竹叶、炙甘草等。

加减：脓液多且黄稠者，可去羌活，加天花粉、漏芦、乳香、没药，以加强清热排脓、祛瘀消滞的作用。

3.3 外治法

（1）滴眼药水：滴眼前按鼻根泪囊区使黏液或脓液自

rulent fluid flow out from the lacrimal punctum, then apply antibiotic eye drop, such as 0. 25% Chloramphenicol Eye Drop, 0. 4% Ciprofloxacin Eye Drop, etc. , 4—6 times a day.

泪点溢出，再用抗生素眼药水滴眼，如 0.25% 氯霉素眼药水、0.4% 环丙沙星眼药水等，每日 4～6 次。

(2) Irrigation of lacrimal duct: Apply 1% Berberine Solution to irrigate and wash the lacrimal duct, once a day or once every second day. Or apply antibiotic solution for irrigation.

(2) 泪道冲洗：可用 1% 黄连水冲洗泪道，每日或隔日 1 次，也可用抗生素药液冲洗。

(3) Probing method of lacrimal duct: For an infant patient, first apply massage at the inferior part of Pt Jingming (BL 1). If it does not work, apply the probing method of lacrimal duct, and then apply the antibiotic eye drop. In the probing method, it is to pay attention to the protection, so as to prevent the lacrimal punctum tearing.

(3) 泪道探通术：若为婴儿患者，一般先行睛明穴下方皮肤按摩，日久无效者，行泪道探通术，术后用抗生素眼药水滴眼。探通时应注意保护，以防泪小点撕裂。

(4) Surgery: If the condition is not cured after conservative treatment, apply dacryocystorhinostomy, or dacryocystectomy, or laser angioplasty of lacrimal duct, according to the condition.

(4) 手术治疗：经保守治疗不愈者，应根据病情选择泪囊鼻腔吻合术，或泪囊摘除术，或泪道激光成形术等。

4 Speculative map

4 思辨导图

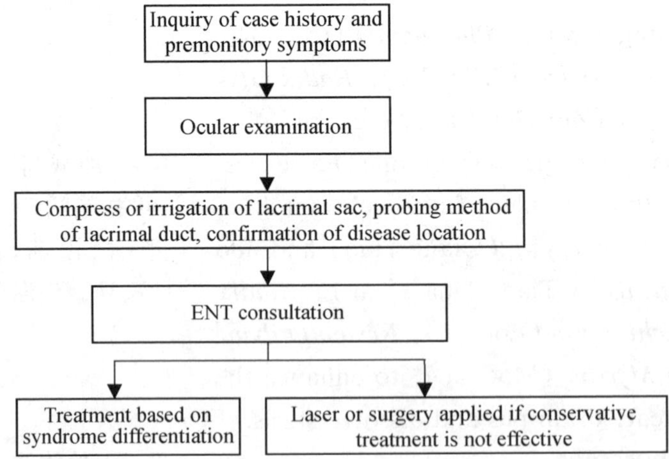

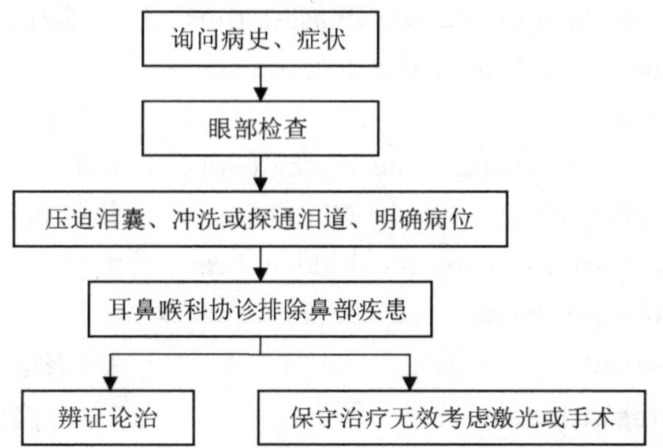

Acute dacryocystitis

急性泪囊炎

Acute dacryocystitis is an acute infection on the basis of chronic dacryocystitis. The common pathogenic bacterium is streptococcus. The major clinical manifestations are sudden onset of redness, swelling, hotness and pain at the lacrimal sac region, and then ulceration with pus.

急性泪囊炎属于慢性泪囊炎基础上的急性感染。最常见的致病菌为链球菌，泪囊区局部的突发红、肿、热、痛，继而溃破出脓是其主要的临床表现。

In traditional Chinese medicine, it is called "eye leakage sore". It is believed that the etiology and pathogenesis are as that qi and blood are insufficient, so the Zheng (Anti-Pathogenic) Qi cannot prevail over the Xie (Pathogenic) Qi. The Xie (Pathogenic) Qi stays inside and the hidden pathogenic heat goes upwards to disturb the lacrimal aperture.

中医学名之为"漏睛疮"；并认为，气血不足，正不胜邪，邪气留恋，蕴伏之热邪上扰泪窍是为其病机。

1 Etiology and pathogenesis

1 病因病机

1.1 Accumulated heat in Heart Meridian. Due to chronic dacryocystitis, the heat-toxin is accumulated inside and the exogenous wind attacks the body, leading to accumulated wind-heat.

1.1 心经蕴热，或素有漏睛，热毒内蕴，复感风邪，风热搏结所致。

1.2 Excessive heat-toxin in heart and spleen. It causes stagnation of qi and blood, and disharmony

1.2 心脾热毒壅盛，致气血凝滞，营卫不和，结聚成疮，

of Ying (Nutrient) and Wei (Defense) Phases, thus forming sores, purulence and ulcer due to excessive internal heat corroding.

热盛内腐成脓而溃。

1.3 Insufficiency of qi and blood. The Zheng (Anti-Pathogenic) Qi cannot prevail over the Xie (Pathogenic) Qi, which retains to cause the hidden heat flaming upwards to disturb the lacrimal aperture.

1.3 气血不足，正不胜邪，邪气留恋，蕴伏之热邪上扰泪窍。

2 Diagnostic essentials

2 诊断要点

2.1 Clinical manifestations

2.1 临床表现

Sudden onset of redness, swelling, burning sensation and pain at the inner canthus, frequent lacrimation with warm tears, accompanied by aversion to cold, fever, headache, etc. in severe condition.

内眦处突发皮肤红肿、灼热、疼痛，热泪频流。重者可伴恶寒、发热、头痛等症。

2.2 Ocular examinations

2.2 眼部检查

Redness, swelling and burning-hotness of skin of inner canthus closing to the nose root, and growing swollen nodule and pain worsened by pressure. Redness and swelling at the face and nose bridge on the affected side in severe condition, severe redness and swelling of eyelids which fail to open, and congestion and edema of bulbar conjunctiva. Fluctuation palpated in the center of nodule, purulence and ulcer. Unhealed sores for long time after redness and swelling are diminishing, forming fistula. Nodules palpated at the area anterior to the ear and the mandibular area in some patients with tenderness.

内眦近鼻根处皮肤红肿灼热，肿核隆起渐大，疼痛拒按；重者患侧鼻梁及颜面均红肿，甚至眼睑红肿难以睁开，球结膜充血水肿；或肿核中央有波动感，形成脓肿甚而溃破；或见红肿消退，疮口经久未敛，形成瘘管。部分患者耳前及颌下可触及肿核，并有压痛。

2.3 Special examinations

2.3 特殊检查

Blood routine examination shows the increase of total white blood cells and neutrophile granulocyte rate.

血常规检查显示白细胞总数及中性粒细胞比例增高。

3 Therapeutic methods

3 治疗方法

3.1 Therapeutic principles

3.1 治疗原则

The dispersing method is applied for the un-

未成脓时以消散为主，

formed purulence, while the incision and drainage method is applied for the formed purulence. In traditional Chinese medicine, the treatment is to focus on the accumulated pathogenic heat in Heart and Spleen Meridians.

已成脓者切开排脓。中医临症多以心脾两经积邪郁热论治。

3.2 Treatment based on syndrome differentiation

3.2 辨证论治

(1) **Upward attack of wind-heat**

(1) **风热上攻**

Main symptoms: Frequent lacrimation with warm tears, redness, swelling and pain at the inner canthus, prominence with palpated nodule, more severe pain by pressure, headache, aversion to cold, fever, red tongue body with thin-yellow tongue coating, and superficial-rapid pulse.

主症:患眼热泪频流,内眦部红肿疼痛,其下方隆起,可扪及肿核,疼痛拒按;头痛,或见恶寒发热。舌红苔薄黄,脉浮数。

Therapeutic methods: Eliminate wind, clear heat, subside swell and dissolve stasis.

治法:疏风清热,消肿散结。

Herbal formulas and drugs: The major formula is *Fairy Formula Life-Saving Drink* (Xian Fang Huo Ming Yin). The commonly-used herbal drugs are *Flos Lonicerae* (Jin Yin Hua), *Radix Trichosanthis* (Tian Hua Fen), *Radix Angelicae Sinensis* (Dang Gui), *Radix Paeoniae Rubra* (Chi Shao), *Resina Olibani* (Ru Xiang), *Myrrha* (Mo Yao), *Squama Manitis* (Chuan Shan Jia), *Spina Gleditsiae* (Zao Jiao Ci), *Radix Angelicae Dahuricae* (Bai Zhi), *Bulbus Fritillariae Thumbergii* (Zhe Bei Mu), etc.

方药:代表方为仙方活命饮,常用药如金银花、天花粉、当归、赤芍、乳香、没药、穿山甲、皂角刺、白芷、浙贝母等。

Modification according to symptoms: Increase the dosage of *Radix Angelicae Dahuricae* (Bai Zhi), *Bulbus Fritillariae Thumbergii* (Zhe Bei Mu) and *Radix Trichosanthis* (Tian Hua Fen), to enhance the action to subside swell and dissolve stasis.

加减:常于方中加重白芷、浙贝母、天花粉的量,以加强消肿散结之功。

(2) **Flaming and excess of heat-toxin**

(2) **热毒炽盛**

Main symptoms: Redness, swelling and hotness at the sick area, hard nodule which is painful by

主症:患处红肿焮热,核硬拒按,疼痛难忍,热泪频

pressure, intolerable pain, frequent lacrimation with warm tears, redness and swells moving to face and eyelids, nodule and tenderness at the area anterior to ear or the mandibular area, accompanied by headache, feverish sensation in body, restlessness, thirst, constipation, red urine and astringent urination, red tongue body with yellow-dry tongue coating, and surging-rapid pulse.

流,甚而红肿漫及颜面胞睑;耳前或颌下有肿核及压痛,可兼头痛身热,心烦口渴,大便燥结,小便赤涩。舌质红,苔黄燥,脉洪数。

Therapeutic methods: Clear heat, relieve toxin, subside swell and dissolve stasis.

治法:清热解毒,消瘀散结。

Herbal formulas and drugs: The major formula is *Coptis Detoxifying Decoction* (Huang Lian Jie Du Tang) plus *Five Ingredients Detoxifying Drink* (Wu Wei Xiao Du Yin). The commonly-used herbal drugs are *Rhizoma Coptidis* (Huang Lian), *Radix Scutellariae* (Huang Qin), *Cortex Phellodendri* (Huang Bo), *Fructus Gardeniae* (Zhi Zi), *Flos Lonicerae* (Jin Yin Hua), *Flos Chrysanthemi* (Ju Hua), *Herba Taraxaci* (Pu Gong Ying), *Herba Violae* (Zi Hua Di Ding), *Radix Semiaquilegiae* (Zi Bei Tian Kui), etc.

方药:代表方为黄连解毒汤合五味消毒饮,常用药如黄连、黄芩、黄柏、栀子、金银花、菊花、蒲公英、紫花地丁、紫背天葵等。

Modification according to symptoms: ① For constipation, add *Radix et Rhizoma Rhei* (Da Huang) to dredge fu organs and reduce heat. ②For severe redness, swelling, hotness and pain at the sick area, add *Radix Curcumae* (Yu Jin), *Resina Olibani* (Ru Xiang) and *Myrrha* (Mo Yao), to activate blood, dissolve stasis, subside swell and stop pain. ③ For nearly-formed purulence, add *Spina Gleditsiae* (Zao Jiao Ci), *Squama Manitis* (Chuan Shan Jia) and *Radix Angelicae Dahuricae* (Bai Zhi), to promote purulence and ulceration.

加减:①若大便燥结者,可加大黄以通腑泻热;②患处红肿热痛甚者,加郁金、乳香、没药以助活血散瘀,消肿止痛;③欲成脓而未溃者,可加皂角刺、穿山甲、白芷以促使脓成溃破。

(3) **Zheng (Anti-Pathogenic) Qi deficiency with Xie (Pathogenic) Qi retention**

(3) **正虚邪留**

Main symptoms: Slight redness, swelling and tenderness at the sick area, repeated attacks without ulceration, or unhealed sores after ulceration, thin and scanty purulent fluid, accompanied by aversion to cold, chills in limbs, pale complexion, low spirit, poor appetite, pale tongue body with thin tongue coating, and thready-weak pulse.

Therapeutic methods: Reinforce qi, nourish blood, support the interior and drain the toxic pus.

Herbal formulas and drugs: The major formula is *Interior-Supporting and Detoxifying Powder* (Tuo Li Xiao Du San). The commonly-used herbal drugs are *Radix Ginseng* (Ren Shen), *Radix Astragali* (Huang Qi), *Rhizoma Atractylodis Macrocephalae* (Bai Zhu), *Sclerotium Poriae* (Fu Ling), *Radix Angelicae Sinensis* (Dang Gui), *Radix Paeoniae Alba* (Bai Shao), *Rhizoma Ligustici Chuanxiong* (Chuan Xiong), *Flos Lonicerae* (Jin Yin Hua), *Fructus Forsythiae* (Lian Qiao), *Radix Angelicae Dahuricae* (Bai Zhi), *Pericarpium Citri Tangerinae* (Chen Pi), etc.

Modification according to symptoms: ① For redness, pain and nodule, add *Flos Chrysanthemi Indici* (Ye Ju Hua), *Herba Taraxaci* (Pu Gong Ying) and *Radix Curcumae* (Yu Jin), to clear heat, subside swell, activate blood and stop pain. ② For unhealed sores after ulceration and pale-white complexion, add *Radix Scrophulariae* (Xuan Shen), *Radix Trichosanthis* (Tian Hua Fen) and *Radix Ampelopsis* (Bai Lian), to nourish yin, clear heat, engender muscles and drain purulence.

3.3 Other therapies

3.3.1 External therapies

(1) Wet-warm compress: For the disease of

主症：患处微红微肿，稍有压痛，时有反复，但不溃破；或溃后漏口难敛，脓液稀少不绝；可伴畏寒肢冷，面色苍白，神疲食少。舌淡苔薄，脉细弱。

治法：补气养血，托里排毒。

方药：代表方为托里消毒散，常用药如人参、黄芪、白术、茯苓、当归、白芍、川芎、金银花、连翘、白芷、陈皮等。

加减：①红痛有肿核，可加野菊花、蒲公英、郁金以助清热消肿，活血止痛；②溃后漏口不敛已久，面色苍白者，宜加玄参、天花粉、白蔹以养阴清热，生肌排脓。

3.3 其他疗法

3.3.1 外治

(1) 湿热敷：早期局部宜

early stage, apply the wet-warm compress, 2 to 3 times a day, to promote rapid purulence.

用湿热敷，每日 2～3 次，促使快速成脓。

(2) Eye drop: Apply antibiotic eye drop, several times a day.

（2）滴眼药水：可用抗生素眼药水滴眼，每日数次。

(3) Medicated compress: For unformed purulence, apply *Purple Gold Ingot* (Zi Jin Ding) with water for external use, or apply *Perfect Golden-Yellow Powder* (Ru Yi Jin Huang San) for external compress, or smash fresh *Folium Hibisci* (Fu Rong Ye), *Flos Chrysanthemi Indici* (Ye Ju Hua), *Herba Portulacae* (Ma Chi Xian) and *Herba Violae* (Zi Hua Di Ding) in equal amount, and apply the herbal paste to clear heat, relieve toxin and dissolve stasis. It should be careful in application of the drugs for external use to avoid them entering the eyes.

（3）药物敷：未成脓者，可用紫金锭磨水外涂，或以如意金黄散调和外敷，或用新鲜芙蓉叶、野菊花、马齿苋、紫花地丁等量，洗净捣烂外敷，以清热解毒，促其消散。各外用药注意勿入眼内。

(4) For formed purulence, it is advisable to incise and drain the pus and to place a drain at the incision and replace it every day, till the complete drainage of pus and heal of wound.

（4）已成脓者，应及时切开排脓，并放置引流条，每日换药，待脓尽伤口愈合。

(5) If the fistula is formed, it is advisable to apply dacryocystectomy and fistulectomy.

（5）若已成漏者，可行泪囊摘除术并切除瘘管。

3.3.2 Internal therapies

3.3.2 内治

(1) According to the condition, promptly select the effective antibiotics in oral administration, or intravenous injection, or intramuscular injection, so as to prevent the condition from worsening.

（1）根据病情及时选择口服或静脉给药或肌肉注射有效抗生素。以免病情加重。

(2) Patent herbal medicines: ①For upward-attack of wind-heat, apply *Coptis Upper-Purifying Bolus* (Huang Lian Shang Qing Wan) for oral administration, 1 bolus each time, and 2 to 3 times a day. ②For flaming and excess of heat-toxin, apply *Bezoare Toxin-Relieving Bolus* (Niu Huang Jie Du Wan) for oral administration, 1 bolus each time, and 3 times a day. ③For Zheng (Anti-Pathogenic) Qi de-

（2）中成药治疗：①黄连上清丸，适用于风热上攻证，口服，每次 1 丸，每日 2～3 次；②牛黄解毒丸，适用于热毒炽盛证，口服，每次 1 丸，每日 3 次；③十全大补丸或人参养荣丸，适用于正虚邪留证，口服水蜜丸，每次 6

ficiency with Xie (Pathogenic) Qi retention, apply *Ten Perfections Reinforcing Bolus* (Shi Quan Da Bu Wan) or *Ginseng Nourishing-Flourihing Bolus* (Ren Shen Yang Rong Wan) for oral administration, 6g each time, and 2 to 3 times a day.

克,每日 2~3 次。

4 Speculative map

4 思辨导图

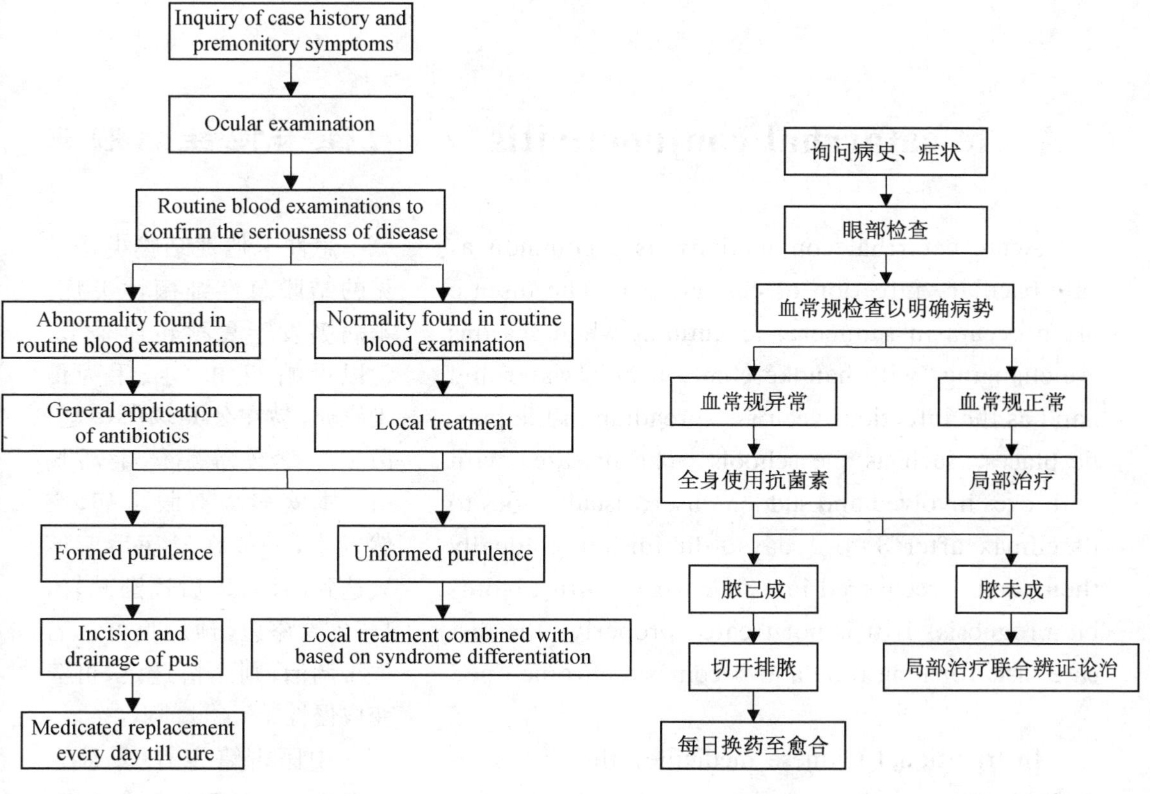

Chapter 3 Sclera-Conjunctiva Diseases

第3章 白睛疾病

Acute catarrhal conjunctivitis

急性卡他性结膜炎

Acute catarrhal conjunctivitis is a common acute bacillary infection of conjunctiva. The disease often occurs in summer and autumn when seasons are changing, with handkerchief, towel, water and hand as the infectious vectors, spreading in the public places, such as the schools. The disease, with both eyes involved and sudden onset, usually goes to its climax after 3 to 4 days, diminishes gradually then, and is recovered in 1 to 2 weeks with favorable prognosis. If it is not treated properly, the disease lasts for long time and becomes a chronic one.

In traditional Chinese medicine, the disease is called "storm wind" or "storm wind-heat attacking circumocular area". In *Standards of Diagnosis and Treatment* (Zheng Zhi Zhun Sheng), it is called "storm wind-heat", which has been used to nowadays. The major clinical manifestations are redness of eye white, excessive, thick and sticky eye discharge, and alternate itching and pain. Its major cause is invasion of pathogenic wind-heat. If there is the accumulated heat in the Lung Meridian as

急性卡他性结膜炎是常见的结膜急性细菌性炎症。本病多发于夏秋转换季节，常以手帕、毛巾、水、手为传染媒介，易在公共场所蔓延，散发于学校等集体生活场所。本病多为双眼患病，突然发生，一般在发病后三四天达到高潮，以后逐渐减轻，1～2周痊愈，预后良好。若失于调治，则病情迁延，可演变成慢性。

中医古籍先有"暴风"、后有"暴风客热外障"之称，自《证治准绳》名之"暴风客热"后，沿用至今。临床以白睛红赤、眵多黏稠、痒痛交作为主要特征。感风热之邪为其主要病因；若素有肺经蕴热，则病更甚。

well, the conditional is more serious.

1 Etiology and pathogenesis

The pathogenic wind-heat invades the body suddenly, retains in the Lung Meridian and attack upwards the eye white. If there is the accumulated heat in the Lung Meridian, the condition is more serious.

1 病因病机

骤感风热之邪，风热相搏，客留肺经，上犯白睛而发；若素有肺经蕴热，则病变更甚。

2 Diagnostic essentials

2.1 Clinical manifestations

Itching, discomfort and burning sensation in the sick eye, excessive tears, purulent discharge, and blurring of vision.

2.2 Ocular examinations

In mild condition, conjunctival congestion can be seen at palpebral conjunctiva and formix. In severe condition, congestion can be seen at both palbebral conjunctiva and bulbar conjunctiva, swelling and distension at eyelids, and bulbar conjunctiva edema in some cases, and large amount and yellow-white discharge in conjunctival sac.

2 诊断要点

2.1 临床表现

患眼痒涩不适，异物感，灼热感、泪多，伴脓性分泌物，视物模糊感。

2.2 眼部检查

轻者仅见睑结膜及穹隆部结膜充血，严重者睑、球结膜均充血，部分有眼睑肿胀、球结膜水肿，结膜囊内大量黄白色分泌物。

3 Therapeutic methods

3.1 Therapeutic principles

The external treatment is the major one, by applying antibiotic eye drop or eye drop composed of heat-clearing and toxin-relieving herbal drugs. In traditional Chinese medicine, due to qi wheel pertaining to lung, it is advisable to remove the wind-heat from the Lung Meridian. Clinically, it is necessary to treat the condition according to the seriousness of wind and heat.

3.2 Treatment based on syndrome differentiation

(1) **More severe wind than heat**

3 治疗方法

3.1 治疗原则

外治为主，应滴用抗生素眼药水或清热解毒眼药水。中医因气轮属肺，以驱肺经风热为要，临证辨风热孰轻孰重而治之。

3.2 辨证论治

(1) **风重于热**

Main symptoms: Itching and sharp-stabbing pain, photophobia, lacrimation, excessive, sticky and thick eye discharge, redness at eye white, slight swelling of eyelids, accompanied by headache, nasal obstruction, aversion to cold, red tongue body with thin-white or slightly yellow tongue coating, and superficial-rapid pulse.

主症：痒涩刺痛，羞明流泪，眵多黏稠，白睛红赤，胞睑微肿；可兼见头痛，鼻塞，恶风。舌质红，苔薄白或微黄，脉浮数。

Therapeutic methods: Eliminate wind and clear heat.

治法：疏风清热。

Herbal formulas and drugs: The major formula is *Lonicera and Forsythia Powder* (Yin Qiao San). The commonly-used herbal drugs are *Flos Lonicerae* (Jin Yin Hua), *Fructus Forsythiae* (Lian Qiao), *Radix Platycodi* (Jie Geng), *Fructus Arctii* (Niu Bang Zi), *Herba Schizonepetae* (Jing Jie), *Rhizoma Phragmitis* (Lu Gen), *Semen Armeniacae Amarum* (Ku Xing Ren), etc.

方药：代表方为银翘散，常用药如金银花、连翘、桔梗、牛蒡子、荆芥、芦根、杏仁等。

Modification according to symptoms: For obvious redness at eye white, add *Flos Chrysanthemi Indici* (Ye Ju Hua), *Herba Taraxaci* (Pu Gong Ying), *Radix Arnebiae seu Lithospermi* (Zi Cao) and *Cortex Moutan Radicis* (Mu Dan Pi), to clear heat, relieve toxin, cool blood and reduce redness.

加减：若白睛红赤明显，可加野菊花、蒲公英、紫草、牡丹皮以清热解毒，凉血退赤。

(2) **More severe heat than wind**

(2) **热重于风**

Main symptoms: More severe pain of eye, aversion to heat, photophobia, excessive, yellow and thick eye discharge, warm and watery tears, redness and swelling of eyelids, redness and edema of eye white, accompanied by thirst, yellow urine, constipation, red tongue body with yellow tongue coating, and rapid pulse.

主症：目痛较甚，怕热畏光，眵多黄稠。热泪如汤，胞睑红肿，白睛红赤浮肿；可兼见口渴，尿黄，便秘。舌红，苔黄，脉数。

Therapeutic methods: Clear heat and eliminate wind.

治法：清热疏风。

Herbal formulas and drugs: The major formula

方药：代表方为泻肺饮，

is *Lung-Reducing Drink* (Xie Fei Yin). The commonly-used herbal drugs are *Gypsum Fibrosum* (Shi Gao), *Radix Scutellariae* (Huang Qin), *Cortex Mori Radicis* (Sang Bai Pi), *Fructus Gardeniae* (Zhi Zi), *Rhizoma seu Radix Notopterygii* (Qiang Huo), *Herba Schizonepetae* (Jing Jie), *Radix Ledebouriellae* (Fang Feng), *Radix Angelicae Dahuricae* (Bai Zhi), *Fructus Forsythiae* (Lian Qiao), *Fructus Aurantii* (Zhi Ke), *Radix Glycyrrhizae Praeparata* (Zhi Gan Cao), etc.

常用药如石膏、黄芩、桑白皮、栀子、羌活、荆芥、防风、白芷、连翘、枳壳、炙甘草等。

Modification according to symptoms: Apply larger dosage of *Cortex Mori Radicis* (Sang Bai Pi) and add *Radix Platycodi* (Jie Geng) and *Semen Descurainiae* (Ting Li Zi) to reduce lung, promote water flow and subside swell. Add *Radix Rehmanniae Cruda* (Sheng Di Huang) and *Cortex Moutan Radicis* (Mu Dan Pi), to clear heat, relieve toxin, cool blood and remove redness. For constipation, add *Radix et Rhizoma Rhei* (Da Huang) to dredge fu organs and reduce heat.

加减：重用桑白皮，酌加桔梗、葶苈子以泻肺利水消肿；可加生地、牡丹皮以清热解毒、凉血退赤；便秘者，可加生大黄以通腑泻热。

(3) **Same seriousness of wind and heat**

(3) **风热并重**

Main symptoms: Alternate hotness, pain and itching at the sick eye, aversion to heat, photophobia, warm tears, eye discharge, redness and edema of eye white, accompanied by headache, nasal obstruction, aversion to cold, fever, thirst with desire to drink water, constipation, red urine, red tongue body with yellow tongue coating, and rapid pulse.

主症：患眼掀热疼痛，刺痒交作，怕热畏光，泪热眵结，白睛赤肿；兼见头痛鼻塞，恶寒发热，口渴思饮，便秘溲赤。舌红，苔黄，脉数。

Therapeutic methods: Eliminate wind, clear heat, and relieve both the exterior and interior symptoms.

治法：疏风清热，表里双解。

Herbal formulas and drugs: The major formula is *Ledebouriella Wondrous Panacea Powde* (Fang Feng Tong Sheng San). The commonly-used herbal

方药：代表方为防风通圣散，常用药如防风、荆芥、薄荷、大黄、芒硝、滑石、栀

drugs are *Radix Ledebouriellae* (Fang Feng), *Herba Schizonepetae* (Jing Jie), *Herba Menthae* (Bo He), *Radix et Rhizoma Rhei* (Da Huang), *Natrii Sulfas* (Mang Xiao), *Talcum* (Hua Shi), *Fructus Gardeniae* (Zhi Zi), *Gypsum Fibrosum* (Shi Gao), *Radix Platycodi* (Jie Geng), *Fructus Forsythiae* (Lian Qiao), *Radix Scutellariae* (Huang Qin), *Rhizoma Ligustici Chuanxiong* (Chuan Xiong), *Radix Angelicae Sinensis* (Dang Gui), *Radix Paeoniae Rubra* (Chi Shao), *Rhizoma Atractylodis Macrocephalae* (Bai Zhu), *Radix Glycyrrhizae Praeparata* (Zhi Gan Cao), etc.

子、石膏、桔梗、连翘、黄芩、川芎、当归、赤芍、白术、炙甘草等。

Modification according to symptoms: For excessive heat-toxin, subtract the pungent and warm drugs of *Herba Ephedrae* (Ma Huang), *Rhizoma Ligustici Chuanxiong* (Chuan Xiong) and *Radix Angelicae Sinensis* (Dang Gui), and add *Herba Taraxaci* (Pu Gong Ying), *Flos Lonicerae* (Jin Yin Hua) and *Flos Chrysanthemi Indici* (Ye Ju Hua), to clear heat and relieve toxin. For severe itching, add *Fructus Viticis* (Man Jing Zi) and *Periostracum Cicadae* (Chan Tui), to eliminate wind and stop itching.

加减：若热毒偏盛者，去麻黄、川芎、当归辛温之品，宜加蒲公英、金银花、野菊花以清热解毒；若刺痒较重者，加蔓荆子、蝉蜕以祛风止痒。

3.3 Local therapy

(1) Antibiotic eye drugs: 0.3% Tobramycin Eye Drop or 0.3% Levofloxacin Eye Drop, and Erythromycin Eye Ointment applied at night.

(2) Eye drop made of heat-clearing and toxin-relieving drug: 0.5% Bear Gall Eye Drop, 6 times a day, or twice every hour for serious condition.

(3) Fumigation and wash by herbal decoction: According to the patterns, select the heat-clearing and toxin-relieving drugs, such as 30g *Herba Taraxaci* (Pu Gong Ying), 30g *Flos Chrysanthemi Indici* (Ye Ju Hua), 10g

3.3 局部治法

（1）抗生素眼药：0.3%妥布霉素、0.3%左氧氟沙星眼药水，晚上涂红霉素眼膏等。

（2）清热解毒眼药：0.5%熊胆眼药水，每日6次，症状严重者可1小时2次。

（3）煎药熏洗：可根据证型辨证处方或选用蒲公英30克，野菊花30克，黄连10克等清热解毒之品，煎水熏洗

Rhizoma Coptidis (Huang Lian), etc., and decoct them for fumigating and washing the sick eye, 2—3 times a day.

患眼，每日2～3次。

3.4 Other therapies

(1) *Coptis Upper-Purifying Bolus* (Huang Lian Shang Qing Wan), 6g each time and twice a day.

(2) *Eye-Brightening and Upper-Purifying Bolus* (Ming Mu Shang Qing Wan), 6g each time and twice a day.

(3) *Primary Purification Capsules* (Yi Qing Jiao Nang), 2 capsules each time and 3 times a day.

3.4 其他疗法

(1) 黄连上清丸，每服6克，每日2次。

(2) 明目上清丸，每服6克，每日2次。

(3) 一清胶囊，每服2粒，每日3次。

4 Speculative map

4 思辨导图

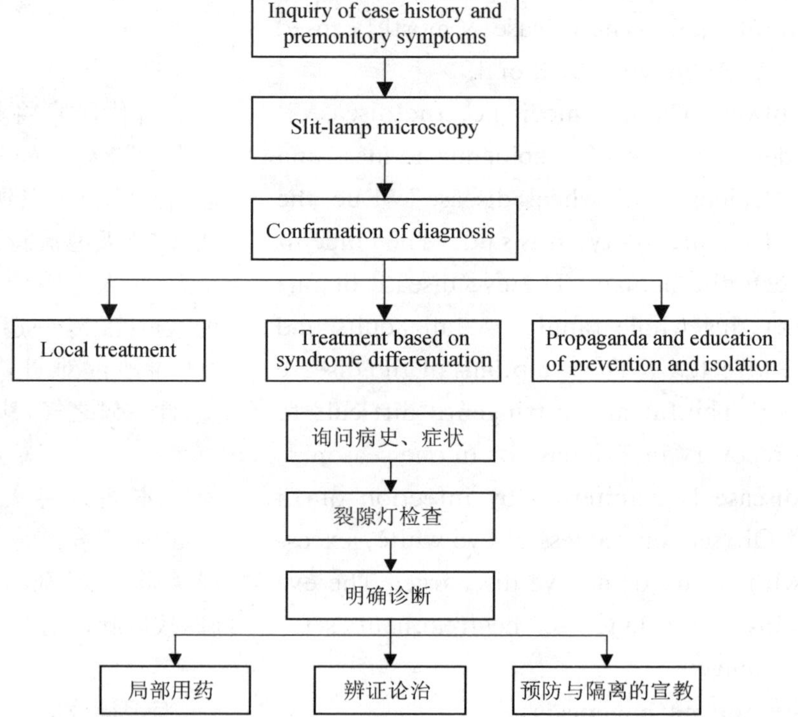

Epidemic viral keratoconjunctivitis

流行性病毒性角结膜炎

Epidemic viral keratoconjunctivitis is a kind of seasonal and infectious disease with quick onset and strong toxicity. It often occurs in spring and autumn, with an incubation period of 2 to 14 days. The both eyes are affected simultaneously, or one eye is affected after another. Usually it is cured in 1 to 2 weeks. In some cases, the shallow layer substrate of cornea is damaged in the late stage, thus the disease may last for longer time, several months or even several years. The disease is mostly caused by infection of Adenovirus 3, 8 or 19.

流行性角结膜炎是一种发病急、毒力强的季节性传染病。多发于春秋两季，潜伏期 2～14 日，双眼同时或先后发病，一般约 1～2 周痊愈。部分后期出现角膜浅基质层损害，则持续时间较长，可达数月或数年之久。常见为腺病毒 3，8，19 型感染。

In traditional Chinese medicine, the disease is called "epidemic red eyes", "epidemic redness and heat" and "epidemic qi wheel disease". Due the knowledge of its infectivity, it is said: "The epidemic toxin infects the human. The eye disease of one person infects his whole family, so all adults and children are affected." The symptoms of the disease are "swelling, painful and astringent, difficult to open eyes, recovery in five days or in one season".

古代医家将其称为"天行赤目""天行赤热""天行气运"；并已经认识到了其传染性，谓："天地流行毒气，能传于人，一人害眼传于一家，不论大小皆传一遍。"其症为"肿痛沙涩难开，或五日而愈，此一候之气，其病安矣"。

The disease is manifested by infection of Li (Epidemic) Qi, sudden redness of eye white, excessive tears with scanty or no eye discharge. The eye white pertains to the lung, so the treatment is focused on the lung.

本病以感天行疫疠之气，白睛突发红赤，泪多眵少或无眵为特征。因白睛属肺，故以肺调治。

1 Etiology and pathogenesis

1 病因病机

The disease is mostly caused by the invasion of Li (Epidemic) Qi which attacks upwards the eye white, or by the accumulated heat in lung and stom-

本病多因疫疠之气上犯白睛；或因肺胃积热，相召疫疠之气，内外合邪，热毒炽

ach, with combination of Li (Epidemic) Qi, forming the excessive heat-toxin which attacks upwards the eyes, or by infection of eyes due to excessive eye discharge.

盛，上攻于目而成。或因患者的眵泪相染所致。

2 Diagnostic essentials

2 诊断要点

2.1 Case history

2.1 病史

There is a history of being infected, such as the patients of similar diseases nearby, or staying in the public place without preventive measures of hygiene.

被传染史，如周围有类似病患者或久处公共场所而卫生防范有所不及。

2.2 Clinical manifestations

2.2 临床表现

Burning sensation, foreign-body sensation, excessive tears and photophobia of the sick eye, or visual disturbance if the cornea is involved.

患眼灼热感、异物感，泪多，畏光，累及角膜可有视力影响。

2.3 Ocular examinations

2.3 眼部检查

(1) Congestion and edema can be seen at the eyelids and conjunctiva, or even flake-like bleeding under the conjuctiva.

(2) Preauricular or mandibular lymph nodes enlargement can be palpated.

(3) In the fluorescent staining examination, the spotted infiltration can be seen under the corneal epithelium, while the dotted nebula is left in the late stage.

（1）眼睑、结膜充血水肿，甚者结膜下片状出血。

（2）耳前或颌下淋巴结肿大。

（3）荧光染色角膜上皮下星点状侵润，后期可遗留星翳。

3 Therapeutic methods

3 治疗方法

3.1 Therapeutic principles

3.1 治疗原则

The disease is caused by the invasion of Li (Epidemic) Qi, so the wind-eliminating and heat-clearing method is the basic method clinically, by focusing on the lung and treating both the internal and the external.

本病系感受疫疠之气所致，临证以祛风清热为基本治法，从肺论治，内外兼顾。

3.2 Treatment based on syndrome differentiation

(1) Early stage of epidemic disease

Main symptoms: Dryness, burning pain, photophobia, lacrimation with thin-clear eye discharge, redness or bleeding of eye white, redness and swelling of eyelids at the sick eye, preauricular or mandibular lymph nodes palpated, red tongue body with thin-yellow tongue coating, and superficial-rapid pulse.

Therapeutic methods: Eliminate wind and clear heat.

Herbal formulas and drugs: The major formula is *Wind-Eliminating and Heat-Clearing Drink* (Qu Feng San Re Yin Zi). The commonly-used herbal drugs are *Rhizoma seu Radix Notopterygii* (Qiang Huo), *Radix Ledebouriellae* (Fang Feng), *Herba Menthae* (Bo He), *Fructus Forsythiae* (Lian Qiao), *Fructus Arctii* (Niu Bang Zi), *Radix et Rhizoma Rhei* (Da Huang), *Fructus Crataegi* (Shan Zha), *Radix Paeoniae Rubra* (Chi Shao), *Radix Angelicae Sinensis* (Dang Gui), *Rhizoma Ligustici Chuanxiong* (Chuan Xiong), *Radix Glycyrrhizae Praeparata* (Zhi Gan Cao), etc.

Modification according to symptoms: If the bleeding of eye white is extensive, add *Radix Rehmanniae Cruda* (Sheng Di Huang) and *Cortex Moutan Radicis* (Mu Dan Pi), to cool blood and clear heat.

(2) Flaming and excessive heat-toxin

Main symptoms: Redness and swelling of eye white, redness and swelling of eyelids, bleeding of eye white, dotted nebula of eye black, photophobia, sharp-stabbing pain, warm and excessive tears,

3.2 辨证论治

(1) 初感疫疠

主症：患眼沙涩灼痛，畏光流泪，眵多清稀，白睛红赤、溢血，胞睑红肿，耳前、颌下可扪及肿核。舌质红，苔薄黄，脉浮数。

治法：疏风清热。

方药：代表方为驱风散热饮子，常用药如羌活、防风、薄荷、连翘、牛蒡子、大黄、山楂、赤芍、当归、川芎、炙甘草等。

加减：若白睛溢血广泛者，加生地黄、牡丹皮以凉血清热。

(2) 热毒炽盛

主症：白睛赤肿，胞睑红肿，白睛溢血，黑睛星翳，羞明刺痛，热泪如汤，口渴引饮，溲赤便结。舌质红，苔

thirst with desire to drink water, dark urine, constipation, red tongue body with yellow tongue coating, and rapid pulse.

黄，脉数。

Therapeutic methods: Reduce fire and relieve toxin.

治法：泻火解毒。

Herbal formulas and drugs: The major formula is *Lung-Reducing Drink* (Xie Fei Yin). The commonly-used herbal drugs are *Gypsum Fibrosum* (Shi Gao), *Radix Scutellariae* (Huang Qin), *Cortex Mori Radicis* (Sang Bai Pi), *Fructus Gardeniae* (Zhi Zi), *Rhizoma seu Radix Notopterygii* (Qiang Huo), *Herba Schizonepetae* (Jing Jie), *Radix Ledebouriellae* (Fang Feng), *Radix Angelicae Dahuricae* (Bai Zhi), *Fructus Forsythiae* (Lian Qiao), *Fructus Aurantii* (Zhi Ke), *Radix Glycyrrhizae Praeparata* (Zhi Gan Cao), etc.

方药：代表方为泻肺饮，常用药如石膏、黄芩、桑白皮、栀子、羌活、荆芥、防风、白芷、连翘、枳壳、炙甘草等。

Modification according to symptoms: For nebula of eye black, add *Periostracum Cicadae* (Chan Tui), *Semen Celosiae* (Qing Xiang Zi), *Fructus Tribuli* (Bai Ji Li) and *Radix Gentianae* (Long Dan).

加减：若黑睛生翳者，加蝉蜕、青葙子、白蒺藜、龙胆草。

3.3 Local therapy

1% Baicallin Eye Drop, or 0.1% Idoxuridine Eye Drop, or Acyclovir Eye Drop, 3 to 4 times a day, or more frequent application according to the condition.

3.3 局部治法

1% 黄芩甙眼药水或 0.1%疱疹净、无环鸟苷眼药水滴眼，每日 3～4 次，也可依据病情频频滴眼。

3.4 Other therapy

Apply Antiviral Oral Liquid, the patent herbal medicine, 1 bottle each time and 3 times a day.

3.4 其他疗法

可用中成药抗病毒口服液，每次 1 支，每日 3 次。

4 Speculative map

4 思辨导图

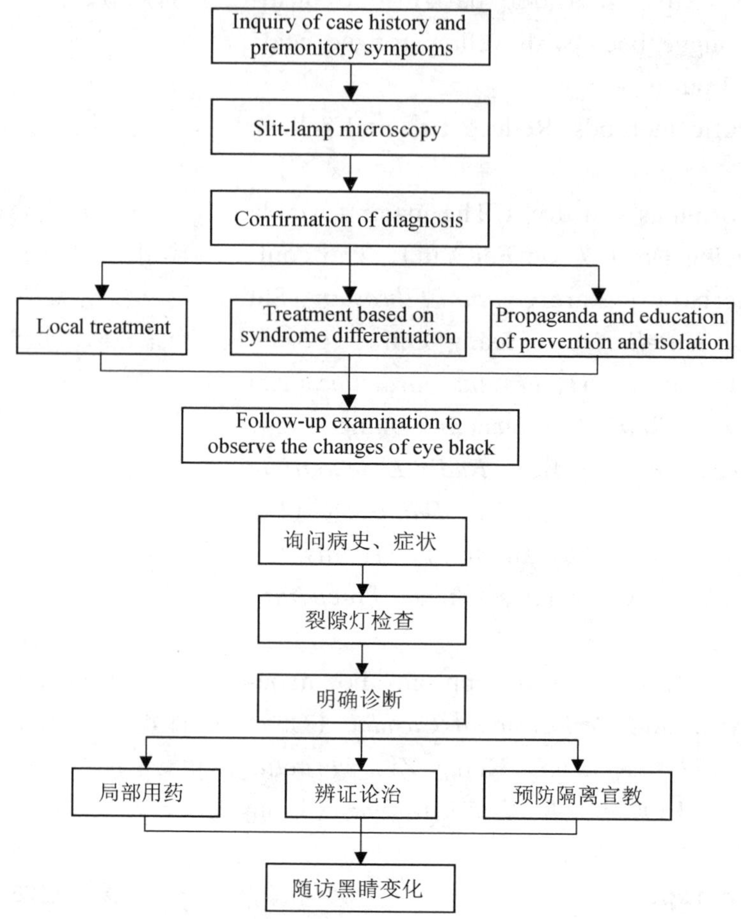

Vernal catarrhal conjunctivitis

Vernal catarrhal conjunctivitis is a kind of immune eye disease, the result of the combined action of type I and type IV reactions. The allergens are pollen, microorganism, animal feather, etc. More severe in spring and milder in winter, the disease has the periodical attacks, more common in male juveniles. The both eyes are affected usually. The disease may last for long time of several years or even

春季卡他性结膜炎

春季卡他性结膜炎是一种免疫性眼病。属Ⅰ、Ⅳ型变态反应共同作用的结果，过敏原为花粉、微生物、动物羽毛等，春剧冬缓，呈周期性发作，多见于青少年男性，常双眼发病，其病程可长达数年或数十年之久，随年龄增

several decades, and be relieved or cured with the age.

长逐渐减轻或痊愈。

In traditional Chinese medicine, the disease is called "seasonal-attacking disease", manifested by intolerable itching of eyes, redness of eye white and come-in-time attack. Because of the weakness of the lung and Wei (Defense) Phase, the exogenous wind-heat attacks upward the eye white, traveling between the skin and muscle of the eyelids. Generally speaking, the accumulated damp-heat in spleen and stomach and the attacking pathogenic wind combine to retain in the eyelid and eye white, to cause the disease. Or the insufficiency of the liver blood induces the internal wind, which attack upwards the eye to cause the disease.

古代医家称之为"时复症",并指出以目痒难忍,白睛红赤,至期而发为特征;因肺卫不固,风热外侵,上犯白睛,往来于胞睑肌肤腠理之间而致病。一般认为,脾胃湿热内蕴,复感风邪,风湿热邪相搏,滞于胞睑、白睛而致病;或肝血不足,虚风内动,上犯于目而致病。

1 Etiology and pathogenesis

1 病因病机

1.1 Because of weakness of lung and Wei (Defense) Phase, the exogenous wind-heat attacks upwards, traveling between the muscle wheel and qi sheel.

1.1 肺卫不固,风热外侵上犯,往来于肉轮与气轮之间。

1.2 Due to internal accumulation of damp-heat in spleen and stomach and the attack of the exogenous wind, the pathogenic wind, damp and heat merge to retain inside the qi wheel and muscle wheel.

1.2 脾胃湿热内蕴,复感风邪,风湿热邪相搏,滞于气轮与肉轮之中。

1.3 Insufficiency of liver blood induces the internal wind, which attacks upward the eye to cause the disease.

1.3 肝血不足,虚风内动,上犯于目而为患。

2 Diagnostic essentials

2 诊断要点

2.1 Case history

2.1 病史

Repeated attacks, more severe in spring and milder in winter.

反复发作,春剧冬缓。

2.2 Clinical manifestations

2.2 临床表现

Severe and intolerable itching of both eyes,

双眼奇痒难忍,灼热不

burning and uncomfortable sensation, foreign-body sensation, sharp-stabbing pain, photophobia, lacrimation, whitish, sticky and silk-like eye discharge.

适，异物感，刺痛甚则畏光流泪，有白色黏丝样分泌物。

2.3 Ocular examinations

(1) Palpebral conjunctiva type: Obscurity and congestion of conjunctival vessels of upper eyelid, flat particles seen in the inner surface of eyelid, ranging like the paving pebbles.

(2) Corneal limbus type: Bulbar conjunctiva congestion, yellow-white glutinous prominent nodules seen at the corneal margin, in mutual fusion, surrounding the corneal margin.

(3) Mixed type: Simultaneous existence of both above two conditions.

2.3 眼部检查

（1）睑结膜型：上睑结膜血管模糊充血，睑内面见扁平颗粒，状如铺路卵石样排列。

（2）角膜缘型：球结膜充血见角膜边缘黄白色胶样隆起结节，或相互融合，包绕角膜缘。

（3）混合型：上述两种情况同时存在。

3 Therapeutic methods

3.1 Therapeutic principles

The endogenous cause is the allergic constitution, while the exogenous cause is just the inducing factor. Therefore, it is advisable in the internal therapy to consider the general condition according to the pulse and symptoms, besides to eliminate wind, stop itching and relieve symptoms. The therapeutic principles are to regulate and adjust the lung and spleen, to eliminate wind, dissolve damp and stop itching. It is better to start the treatment before the attack of the disease.

3 治疗方法

3.1 治疗原则

本病内因在于体质过敏，外因仅为诱发的因素，故内治除祛风止痒、缓解症状外，尚应根据患者全身脉症给以综合考虑。临证以调节肺脾为本，驱风除湿止痒论治。本病的治疗最好在发作前即开始。

3.2 Treatment based on syndrome differentiation

(1) **Attack of exogenous wind-heat**

Main symptoms: Intolerable itching of eye, burning sensation, slight pain, whitish, sticky and silk-like eye discharge, pebble-like particles in the inner surface of eyelid, turbidity and redness of eye

3.2 辨证论治

（1）**外感风热**

主症：眼痒难忍，灼热微痛，有白色黏丝样眼眵，胞睑内面遍生状如小卵石样颗粒，白睛污红。舌淡红，苔薄

white, light-red tongue body with thin-white tongue coating, and superficial-rapid pulse.

白,脉浮数。

Therapeutic methods: Eliminate wind and stop itching.

治法:祛风止痒。

Herbal formulas and drugs: The major formula is *Wind-Dispelling Powder* (Xiao Feng San). The commonly-used herbal drugs are *Herba Schizonepetae* (Jing Jie), *Herba Menthae* (Bo He), *Radix Ledebouriellae* (Fang Feng), *Bombyx Batryticatus* (Jiang Can), *Periostracum Cicadae* (Chan Tui), *Pericarpium Citri Tangerinae* (Chen Pi), *Cortex Magnoliae Officinalis* (Hou Pu), *Radix Codonopsis Pilosulae* (Dang Shen), *Sclerotium Poriae* (Fu Ling), *Rhizoma Ligustici Chuanxiong* (Chuan Xiong), etc.

方药:代表方为消风散,常用药如荆芥、薄荷、防风、僵蚕、蝉蜕、陈皮、厚朴、党参、茯苓、川芎等。

Modification according to symptoms: For severe itching, add *Folium Mori* (Sang Ye), *Flos Chrysanthemi* (Ju Hua) and *Fructus Tribuli* (Bai Ji Li) to enhance the action to eliminate wind and stop itching. For severe redness and burning sensation of eye white, add *Cortex Moutan Radicis* (Mu Dan Pi), *Radix Paeoniae Rubra* (Chi Shao) and *Radix Curcumae* (Yu Jin), to cool blood, dissolve stasis and relieve redness.

加减:痒甚者,酌加桑叶、菊花、刺蒺藜以增祛风止痒之功;若白睛红赤、灼热明显者,可加牡丹皮、赤芍、郁金以凉血消滞退赤。

(2) **Damp-heat combined with wind**

(2) **湿热夹风**

Main symptoms: Severe and intolerable itching of the sick eye, more severe itching after exposing to the wind and sun or wiping eyes, excessive tears, thick, sticky and silk-like eye discharge, pebble-like particles in the inner surface of eyelid, turbidity and yellowness of eye white, glutinous nodule occurring at the juncture of eye black and white, red tongue body with yellow-sticky tongue coating, and rapid pulse.

主症:患眼奇痒难忍,风吹日晒、揉拭眼部后加剧,泪多眵稠呈黏丝状,睑内面遍生颗粒,状如小卵石排列,白睛污黄,黑白睛交界处呈胶样结节隆起。舌质红,苔黄腻,脉数。

Therapeutic methods: Clear heat, dissolve damp, eliminate wind and stop itching.

治法：清热除湿，祛风止痒。

Herbal formulas and drugs: The major formula is *Dampness-Dispersing Decoction* (Chu Shi Tang). The commonly-used herbal drugs are *Sclerotium Poriae* (Fu Ling), *Talcum* (Hua Shi), *Semen Plantaginis* (Che Qian Zi), *Radix Scutellariae* (Huang Qin), *Rhizoma Coptidis* (Huang Lian), *Radix Ledebouriellae* (Fang Feng), *Herba Schizonepetae* (Jing Jie), *Fructus Aurantii* (Zhi Ke), *Pericarpium Citri Tangerinae* (Chen Pi), *Radix Glycyrrhizae Praeparata* (Zhi Gan Cao), etc.

方药：代表方为除湿汤，常用药如茯苓、滑石、车前子、黄芩、黄连、防风、荆芥、枳壳、陈皮、炙甘草等。

Modification according to symptoms: Add *Cortex Dictamni* (Bai Xian Pi), *Fructus Kochiae* (Di Fu Zi) and *Herba Artemisiae Scopariae* (Yin Chen Hao) to enhance the action to dissolve damp and stop itching. For pebble-like particles or glutinous nodules in the inner surface of eyelid, add *Radix Curcumae* (Yu Jin) and *Rhizoma Ligustici Chuanxiong* (Chuan Xiong) to dissolve stasis.

加减：常于方中加白鲜皮、地肤子、茵陈蒿以增强除湿止痒之力；睑内面遍生状如小卵石样颗粒及有胶样结节隆起者，可加郁金、川芎以消郁滞。

(3) **Blood deficiency leading to wind**

(3) **血虚生风**

Main symptoms: Mild and sporadic itching of eye, slight turbidity and redness of eye white, lusterless or sallow-yellow complexion, pale tongue body, and thready pulse.

主症：眼痒势轻，时作时止，白睛微显污红；面色少华或萎黄。舌淡，脉细。

Therapeutic methods: Nourish blood and eliminate wind.

治法：养血息风。

Herbal formulas and drugs: The major formula is *Four Agents Decoction* (Si Wu Tang). The commonly-used herbal drugs are *Radix Angelicae Sinensis* (Dang Gui), *Radix Rehmanniae Praeparata* (Shu Di Huang), *Rhizoma Ligustici Chuanxiong* (Chuan Xiong), *Radix Paeoniae Alba* (Bai Shao), etc.

方药：代表方为四物汤，常用药如当归、熟地黄、川芎、白芍等。

Modification according to symptoms: Add *Fructus Tribuli* (Bai Ji Li) and *Radix Ledebouriellae*

加减：宜加白蒺藜、防风以增祛风止痒之功；加炒白

(Fang Feng) to enhance the action of eliminate wind and stop itching. Add *Rhizoma Atractylodis Macrocephalae* (Bai Zhu), *Sclerotium Poriae* (Fu Ling) and *Radix Codonopsis Pilosulae* (Dang Shen) to strengthen the spleen and benefit qi so as to produce qi and blood.

术、茯苓、党参以健脾益气，使气血生化有源。

3.3 Local therapy

(1) Steroids eye drops (Tobradex Eye Drop) are applied to effectively relieve the symptoms and signs, 3 times a day and 1 drop each time.

(2) 2% to 4% Sodium Cromoglycate Eye Drop is applied 3 times a day and 1 drop each time.

(3) 0.1% Epinephrine Solution is applied in combination, so as to relieve local vessel congestion.

(4) 2% Cyclosporine Eye Drop is applied to regulate the immunity.

3.3 局部治疗

（1）激素类眼液（典必殊眼药水）可有效地缓解症状、体征。眼液每日3次，每次1滴。

（2）用2%～4%色苷酸钠眼液，每日3次，每次1滴。

（3）必要时配合用0.1%肾上腺素溶液，可减轻局部血管充血。

（4）可用2%环孢霉素眼用溶液滴眼，调节免疫。

3.4 Supplementary therapies

(1) Cold compress: The application of local cold compress may reduce the tissue reaction and relieve symptoms.

(2) Acupuncture: The points are Chengqi (ST 1), Guangming (GB 37), Waiguan (TE 5), Hegu (LI 4), Zusanli (ST 36), etc., to regulate the immunity. The treatment is given once a day, and 10 sessions of treatment make up a course.

(3) For the cases with severe condition, 0.25g Aspirin is taken orally, 3 times a day, and 2 to 4 weeks make up a course. Or 25 mg Indomethacin is taken orally, 3 times a day, and 2 weeks make up a course.

(4) Eye drop made of heat-clearing and toxin-relieving drug, 0.5% Bear Gall Eye Drop is applied.

3.4 辅助疗法

（1）冷敷：局部冷敷可减少组织反应，改善症状。

（2）针刺：选取承泣、光明、外关、合谷、足三里等穴调节免疫，每日1次，10次为1个疗程。

（3）病情严重者，可口服阿司匹林0.25g，每日3次，2～4周为1个疗程；或口服消炎痛25 mg，每日3次，2周为1个疗程。

（4）滴用清热解毒类眼药水，如0.5%熊胆眼药水。

4 Speculative map

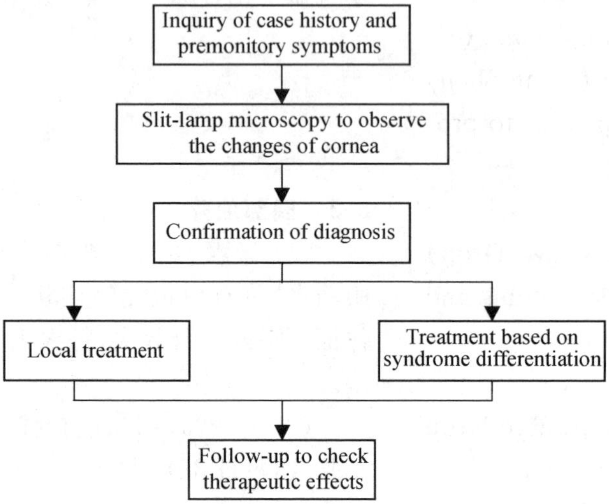

Inquiry of case history and premonitory symptoms
↓
Slit-lamp microscopy to observe the changes of cornea
↓
Confirmation of diagnosis
↓
Local treatment | Treatment based on syndrome differentiation
↓
Follow-up to check therapeutic effects

4 思辨导图

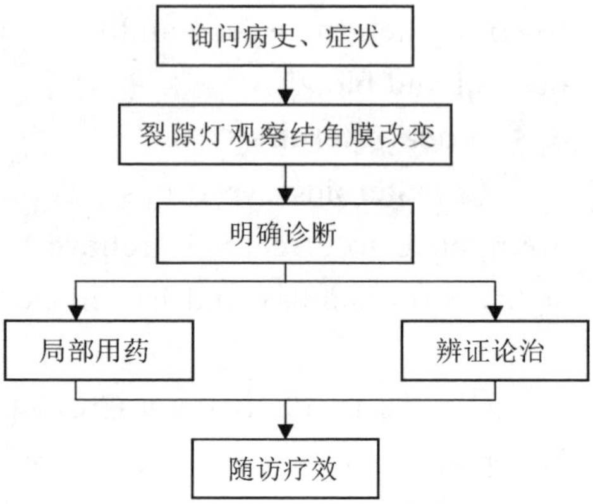

询问病史、症状
↓
裂隙灯观察结角膜改变
↓
明确诊断
↓
局部用药 | 辨证论治
↓
随访疗效

Phlyctenular keratoconjunctivitis

Phlyctenular keratoconjunctivitis is a kind of localized disease of eye due to the allergic reaction of conjunctiva and cornea on the endogenous micro-protein. But the exact cause is not confirmed yet. The single eye is affected mostly.

In traditional Chinese medicine, the disease is called "eye white particles" or "eye white ulcer", manifested by corn-like small blisters on the surface of eye white with red-colored vessels around. The location of the disease is the eye white, pertaining to the Lung Meridian. The pathogenic dryness-heat attacks the Lung Meridian to disturb the qi activities. Due to insufficiency of the lung yin, the water and fire are disharmonious, leading to upward-flaming of the false fire.

泡性角结膜炎

泡性角结膜炎被认为是结膜、角膜对内源性微生物蛋白质变态反应引起的眼局部病变。但确切的病因不能确定。以单眼发病为多。

本病属中医学"金疳""金疡"的范畴，临床表现可归纳为以白睛表层生玉粒样小疱，周围绕以赤脉为特征。本病病变部位在白睛，属肺经之疾，肺经燥热，气机不宣；肺阴不足，水火不济而致虚火上炎。

1 Etiology and pathogenesis

1.1 Dryness-heat in Lung Meridian. The lung fire is excessive and disturbs the lung's dispersing and spreading function, qi activities stop to cause accumulated heat, which becomes particles.

1.2 Insufficiency of lung yin. The false fire is excessive and attacks the qi wheel, causing blood vessel blockage at the eye white.

1.3 Disharmony of spleen and stomach. The earth fails to promote the metal, so the lung-metal loses the nourishment, leading to qi activity stoppage. As a result, qi stagnation and blood stasis occur at the qi wheel.

2 Diagnostic essentials

2.1 Clinical manifestations

Slight discomfort at the eye, blister-like nodules occurring at the cornea, photophobia and lacrimation.

2.2 Ocular examinations

(1) Phlyctenular conjunctivitis: Miliary and grey-red nodules at the bulbar conjunctiva, congestion of nearby conjunctiva, absence of tenderness, moveable nodules by pushing, and self-cured after rupture.

(2) Phlyctenular keratitis: Blebs occurring at the cornea, and superficial nebula due to invasion of blood vessel nebula in prognosis.

(3) Phlyctenular keratoconjunctivitis: Blebs occurring at the corneal limbus, smaller blebs occurring singly or in clusters with mutual fusion.

3 Therapeutic methods

3.1 Therapeutic principles

Find out the possible causes and treat it accord-

1 病因病机

1.1 肺经燥热，肺火偏盛，宣发失司，气机郁滞，聚而为疳。

1.2 肺阴不足，虚火偏盛，气轮受邪，白睛血络滞而不行。

1.3 脾胃失调，土不生金，肺金失养，气机不畅，气血凝滞气轮而成。

2 诊断要点

2.1 临床症状

眼部仅有轻微的不适，疱样结节位于角膜可出现畏光流泪。

2.2 眼部检查

（1）疱性结膜炎：球结膜呈灰红色粟粒样结节，周围结膜充血，按压无痛，推知可移，溃破后自愈。

（2）疱性角膜炎：疱疹位于角膜，预后伴随血管翳侵入角膜留有浅层翳障。

（3）疱性角结膜炎：位于角膜缘，疱疹较小，可单发也可多发成串，相互融合。

3 治疗方法

3.1 治疗原则

查找可能存在的病因，

ing to the cause. In traditional Chinese medicine, it is advisable to treat the lung as the major method, to disperse the lung and benefit qi so as to dissolve the stasis in the early stage, and to moisturize the lung and inhibit the false fire so as to smooth the qi and blood flow in the late stage.

对因治疗。中医临证以治肺为主,病初宣肺利气以散结,病后润肺以抑虚火,使气血得以畅行。

3.2 Treatment based on syndrome differentiation

3.2 辨证论治

(1) **Dryness-heat in Lung Meridian**

(1) **肺经燥热**

Main symptoms: Dryness and pain of eye, warm tears with dry eye discharge, small blebs at the superficial layer of eye white with thick and red vessels nearby, thirst, dryness in nose, constipation, dark urine, red tongue body with thin-yellow tongue coating, and rapid pulse.

主症:目涩疼痛,泪热眵结;白睛浅层生小疱,其周围赤脉粗大;或有口渴鼻干,便秘溲赤。舌质红,苔薄黄,脉数。

Therapeutic methods: Reduce lung and dissolve stasis.

治法:泻肺散结。

Herbal formulas and drugs: The major formula is *Lung-Reducing Decoction* (Xie Fei Tang). The commonly-used herbal drugs are *Cortex Mori Radicis* (Sang Bai Pi), *Cortex Lycii Radicis* (Di Gu Pi), *Radix Scutellariae* (Huang Qin), *Rhizoma Anemarrhenae* (Zhi Mu), *Radix Ophiopogonis* (Mai Dong), *Radix Platycodi* (Jie Geng), etc.

方药:代表方为泻肺汤,常用药如桑白皮、地骨皮、黄芩、知母、麦门冬、桔梗等。

Modification according to symptoms: Add *Radix Paeoniae Rubra* (Chi Shao) and *Cortex Moutan Radicis* (Mu Dan Pi), to cool blood, activate blood and relieve redness. Add *Fructus Forsythiae* (Lian Qiao), so enhance the action to clear heat and dissolve stasis. For the blebs occurring at the edge of eye black, add *Spica Prunellae* (Xia Ku Cao) and *Semen Cassiae* (Jue Ming Zi), to purify liver and reduce fire. For constipation, add *Radix et Rhizoma Rhei* (Da Huang), to reduce fu organs and clear

加减:常于方中加赤芍、牡丹皮以凉血活血退赤,加连翘以增清热散结之功;若小疱位于黑睛边缘者,加夏枯草、决明子以清肝泻火;大便秘结者,可加大黄以泻腑清热。

heat.

(2) **Insufficiency of lung yin**

Main symptoms: Dull pain and slightly astringent felling, dry eye discharge, small blebs at the eye white with light-red vessels nearby, repeated attacks, dry cough, dry throat, red tongue body with scanty or with no tongue coating, and thready-rapid pulse.

Therapeutic methods: Nourish yin and moisturize lung.

Herbal formulas and drugs: The major formula is *Yin-Nourishing and Lung-Cleaning Decoction* (Yang Yin Qing Fei Tang). The commonly-used herbal drugs are *Radix Rehmanniae Cruda* (Sheng Di Huang), *Radix Ophiopogonis* (Mai Dong), *Radix Scrophulariae* (Xuan Shen), *Bulbus Fritillariae Cirrhosae* (Chuan Bei Mu), *Cortex Moutan Radicis* (Mu Dan Pi), *Herba Menthae* (Bo He), *Radix Paeoniae Alba* (Bai Shao), *Radix Glycyrrhizae Praeparata* (Zhi Gan Cao), etc.

Modification according to symptoms: Add *Spica Prunellae* (Xia Ku Cao) and *Fructus Forsythiae* (Lian Qiao) to enhance the action to clear heat and eliminate Xie (Pathogenic) Qi.

(3) **Deficiency of lung and spleen**

Main symptoms: Small blebs at the eye white with red vessels nearby, intractable condition which is difficult to cure, repeated attacks, fatigue, lassitude, poor appetite, abdominal discomfort, pale tongue body with thin-white tongue coating, and thread-weak pulse.

Therapeutic methods: Benefit qi and strengthen spleen.

Herbal formulas and drugs: The major formula

(2) **肺阴不足**

主症:隐涩微疼,眼眵干结,白睛生小疱,周围赤脉淡红,反复再发;可有干咳咽干。舌质红,少苔或无苔,脉细数。

治法:滋阴润肺。

方药:代表方为养阴清肺汤,常用药如生地黄、麦门冬、玄参、川贝母、牡丹皮、薄荷、白芍、炙甘草等。

加减:常于方中加夏枯草、连翘以增清热散邪之功。

(3) **肺脾亏虚**

主症:白睛小疱周围赤脉轻微,日久难愈,或反复发作;疲乏无力,食欲不振,腹胀不舒。舌质淡,苔薄白,脉细无力。

治法:益气健脾。

方药:代表方为参苓白

is Ginseng, Poria and Atractylodes Powder (Shen Ling Bai Zhu San). The commonly-used herbal drugs are *Radix Ginseng* (Ren Shen), *Rhizoma Atractylodis Macrocephalae* (Bai Zhu), *Sclerotium Poriae* (Fu Ling), *Semen Coicis* (Yi Yi Ren), *Rhizoma Dioscoreae* (Shan Yao), *Semen Dolichoris* (Bian Dou), *Semen Nelumbinis* (Lian Zi Rou), *Fructus Amomi* (Sha Ren), *Pericarpium Citri Tangerinae* (Chen Pi), *Radix Platycodi* (Jie Geng), *Radix Glycyrrhizae Praeparata* (Zhi Gan Cao), etc.

Modification according to symptoms: Add *Cortex Mori Radicis* (Sang Bai Pi) and *Radix Paeoniae Rubra* (Chi Shao) to relieve redness of eye and relieve pain of eye.

3.3 Local therapy

(1) 0.5% Cortisone Acetate Eye Drop or 0.025% Dexamethasone Eye Drop is applied. Antibiotics, such as 0.3% Ofloxacin Eye Drop or Ointment, are combined, 3 to 4 times a day respectively.

(2) 0.5% Bear Gall Eye Drop is applied 3 to 6 times a day.

4 Speculative map

Inquiry of case history and premonitory symptoms
↓
Slit-lamp microscopy to observe the blebs
↓
Confirmation of diagnosis
↓
Local treatment | Treatment based on syndrome differentiation

术散，常用药如人参、白术、茯苓、薏苡仁、山药、扁豆、莲子肉、砂仁、陈皮、桔梗、炙甘草等。

加减：可加桑白皮、赤芍以缓目赤、止目痛。

3.3 局部治疗

（1）0.5%醋酸可的松滴眼液或0.025%地塞米松滴眼液。配合抗生素类药物，如0.3%氧氟沙星眼药水或眼膏等，每日各3～4次。

（2）中药0.5%熊胆眼药水，每日3～6次。

4 思辨导图

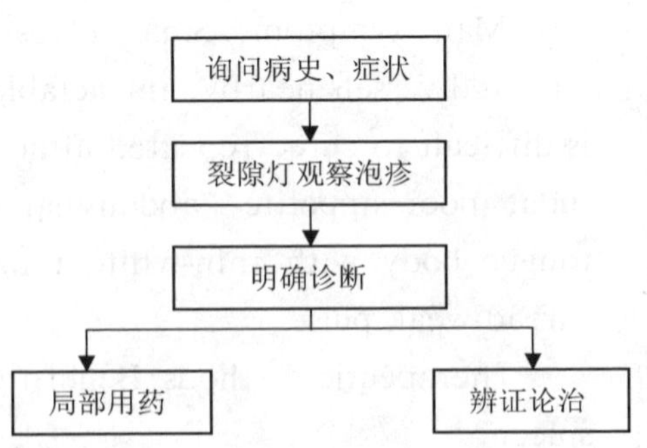

Scleratitis

巩膜炎

Scleratitis pertains to the granulomatous proliferation response, featured by long course of disease and repeated attacks. It often occurs at the space between the corneal limbus and muscular attachment, more commonly seen in females. Two types of episcleritis and anterior scleritis seen in the clinic, the former has a favorable prognosis, pertaining to the self-limited type, while the latter involves the nearby tissues to cause the disorders there and has an unfavorable prognosis. The causative factors are complicated, mostly believed that it is an autoimmune connective tissue disease.

巩膜炎属于肉芽肿性增殖反应。其特点病程长,反复发作。常发生于角膜缘至肌附着点间,好发于女性。临床常见表层巩膜炎和前部巩膜炎两种类型,病因复杂,多认为属于自身免疫性结缔组织疾病,前者预后良好属于自限性类型,而后者可累及邻近组织出现变症。预后不佳。

In traditional Chinese medicine, the disease is called "fire-type particles" or "fire-type ulcer", manifested by purple-red and limited prominence at the inner layer of eye white, with pain which is worsened by pressure. The pathogenesis is the hyperactivity of lung heat, causing the accumulated fire which fails to be dispersed and spread, or the pathogenic wind, damp and heat attacking the upper along the meridian, or the accumulated heat in the Lung Meridian, consuming yin and causing false fire to flame upwards.

本病属中医学"火疳""火疡"的范畴;临床有白睛里层呈紫红色局限性隆起且疼痛拒按的表现;病机为肺热亢盛,火郁不得宣泄;或风湿热邪循经上犯;反复者为肺经郁热,日久伤阴,虚火上炎。

1 Etiology and pathogenesis

1 病因病机

1.1 Hyperactivity of heat in lung. It disturbs the qi activities, so as to cause qi stagnation and blood stasis, becoming the particles as a result.

1.1 肺热亢盛,气机不利,以致气滞血瘀,滞结为疳。

1.2 Internal accumulated heat-toxin in heart and lung. The accumulated fire fails to be dispersed and spread, so going upwards to the qi wheel.

1.2 心肺热毒内蕴,火郁不得宣泄,上逼气轮所致。

1.3 Original Bi (Obturation) Pattern. Pathogenic wind-damp attacks the meridians and stays for long time to change into heat. All the pathogenic wind, damp and heat attack upwards the qi wheel along the meridian, to cause the disease.

1.3 素有痹证,风湿久郁经络,郁久化热,风湿热邪循经上犯于气轮而发病。

1.4 Accumulated heat in Lung Meridian. It retains in Lung Meridian to consume yin, so as to cause the false fire which attacks upwards the qi wheel.

1.4 肺经郁热,日久伤阴,虚火上攻气轮。

2 Diagnostic essentials

2 诊断要点

2.1 Clinical manifestations

2.1 临床表现

Astrigent feeling and pain of the sick eye, photophobia and lacrimation in mild condition, severe eye pain which radiates to the orbit, or more severe pain when the eyeball is rotating, and blurring of vision in serious condition.

轻者患眼涩痛,畏光流泪。重者目痛剧烈,痛连目眶四周,或眼珠转动时疼痛加剧,视物不清。

2.2 Ocular examination

2.2 眼部检查

Dark-red colour and diffusing congestion at the superficial layer of sclera, and limited and tender nodules which is fixed by pushing and worsened by pressure.

巩膜表层暗红色弥漫性充血,局限性压痛性结节,推之不移、拒按。

3 Therapeutic methods

3 治疗方法

3.1 Therapeutic principles

3.1 治疗原则

The ideal method is to find out the causative factor and to treat the disease aiming at the causative factor. But it is actually difficult to find out the causative factor, so it is advisable to apply the comprehensive treatment. Clinically, to identify the true fire or false of the Lung Meridian is the major method.

理想的方法是寻找病因,并针对病因进行治疗;但实际查找病因较为困难,多采取综合治疗。临证以辨识肺经虚实之火为要。

3.2 Treatment based on syndrome differentiation

3.2 辨证论治

(1) **Accumulated fire in Lung Meridian**

(1) **肺经郁火**

Main symptoms: Moderate onset of disease, pain of sick eye, photophobia with desire to close eye,

主症:发病稍缓,患眼疼痛,羞明欲闭,白睛局部紫红

purple-red and prominent nodules at the eye white, severe pain occurring by touching, dry mouth, sore throat, cough, constipation, red tongue body with thin-yellow tongue coating, and rapid pulse.

色结节隆起，触之痛甚，可伴口干咽痛，咳嗽便秘。舌质红，苔薄黄，脉数。

Therapeutic methods: Purify lung and reduce heat.

治法：清肺泻热。

Herbal formulas and drugs: The major formula is *White Lung-Reducing Powder* (Xie Bai San). The commonly-used herbal drugs are *Cortex Mori Radicis* (Sang Bai Pi), *Cortex Lycii Radicis* (Di Gu Pi), *Radix Glycyrrhizae* (Gan Cao), etc.

方药：代表方为泻白散，常用药如桑白皮、地骨皮、甘草等。

Modification according to symptoms: Add *Semen Descurainiae* (Ting Li Zi) and *Semen Armeniacae Amarum* (Ku Xing Ren), to enhance the action to reduce lung, clear heat and dissolve stasis. Add *Flos Carthami* (Hong Hua) and *Radix Curcumae* (Yu Jin), to activate blood, dissolve stasis and relieve accumulation.

加减：可加葶苈子、苦杏仁以增强泻肺之力，清热散结；加红花、郁金以活血化瘀，散结消滞。

(2) **Accumulated fire-toxin**

(2) **火毒蕴结**

Main symptoms: Abupt onset, severe pain of sick eye which is difficult to open, photophobia, lacrimation, eye pain which is worsened by pressure, blurring of vision, big and promiment nodules at the eye white, or cluster-like nodules with red-purple blood vessels nearby, bitter taste in mouth, dry throat, coarse breathing, restlessness, constipation, dark urine, red tongue with yellow tongue coating, and rapid-forceful pulse.

主症：发病较急，患眼疼痛难睁，羞明流泪，目痛拒按，视物不清，白睛结节大而隆起，或连缀成环，周围血脉紫赤怒张；伴见口苦咽干，气粗烦躁，便秘溲赤。舌红，苔黄，脉数有力。

Therapeutic methods: Reduce fire, relieve toxin, cool blood and dissolve stasis.

治法：泻火解毒，凉血散结。

Herbal formulas and drugs: The major formula is *Yin-Returning and Tribulation-Relieving Decoction* (Huan Yin Jiu Ku Tang). The commonly-used herbal drugs are *Rhizoma Coptidis* (Huang Lian), *Radix Scutellariae* (Huang Qin), *Cortex Phellodendri*

方药：代表方为还阴救苦汤，常用药如黄连、黄芩、黄柏、龙胆草、连翘、羌活、防风、细辛、藁本、柴胡、桔梗、知母、生地黄、川芎、当归、升

(Huang Bo), *Radix Gentianae* (Long Dan), *Fructus Forsythiae* (Lian Qiao), *Rhizoma seu Radix Notopterygii* (Qiang Huo), *Radix Ledebouriellae* (Fang Feng), *Herba Asari* (Xi Xin), *Rhizoma Ligustici* (Gao Ben), *Radix Bupleuri* (Chai Hu), *Radix Platycodi* (Jie Geng), *Rhizoma Anemarrhenae* (Zhi Mu), *Radix Rehmanniae Cruda* (Sheng Di Huang), *Rhizoma Ligustici Chuanxiong* (Chuan Xiong), *Radix Angelicae Sinensis* (Dang Gui), *Rhizoma Cimicifugae* (Sheng Ma), *Rhizoma Atractylodis* (Cang Zhu), *Radix Glycyrrhizae Praeparata* (Zhi Gan Cao), etc.

麻、苍术、炙甘草等。

Modification according to symptoms: Subtract the warm-dry drugs accordingly, and add *Gypsum Fibrosum Cruda* (Sheng Shi Gao), to enhance the action to clear heat and reduce fire.

加减：方中温燥之药应酌情减少，并加生石膏以增强清热泻火之功。

(3) **Pathogenic wind, damp and heat attacking eye**

(3) **风湿热邪攻目**

Main symptoms: Quick onset of disease, distension, pain and tenderness of eyeball, photophobia, lacrimation, blurring of vision, purple-red and prominent nodules at the eye white with red vessels nearby, aching and pain of joints, swelling and distension of joints, heavy and aching sensation in body, prolonged and intractable disease which is difficult to be cured, white-sticky tongue coating, and rolling or soft pulse.

主症：发病较急，眼珠胀闷而疼，且有压痛感，羞明流泪，视物不清；白睛有紫红色结节样隆起，周围有赤丝牵绊；常伴有骨节酸痛，肢节肿胀，身重酸楚，病程缠绵难愈。舌苔白腻，脉滑或濡。

Therapeutic methods: Eliminate wind, dissolve damp, clear heat and relieve accumulation.

治法：祛风化湿，清热散结。

Herbal formulas and drugs: The major formula is *Wind-Eliminating, Damp-Dissolving and Blood-Activating Decoction* (San Feng Chu Shi Huo Xue Tang). The commonly-used herbal drugs are *Rhizoma seu Radix Notopterygii* (Qiang Huo), *Radix*

方药：代表方为散风除湿活血汤，常用药如羌活、独活、防风、鸡血藤、忍冬藤、当归、川芎、赤芍、红花、前胡、枳壳、炙甘草等。

Angelicae Pubescentis (Du Huo), *Radix Ledebouriellae* (Fang Feng), *Caulis Spatholobi* (ji xue teng), *Caulis Lonicerae* (Ren Dong Teng), *Radix Angelicae Sinensis* (Dang Gui), *Rhizoma Ligustici Chuanxiong* (Chuan Xiong), *Radix Paeoniae Rubra* (Chi Shao), *Flos Carthami* (Hong Hua), *Radix Peucedani* (Qian Hu), *Fructus Aurantii* (Zhi Ke), *Radix Glycyrrhizae Praeparata* (Zhi Gan Cao), etc.

Modification according to symptoms: For fire-type particles with obvious redness, subtract some pungent, warm and wind-eliminating drugs, and add *Cortex Moutan Radicis* (Mu Dan Pi) and *Radix Salviae Miltiorrhizae* (Dan Shen) to cool blood, activate blood and dissolve stasis, or add *Cortex Mori Radicis* (Sang Bai Pi) and *Cortex Lycii Radicis* (Di Gu Pi) to purify lung and reduce heat. For aching and pain of joints, and swelling and distension of joints, add *Herba Siegesbeckiae* (Xi Xian Cao), *Radix Gentianae Macrophyllae* (Qin Jiao), *Caulis Trachelospermi* (Luo Shi Teng) and *Cortex Erythriniae* (Hai Tong Pi), to eliminate wind-damp and dredge meridians and collaterals.

加减：火疳红赤甚者，可去方中部分辛温祛风之品，选加牡丹皮、丹参以凉血活血消瘀，加桑白皮、地骨皮以清泻肺热；②若骨节酸痛，肢节肿胀者，可加豨签草、秦艽、络石藤、海桐皮等以祛风湿、通经络。

(4) **Insufficiency of lung yin**

Main symptoms: Repeated attacks of disease in the late stage, aching, pain and dryness of eye, lacrimation, blurring of vision, not very prominent nodules at eye white in deep-purple color, inobvious tenderness, dry mouth and throat, tidal fever, flushed cheeks, constipation, red tongue body with scanty fluid, and thready-rapid pulse.

Therapeutic methods: Nourish yin, purify lung and dissolve stasis.

Herbal formulas and drugs: The major formula is *Yin-Nourishing and Lung-Cleaning Decoction*

(4) **肺阴不足**

主症：病情反复发作，病至后期，眼感酸痛，干涩流泪，视物欠清，白睛结节不甚高隆，色紫暗，压痛不明显；口咽干燥，或潮热颧红，便秘不爽。舌红少津，脉细数。

治法：养阴清肺，兼以散结。

方药：代表方为养阴清肺汤，常用药如生地黄、麦门

(Yang Yin Qing Fei Tang). The commonly-used herbal drugs are *Radix Rehmanniae Cruda* (Sheng Di Huang), *Radix Ophiopogonis* (Mai Dong), *Radix Scrophulariae* (Xuan Shen), *Bulbus Fritillariae Cirrhosae* (Chuan Bei Mu), *Cortex Moutan Radicis* (Mu Dan Pi), *Herba Menthae* (Bo He), *Radix Paeoniae Alba* (Bai Shao), *Radix Glycyrrhizae Praeparata* (Zhi Gan Cao), etc.

冬、玄参、川贝母、牡丹皮、薄荷、白芍、炙甘草等。

Modification according to symptoms: For severe yin deficiency and fire hyperactivity, add *Rhizoma Anemarrhenae* (Zhi Mu) and *Cortex Lycii Radicis* (Di Gu Pi), to enhance the action to nourish yin and reduce fire. For intractable nodules at eye white for long time, apply *Radix Paeoniae Rubra* (Chi Shao) instead of *Radix Paeoniae Alba* (Bai Shao), and add *Radix Salviae Miltiorrhizae* (Dan Shen), *Radix Curcumae* (Yu Jin), *Spica Prunellae* (Xia Ku Cao) and *Concha Arcae* (Wa Leng Zi) accordingly, to clear heat and dissolve stasis.

加减：若阴虚火旺甚者，加知母、地骨皮以增滋阴降火之力；若白睛结节日久，难以消退者，以赤芍易方中白芍，酌加丹参、郁金、夏枯草、瓦楞子以清热消瘀散结。

3.3 Local therapy

3.3 局部治疗

3.3.1 Steroids: 0.5% Cortisone Acetate Eye Drop or 0.025% Dexamethasone Eye Drop is applied 4 to 6 times a day, or 1% Prednisone Eye Drop is applied 4 to 6 times a day. If iridocyclitis is complicated, antibiotic eye drop or heat-clearing and toxin-relieving eye drop is applied.

3.3.1 激素治疗：0.5%醋酸可的松滴眼液或0.025%地塞米松滴眼液，每日4～6次，或1%强的松龙滴眼液，每日4～6次滴眼。若并发瞳神紧小者，可同时选用抗生素眼液或清热解毒眼药水。

3.3.2 Suppplementary treatment

(1) Local heat compress or wet-heat compress with the herbal decoction is applied to relieve symptoms of eyes, promote qi and blood flow and shorten the course of disease.

(2) Mydriasis: If it is necessary, 1% Atropine Eye Drop or Ointment is applied for mydriasis, so as to pre-

3.3.2 辅助治疗

(1) 局部热敷或用内服药渣再煎水湿热敷，对减轻眼部症状，促进气血流畅，缩短病程有辅助作用。

(2) 散瞳：需及时滴1%阿托品滴眼液或眼膏扩瞳，以

vent the complications.

防并发症。

3.4 Other therapy

3.4 其他疗法

(1) Acupuncture: The points of Cuanzhu (BL 2), Jingming (BL 1), Sizhukong (TE 23), Chengqi (ST 1), Sibai (ST 2), Taiyang (EX-HN 5), Hegu (LI 4), Quchi (LI 11), Baihui (GV 20), etc. are selected. In each treatment, 3 to 5 points are applied alternately with reducing methods. For the excess heat pattern, the blood-letting method is applied on the points of Hegu (LI 4) and Taiyang (EX-HN 5). The treatment is given once a day, the needles are retained for 30 minutes, and the 10-day treatments make up a course.

(1) 针刺治疗:取攒竹、睛明、丝竹空、承泣、四白、太阳、合谷、曲池、百会等,每次选3～5穴,交替轮取,泻法为主;实热证明显者可于合谷、太阳点刺放血。每日1次,每次留针30分钟,10日为1个疗程。

(2) Oral administration of western medicine: For the cases with a more severe condition, the nonsteroidal anti-inflammatory drugs, such as Indomethacin, Phenylbutazone, etc., can be added. For the cases with a very severe condition, the glucocorticosteroids are added.

(2) 口服西药:对病情较严重者,应加服消炎痛、保泰松等非皮质类固醇消炎药;病情严重者,应加服糖皮质类固醇激素制剂。

4 Speculative map

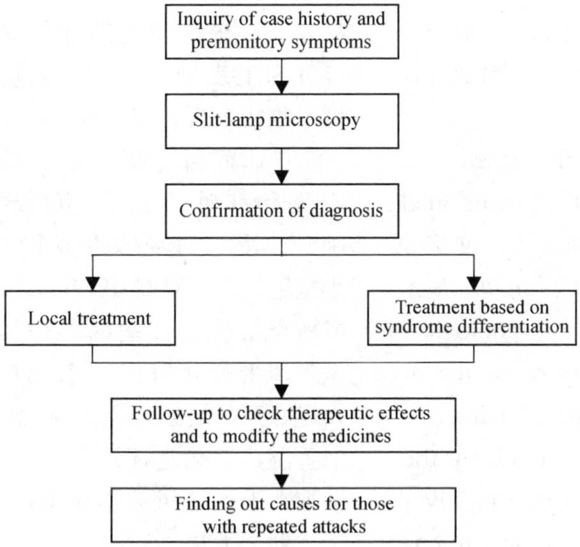

Inquiry of case history and premonitory symptoms
↓
Slit-lamp microscopy
↓
Confirmation of diagnosis
↓
Local treatment | Treatment based on syndrome differentiation
↓
Follow-up to check therapeutic effects and to modify the medicines
↓
Finding out causes for those with repeated attacks

4 思辨导图

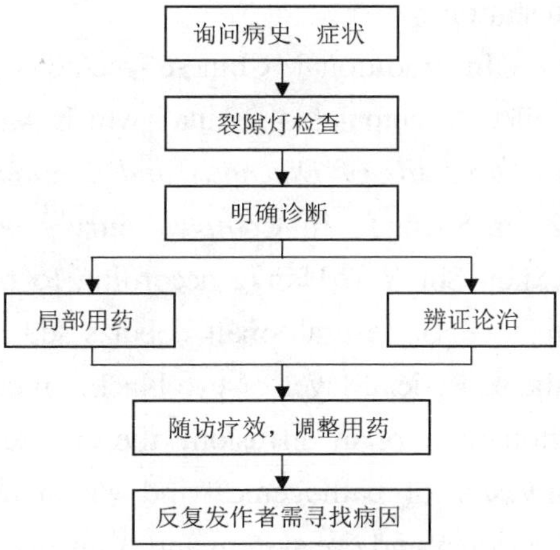

询问病史、症状
↓
裂隙灯检查
↓
明确诊断
↓
局部用药 | 辨证论治
↓
随访疗效,调整用药
↓
反复发作者需寻找病因

Chapter 4 Cornea Diseases

第 4 章 黑睛疾病

Viral keratitis

病毒性角膜炎

Viral keratitis is a kind of corneal immune reaction caused by infection of herpes simplex virus (HSV) of type I. The single eye is affected mostly, or the both eyes are affected simultaneously, or one eye is affected after another. After the first affection, the virus may lurk in the trigeminal ganglion and the corneal tissues for long time, so the repeated attacks of the disease occur when the body immunity is low. According to the affected areas, it is divided into epithelial type, matrix type and endothelial type, with different clinical manifestations.

In traditional Chinese medicine, the disease is called "accumulated nebula" which was first mentioned in *Standards of Diagnosis and Treatment* (Zheng Zhi Zhun Sheng). In *Complete Survey on Ophthalmology* (Shen Shi Yao Han), according to the morphological features of several small nebulas suddenly occurring at the superficial layer of eye black, in cluster, or in conglobation, or in diffusion, the disease is caused by the invasion of pathogenic wind which disturbs the Liver Meridian and eye system and transforms into heat to enter in the interior, manifested by astringent sensation

病毒性角膜炎为单纯疱疹病毒(herpes simplex virus, HSV)Ⅰ型感染而引发的角膜免疫反应。常单眼为患,亦可双眼同时或先后发生。由于病毒初次感染后在三叉神经节及角膜组织内可以长期潜伏,因而在机体抵抗力下降时易复发。根据侵犯的部位又可分为上皮型、基质型、内皮型。临床表现各有不同。

中医病名为聚星障,首载于《证治准绳》。其后《审视瑶函》依据黑睛浅层骤生多个细小星翳,其形或联缀,或团聚或散漫等变化多端的形态辨识为风邪侵扰肝经目系化热入里,患眼沙涩疼痛、羞明、流泪等湿热互患之证候与病机,治疗上沿用祛风清热除湿,扶正祛邪之大法。

and pain of eye, photophobia and lacrimation due to accumulated damp-heat. In the treatment, it is to apply the wind-eliminating, heat-clearing and damp-dissolving method and the Zheng (Anti-Pathogenic) Qi-strengthening and Xie (Pathogenic) Qi-removing method.

1 Etiology and pathogenesis

1.1 Invasion of exogenous pathogenic wind: It attacks the meridian and transforms into heat, disturbing upwards the wind wheel to cause nebula at the eye black.

1.2 Body constitution of internal damp-heat: Damp-heat blocks the spleen-earth, so the earth counter-acts on the wood, leading to abnormal fumigation and steaming on eye black.

1.3 Deficiency of both qi and yin: The pathogenic toxin avails the body of the opportunity of deficiency, leading to repeated attacks of the disease which lasts for long time and is difficult to be cured.

2 Diagnostic essentials

2.1 Clinical manifestations

Common cold in the early stage, or repeated attacks of the disease, astringent sensation and pain of eye, photophobia, lacrimation, difficulty to open eyes, and visual decrease of different degrees.

2.2 Ocular examinations

(1) Conjunctival ciliary congestion or mixed congestion.

(2) Slit-lamp microscopy

① Epithelial type: starred or dotted nebula at cornea, in cluster, or in arborization, or in geography, fluorescent staining positive. ② Matrix type: Nebula and edema at deep layer of cornea, in disc-shape, with depressed sensation at the diseased area, even corneal perforation. ③ Endothelial type: Corneal edema,

1 病因病机

1.1 风邪外袭，循经化热，上犯风轮，黑睛生翳而发病。

1.2 素体湿热内蕴，久困脾土，土反侮木，熏蒸黑睛。

1.3 气阴两虚，邪毒复陷，病情反复，或迁延难愈。

2 诊断要点

2.1 临床表现

初发有感冒史，或眼部反复发作史。眼部沙涩疼痛，畏光流泪，眼睑难睁，伴有不同程度视力下降。

2.2 眼部检查

(1) 程度不同的球结膜睫状充血或混合性充血。

(2) 裂隙灯显微镜下

①上皮型：角膜星点状混浊，相互融合成簇状或树枝状或地图状，荧光染色阳性；②基质型：角膜深层混浊水肿，状如圆盘，病变区知觉减退，可致角膜穿孔；③内皮型：角

thickening, aqueous flare, KP(+) complicated by iridocyclitis, leading to corneal diseases and intraocular pressure elevation.

膜水肿、增厚、房水闪辉、KP(+)并发瞳神紧小症,导致角膜病变、眼压升高。

3 Therapeutic methods

3 治疗方法

3.1 Therapeutic principles

3.1 治疗原则

It is to treat the virus in the early stage, while to apply both traditional Chinese medicine and western medicine in the late stage or for those with repeated attacks. It is also need to pay attention to the immunity adjustment.

初发以抗病毒为主,后期或复发者采用中西医结合治疗,注重免疫调节。

3.2 Treatment based on syndrome differentiation

3.2 辨证论治

(1) **Invasion of exogenous pathogenic wind, transforming to heat along meridian**

(1) **风邪外袭,循经化热**

Main symptoms: Aversion to cold, fever, nasal obstruction, sore throat, astringent sensation and pain of the sick eye, photophobia, lacrimation, conjunctival ciliary congestion, dotted or starred nebula at the superficial layer of cornea, more or less, sparse or dense, red tongue body with thin-yellow tongue coating, superficial-rapid or wiry-rapid pulse.

主症:恶风发热,鼻塞、咽痛;患眼涩痛,畏光、流泪,球结膜睫状充血,角膜浅层点状星翳,或多或少,或疏散或密聚。舌质红,苔薄黄,脉浮数或弦数。

Therapeutic methods: Eliminate wind, clear heat, purify liver and reduce fire.

治法:疏风散热,清肝泻火。

Herbal formulas and drugs: The major formula is *Notoptreygium Wind-Eliminating Decoction* (Qiang Huo Sheng Feng Tang) plus *Gentian Liver-Draining Decoction* (Long Dan Xie Gan Tang). The commonly-used herbal drugs are *Rhizoma seu Radix Notopterygii* (Qiang Huo), *Radix Angelicae Dahuricae* (Bai Zhi), *Radix Bupleuri* (Chai Hu), *Radix Platycodi* (Jie Geng), *Herba Schizonepetae* (Jing Jie), *Radix Gentianae* (Long Dan Cao), *Fructus Gardeniae* (Zhi Zi), *Radix Scutellariae* (Huang Qin), *Radix Angelicae Sinensis* (Dang Gui), *Radix Rehmanniae Cruda* (Sheng Di Huang),

方药:代表方为羌活胜风汤合龙胆泻肝汤,常用药如羌活、白芷、柴胡、桔梗、荆芥、龙胆草、栀子、黄芩、当归、生地等。

etc.

Modification according to symptoms: For difficulty to open eyes, photophobia and excessive tears, add *Fructus Viticis* (Man Jing Zi), *Radix Ledebouriellae* (Fang Feng) and *Folium Mori* (Sang Ye), to purify liver and brighten eyes. For more obvious corneal congestion and edema, add *Cortex Moutan Radicis* (Mu Dan Pi), *Radix Isatidis* (Ban Lan Gen), *Folium Isatidis* (Da Qing Ye) and *Radix Arnebiae seu Lithospermi* (Zi Cao), to cool blood and relieve toxin. For yellow and red urine, add *Herba Dianthi* (Qu Mai) and *Herba Polygoni Avicularis* (Bian Xu), to promote urination.

加减：眼睑难睁、怕光、多泪者，加蔓荆子、防风、桑叶以清肝明目；角膜水肿，充血明显者可加牡丹皮、板蓝根、大青叶、紫草凉血解毒；小便黄赤者，可加瞿麦、萹蓄以清利小便。

(2) **Stickiness and stagnation of damp-heat, conflict between the Zheng (Anti-Pathogenic) and Xie (Pathogenic) Qi**

(2) **湿热黏滞，正邪相搏**

Main symptoms: Warm and sticky tears from the sick eye, mixed congestion of bulbar conjunctiva, corneal nebula in geography, or nebula at the deep layer of cornea in disc-shape, swelling and white-color, or prolonged disease with repeated attacks, accompanied by heavy sensation in head, stuffy chest, stickiness in mouth, poor appetite, abdominal distension, loose feces, red tongue body with yellow-sticky tongue coating, and soft-rapid pulse.

主症：患眼泪热胶黏，球结膜混合型充血，角膜翳障，状若地图，或角膜深层翳如圆盘，肿胀色白；或病情缠绵，反复发作；伴头重胸闷，口黏纳呆，腹满便溏。舌质红，苔黄腻，脉濡数。

Therapeutic methods: Clear heat, dissolve damp, strengthen Zheng (Anti-pathogenic) Qi and remove Xie (Pathogenic) Qi.

治法：清热化湿，扶正祛邪。

Herbal formulas and drugs: The major formula is *Three Seeds Decoction* (San Ren Tang). The commonly-used herbal drugs are *Semen Armeniacae Amarum* (Ku Xing Ren), *Semen Amomi Cardamomi* (Bai Dou Kou Ren), *Semen Coicis* (Yi Yi Ren), *Rhizoma Pinelliae* (Ban Xia), *Cortex Magnoliae Officinalis* (Hou Pu), *Talcum* (Hua Shi), *Herba Lophatheri* (Dan Zhu Ye),

方药：代表方为三仁汤，常用药如苦杏仁、白豆寇仁、薏苡仁、半夏、厚朴、滑石、淡竹叶、通草等。

Medulla Tetrapanacis (Tong Cao), etc.

Modification according to symptoms: For focal turbidity, add *Radix Scutellariae* (Huang Qin), *Semen Dolichoris Album* (Bai Bian Dou) and *Cortex Magnoliae Officinalis* (Hou Pu), to clear heat and dissolve damp. For severe congestion and pain, add *Rhizoma Coptidis* (Huang Lian), *Folium Isatidis* (Da Qing Ye), *Radix Paeoniae Rubra* (Chi Shao) and *Herba Violae* (Zi Hua Di Ding), to clear heat and relieve toxin. For prolonged disease, add *Radix Astragali* (Huang Qi), *Radix Ophiopogonis* (Mai Dong), *Radix Codonopsis Pilosulae* (Dang Shen), *Radix Ledebouriellae* (Fang Feng) and *Radix Glycyrrhizae* (Gan Cao), to benefit and nourish yin so as to strengthen Zheng (Anti-Pathogenic) Qi.

加减：病灶污秽者，加黄芩、白扁豆、厚朴清热除湿；充血、疼痛为甚者，加黄连、大青叶、赤芍、紫花地丁以清热解毒；病程迁延者，加黄芪、麦门冬、党参、防风、甘草益气养阴以扶正。

(3) **Deficiency of both qi and yin, deep retention of pathogenic toxin**

(3) **气阴两虚，邪毒复陷**

Main symptoms: Dry, astringent and uncomfortable sensation inside eye, mild photophobia, slight ciliary congestion, repeated attacks of corneal nebula which lasts for long time and is difficult to be cured, alternate new and old nebulas, accompanied by dry throat, fatigue, catching cold easily, red tongue body with scanty fluid, thready or thready-rapid pulse.

主症：眼内干涩不适，怕光较轻，睫状充血轻微，角膜翳障时发，迁延不愈；新旧翳障相间，或伴咽干咽燥；易疲劳感，易感冒。舌红少津，脉细或细数。

Therapeutic methods: Benefit qi, nourish yin, relieve toxin and remove nebula.

治法：益气养阴，解毒退翳。

Herbal formulas and drugs: The major formula is *Jade Screen Powder* (Yu Ping Feng San) plus *Crude and Prepared Rehmannia Pills* (Sheng Shu Di Huang Wan). The commonly-used herbal drugs are *Radix Astragali* (Huang Qi), *Rhizoma Atractylodis Macrocephalae* (Bai Zhu), *Radix Ledebouriellae* (Fang Feng), *Radix Rehmanniae Praeparata* (Shu Di Huang), *Radix Rehmanniae Cruda* (Sheng Di Huang), *Herba Dendrobii* (Shi Hu), *Radix Achyranthis Bidentatae* (Niu Xi), *Fructus*

方药：代表方为玉屏风散合生熟地黄丸，常用药如黄芪、白术、防风、熟地黄、生地黄、石斛、牛膝、枳壳、苦杏仁、羌活、菊花等。

Aurantii (Zhi Ke), *Semen Armeniacae Amarum* (Ku Xing Ren), *Rhizoma seu Radix Notopterygii* (Qiang Huo), *Flos Chrysanthemi* (Ju Hua), etc.

Modification according to symptoms: Add *Flos Chrysanthemi Indici* (Ye Ju Hua), *Folium Isatidis* (Da Qing Ye) and *Cortex Fraxini* (Qin Pi) to clear heat and relieve toxin. For more obvious congestion, add *Rhizoma Anemarrhenae* (Zhi Mu) and *Cortex Phellodendri* (Huang Bo) to nourish yin and reduce fire. Add *Radix Arnebiae seu Lithospermi* (Zi Cao), *Periostracum Cicadae* (Chan Tui) and *Herba Equiseti Hiemalis* (Mu Zei) to remove nebula and brighten eyes.

加减:加野菊花、大青叶、秦皮等清热解毒;充血较明显者,加知母、黄柏以滋阴降火,紫草、蝉蜕、木贼退翳明目。

3.3 Etiological therapy

(1) Antiviral eye drop or gelatin as the preferred treatment: Apply 0.1% Acyclovir Eye Drop, or 0.05% Ancitabine Eye Drop, or Ganciclovir Eye Gelatin, or Recombinant Interferon α2b Eye Drop.

(2) Oral administration of antiviral medicines: Apply Acyclovir Pills, 5 times a day and 200 mg each time continuously for 2 weeks.

(3) Intravenous injection of antiviral medicines for severe cases: Apply 750 mg Acyclovir, once a day continuously for 7 to 10 days.

3.3 病因治疗

(1) 首选抗病毒滴眼液或凝胶:0.1%阿昔洛韦滴眼液,或0.05%环胞苷滴眼液、更昔洛韦眼用凝胶、重组人干扰素α2b滴眼液。

(2) 抗病毒药物口服,阿昔洛韦片,每日5次,每次200 mg,连服2周。

(3) 严重者,静脉滴注抗病毒药物:阿昔洛韦750 mg,每日1次,用药7～10日。

3.4 Supplementary therapies

(1) Mydriasis: It is to avoid complicated iridocyclitis. Apply 1% Atropine Sulfate Eye Drop or Eye Gelatin, or apply Tropicamide Eye Drop for a short-term effect.

(2) Fumigation or wet-warm compress with herbal decoction: The herbal drugs are *Flos Lonicerae* (Jin Yin Hua), *Fructus Forsythiae* (Lian Qiao), *Herba Taraxaci* (Pu Gong Ying), *Folium Isatidis* (Da Qing Ye), *Herba Menthae* (Bo He),

3.4 辅助治疗

(1) 散瞳:避免并发瞳神紧小症。1%硫酸阿托品滴眼液或眼用凝胶,短效剂选用托吡卡胺滴眼液。

(2) 中药煎剂熏洗或湿热敷:金银花、连翘、蒲公英、大青叶、薄荷、紫草、柴胡、秦皮、黄芩等过滤药汁后,待微温时冲洗眼部;或以毛巾浸

Radix Arnebiae seu Lithospermi (Zi Cao), *Radix Bupleuri* (Chai Hu), *Cortex Fraxini* (Qin Pi), *Radix Scutellariae* (Huang Qin), etc. After filtration and cooling, the decoction is applied to wash the eye. Or a towel is soaked in the decoction when it is warm and compressed on the eye, 2 to 3 times a day.

泡后湿热敷眼部,每日2～3次。

(3) Patent herbal medicines: Apply Instant Granules of Resisting Virus for those caused by pathogenic wind-heat, and apply *Bezoare Toxin-Relieving Bolus* (Niu Huang Jie Du Wan) for those caused by liver fire.

(3) 中成药治疗:风热所致者可用抗病毒冲剂,肝火所致者可用牛黄解毒丸。

(4) Disciform corneal diseases: For those with unobvious fluorescent staining, add glucocorticoids for local area on the basis of enough antiviral medicines, as 0.02% Fluorometholone Eye Drop. But it is necessary to observe carefully the focal changes.

(4) 盘状角膜病变,荧光染色不明显者,可在足量抗病毒药物治疗前提下,局部加用糖皮质激素,如滴用0.02%氟米龙滴眼液等,但需密切观察病灶变化。

(5) Acupuncture: The points are Jingming (BL 1), Sibai (ST 2), Sizhukong (TE 23), Cuanzhu (BL 2), Hegu (LI 4), Zusanli (ST 36), Guangming (GB 37), Ganshu (BL 18), etc. In each treatment, 2 local points and 2 distant points are selected to apply in alternation, with reinforcing or reducing methods according to the deficiency or excess pattern of the disease.

(5) 针刺治疗:可选用睛明、四白、丝竹空、攒竹、合谷、足三里、光明、肝俞等穴,每次局部取2穴,远端取2穴,交替使用,根据病情虚实酌情使用补泻手法。

3.5 Treatment for complications

For those with risk of corneal perforation, apply the amniotic membrane transplantation and conjunctival flap covering surgery. For those with the corneal leukoma, that influences the vision, left after the cure of disease, apply deep lamellar endothelial keratoplasty.

3.5 并发症治疗

有角膜穿孔危险者选用羊膜移植术、结膜瓣遮盖术;病愈后遗留白斑影响视力者可采用深板层角膜移植术等。

4 Speculative map

Inquiry of case history and premonitory symptoms
↓
Visual examination and slit-lamp microscopy
↓
Confirmation of diagnosis
↓
Local antiviral treatment | Treatment based on syndrome differentiation
↓
Follow-up to check therapeutic effects and modify medicines
↓
Prevention of recurrence

4 思辨导图

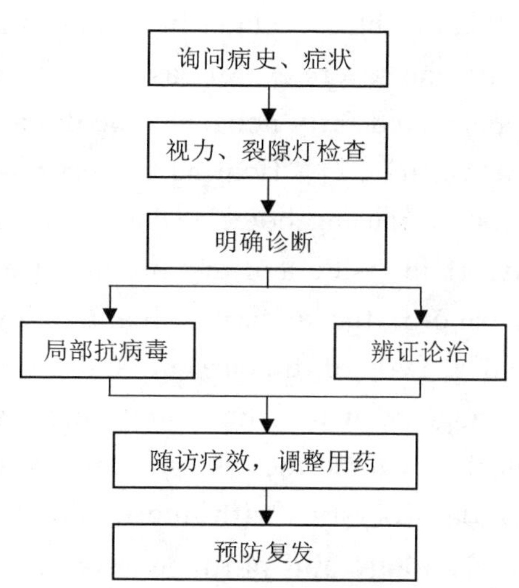

Bacterial keratitis

Bacterial keratitis is a kind of acute purulent keratitis due to bacterial infection, often seen in the condition of traumatic injury of cornea or after corneal foreign body removal. The factors, such as contact lens, trichiasis, xerophthalmia, etc., which influence the integrity of the corneal epithelium are the incentives of the disease. The commonly-seen bacteria are staphylococcus, pneumococcus, streptococcus, pseudomonas aeruginosa, bifidobacterium, etc. existing in the natural environment. The treacherous condition is pseudomonas aeruginosa infection which rapidly causes corneal ulcers, even

细菌性角膜炎

细菌性角膜炎指细菌感染引起的急性化脓性角膜炎症，常见于角膜外伤或角膜异物剔除术后，接触镜、倒睫、干眼等影响角膜上皮完整的因素均是造成此病的诱因。常见致病菌为自然环境下生存的葡萄球菌、肺炎球菌、链球菌、绿脓杆菌、双歧杆菌等，较为凶险的绿脓杆菌感染可迅速地导致角膜溃疡，甚至穿孔、眼内炎。延误

perforation and entophthalmia. The delayed or improper treatment may cause retained scar to further influence the vision.

或不当处理均可遗留瘢痕而影响视力。

In traditional Chinese medicine, the disease is called eye black nebula in creamy shape, while the acute and severe eye disease with hypopyon is called "coagulated fatty nebula". The disease is manifested by "fattiness", "floating", "crispiness", "tenderness", "causing hole, leakage, iridoptosis, ulcerative fluid inside and dry prominence outside". Furthermore, the disease is featured by quick change and growth of the urgent and risky disease. The pathogenic wind, heat and toxin attack the eye black to caused the disease in the condition of original dacryocystitis with internal hidden toxin.

中医学将此类表现为黑睛生翳,状如凝脂,伴有黄液上冲的急重眼病归属于"凝脂翳"。并用黑睛面"肥""浮""脆""嫩""甚则为窟、为漏、为蟹睛,内溃睛膏,外为枯凸",且善变而速长的表象,归纳了病变急危的特征,强调风热邪毒触染黑睛;或素有漏睛,邪毒内伏,乘伤侵袭致病。

1 Etiology and pathogenesis

1 病因病机

1.1 Injury of wind wheel, pathogenic wind, heat and toxin attacking eye black: Due to original dacryocystitis with internal hidden toxin, the wind wheel is infected.

1.1 风轮受袭,风热邪毒乘袭于黑睛;或素有漏睛,伏邪壅盛,风轮不慎被染。

1.2 Qi and yin deficiency after chronic disease: Due to insufficiency of Zheng (Anti-Pathogenic) Qi and retention of exogenous pathogens, the wind wheel is attacked by the pathogens which cause prolonged and incurable ulcers.

1.2 久病之后气虚阴伤:正气不足,外邪滞留,或致风轮受邪溃陷,缠绵不愈。

2 Diagnostic essentials

2 诊断要点

2.1 Case history of traumatic injury of cornea, or dacryocystitis or contact lens.

2.1 角膜外伤或泪囊炎或佩戴接触镜等病史。

2.2 Clinical manifestations

2.2 临床表现

Sudden pain occurring at the eye, photophobia, lacrimation, accompanied by purulent discharge, and visual decrease of different degrees.

眼部突然疼痛,畏光流泪,伴脓性分泌物,视力不同程度下降。

2.3 Ocular examinations

Spasm and edema of eyelid, and mixed congestions of cornea; yellow-white compact and infiltrative focus at the cornea, with fuzzy boundary and covered by necrotic tissue; the positive fluorescent staining, complicated by anterior chamber inflammatory exudation or hypopyon.

3 Therapeutic methods

3.1 Therapeutic principles

For the disease caused by heat-toxin burning fluid to form up purulence and ulcers, apply the therapeutic principles "to reduce it for excess" and "to cool it for heat", by focusing on the liver to eliminate the pathogens and brighten the eyes and to prevent the progression of disease.

3.2 Treatment based on syndrome differentiation

(1) **Heat-toxin accumulation and excess**

Main symptoms: Pain at head and eyes, photophobia, lacrimation, visual decrease, redness of eye white, star-like and grey-white nebula with fuzzy boundary and covered by thin fatty tissue at the eye black, accompanied by fever, thirst, dark urine, constipation, red tongue body with yellow tongue coating, and rapid pulse.

Therapeutic methods: Clear heat and relieve toxin.

Herbal formulas and drugs: The major formula is *Lonicera Detoxifying Decoction* (Yin Hua Jie Du Tang). The commonly-used herbal drugs are *Flos Lonicerae* (Jin Yin Hua), *Herba Violae* (Zi Hua Di Ding), *Rhizoma Coptidis* (Huang Lian), *Fructus Forsythiae* (Lian Qiao), *Spica Prunellae* (Xia Ku

2.3 眼部检查

眼睑痉挛水肿，结膜混合性充血。角膜黄白色致密浸润病灶，边界模糊，上覆坏死组织；荧光素染色阳性，并发前房炎性渗出或积脓。

3 治疗方法

3.1 治疗原则

针对热毒灼津，蓄腐成脓而溃的病变，采用“实者泻之”“热者寒之”的治疗原则，多从肝论治，驱邪明目，以防其变化。

3.2 辨证论治

（1）**热毒壅盛**

主症：头目疼痛，羞明流泪，视力减退，抱轮红赤，黑睛生翳如星，色呈灰白，边缘不清，上覆薄脂；可伴发热口渴、溲赤便秘。舌质红，苔黄，脉数。

治法：清热解毒。

方药：代表方为银花解毒汤，常用药如金银花、紫花地丁、黄连、连翘、夏枯草、茯苓、牡丹皮等。

Cao), *Sclerotium Poriae* (Fu Ling), *Cortex Moutan Radicis* (Mu Dan Pi), etc.

Modification according to symptoms: For the disease in the early stage, add *Fructus Viticis* (Man Jing Zi), *Herba Schizonepetae* (Jing Jie) and *Radix Ledebouriellae* (Fang Feng) to eliminate wind and clear heat. For severe redness, hotness, swelling and pain of eye, add *Cortex Moutan Radicis* (Mu Dan Pi), *Radix Scrophulariae* (Xuan Shen), *Resina Olibani* (Ru Xiang) and *Myrrha* (Mo Yao) to cool blood and dissolve stasis. Add *Radix Trichosanthis* (Tian Hua Fen), *Gypsum Fibrosum Cruda* (Sheng Shi Gao) and *Natrii Sulfas* (Mang Xiao) to enhance the actions to clear heat, produce fluid, reduce fire and unblock the fu organs.

加减：如疾病初起者，可加蔓荆子、荆芥、防风疏风清热；眼赤热肿痛较重者，可加牡丹皮、玄参、乳香、没药以凉血化瘀；加天花粉、生石膏、芒硝，以增清热生津、泻火通腑之功。

(2) **Zheng (Anti-Pathogenic) Qi deficiency and Xie (Pathogenic) Qi retention**

(2) **正虚邪恋**

Main symptoms: Decrease of eye pain and photophobia, dry and astringent sensation inside eye, slight redness at eye white, ulcers at eye black, thinner fatty tissue which is unhealed for long time, accompanied by dry mouth and throat, lassitude, loose feces, red tongue body and thready-rapid pulse, or pale tongue body and weak pulse.

主症：眼痛羞明减轻，眼内干涩，抱轮微红，黑睛溃陷，凝脂减薄，但日久不敛；常伴口燥咽干，体倦便溏。舌红脉细数，或舌淡脉弱。

Therapeutic methods: Strengthen Zheng (Anti-Pathogenic) Qi and eliminate Xie (Pathogenic) Qi.

治法：扶正祛邪。

Herbal formulas and drugs: For yin deficiency, the major formula is *Yin-Nourishing and Nebula-Removing Decoction* (Zi Yin Tui Yi Tang) or *Sea Treasure and Rehmannia Powder* (Hai Zang Di Huang San). The commonly-used herbal drugs are *Rhizoma Anemarrhenae* (Zhi Mu), *Radix Scrophulariae* (Xuan Shen), *Radix Rehmanniae Cruda* (Sheng Di Huang), *Radix Rehmanniae Praeparata*

方药：偏于阴虚者以滋阴退翳汤或海藏地黄散为代表方；常用药如知母、玄参、生熟地黄、当归、麦门冬、白蒺藜、菊花、青葙子、蝉蜕、谷精草、木贼、黄连等。偏于气虚者以托里消毒散去陈皮，加蝉蜕、木贼、白蒺藜等。

(Shu Di Huang), *Radix Angelicae Sinensis* (Dang Gui), *Radix Ophiopogonis* (Mai Dong), *Fructus Tribuli* (Bai Ji Li), *Flos Chrysanthemi* (Ju Hua), *Semen Celosiae* (Qing Xiang Zi), *Periostracum Cicadae* (Chan Tui), *Eriocaulon Buergerianum* (Gu Jing Cao), *Herba Equiseti Hiemalis* (Mu Zei), *Rhizoma Coptidis* (Huang Lian), etc. For qi deficiency, the major formula is *Interior-Supporting and Detoxifying Powder* (Tuo Li Xiao Du San), by subtracting *Pericarpium Citri Tangerinae* (Chen Pi) and adding *Periostracum Cicadae* (Chan Tui), *Herba Equiseti Hiemalis* (Mu Zei), *Fructus Tribuli* (Bai Ji Li), etc.

3.3 Etiological therapies

Apply the medicines according to the pathogenic bacteria and drug sensitivity results. The application of the medicines should be maintained for a period of time after the control of the condition.

(1) Frequent application of high-concentration spectrum antibiotics: 0.5% Ofloxacin Eye Drop is applied once every 15 to 30 minutes. For severe cases, it is applied once every 5 minutes in the first 30 minutes, and less frequently after the control of the condition. The antibiotic eye ointment is applied at night.

(2) For the cases with severe infection complicated with panophthalmitis, or the cases of secondary condition due to perforating wound of eye, the general antibiotic treatment is applied.

3.4 Supplementary therapies

(1) Mydriasis for prevention of complicated iris inflammatory reaction: Tropicamide Eye Drop is applied.

(2) Acupuncture: The points are Hegu (LI 4),

3.3 病因治疗

原则上根据病原菌及药敏结果用药。病情控制后，需维持一段时间。

(1) 高浓度广谱抗生素眼液频点：如0.5%氧氟沙星每15～30分钟一次。严重者可在前30分钟内，每5分钟一次，病情控制后，逐渐减少用药次数。抗生素眼膏夜间使用。

(2) 感染严重，可能并发全眼球炎者，或继发于眼球穿通伤后患者，予以全身抗生素治疗。

3.4 辅助治疗

(1) 散瞳以预防并发的虹膜炎性反应：托品卡胺眼药。

(2) 针灸：取合谷、曲池、

Quchi (LI 11), Taiyang (EX-HN 5), Cuanzhu (BL 2), Taichong (LR 3), etc., to relieve pain of eye.

太阳、攒竹、太冲等穴缓解眼部疼痛。

(3) Patent herbal medicines: For those with manifestations of wind-heat, apply *Lonicera and Forsythia Toxin-Relieving* (Yin Qiao Jie Du Pian). For those with severe heat-toxin, apply *Bezoare Toxin-Relieving Bolus* (Niu Huang Jie Du Wan).

(3) 中成药:有风热表现者可用银翘解毒片,热毒较重者用牛黄解毒丸。

3.5 Treatment for complications

3.5 并发症治疗

(1) Apply focal debridement and conjunctival flap covering surgery.

(1) 病灶清创联合结膜瓣遮盖术。

(2) For those with cornea to be ulcerated, apply lamellar keratoplasty or penetrating lamellar keratoplasty.

(2) 角膜将要溃破者,可采取板层角膜移植术或穿透性角膜移植术。

(3) For those with ulcerated cornea and eyeball proptosis, apply evisceration of eye.

(3) 角膜已经溃穿者,眼球内容物脱出,则须行眼内容物剜出术。

4 Speculative map

4 思辨导图

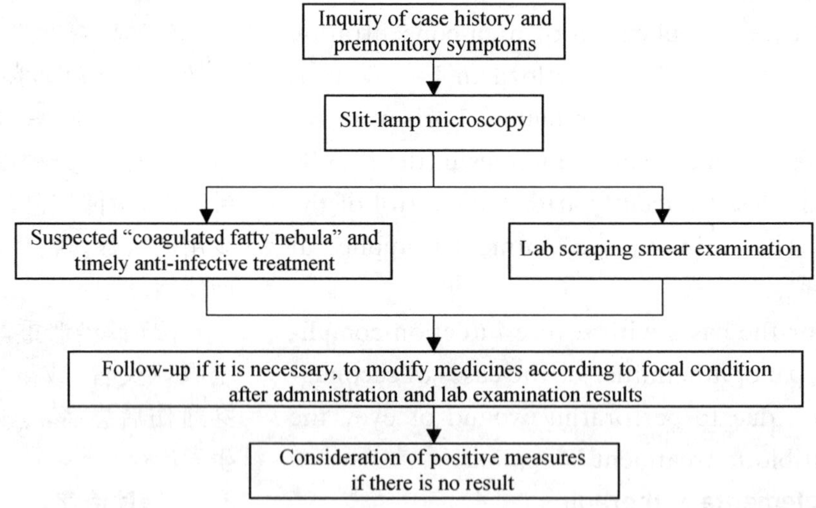

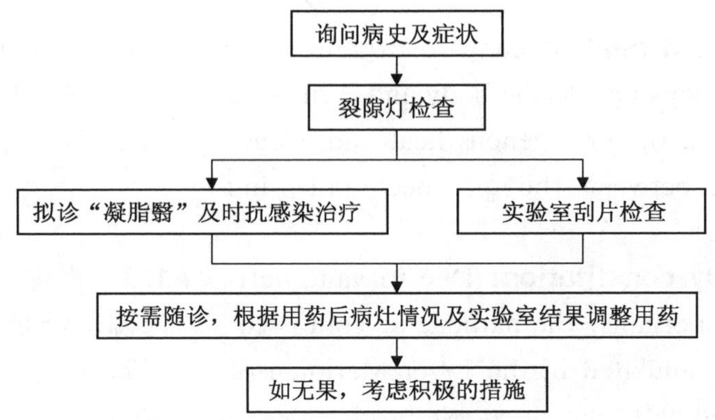

Mooren's Ulcus

蚕蚀性角膜溃疡

Mooren's Ulcus is a kind of chronic, progressive, spontaneous and marginal corneal ulcer, without confirmed causes. Possibly, the endogenous and exogenous incentives cause antigenic changes of cornea and conjunctiva, to touch off the immune stress reaction of the organism, leading to the progressive solution of cornea, conjunctiva and sclera. The both eyes may be affected one after the other.

蚕蚀性角膜溃疡是一种慢性、进行性、自发性、边缘性角膜溃疡。确切的病因不清，可能为内外诱因导致角膜与结膜的抗原性改变，触发机体的免疫应急反应，导致角膜、结膜、巩膜进行性溶解，双眼可先后发病。

In traditional Chinese medicine, the disease is called "petal nebula", manifested by eye pain, white-colored nebula suddenly occurring at the eye black, in basin-like and petal shape, nebula of whole eye blackoccurring, extensive scarring, and visual decrease, intractable and incurable.

本病相当于中医的“花翳白陷”，主症为，发病时眼痛，黑睛骤生白翳，四周高起，中间低陷，状如花瓣，最终花翳侵及整个黑睛，广泛结瘢而严重影响视力，顽固难愈。

1 Etiology and pathogenesis

1 病因病机

1.1 Invasion of exogenous wind-heat: It attacks the lung first and then the liver, because the metal is excessive and over-acts on the wood. The pathogenic heat attacks the wind wheel upwards along the

1.1 风热外袭，肺先受之，金盛克木，肺疾犯肝，邪热循经而上攻风轮。

meridian.

1.2 Accumulated heat in zang-fu organs: The exogenous pathogens invade the body and transform into heat, so both the endogenous heat and exogenous heat fight between the qi wheel and wind wheel.

1.2 脏腑积热，复感外邪，入里化热，邪热炽盛，内外相搏于气轮风轮间。

1.3 Weak body constitution: Due to yang deficiency of zang-fu organs, the pathogenic cold is coagulated and accumulated in the Liver Meridian of Foot-Jueyin, leading to nebula at eye black.

1.3 素体羸弱，脏腑阳虚，寒邪凝结足厥阴肝经，导致黑睛生翳。

2 Diagnostic essentials

2 诊断要点

2.1 History of chronic and progressive features.

2.1 慢性、进行性病史。

2.2 Pain, photophobia, lacrimation and blurred vision of the sick eye.

2.2 患眼疼痛、畏光、流泪，视物模糊。

2.3 Conjunctival and ciliary congestion, white and groove-like ulcers at the margin of cornea, gradually broadening and deepening, repeated occurrence of neovascularization; positive fluorescent staining at the ulcerative area during attacks.

2.3 球结膜睫状充血，角膜边缘片状白色伴沟形溃疡，逐渐扩展加深，反复呈现伴新生血管长入。发作时溃疡处荧光素染色呈阳性。

3 Therapeutic methods

3 治疗方法

3.1 Therapeutic principles

3.1 治疗原则

In the stage of attack, rapidly apply glucocorticoid or immunosuppressive agent to control the condition. In the stage of remission, apply the herbal medicine to regulate the body according to pattern identification, so as to improve the immune stress response. According to the theory of five wheels, the eye white pertains to the lung, while the eye black pertains to the liver. The lung disease involves the liver, so the pathogenic heat attack the eye black upwards along the meridian. Or the accumulated heat in the lung and liver causes ulcers of eye black, so it is advisable to apply the method to clear and

发病时快速用糖皮质激素或免疫抑制剂控制，缓解期中药辨证调理，改善免疫应急。按五轮学说，白睛属肺，黑睛属肝，肺疾犯肝，邪热循经而上攻黑睛；或肺肝积热，黑睛溃陷，故以清泻肺肝之热为要，佐以调理气机。

reduce heat in the lung and liver, and to assist the method to regulate and adjust qi activities.

3.2 Treatment based on syndrome differentiation

(1) Wind-heat in lung and liver

Main symptoms: Blurring of vision, astringent sensation, pain, photophobia, lacrimation, redness of eye white, sudden occurrence of white nebula at the margin of eye black, gradually broadening in a basin shape, redness of tip and edges of tongue, thin-yellow tongue coating, and superficially-rapid pulse.

Therapeutic methods: Eliminate wind and clear heat.

Herbal formulas and drugs: The major formula is *Liver-Restoring Powder in Addition* (Jia Wei Xiu Gan San). The commonly-used herbal drugs are *Rhizoma seu Radix Notopterygii* (Qiang Huo), *Herba Ephedrae* (Ma Huang), *Herba Schizonepetae* (Jing Jie), *Herba Menthae* (Bo He), *Radix Ledebouriellae* (Fang Feng), *Fructus Gardeniae* (Zhi Zi), *Radix Scutellariae* (Huang Qin), *Fructus Forsythiae* (Lian Qiao), *Radix et Rhizoma Rhei* (Da Huang), *Flos Chrysanthemi* (Ju Hua), *Herba Equiseti Hiemalis* (Mu Zei), *Fructus Tribuli* (Bai Ji Li), *Radix Angelicae Sinensis* (Dang Gui), *Rhizoma Ligustici Chuanxiong* (Chuan Xiong), *Radix Paeoniae Rubra* (Chi Shao), *Radix Glycyrrhizae* (Gan Cao), etc.

Modification according to symptoms: For redness at eye white, add *Cortex Mori Radicis* (Sang Bai Pi) to enhance the action to clear heat in lung. For gradual growth of nebula at eye black, add *Radix Gentianae* (Long Dan Cao), to enhance the ac-

3.2 辨证论治

(1) 肺肝风热

主症：患眼视物模糊，碜涩疼痛，畏光流泪，抱轮红赤，黑睛边际骤生白翳，渐渐扩大，四周高起，中间低陷。舌边尖红，苔薄黄，脉浮数。

治法：疏风清热。

方药：代表方为加味修肝散，常用药如羌活、麻黄、荆芥、薄荷、防风、栀子、黄芩、连翘、大黄、菊花、木贼、白蒺藜、当归、川芎、赤芍、甘草等。

加减：白睛混赤者，可加桑白皮以助清肺热；黑睛生翳渐大者，加龙胆草以助清肝热。

tion to clear heat in liver.

(2) **Excessive heat in fu organs**

Main symptoms: Visual decrease, severe pain at head and eye, astringent sensation, photophobia, frequent lacrimation with warm tears, redness and swelling of eyelid, redness at eye white, yellow-colored and ulcerative nebula at eye black, rapidly attacking the whole eye black from periphery and covering the pupil, or hypopyon, iridocyclitis, mostly accompanied by fever, thirst, yellow urine, constipation, red tongue body with yellow tongue coating, and rapid-forceful pulse.

Therapeutic methods: Unblock fu organs and reduce heat.

Herbal formulas and drugs: The major formula is *Liver-Draining Decoction* (Xie Gan Tang). The commonly-used herbal drugs are *Radix Gentianae* (Long Dan Cao), *Radix Scutellariae* (Huang Qin), *Fructus Gardeniae* (Zhi Zi), *Radix et Rhizoma Rhei* (Da Huang), *Radix Bupleuri* (Chai Hu), *Herba Schizonepetae* (Jing Jie), *Radix Ledebouriellae* (Fang Feng), *Radix Angelicae Sinensis* (Dang Gui), *Pericarpium Citri Reticulatae Viride* (Qing Pi), *Herba Equiseti Hiemalis* (Mu Zei), *Fructus Tribuli* (Bai Ji Li), *Semen Cassiae* (Jue Ming Zi), etc.

Modification according to symptoms: For severe redness at eye white, add *Cortex Moutan Radicis* (Mu Dan Pi), *Radix Paeoniae Rubra* (Chi Shao) and *Spica Prunellae* (Xia Ku Cao) to clear heat, cool blood and relieve redness. For hypopyon, add *Fructus Gardeniae* (Zhi Zi), *Gypsum Fibrosum Cruda* (Sheng Shi Gao) and *Radix Trichosanthis* (Tian Hua Fen) in larger dose to clear heat and reduce fire.

(2) **腑热炽实**

主症：患眼视力下降，头目剧痛，碜涩畏光，热泪频流，胞睑红肿，白睛混赤，黑睛生翳色黄溃陷，从四周蔓生，迅速侵蚀整个黑睛，遮掩瞳神，或见黄液上冲、瞳神紧小；多伴发热口渴，溲黄便结。舌红苔黄，脉数有力。

治法：通腑泻热。

方药：代表方为泻肝汤，常用药如龙胆草、黄芩、栀子、大黄、柴胡、荆芥、防风、当归、青皮、木贼、白蒺藜、决明子等。

加减：白睛混赤严重者，可加牡丹皮、赤芍、夏枯草以清热凉血退赤；伴黄液上冲者，可加用且重用栀子、生石膏、天花粉以清热泄火。

(3) **Yang deficiency and cold coagulation**

Main symptoms: Visual decrease, dark-red colour of eye white, nebula with rodent ulcer at the margin of eye black, prolonged and incurable disease, accompanied by chills in four limbs, pale tongue body with no tongue coating or with white-slippery tongue coating, and deep-thready pulse.

Therapeutic methods: Warm yang and eliminate cold.

Herbal formulas and drugs: The major formula is *Angelica Counterflow Cold Decoction* (Dang Gui Si Ni Tang). The commonly-used herbal drugs are *Radix Angelicae Sinensis* (Dang Gui), *Ramulus Cinnamomi* (Gui Zhi), *Herba Asari* (Xi Xin), *Radix Paeoniae Alba* (Bai Shao), *Fructus Ziziphi Jujubae* (Da Zao), *Radix Glycyrrhizae Praeparata* (Zhi Gan Cao), *Rhizoma Zingiberis* (Gan Jiang), etc.

Modification according to symptoms: Add *Radix Salviae Miltiorrhizae* (Dan Shen) and *Flos Carthami* (Hong Hua) to activate blood and dredge vessels. For sudden occurrence of redness and itching, add *Herba Equiseti Hiemalis* (Mu Zei), *Periostracum Cicadae* (Chan Tui) and *Radix Ledebouriellae* (Fang Feng), to remove nebula and brighten eyes.

(3) **阳虚寒凝**

主症：患眼视力下降，白睛暗赤，黑睛缘生翳溃陷，状如蚕蚀，迁延不愈；或兼四肢不温；舌淡无苔或白滑苔，脉沉细。

治法：温阳散寒。

方药：代表方为当归四逆汤，常用药如当归、桂枝、细辛、白芍、大枣、炙甘草、干姜等。

加减：常于方中加丹参、红花以活血通脉；如赤痒突起者，加木贼、蝉蜕、防风以退翳明目。

3.3 Etiological therapies

Apply hormonal collagen enzyme inhibitors or immunosuppressive agent eye drop.

(1) Apply 0.02% to 1% Fluorometholone Eye Drop, or 2% Cysteic Acid Eye Drop, or 1% to 2% Cyclosporin A Eye Drop.

(2) For those with intractable condition, add

3.3 病因治疗

激素类胶原酶抑制剂或免疫抑制剂滴眼液。

(1) 0.02%～1%氟米龙滴眼液，2%半胱氢酸滴眼液，或1%～2%环孢霉素A油制剂。

(2) 病情顽固者可全身

50 mg cyclophosphamide to apply generally, three times a day by oral administration.

(3) Apply generally glucocorticoids, such as prednisone pills by gradually decrease of dose after the control of the condition.

加用环磷酰胺 50 毫克,每日 3 次口服。

(3) 全身应用糖皮质激素,如强的松片,待病情控制后逐渐减量。

3.4 Supplementary therapies

(1) Prevention of infection: 0.5% Levofloxacin Eye Drop or 0.3% Tobramycin Eye Drop, 3 to 4 times a day.

(2) Mydriatic Eye Drop or Eye Gelatin: Apply 1% Atropine Eye Drop or Eye Gelatin, to prevent papillary synechia caused by inflammation.

(3) Fumigation and wet-warm compress with herbal decoction: The herbal drugs are *Flos Lonicerae* (Jin Yin Hua), *Herba Taraxaci* (Pu Gong Ying), *Rhizoma Coptidis* (Huang Lian), *Radix Angelicae Sinensis* (Dang Gui), *Radix Ledebouriellae* (Fang Feng), *Semen Armeniacae Amarum* (Ku Xing Ren), *Radix Gentianae* (Long Dan Cao), etc. After filtration and cooling, apply the herbal decoction to wash or apply wet-warm compress on the eye, 3 to 4 times a day.

(4) Patent herbal medicines: For those with manifestations of wind-heat, apply *Lonicera and Forsythia Toxin-Relieving* (Yin Qiao Jie Du Pian). For those with severe heat-toxin, apply *Bezoare Toxin-Relieving Bolus* (Niu Huang Jie Du Wan).

(5) Surgery: Apply the improved circular cutting and scorching method on the ulcerative surface. Apply promptly the keratoplasty for corneal rupture or forthcoming corneal rupture.

3.4 辅助治疗

(1) 预防感染:0.5%左氧氟沙星滴眼液或0.3%妥布霉素滴眼液等,每日 3～4 次。

(2) 散瞳眼液或眼用凝胶:1%阿托品滴眼液或眼用凝胶,以防炎症导致瞳孔粘连。

(3) 中药煎剂熏眼及湿热敷:金银花、蒲公英、黄连、当归尾、防风、杏仁、龙胆草等水煎,过滤药汁,待温度适宜时熏眼,或作湿热敷,每日 3～4 次。

(4) 中成药治疗:有风热表现者可用银翘解毒片口服,热毒重者口服牛黄解毒丸。

(5) 手术:溃疡面可采用改良割烙术,角膜溃破或即将溃破者可及时行角膜移植术。

4 Speculative map

4 思辨导图

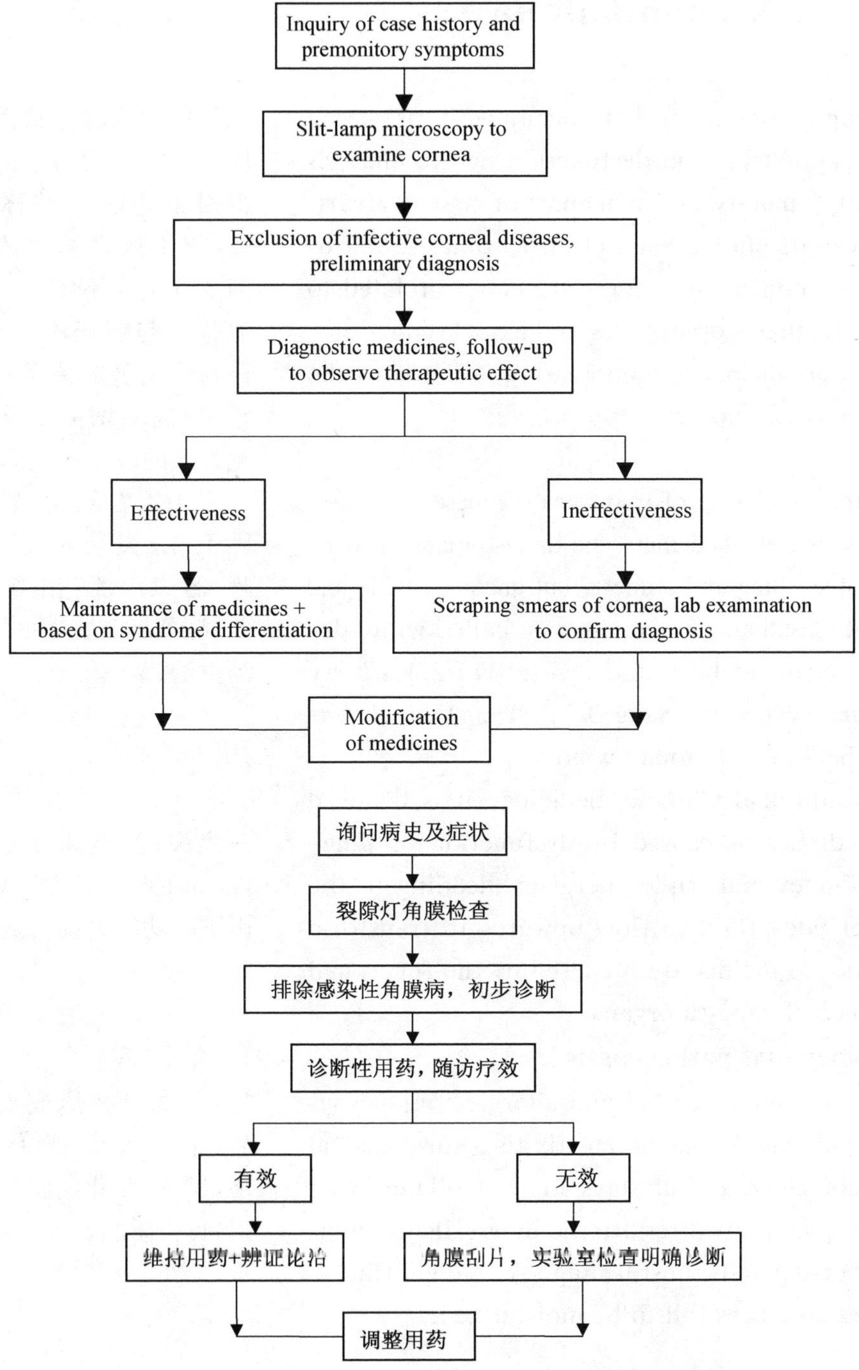

Xerophthalmia

干　眼　症

Xerophthalmia, or keratoconjunctivitis sicca, is a disease of tear film dysfunction due to changes of quantity, quality and dynamics of tears by various causes. Its etiology and classification are not uniform. Its clinical symptoms are closely related to ametropia, presbyopia, drug-induced lesion, etc. Recently, its incidence is increasing, related to the change of visual modes.

各种原因导致泪液量和质以及泪液动力学的改变使得泪膜功能异常称为干眼症，或干燥性结角膜炎。病因及分类尚不统一。其临床症状又与屈光不正、老视及药物性损害等关系密切。近年，发病率增高似乎又与视觉方式的改变相关。

In ancient classics of traditional Chinese medicine, the disease is described that "the disease manifested by absence of swelling and redness, but uncomfortable and astringent sensation, blurred vision, is called white-dry eye". It is said to be treated with *White Mulberry Radix-Bark Decoction* (Sang Bai Pi Tang) which acts to clear heat and eliminate wind.

中医古籍中描述的"不肿不赤，爽快不得，沙涩昏朦，名曰白涩"相当于本病，并提出以清热疏风之桑白皮汤主治。

In traditional Chinese medicine, it is believed that the disease is caused by dysfunction of lung, spleen, kidney and triple energizer, leading to the failure of body fluid to flow upwards to transform into tears. So the disease is caused by the functional disturbance of zang-fu organs.

中医学认为肺、脾、肾、三焦失运，至津液不能上承以为泪液之故，即认为本病由脏腑功能失调所致。

1　Etiology and pathogenesis

1　病因病机

1.1　After acute catarrhal and allergic conjunctivitis or epidemic keratoconjunctivitis, the residual heat is not cleared, but stays in the collaterals of lung and spleen. As a result, the lung fails to dominate dispersing and transforming. As the yin fluid is consumed, the eyes fail to be moisturized.

1.1　暴风客热或天行赤眼后，余热未清，隐伏肺脾之络，肺失宣化，加之阴液受损，目失濡润。

1.2 Due to failure of spleen in transporting, qi and blood fail to be produced and the Qing (Clear) Qi fails to ascend. As a result, the body fluid and blood fail to flow upwards to nourish the head and face, and the eyes fail to be nourished.

1.2 脾失健运，气血运化无源，清气不升，津血不能上荣头面，目窍失养。

1.3 Due to insufficiency of kidney, the kidney's transforming function is disturbed, leading to retention of water and distributive abnormality of water, so that the eyes fail to be moisturized.

1.3 肾阴不足，气化失司，水液潴留，输布异常，目失润泽。

2 Diagnostic essentials

2 诊断要点

2.1 Dry, astringent and uncomfortable sensations at eyes, itching and redness from time to time, frequent blinks, photophobia and eye fatigue.

2.1 眼部干涩不适，时痒时红，频频眨目，畏光疲劳。

2.2 Narrowness of lacrimal rivus, roughness of corneal epithelium, point-like positive of fluorescent staining, and sticky and silk-like discharge inside conjunctival sac.

2.2 泪河变窄，角膜上皮粗糙感，荧光素染色呈细点状阳性，结膜囊囊内黏丝样分泌物。

2.3 Schirmer I Test

Tear volume < 5 mm / 5 minutes. Break-up Time: BUT < 10 seconds.

2.3 Schirmer I 试验

泪液量<5 毫米/5 分钟。泪膜破裂时间:BUT<10 秒。

3 Therapeutic methods

3 治疗方法

3.1 Therapeutic principles

Treat the superficial symptoms by applying local medical therapy, while treat the root cause by pattern identification. Clinically, it is advisable to regulate the qi activities of the lung, spleen and kidney.

3.1 治疗原则

局部用药治其标，综合辨证治其本；临证以调理肺脾肾三脏气机为要。

3.2 Treatment based on syndrome differentiation

3.2 辨证论治

(1) **Lung failing to dominate dispersing and transforming**

(1) **肺失宣化**

Main symptoms: Dry, astringent and burning sensation inside eye, photophobia, lacrimation, absence of redness at eye white, lentigo at eye black,

主症：眼内干涩灼热，畏光流泪，白睛不红，黑睛着色；多兼体瘦面黄。舌淡红，

accompanied by thin body, sallow-yellow complexion, light-red tongue body with thin-white tongue coating, and thready pulse.

苔薄白,脉细。

Therapeutic methods: Eliminate wind, clear heat and disperse lung.

治法:疏风清热宣肺。

Herbal formulas and drugs: The major formula is *White Mulberry Radix-Bark Decoction* (Sang Bai Pi Tang). The commonly-used herbal drugs are *Cortex Mori Radicis* (Sang Bai Pi), *Cortex Lycii Radicis* (Di Gu Pi), *Radix Scutellariae* (Huang Qin), *Flos Inulae* (Xuan Fu Hua), *Sclerotium Poriae* (Fu Ling), *Rhizoma Alismatis* (Ze Xie), *Radix Scrophulariae* (Xuan Shen), *Radix Ophiopogonis* (Mai Dong), *Flos Chrysanthemi* (Ju Hua), *Radix Platycodi* (Jie Geng), *Radix Glycyrrhizae Praeparata* (Zhi Gan Cao), etc.

方药:代表方为桑白皮汤,常用药如桑白皮、地骨皮、黄芩、旋覆花、茯苓、泽泻、玄参、麦门冬、菊花、桔梗、炙甘草等。

Modification according to symptoms: Add *Semen Armeniacae Amarum* (Ku Xing Ren) to enhance the action to disperse the lung qi. For dry and astringe sensation, add *Rhizoma Polygonati Odorati* (Yu Zhu) to nourish yin and produce fluid.

加减:可加杏仁与方中桔梗合用宣肺气;干涩不爽加玉竹养阴生津。

(2) **Spleen failing to dominating transportation and transformation**

(2) **脾失运化**

Main symptoms: Photophobia, lacrimation, dryness and astringe sensation of eye white, corneal opacity or ulcer, accompanied by thin body, bulging distension or even prominent veins of abdomen, low spirit or restlessness and excitement, poor sleep, or abnormal movements, pale tongue body with thin-sticky tongue coating, and thready-rapid pulse.

主症:患眼畏光流泪,白睛干涩,黑睛混浊或有溃疡;形体消瘦,肚腹膨胀,甚则青筋暴露,精神不振或易烦躁激动,睡眠不宁,或动作异常。舌淡,苔薄腻,脉细数。

Therapeutic methods: Equilibrate and reinforce qi and blood.

治法:平补气血。

Herbal formulas and drugs: The major formula is *Eight Agents Decoction* (Ba Wu Tang). The commonly-used herbal drugs are *Radix Ginseng* (Ren

方药:代表方为八物汤,常用药如人参、黄芪、茯苓、熟地黄、当归、芍药、川芎、菊

Shen), *Radix Astragali* (Huang Qi), *Sclerotium Poriae* (Fu Ling), *Radix Rehmanniae Praeparata* (Shu Di Huang), *Radix Angelicae Sinensis* (Dang Gui), *Radix Paeoniae Alba* (Bai Shao), *Rhizoma Ligustici Chuanxiong* (Chuan Xiong), *Flos Chrysanthemi* (Ju Hua), *Semen Cassiae* (Jue Ming Zi), etc.

花,决明子等。

Modification according to symptoms: For belching and poor appetite, add *Radix Aucklandiae* (Mu Xiang) and *Pericarpium Citri Tangerinae* (Chen Pi) to dilate middle energizer and promote qi flow. Add *Herba Dendrobii* (Shi Hu), *Radix Ophiopogonis* (Mai Dong) and *Radix Rehmanniae Cruda* (Sheng Di Huang) to nourish yin and produce body fluid.

加减:嗳气、饮食不香者,加木香、陈皮宽中行气;②加石斛、麦门冬、生地黄养阴生津。

(3) **Kidney failing to dominate transformation**

(3) **肾失气化**

Main symptoms: Dry and astringent sensation, photophobia, frequent blinks, blurring of vision, milder or more severe condition from time by time, slight redness of pupil, lack of luster of eye black, pale tongue body with thin tongue coating, and thready-weak pulse.

主症:患眼干涩羞明,频频眨眼,视物欠清,时轻时重,抱轮微红,黑睛欠光泽。舌淡,苔薄,脉细弱。

Therapeutic methods: Warm kidney and reinforce qi.

治法:温肾补气。

Herbal formulas and drugs: The major formula is *Golden Chamber Kidney Qi Pills* (Jin Kui Shen Qi Wan). The commonly-used herbal drugs are *Radix Rehmanniae Praeparata* (Shu Di Huang), *Rhizoma Dioscoreae* (Shan Yao), *Fructus Corni* (Shan Zhu Yu), *Rhizoma Alismatis* (Ze Xie), *Sclerotium Poriae* (Fu Ling), *Cortex Moutan Radicis* (Mu Dan Pi), *Ramulus Cinnamomi* (Gui Zhi), *Radix Aconiti Praeparata* (Fu Zi), etc.

方药:代表方为金匮肾气丸,常用药如熟地黄、山药、山茱萸、泽泻、茯苓、牡丹皮、桂枝、附子等。

Modification according to symptoms: For blurring of vision, add *Periostracum Cicadae* (Chan Tui), *Fructus Tribuli* (Bai Ji Li) and *Semen Celosiae* (Qing

加减:视物模糊者,加蝉蜕、白蒺藜、青葙子祛风明目。

Xiang Zi) to eliminate wind and brighten eyes.

3.3 Local therapies

(1) Supplement of tears: Artificial tears without antiseptic substance are applied according to the necessity.

(2) Vitamin A Oil: Eye dropping, 1 to 2 drops each time and 4 times a day.

(3) Steroids or immune suppressor: Apply Flumetholon or Cyclosporin A, 3 to 4 times a day.

(4) Lacrimal punctum block: Apply to decrease lacrimal drainage.

3.4 Supplementary therapies

(1) Apply anti-infective or antiallergic eye drop, such as Ofloxacin Eye Drop or Emedastine Difumarate Eye Drop.

(2) Apply hydrophilic corneal contact lens, but follow-up is needed.

(3) Apply the eye moistening glasses or the eye shield.

(4) Spinal-pinching method in traditional Chinese medicine: From Pt Changqiang (GV 1) to Pt Dazhui (GV 14), the thumbs and index fingers are applied to pinch the skin and muscle bilateral to the spine and move upwards alternately to reach Pt Dazhui (GV 1). The whole manipulation is taken as once. The same manipulation of spinal-pinching method is repeated 6 times. In the fifth and sixth manipulations, the thumbs are applied to pinch the muscles at the costal region about 4 to 5 times, then the thumbs are applied to push-press from Pt Mingmen (GV 4) to Pt Shenshu (BL 23) 2 to 3 times. Such a treatment is given 2 to 3 times a day and continuously for 3 to 5 days. This method acts to regu-

3.3 局部治疗

(1) 补充泪液:按需选用不含防腐剂的人工泪液。

(2) 维生素A油剂点眼,每次1～2滴,每日4次。

(3) 激素或免疫抑制剂:氟美瞳、环胞霉素A,每日3～4次。

(4) 封闭泪小点,减少泪液引流。

3.4 辅助治疗

(1) 抗感染或抗过敏眼液,如氧氟沙星、埃美丁眼液。

(2) 亲水性角膜接触镜,需随访。

(3) 湿房镜或眼罩。

(4) 中医捏脊疗法:从长强至大椎穴操作,以两手指背横压在长强穴部位,向大椎穴推进,同时以两手拇指与食指将皮肤肌肉捏起,交替向上,直至大椎,作为1次。如此连续捏脊6次。在推捏第五六次时,以拇指在肋部将肌肉提起,约提4～5下,捏完后再以两拇指从命门向肾俞左右推压2～3下。每日2～3次,连续3～5日。此法有调理脾胃、调和阴阳、疏通经络的作用。

late the spleen and stomach, harmonize yin and yang, and dredge the meridians and collaterals.

4 Speculative map

4 思辨导图

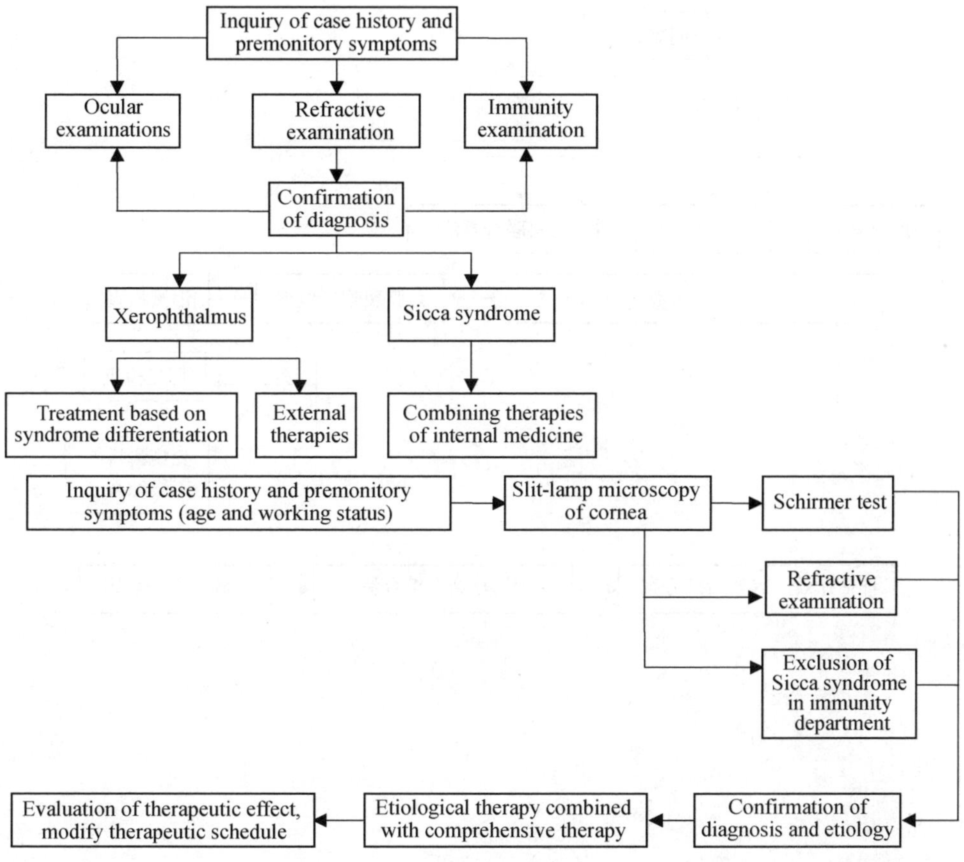

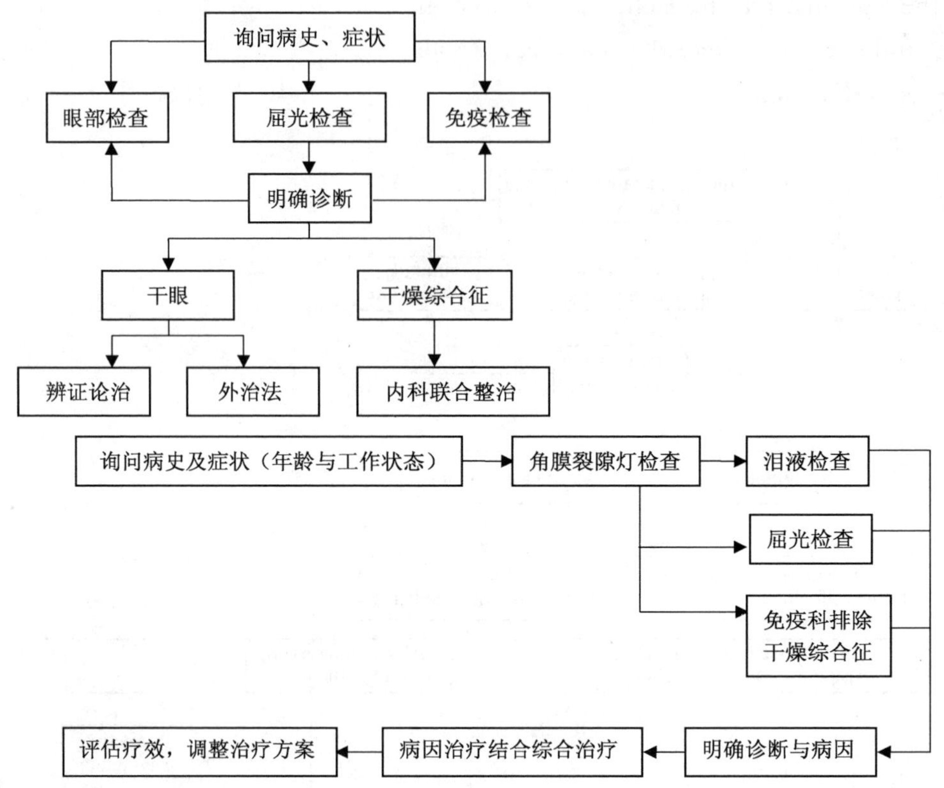
询问病史、症状
眼部检查
屈光检查
免疫检查
明确诊断
干眼
干燥综合征
辨证论治
外治法
内科联合整治
询问病史及症状（年龄与工作状态）
角膜裂隙灯检查
泪液检查
屈光检查
免疫科排除干燥综合征
明确诊断与病因
病因治疗结合综合治疗
评估疗效，调整治疗方案

Chapter 5 Pupil Diseases

第5章 瞳神疾病

Anterior uveitis

前葡萄膜炎

Anterior uveitis is a kind of inflammation occurring at sclera or / and anterior ciliary body, the most commonly-seen uveitis. The possible incidence factors are virus infection, traumatic injury and immune abnormality. Anatomically, the sclera and ciliary body are mutually connected with close relation, and supplied by sclera macrocyclic blood. The rich and slow blood supply is the cause of various endogenous pathogenic factors which lead to iridocyclitis, often seen in young adults, with repeated attacks and incurable condition.

In traditional Chinese medicine of different dynasties, the knowledge to the disease was quite unified. Due to the major symptom of the disease is tight and small pupil, the disease is called "iridocyclitis" in *Standards of Diagnosis and Treatment* (Zheng Zhi Zhun Sheng). The pupil pertains to the water wheel and kidney, while the liver and kidney share a same source. Therefore, the causes of the disease are mostly related to the liver and kidney.

前葡萄膜炎是指发生于虹膜或(和)前部睫状体的炎症,是临床最多见的葡萄膜炎,病毒感染、外伤、免疫异常可能是发病的因素。虹膜和睫状体在解剖上互相连接,关系密切,且同为虹膜大环供血,丰富而缓慢的血供是体内各种致病因子导致虹膜睫状体炎的原因,常见于青壮年,病变多反复,缠绵难愈。

历代中医对此认识较为统一,准确地观察到瞳神紧小为本病的主要症状,《证治准绳》以"瞳神紧小"命名。瞳神为水轮,内应于肾,肝肾同源。故本病之因常责之于肝肾。

1 Etiology and pathogenesis

1.1 The wind-heat in the Liver Meridian or the

1 病因病机

1.1 肝经风热或肝胆火邪

pathogenic fire in the liver and gallbladder attacks the upper, so that the pupil becomes contracted and non-spread, leading to the disease.

循经上犯，瞳仁缩而不展发为本病.

1.2 The wind-damp or wind-damp transforming into heat causes the pupil being steamed and fumigated, leading to the disease.

1.2 罹患风湿或风湿郁而化热，熏蒸瞳神所致。

1.3 The chronic diseases damage yin, to cause yin deficiency of liver and kidney and up-flaming of false fire, so that the pupil loses its nourishment. The false fire heats and burns the pupil, so that the pupil becomes contracted and dispread, leading to the disease. Due to the contracted and non-spread pupil, it is adhesive to the crystalline lens, leading to papillary metamorphosis. Or due to some eye diseases in which the pathogens enter in the deep part of eye or due to traumatic injury which damages the pupil, the disease is caused.

1.3 久病伤阴，肝肾阴亏，虚火上炎，黄仁失养，更因虚火煎灼，黄仁或展而不缩为瞳神紧小；或展缩失灵，与晶珠粘连成瞳神干缺。亦可因某些眼病病邪深入或外伤损及黄仁而成本病。

2 Diagnostic essentials

2 诊断要点

2.1 Clinical manifestations

Sudden onset of redness and pain of eyes, photophobia, lacrimation, decrease of vision, or accompanied by aching and pain of joints.

2.1 临床表现

突发眼红、疼痛、畏光流泪，视力下降。或伴有关节酸楚疼痛。

2.2 Ocular examinations

(1) Decrease of vision in various degrees.

(2) Conjunctival mixed hemorrhage, in which the dust-like, dot-like or suet-like deposits at the inferior back wall of cornea can be seen. The dust-like deposits at the inferior back wall of cornea is often seen in nongranulomatous inflammation, while the suet-like deposits at the inferior back wall of cornea in granulomatous inflammation.

(3) Aqueous flare or aqueous turbidity (positive Tyndall phenomenon) is caused by large amount of

2.2 眼部检查

(1) 视力不同程度下降。

(2) 球结膜混合充血，角膜下方后壁可见粉尘状或小点状或羊脂状沉着物。微尘状角膜后沉着物多见于非肉芽肿性炎症，而羊脂状角膜后沉着物多见于肉芽肿性炎症。

(3) 房水闪辉或浑浊（丁道尔现象阳性），房水渗出严

polymorphonuclear leukocyte deposits to lead to hypopyon when the aqueous humor leakage is severe. Occasionally, the hyphema is caused by large amount of red blood cells entering into the anterior chamber.

重时，由于大量多形核白细胞沉积而出现前房积脓；偶尔由于红细胞大量进入前房而形成前房积血。

(4) Unclear texture of pupil, miosis or insensitivity to light. If the treatment is improper, the inflammatory adhesion between the pupil and crystalline lens may occur, so as to lead to plum blossom-like lock or even membrane-like lock.

（4）瞳孔纹理不清，缩小，对光反应不敏感。处理不当瞳孔可与晶状体发生炎性粘连而呈梅花状甚至膜样锁闭。

(5) Pigment adhesion at the surface of crystalline lens or lenticular opacity can be seen.

（5）晶状体表面色素附着或出现晶状体混浊。

(6) If the opacity is located at the posterior part of vitreous body and the grey-white retinal opacity can be seen at the fundus, and the vision decreases obviously, it is possible to be intermediate, posterior or panuveitis and need to be diagnosed definitively.

（6）当混浊位于玻璃体后部，眼底见视网膜灰白色混浊，视力下降明显，则可能为中间或后部或全葡萄膜炎，需明确诊断。

2.3 Auxiliary examinations

2.3 辅助检查

(1) Blood routine examination, blood glucose examination, ESR examination and RF examination.

（1）血常规、血糖、血沉、类风湿因子检查。

(2) Syphilis serum antibody test.

（2）梅毒抗体试验。

(3) HLA-B27 antigen examination, to find ankylosing spondylitis or HLA-B27 related uveitis.

（3）查 HLA-B27 抗原，有助于发现关节强直性脊柱炎或者 HLA-B27 相关性葡萄膜炎。

(4) Chest X-ray examination and fiber colonscopy, to find pulmonary and intestinal tuberculosis.

（4）胸部 X 线检查及纤维结肠镜检查，有助于发现肺及肠道结核病。

(5) Ocular B-ultrasonic examination and ocular OCT to exclude posterior uveitis.

（5）眼部 B 超和眼部 OCT 排除后部葡萄膜炎。

(6) Ocular UBM examination to exclude intermediate uveitis.

（6）眼部 UBM 检查排除中间葡萄膜炎。

3 Therapeutic methods

3.1 Therapeutic principles

Apply a thorough treatment aiming at the causative factors. If the causative factors are not confirmed, it is advisable to apply the drug mydriasis to reduce the complications, the symptomatic treatment with local steroids to avoid injury of ocular tissues and to achieve a better effect. Usually, it is not advisable to apply large amount of steroids for whole body in the treatment of anterior uveitis. The therapeutic principles are to reduce the Liver Meridian for excess pattern, and to reinforce the Kidney Meridian for deficiency pattern.

3.2 Treatment based on syndrome differentiation

(1) **Wind-heat in liver meridian**

Main symptoms: Quick onset of disease, blurring of vision, ciliary hyperemia, iridocyclitis, headache, fever, dry mouth, red tongue body with thin-white or thin-yellow tongue coating, and superficial-rapid pulse.

Therapeutic methods: Eliminate wind and clear heat.

Herbal formulas and drugs: The major formula is *New-Made Bupleurum and Coptis Decoction* (Xin Zhi Chai Lian Tang). The commonly-used herbal drugs are *Radix Gentianae* (Long Dan Cao), *Fructus Gardeniae* (Zhi Zi), *Radix Scutellariae* (Huang Qin), *Rhizoma Coptidis* (Huang Lian), *Herba Schizonepetae* (Jing Jie), *Radix Ledebouriellae* (Fang Feng), *Fructus Viticis* (Man Jing Zi), *Radix Bupleuri* (Chai Hu), *Radix Paeoniae Rubra* (Chi Shao), *Radix Glycyrrhizae Praeparata* (Zhi Gan Cao), etc.

3 治疗方法

3.1 治疗原则

针对病因，进行彻底治疗；病因不明确时，药物散瞳，减少并发症，局部激素对症治疗，避免眼组织遭受破坏，争取较好的后果。一般前葡萄膜炎不建议全身大量激素治疗。临证以泻肝经之实，补肾经之虚为主要原则。

3.2 辨证论治

（1）肝经风热

主症：起病急，视物模糊，抱轮红赤，瞳神紧小，头痛发热，口干舌红，苔薄白或薄黄，脉浮数。

治法：祛风清热。

方药：代表方为新制柴连汤，常用药如龙胆草、栀子、黄芩、黄连、荆芥、防风、蔓荆子、柴胡、赤芍、炙甘草等。

Modification according to symptoms: For severe pain, add *Radix Rehmanniae Cruda* (Sheng Di Huang), *Cortex Moutan Radicis* (Mu Dan Pi), *Radix Salviae Miltiorrhizae* (Dan Shen) and *Fructus Leonuri* (Chong Wei Zi).

加减：痛甚者，加生地黄、牡丹皮、丹参、茺蔚子。

(2) **Fire flaming in liver and gallbladder**

(2) **肝胆火炽**

Main symptoms: Severe condition, ciliary hyperemia, aqueous humor turbidity, iridocyclitis, contracted and non-spread pupil, bitter taste in mouth, dry throat, restlessness, anger, red tongue body with yellow tongue coating, and wiry-rapid pulse.

主症：病情重，抱轮红赤，神水混浊，瞳神缩小且展缩失灵。全身多见口苦咽干，烦躁易怒，舌红苔黄，脉弦数。

Therapeutic methods: Purify and reduce liver and gallbladder.

治法：清泻肝胆。

Herbal formulas and drugs: The major formula is *Gentian Liver-Draining Decoction* (Long Dan Xie Gan Tang). The commonly-used herbal drugs are *Radix Gentianae* (Long Dan Cao), *Radix Scutellariae* (Huang Qin), *Rhizoma Coptidis* (Huang Lian), *Fructus Gardeniae* (Zhi Zi), *Semen Plantaginis* (Che Qian Zi), *Rhizoma Alismatis* (Ze Xie), *Radix Angelicae Sinensis* (Dang Gui), *Radix Rehmanniae Cruda* (Sheng Di Huang), *Radix Bupleuri* (Chai Hu), *Radix Glycyrrhizae Praeparata* (Zhi Gan Cao), etc.

方药：代表方为龙胆泻肝汤，常用药如龙胆草、黄芩、黄连、栀子、车前子、泽泻、当归、生地黄、柴胡、炙甘草等。

Modification according to symptoms: For severe pain, add *Cortex Moutan Radicis* (Mu Dan Pi), *Radix Paeoniae Rubra* (Chi Shao) and *Flos Carthami* (Hong Hua). For thirst, constipation and hypopyon, add *Gypsum Fibrosum* (Shi Gao), *Rhizoma Anemarrhenae* (Zhi Mu) and *Radix et Rhizoma Rhei* (Da Huang) to reduce the excess pattern.

加减：痛甚者，加牡丹皮、赤芍、红花；口渴便秘，黄液上冲，加石膏、知母、大黄泻实。

(3) **Wind-damp combined with heat**

(3) **风湿挟热**

Main symptoms: Prolonged course of disease which is lingering with repeated attacks, slow or

主症：发病程较长，病情缠绵，且易反复，发病或缓或

quick onset of disease, commonly seen in the diseases of rheumatism and gout, ocular symptoms of distending pain at the eyeball and supraorbital ridge, distension, swelling, aching and pain of joints, blurring of vision, acute or chronic iridocyclitis, aqueous humor turbidity, unclear texture of pupil, yellow-sticky tongue coating, and wiry-rapid or soft-rapid pulse.

急，多见于有风湿、痛风等症。眼珠及眉棱骨胀痛之眼症及肢节肿胀、酸楚疼痛目赤痛，眉棱骨胀痛，视物昏矇，瞳神紧小或偏缺不圆，神水混浊，黄仁纹理不清。舌苔黄腻，脉弦数或濡数。

Therapeutic methods: Eliminate wind, dissolve damp and clear heat.

治法：祛风除湿清热。

Herbal formulas and drugs: The major formula is *Yang-Inhibiting Liqueur and Coptis Powder* (Yi Yang Jiu Lian San). The commonly-used herbal drugs are *Radix Scutellariae* (Huang Qin), *Rhizoma Coptidis* (Huang Lian), *Cortex Phellodendri* (Huang Bo), *Fructus Gardeniae* (Zhi Zi), *Radix Rehmanniae Cruda* (Sheng Di Huang), *Rhizoma Anemarrhenae* (Zhi Mu), *Crystalline Mirabilite* (Han Shui Shi), *Rhizoma seu Radix Notopterygii* (Qiang Huo), *Radix Ledebouriellae* (Fang Feng), *Fructus Viticis* (Man Jing Zi), *Radix Angelicae Dahuricae* (Bai Zhi), *Radix Peucedani* (Qian Hu), *Radix Ledebouriellae* (Fang Ji), *Radix Glycyrrhizae Praeparata* (Zhi Gan Cao), etc.

方药：代表方为抑阳酒连散，常用药如黄芩、黄连、黄柏、栀子、生地黄、知母、寒水石、羌活、防风、蔓荆子、白芷、前胡、防己、炙甘草等。

(4) **False fire upward-flaming**

(4) **虚火上炎**

Main symptoms: Chronic inflammation with repeated attacks, mild condition or late stage of condition, various degrees of condition, dryness and discomfort at eyes, blurring of vision, ciliary hyperemia, dust-like deposits at the posterior wall of pupil, aqueous humor turbidity, mild iris atrophy, chronic iridocyclitis, crystalline opacity, accompanied by dizziness, insomnia, restlessness and feverish sensation at palms and soles, dry mouth and throat, red tongue body with scanty tongue coating, and thready-rapid pulse.

主症：多见于慢性炎症反复发作，病势较缓或病至后期，病势较缓，时轻时重，眼干涩不适，视物昏花，或见抱轮红赤，黑晶后壁可有粉尘状沉着物，可见神水混浊，黄仁轻度萎缩，瞳神干缺，晶珠混浊；可兼头晕失眠，五心烦热，口燥咽干，舌红少苔，脉细数。

Therapeutic methods: Nourish yin and subdue fire.

治法：滋阴降火。

Herbal formulas and drugs: The major formula is Anemarrhena, Phellodendron, and *Rehmannia Decoction* (Zhi Bai Di Huang Tang). The commonly-used herbal drugs are *Radix Rehmanniae Praeparata* (Shu Di Huang), *Fructus Corni* (Shan Zhu Yu), *Rhizoma Dioscoreae* (Shan Yao), *Rhizoma Alismatis* (Ze Xie), *Cortex Moutan Radicis* (Mu Dan Pi), *Sclerotium Poriae* (Fu Ling), *Rhizoma Anemarrhenae* (Zhi Mu), *Cortex Phellodendri* (Huang Bo), etc.

方药：代表方为知柏地黄汤，常用药如熟地黄、山茱萸、山药、泽泻、牡丹皮、茯苓、知母、黄柏等。

Modification according to symptoms: For blurring of vision, add *Fructus Lycii* (Gou Qi Zi) and *Flos Chrysanthemi* (Ju Hua) to benefit essence and brighten eyes.

加减：视物模糊者，加枸杞子、菊花益精明目。

3.3 Local therapies

3.3 局部治疗

(1) Immediate mydriasis: Apply atropine, the cycloplegic, to prevent posterior synechia of iris, to relieve spasm of ciliary muscle and sphincter pupillae muscle, decrease edema, congestion and pain, so as to promote the inflammatory absorption and alleviate the patient's pains.

（1）立即散瞳，使用睫状肌麻痹剂阿托品，防止虹膜后粘连，解除睫状肌、瞳孔括约肌的痉挛，减轻水肿、充血及疼痛，促进炎症恢复和减轻患者痛苦。

(2) Rapid anti-inflammatory treatment: Apply the glucocorticosterioid eye drop, to prevent the ocular tissue damage and occurrence of complications. Apply non-steroidal anti-inflammatory eye drop, to treat the causative factors and complications.

（2）迅速抗炎，使用糖皮质激素滴眼剂，以防止眼组织破坏和并发症的发生。非甾体消炎药滴眼液点眼；针对病因及并发症的治疗。

(3) Subconjunctival injection: Apply the glucocorticosterioid injection and mydriatics to treat.

（3）结膜下注射：糖皮质激素及散瞳剂治疗。

(4) Characteristic treatment: Apply the herbal dredge left after oral administration for local hot medicated compress.

（4）特色疗法：可用内服中药的药渣作局部熨敷。

3.4 Other therapies

3.4 其他疗法

(1) Apply non-steroidal anti-inflammatory drug to

（1）非甾体消炎药可以

assist the decrease of inflammatory reaction.

(2) Acupuncture: The commonly-used points are Jingming (BL 2), Cuanzhu (BL 2), Sizhukong (TE 23), Ganshu (BL 18), Zusanli (ST 36), Hegu (LI 4), etc. In each treatment, apply 2 local points and 1 to 2 distant points.

帮助减轻炎症反应。

（2）针灸治疗。常用穴为睛明、攒竹、丝竹空、肝俞、足三里、合谷等。每次局部取2穴，远端配1～2穴。

4 Speculative map

4 思辨导图

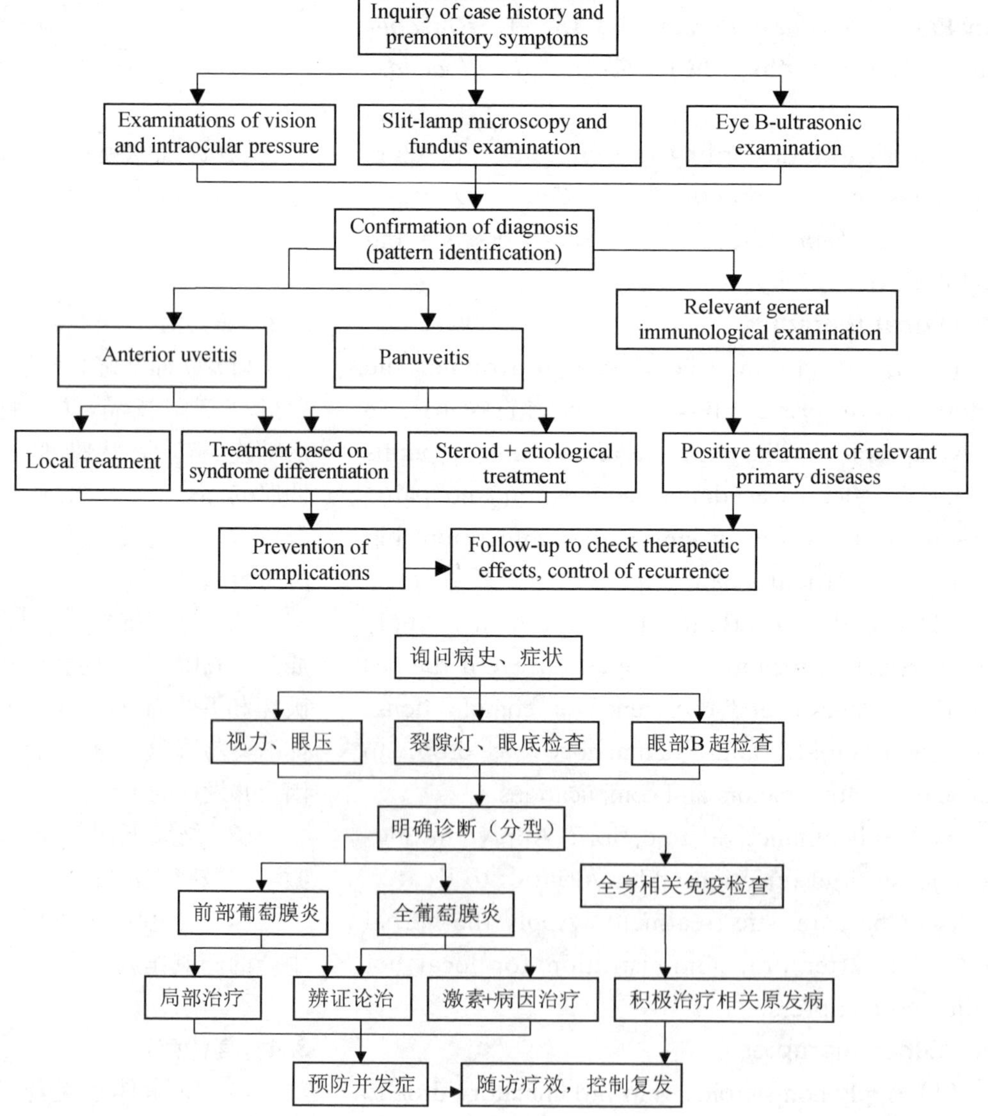

Acute angle-closure glaucoma

急性闭角型青光眼

Acute angle-closure glaucoma (AACG) is a kind of optic damage disease in which the intraocular pressure increases due to acute aqueous humor drainage disturbance, induced by papillary block. It is often seen in the old people over 50, and morbidity in females is double of that in males. The shallow anterior chamber and short eye axis are the major anatomical factors of the disease. There is also chronic angle-closure glaucoma in the clinic.

急性闭角型青光眼是由瞳孔阻滞诱发的急性房水引流障碍导致眼压升高而损害视神经的疾病。多见于50岁以上的老年人，女性患者发病率常为男性患者的2倍。其浅前房、短眼轴是发病的主要解剖因素。临床上也有慢性闭角类型。

According to the manifestations of headache, redness, distension and pain of eyes, sudden decrease of vision, pupil dilation and greenness, etc. occurring in the attack of the disease, it is called "green wind glaucoma" in traditional Chinese medicine. Its major pathogenesis is described as wind-fire of liver and gallbladder upward-attacking the head and eyes, emotional outburst, upward-going of qi and fire, accumulation of phlegm and stasis, and blockage of eye collaterals.

根据发作时的头痛、眼红、胀痛、视力锐减、瞳孔散大色青等表现，中医学将其命名为"绿风内障"。肝胆风火上攻头目，情志过激、气火上逆，痰火互结、玄府塞闭为其主要病机。

1 Etiology and pathogenesis

1 病因病机

1.1 Pathogenic heat attacks the internal to cause hyperactivity of fire-heat in liver and gallbladder. The extreme heat produces the wind, and the wind-fire attacks to eyes to cause the blockage of eye collaterals. The aqueous humor drainage is disturbed and accumulated inside the eyes to cause the disease.

1.1 邪热犯内，肝胆火热亢盛，热极生风，风火攻目，目中玄府闭塞，神水排出受阻，积于眼内所致。

1.2 Emotional outburst causes qi stagnation which produces the fire. Qi and fire go upwards to block the eye collaterals, so that the aqueous humor drain-

1.2 情志过激，气郁生火，气火上逆，壅塞目中玄府，神水排出不畅，蓄积于目中。

age is disturbed and accumulated inside the eyes to cause the disease.

1.3 The damp in the spleen transforms into the phlegm which further transforms into heat. The heat and phlegm is accumulated to block the eye collaterals, so that the aqueous humor drainage is disturbed and accumulated inside the eyes to cause the disease.

1.3 脾湿生痰，痰郁化热，痰火郁结，阻塞玄府，神水滞留目内遂致。

2 Diagnostic essentials

2 诊断要点

2.1 Subjective symptoms

2.1 自觉症状

Blurring of vision, halo vision, frontal pain on the same side of the sick eye, aching and distension at the root of nose, relieved and removed symptoms after rest. Severe distension and pain at the sick eye during the attack, photophobia, lacrimation, sudden decrease of vision, accompanied by the general symptoms of headache on the same side, nausea, vomiting, etc.

视物模糊，虹视，患眼同侧额部疼痛及鼻根酸胀，休息后缓解或消除。发作时患眼剧烈胀痛，羞明流泪，视力骤降。常伴同侧头痛、恶心、呕吐等全身症状。

2.2 Ocular examinations

2.2 眼部检查

Mixed congestion of bulbar conjunctiva; fog-like edema at cornea; more shallowness of anterior chamber; papillary dilation and loss of light reaction; increase of intraocular pressure, over 40 mmHg.

球结膜混合充血；角膜雾状水肿；前房较浅；瞳孔散大，光反应消失；眼压升高，多在40 mmHg以上。

2.3 Auxiliary examinations

2.3 辅助检查

(1) Ultrasound biomicroscopy (UBM) indicates angle crowdedness even closure, ciliary edema or forward rotation, etc.

（1）超声生物显微镜（UBM）显示房角结构拥挤，甚至关闭，睫状体水肿或旋前等。

(2) Gonioscopy indicates angle narrowness or closure.

（2）房角镜检查显示窄闭房角。

3 Therapeutic methods

3 治疗方法

3.1 Therapeutic principles

3.1 治疗原则

The disease attacks quickly, so greatly damages

本病发病急，对视力危

the vision, even causes blindness. It is necessary to save the sight above all, so it is advisable to apply the comprehensive treatment. In traditional Chinese medicine, it is often caused by wind, fire, heat and phlegm and treated by focusing on the liver.

害极大,甚至可致失明,以挽救视力为先,临证宜综合治疗。中医辨证多以风、火、热、痰为患,从肝论治。

3.2 First aid measures

(1) Miosis: Apply 1% to 2% Pilocarpine Eye Drop once every 15 minutes. After the pupil narrowness, keep the application 3 to 4 times a day.

(2) Steroids: Apply local or general glucocorticoids, to reduce the reactive edema of ciliary body and rapidly decrease the intraocular pressure.

(3) Hypertonic dehydrant: Apply 20% mannitol solution, 1 to 1.5g / kg, by rapid intravenous injection, to decrease the intraocular pressure in a short period of time through high permeability to subtract the water inside the vitreous body..

(4) Carbonic anhydrase inhibitors: Apply acetazolamide or methazolamide for oral administration, to subtract the aqueous humor so as to decrease the intraocular pressure.

(5) Surgery: Select the surgical methods according to the recovery of intraocular pressure and the scope of chamber angle adhesion after the above-mentioned drug treatments. ① For those with chamber angle opening or adhesion less than 1 / 3, apply peripheral iridectomy or laser iridotomy. ② For those with extensive adhesion of chamber angle, apply glaucoma trabeculectomy, or glaucoma drainage nail surgery, etc. ③ Apply Phaco + IOL, to relieve the crowdedness of chamber angle.

3.2 急救措施

(1) 缩瞳:1%～2%毛果芸香碱眼药水,每15分钟1次,瞳孔回缩小后,维持每日3～4次。

(2) 激素:局部或全身应用糖皮质激素制剂,以减轻睫状体反应性水肿,有利快速降低眼压。

(3) 高渗脱水剂:20%甘露醇溶液1～1.5g/kg,每天静脉快速滴注,通过高渗透压减少玻璃体中的水分来达到短期降低眼压的作用。

(4) 碳酸酐酶抑制剂:可选用乙酰唑胺或尼目克斯等口服,以减少房水产生而降低眼压。

(5) 手术治疗:经上述药物治疗,根据眼压恢复情况及房角粘连的范围来选择手术方式。①房角开放或粘连不超过1/3者,行周边虹膜切除术或激光虹膜切开术;②房角广泛粘连者,需行青光眼小梁滤过性手术,或青光眼引流钉等手术;③可考虑施行Phaco+IOL术,解决房角拥挤状况。

3.3 Treatment based on syndrome differentiation

(1) **Wind-fire attacking eyes**

Main symptoms: Quick onset of disease, distension and pain of eye, headache on same side, sudden decrease of vision, redness of eye, fog-like turbidity of cornea, papillary dilation, red tongue body with yellow tongue coating, and rapid pulse.

Therapeutic methods: Clear heat and reduce fire, soothe liver and eliminate wind.

Herbal formulas and drugs: The major formula is *Green Wind Antelope Horn Drink* (Lu Feng Ling Yang Yin). The commonly-used herbal drugs are *Cornu Antelopis* (Ling Yang Jiao), *Radix Scrophulariae* (Xuan Shen), *Rhizoma Anemarrhenae* (Zhi Mu), *Radix Scutellariae* (Huang Qin), *Sclerotium Poriae* (Fu Ling), *Semen Plantaginis* (Che Qian Zi), *Radix et Rhizoma Rhei* (Da Huang), *Radix Ledebouriellae* (Fang Feng), *Herba Asari* (Xi Xin), *Radix Platycodi* (Jie Geng), etc.

(2) **Up-reverse flow of qi-fire**

Main symptoms: Same eye symptoms as the above, instable emotions, and high blood pressure.

Therapeutic methods: Soothe liver and relieve depression, reduce fire and subdue the up-reversed qi.

Herbal formulas and drugs: The major formula is *Peony Bark and Capejasmine Free Wanderer Powder* (Dan Zhi Xiao Yao San) plus *Coptis and Evodia Pills* (Zuo Jin Wan). The commonly-used herbal drugs are *Radix Bupleuri* (Chai Hu), *Radix Angelicae Sinensis* (Dang Gui), *Radix Paeoniae Alba* (Bai Shao), *Sclerotium Poriae* (Fu Ling), *Rhizoma Atractylodis Macrocephalae* (Bai Zhu), *Cortex Moutan*

3.3 辨证论治

(1) **风火攻目**

主症：发病急骤，眼胀痛，同侧头痛，视力骤降，白睛混赤，黑睛雾状混浊，瞳神散大，舌红苔黄脉数。

治法：清热泻火，平肝熄风。

方药：代表方为绿风羚羊饮，常用药如羚羊角、玄参、知母、黄芩、茯苓、车前子、大黄、防风、细辛、桔梗等。

(2) **气火上逆**

主症：眼症同上，情绪不稳定，血压偏高。

治法：疏肝解郁，泻火降逆。

方药：代表方为丹栀逍遥散合左金丸，常用药如柴胡、当归、白芍、茯苓、白术、牡丹皮、栀子、薄荷、煨生姜、黄连、吴茱萸等。

Radicis (Mu Dan Pi), *Fructus Gardeniae* (Zhi Zi), *Herba Menthae* (Bo He), *Rhizoma Zingiberis Recens* (Sheng Jiang) Baked, *Rhizoma Coptidis* (Huang Lian), *Fructus Evodiae* (Wu Zhu Yu), etc.

(3) **Phlegm-fire accumulation and stagnation**

Main symptoms: Same eye symptoms as the above, severe headache, severe vomiting, poor appetite, red tongue body with sticky tongue coating, and rolling-rapid pulse.

Therapeutic methods: Reduce fire and dissolve phlegm.

Herbal formulas and drugs: The major formula is *General's Pain-Stopping Pills* (Jiang Jun Ding Tong Wan). The commonly-used herbal drugs are *Radix Scutellariae* (Huang Qin), *Pericarpium Citri Tangerinae* (Chen Pi), *Rhizoma Pinelliae Praeparata* (Zhi Ban Xia), *Rhizoma Gastrodiae* (Tian Ma), *Radix Platycodi* (Jie Geng), *Radix Angelicae Dahuricae* (Bai Zhi), *Bombyx Batryticatus* (Bai Jiang Can), *Radix et Rhizoma Rhei* (Da Huang), etc.

(3) **痰火郁结**

主症：眼症同上，头痛剧烈，呕吐较重，茶饭不思，舌红苔腻，脉滑数。

治法：降火逐痰。

方药：代表方为将军定痛丸，常用药如黄芩、橘皮、制半夏、天麻、桔梗、白芷、白僵蚕、大黄等。

3.4 Other therapy

Acupuncture therapy may relieve the general symptoms of headache, eye pain, nausea, vomiting, etc., and also acts to protect the visual function.

Major points: Jingming (BL 2), Shangjingming (EX-HN), Fengchi (GB 20), Taiyang (EX-HN 5), Sibai (ST 2), Hegu (LI 4), Shenmen (HT 7) and Baihui (GV 20).

Adjunct points: Quchi (LI 11) and Waiguan (TE 5) for wind-fire attacking eyes, Xingjian (LR 2) and Taichong (LR 3) for up-reverse flow of qi-fire, Fenglong (ST 40) and Zusanli (ST 36) for phlegm-fire accumulation and stagnation, and

3.4 其他疗法

配合针灸治疗可缓解头眼疼痛及恶心、呕吐等全身症状，对视功能有一定保护作用。

主穴：睛明、上睛明、风池、太阳、四白、合谷、神门、百会。

配穴：风火攻目证，选曲池、外关；气火上逆证，选行间、太冲；痰火郁结证，选丰隆、足三里等。恶心呕吐明显者加内关、胃俞。

Neiguan (PC 6) and Weishu (BL 21) for more obvious nausea and vomiting.

The reducing methods of twisting and lifting-thrusting the needles are applied for all the above points. Withdraw the needles or leave the needles for 10 minutes when the obvious needling sensation occurs after manipulating the needles. For severe pain, it is advisable to apply the blood-letting method at points of Dadun (LR 1), Hegu (LI 4), Jiaosun (TE 20) and Taiyang (EX-HN 5).

以上均用捻转提插之泻法，行手法至有明显针感后出针或留针 10 分钟。疼痛严重者，可于大敦、合谷、角孙、太阳穴点刺放血。

4 Speculative map

4. 思辨导图

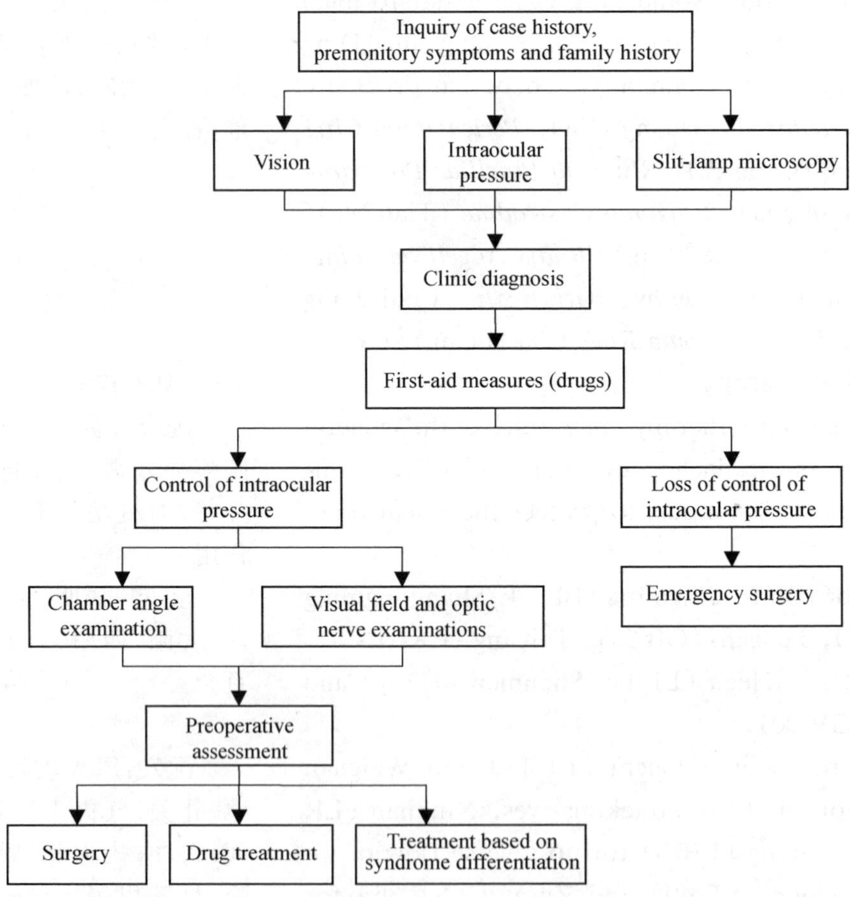

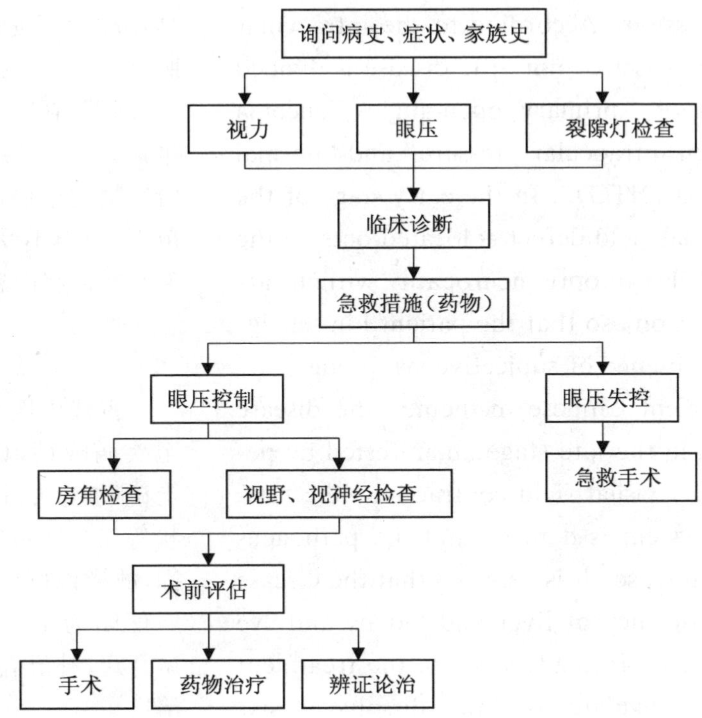

Primary open-angle glaucoma

Primary glaucoma is a kind of eye disease with inheritance tendency, finally causing blindness due to high intraocular pressure or pathological intraocular pressure fluctuation, accompanied by progressive optic nerve damage. The cause of the disease remains unknown. The cause of intraocular pressure increase is aqueous humor outflow obstructing at the trabecular meshwork-Schlemm's canal or at the scleral venous system. It is believed that some of the patients have the genetic cause, such as TIGR gene, OPTN gene, etc. 50% of the glaucoma patients have the family history, slightly more common in males. The disease is featured by an insidious onset

原发性开角型青光眼

原发性青光眼是指高眼压或病理性眼压波动同时伴有进行性视神经损害，最终导致失明的具有遗传倾向的眼病。病因不明，眼压升高的原因是房水的外流受阻于小梁网-Schlemm管或者巩膜静脉系统。目前认为部分患者有基因致病倾向，如TIGR基因、OPTN基因等，50%患者有青光眼家族史。男性略多，起病隐匿，进展缓慢。根据患者是否有眼压升

and slow progression. According to the intraocular pressure if it increases or not, the disease is divided into two types of "primary open-angle glaucoma (POAG) of high intraocular pressure" and "normal tension glaucoma (NTG)". In the early stage of the disease, the visual field defect is located outside the central fixation due to optic neuropathy without affection of the vision, so that the patient himself ignores it due to absence of subjective symptoms.

高,分成"原发性开角型青光眼高眼压型"和"正常眼压性青光眼"两种类型。在病变早期,视神经病变引起的视野缺损位于中心注视以外的范围,视力不受影响,患者缺乏自觉症状而忽略。

In the ancient Chinese medicine, the disease was understood in the late stage, manifested by pedestraian impact, visual field contraction, etc. Because the eye system is damage and the pathogens are firm in the disease, it is believed that the disease is caused by deficiency of liver and kidney and eye collateral blockage. It is advisable in the treatment to soothe liver, regulate qi flow, dissolve stasis, open apertures, reinforce liver, benefit kidney, warm yang and strengthen transportation.

古代中医认识此病均已至疾病晚期,以其临床见行走碰物撞人、视野缩窄呈管状等症,目系损害,邪坚病固,故皆以肝肾亏虚,目中玄府郁闭为论,以疏肝理气行瘀开窍,补肝益肾,温阳助运治之。

1 Etiology and pathogenesis

1 病因病机

1.1 Liver qi stagnation. The vessels and collaterals of eye are blocked, so the aqueous humor becomes stagnant.

1.1 肝郁气滞,目中脉络不利,玄府郁闭,神水瘀滞。

1.2 Congenital insufficiency. Yang qi in the eye collaterals does not flow smoothly, so the phlegm-damp blocks the collaterals and damage the eye system.

1.2 禀赋不足,玄府阳运不济,痰湿阻滞络脉,目系受损。

1.3 Chronic diseases. Due to deficiency of liver and kidney, the eyes lose nourishment and the aqueous humor becomes stagnant.

1.3 久病肝肾亏虚,目窍失养,神水滞涩。

2 Diagnostic essentials

2 诊断要点

2.1 Intraocular pressure $>$ 21 mmHg, or normal intraocular pressure.

2.1 眼压>21 mmHg,或眼压在正常范围。

2.2 Gonioscopy, UBM and other examinations indicate opening of anterior chamber angle.

2.2 房角镜、UBM、检查提示前房角开放。

2.3 Characteristic visual field defect in glaucoma.

2.3 青光眼特征性视野缺损。

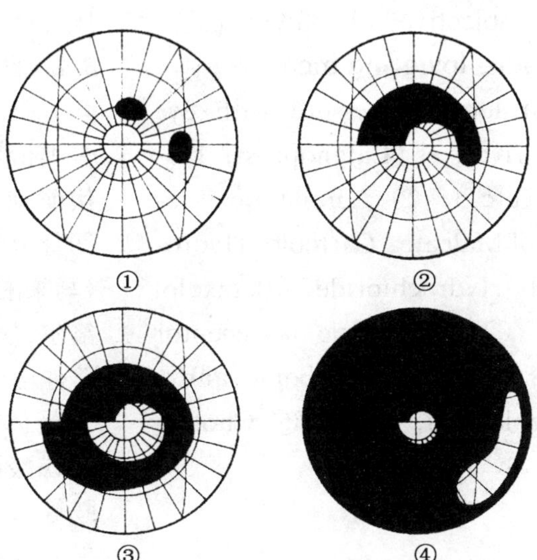

2.4 With OCT, it is possible to find out glaucomatous optic disc change and / or retinal nerve fiber layer defect in the earlier stage.

2.4 借助于OCT可以更早期地查出青光眼性视盘改变和(或)有视网膜神经纤维层缺损。

2.5 24-hour intraocular pressure measurement indicates intraocular pressure difference > 8 mmHg, and double intraocular pressure difference > 5 mmHg, so as to assist the diagnosis.

2.5 24小时眼压测定提示眼压差值>8 mmHg,双眼压差>5 mmHg以协助诊断。

2.6 Visual electrophysiology examination: In Figure VEP, P100 latency is prolonged and the amplitude decreases. In Figure ERG, the amplitude decreases.

2.6 **视觉电生理检查:**图形VEP的P100潜时延长,振幅下降;图形ERG振幅下降。

3 Therapeutic methods

3 治疗方法

3.1 Therapeutic principles

3.1 治疗原则

Decrease the intraocular pressure long and stably, take recheck and follow-up perpetually and regularly, modify the therapeutic program timely, and terminate or delay the visual field deterioration, so

长期而稳定地降低眼压,终身定期复查随访,及时调整治疗方案,终止或延缓视野的恶化,最大可能地保

as to maximize the maintenance of visual function. In the treatment, it is stressed to establish a safe "intraocular pressure of objective" of individuals.

持视功能。治疗上强调设定个体患者安全的"目标眼压"。

3.2 Intraocular pressure lowering measures

(1) Decrease intraocular pressure with eye drugs: ① Prostanoid derivatives (Latanoprost, Travoprost, Bimatoprost, etc.); ② Adrenergic β-receptor blockers (Timolol Maleate, Carteolol Hydrochloride, Levobunolol Hydrochloride, Betaxolol Hydrochloride, etc.); ③ Adrenergic α_2-receptor agonists (Brimonidine, etc.); ④ Carbonic anhydrase inhibitors (Brinzolamide, etc.); ⑤ Choline drugs (Pilocarpine, etc.).

(2) Laser trabeculoplasty: Promote the drainage of Schlemm-trabecular meshwork.

(3) Filtration surgery to increase the external or internal drainage of aqueous humor: ① Trabeculectomy; ② Non-penetrating trabeculectomy.

3.2 降眼压措施

(1) 眼药降压:①前列腺素类衍生物(拉坦前列素、曲伏前列素、贝美前列素等);②肾上腺素能β-受体阻断剂(马来酸噻吗洛尔、盐酸卡替洛尔、盐酸左布诺洛尔、盐酸倍他洛尔等);③肾上腺素能α_2受体激动剂(溴莫尼定);④碳酸酐酶抑制剂(布林佐胺等);⑤拟胆碱类药物(毛果云香碱等)。

(2) 激光小梁成型术,促进小梁网-Schlemm管的引流。

(3) 滤过手术增加房水的外或内引流:①小梁切除术;②非穿透性小梁切除术。

3.3 Treatment based on syndrome differentiation

(1) Liver depression and qi stagnation

Main symptoms: Blurring of vision constantly, slightly distension of eyeballs, slight redness of eyes, or slight dilation of pupil, fundus optic disc ratio > 0.6, or optic disc ratio of both eyes > 0.2, visual field defect, slightly high intraocular pressure, accompanied by emotional depression, restlessness, bitter taste in mouth, red tongue body with yellow tongue coating, and wiry-thready pulse.

Therapeutic methods: Soothe liver and relieve depression.

Herbal formulas and drugs: The major formula

3.3 辨证论治

(1) 肝郁气滞

主症:时有视物昏朦,目珠微胀,轻度抱轮红赤,或瞳神稍大,眼底视盘杯盘比大于0.6,或两眼视盘杯盘比差大于0.2;可见视野缺损,眼压偏高;或兼情志不舒,心烦口苦;舌红,苔黄,脉弦细。

治法:疏肝解郁。

方药:代表方为逍遥散,

is *Free Wanderer Powder* (Xiao Yao San). The commonly-used herbal drugs are *Radix Bupleuri* (Chai Hu), *Radix Angelicae Sinensis* (Dang Gui), *Radix Paeoniae Alba* (Bai Shao), *Sclerotium Poriae* (Fu Ling), *Herba Menthae* (Bo He), *Rhizoma Zingiberis Recens* (Sheng Jiang) Baked, etc.

常用药如柴胡、当归、白芍、茯苓、白术、薄荷、煨生姜等。

(2) **Phlegm-damp occupying eyes**

(2) **痰湿泛目**

Main symptoms: Blurring of vision occasionally in the early stage, or slight dilation of pupil, growing ratio of fundus optic disc, or optic disc ratio of both eyes > 0.2, pale optic disc in severe condition, visual field defect, or tubular visual field, slightly high intraocular pressure, nausea, vomiting, pale tongue body with white-sticky tongue coating, and rolling pulse.

主症：早期偶有视物昏朦，或瞳神稍大，眼底杯盘比渐大，或两眼杯盘比差值大于0.2，严重时视盘苍白，视野缺损，甚或呈管状，眼压偏高；可伴头昏眩晕，恶心欲呕；舌淡，苔白腻，脉滑。

Therapeutic methods: Warm yang, dissolve phlegm, promote flow and remove damp.

治法：温阳化痰，利水渗湿。

Herbal formulas and drugs: The major formula is *Gallbladder-Warming Decoction* (Wen Dan Tang) plus *Poria Five Powder* (Wu Ling San). The commonly-used herbal drugs are *Rhizoma Pinelliae* (Ban Xia), *Pericarpium Citri Tangerinae* (Chen Pi), *Sclerotium Poriae* (Fu Ling), *Polyporus Umbellatus* (Zhu Ling), *Fructus Aurantii Immaturus* (Zhi Shi), *Caulis Bambusae in Taeniam* (Zhu Ru), *Rhizoma Alismatis* (Ze Xie), *Rhizoma Atractylodis Macrocephalae* (Bai Zhu), *Ramulus Cinnamomi* (Gui Zhi), *Radix Glycyrrhizae Praeparata* (Zhi Gan Cao), etc.

方药：代表方为温胆汤合五苓散，常用药如半夏、橘皮、茯苓、猪苓、枳实、竹茹、泽泻、白术、桂枝、炙甘草等。

(3) **Liver and kidney deficiency**

(3) **肝肾亏虚**

Main symptoms: Chronic condition, blurring of vision, slight dilation of pupil, visual field defect, or tubular visual field, pale optic disc, accompanied by dizziness, insomnia, weakness at low back and

主症：患病日久，视物不清，瞳神稍大，视野缺损或呈管状，视盘苍白；可伴头晕失眠，腰膝无力，舌淡苔薄，脉

knees, pale tongue body with thin tongue coating, and thready-deep-weak pulse, or accompanied by pale complexion, chills in limbs, pale tongue body with white tongue coating, and thready-deep pulse.

细沉无力；或面白肢冷，精神倦怠，舌淡苔白，脉细沉。

Therapeutic methods: Reinforce and benefit liver and kidney.

治法：补益肝肾。

Herbal formulas and drugs: The major formula is *Scenery-Residing Pills Modified* (Jia Jian Zhu Jing Wan). The commonly-used herbal drugs are *Semen Plantaginis* (Che Qian Zi), *Radix Angelicae Sinensis* (Dang Gui), *Radix Rehmanniae Praeparata* (Shu Di Huang), *Fructus Schisandrae* (Wu Wei Zi), *Fructus Lycii* (Gou Qi Zi), *Fructus Broussonetiae* (Chu Shi Zi), *Semen Cuscutae* (Tu Si Zi), *Capsicum Annuum* (Chuan Jiao), etc.

方药：代表方为加减驻景丸，常用药如：车前子、当归、熟地黄、五味子、枸杞子、楮实子、菟丝子、川椒等。

4 Speculative map

4 思辨导图

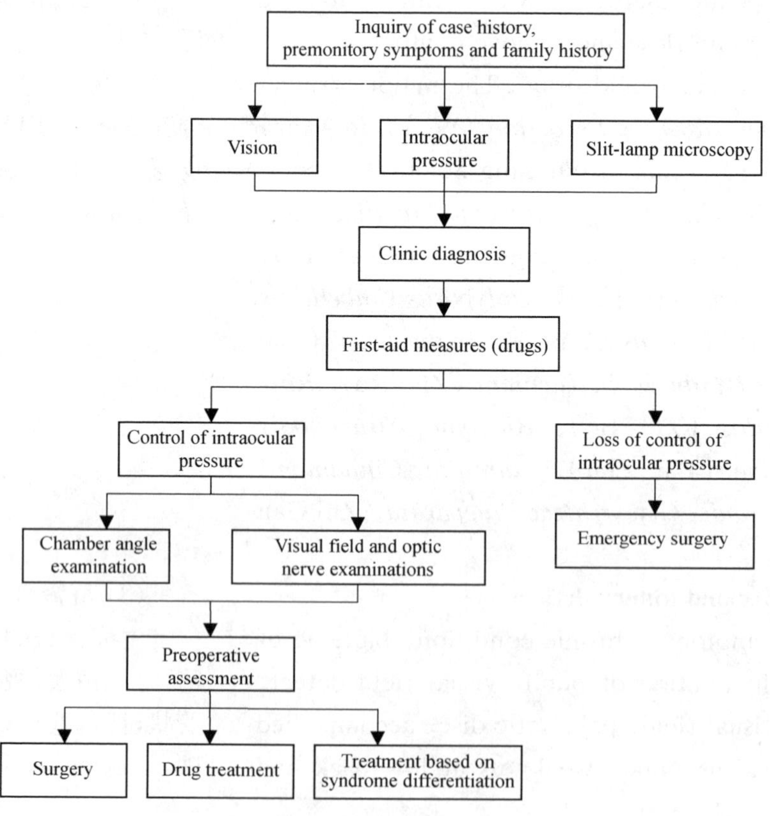

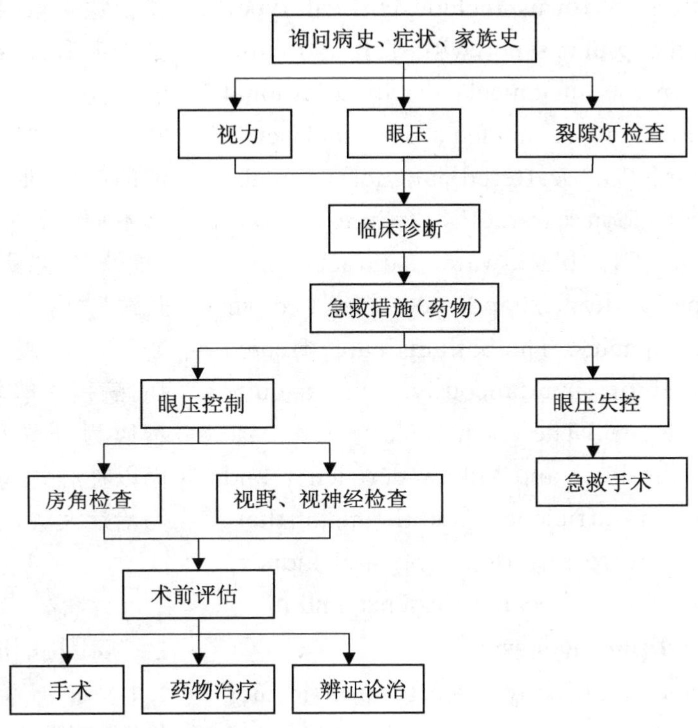

Senile cataract

老年性白内障

Senile cataract is a kind of eye disease with gradual lenticular opacity, slow decrease of vision and blindness along with the ageing.

老年性白内障是指随着年龄的增加,晶状体逐渐混浊,视力缓慢下降,终致失明的眼病。

In traditional Chinese medicine, the crystalline lens, called crystal pearls, are a pair of convex circular hyalosomes. Their pellucidity helps the light entering, and their elasticity acts to regulate the focus. It is believed in traditional Chinese medicine that the factors such as senile metabolism, diseases, etc. make the crystalline lens become opacity, so as to influence the visual quality, so-called senile cata-

中医学称晶状体为晶珠,为一双凸扁圆形类围棋子样透明体,其透明状态有助于光线的进入,其本身的弹性可调节起到清晰调焦的作用,现代中医认识了其原因为老年性的代谢、疾病等因素逐步使其混浊从而影响

ract. The expression forms include cortical type, nuclear type and capsular type, with different clinical symptoms. In the ancient classics of traditional Chinese medicine, it is named "icy cataract", "transverse cataract", "scattered cataract", "jujube cataract", "half-moon cataract", "white cataract with yellow center", "black-water cataract", etc. according to the location, shape, degree and colour of the lenticular opacity. The both eyes are affected one after another or simultaneously, with a quite long course of disease. The essentials of the disease are thought be the liver and kidney deficiency and essence and blood insufficiency, and the major therapeutic methods are to reinforce liver and kidney, nourish yin and blood and benefit essence and qi.

了视觉质量，称为圆翳内障。其表现形式有皮质性、核性、囊模性而产生不同的临床症状。中医古籍曾依据晶珠混浊的部位、形态、程度及颜色等不同，分别命名为"冰翳""横翳""散翳""枣花翳""偃月翳""白翳黄心""黑水凝翳"等，两眼先后或同时发病，病程一般较长，并认识其本质为肝肾亏虚，精血不足而以补肝肾、养阴血、益精气为治疗大法。

1 Etiology and pathogenesis

1 病因病机

1.1 Old age and weak body. Due to insufficiency of liver and kidney and deficiency of qi and yin, the crystalline lens loses the nourishment and become opacity gradually.

1.1 年老体弱，肝肾不足，气阴亏损，晶珠失养而渐趋混浊。

1.2 Spleen qi deficiency. The spleen fails to transport and transform the water, causing endogenous damp which flows upwards to the crystalline lens to cause opacity gradually.

1.2 脾虚气弱，运化失健，或水湿内生，上泛晶珠而混浊。

1.3 Liver depression and qi stagnation. The stagnation transforms to heat which disturbs the upper eyes to cause crystalline opacity.

1.3 肝郁不舒，郁而化热，上扰目窍，致晶珠逐渐混浊。

2 Diagnostic essentials

2 诊断要点

2.1 Over 50 in age, clear near vision and blurred far vision in the early stage, or double vision, and progressive decrease of vision.

2.1 年龄在 50 岁以上，早期或视近尚明而视远模糊，或视一为二，视力渐进性下降。

2.2 Opacity of crystalline lens in different loca-

2.2 晶状体不同部位、不同

tion, different shape and different degree.

2.3 Exclusion of other eye diseases and general diseases.

3 Therapeutic methods

3.1 Therapeutic principles

In the early stage, it is advisable to apply drug treatment and diopter correction to increase the visual quality. If the life or work is influenced, it is advisable to apply surgical treatment. According to pattern identification, the major therapeutic principles are to reinforce liver and kidney, nourish yin and blood and benefit essence and qi.

3.2 Treatment based on syndrome differentiation

(1) **Liver depression and qi stagnation**

Main symptoms: Clear or blurred vision now and then, non-decrease of vision, unserious opacity of crystalline lens, red tongue body with thin-yellow tongue coating, and wiry pulse or wiry-rapid pulse.

Therapeutic methods: Soothe liver, relieve depression and brighten eyes.

Herbal formulas and drugs: The major formula is *Free Wanderer Powder* (Xiao Yao San) plus *Four Agents Decoction* (Si Wu Tang). The commonly-used herbal drugs are *Radix Bupleuri* (Chai Hu), *Radix Angelicae Sinensis* (Dang Gui), *Radix Paeoniae* (Shao Yao), *Sclerotium Poriae* (Fu Ling), *Rhizoma Atractylodis Macrocephalae* (Bai Zhu), *Herba Menthae* (Bo He), *Radix Rehmanniae Cruda* (Sheng Di Huang), *Radix Paeoniae Alba* (Bai Shao), *Rhizoma Ligustici Chuanxiong* (Chuan Xiong), *Rhizoma Zingiberis Recens* (Sheng Jiang) Baked, etc.

形态及不同程度的混浊。

2.3 排除其他眼病和全身性疾病。

3 治疗方法

3.1 治疗原则

初病患者以药物治疗，屈光矫正提高视觉质量。影响生活或工作时，应行手术治疗。辨证以虚为本，补肝肾、养阴血、益精气为主要治则。

3.2 辨证论治

(1) **肝郁不舒**

主症：视物时清时糊，视力未降，晶珠混浊不甚，或目涩胀；时有眉棱骨痛，舌红苔薄黄，脉弦或弦数。

治法：疏肝解郁明目。

方药：代表方为逍遥散加四物汤，常用药如柴胡、当归、芍药、茯苓、白术、薄荷、生地黄、白芍、川芎、煨生姜等。

(2) **Spleen qi deficiency**

Main symptoms: Blurred vision, slow decrease of vision, or clear near vision and blurred far vision, gradual opacity of crystalline lens, accompanied by shortness of breath, dislike of speaking, fatigue of limbs and body, pale tongue body with white tongue coating, and slow-weak pulse.

Therapeutic methods: Benefit qi, strengthen spleen, promote water flow and dissolve damp.

Herbal formulas and drugs: The major formula is *Four Nobles Decoction* (Si Jun Zi Tang). The commonly-used herbal drugs are *Radix Codonopsis Pilosulae* (Dang Shen), *Rhizoma Atractylodis Macrocephalae* (Bai Zhu), *Sclerotium Poriae* (Fu Ling), *Radix Glycyrrhizae Praeparata* (Zhi Gan Cao), etc.

(2) **脾气虚弱**

主症：视物模糊，视力缓降，或视近尚明而视远模糊，晶珠渐混；或伴少气懒言，肢体倦怠；舌淡，苔白，脉缓弱。

治法：益气健脾，利水渗湿。

方药：代表方为四君子汤，常用药如党参、白术、茯苓、炙甘草等。

(3) **Liver and kidney insufficiency**

Main symptoms: Blurred vision, slow decrease of vision, obvious opacity of crystalline lens, accompanied by dizziness, tinnitus, poor sleep, poor memory, aching at low back and weakness at legs, dry mouth, red tongue body with scanty tongue coating, and thready pulse, or accompanied by tinnitus, hearing decrease, tidal fever, nocturnal sweats, vexation, poor sleep, red and dry tongue coating with thin-yellow tongue coating, and thready-wiry-rapid pulse.

Therapeutic methods: Reinforce and benefit liver and kidney, clear heat and brighten eyes.

Herbal formulas and drugs: The major formula is *Eye-Brightening Rehmannia Pills* (Ming Mu Di Huang Wan). The commonly-used herbal drugs are *Radix Rehmanniae Cruda* (Sheng Di Huang), *Radix Rehmanniae Praeparata* (Shu Di Huang), *Fruc-*

(3) **肝肾不足**

主症：视物昏花，视力缓降，晶珠混浊明显；或头昏耳鸣，少寐健忘，腰酸腿软，口干；舌红，苔少，脉细。或见耳鸣耳聋，潮热盗汗，虚烦不寐，舌红少津，苔薄黄，脉细弦数。

治法：补益肝肾，清热明目。

方药：代表方为明目地黄丸，常用药如生熟地黄、山茱萸、山药、牡丹皮、泽泻、茯苓、柴胡、当归、五味子等。

tus Corni (Shan Zhu Yu), *Rhizoma Dioscoreae* (Shan Yao), *Cortex Moutan Radicis* (Mu Dan Pi), *Rhizoma Alismatis* (Ze Xie), *Sclerotium Poriae* (Fu Ling), *Radix Bupleuri* (Chai Hu), *Radix Angelicae Sinensis* (Dang Gui), *Fructus Schisandrae* (Wu Wei Zi), etc.

3.3 Other therapies

(1) Surgical treatment: Apply phacoemulsification plus intraocular lens implantation. Under the operating microscope, apply phacoemulsification instrument to smash and extract the crystalline lens, clean the cortex, and then implant the artificial lens into the sac. This surgical operation, featured by small incision, short operating time, small wound and quick recovery of vision, is one of the most commonly-used surgical methods in the clinic. The artificial lens has been improved constantly in its optical property.

(2) Patent herbal medicines: ① Apply *Lycium, Chrysanthemun and Rehmannia Pills* (Qi Ju Di Huang Wan), Anemarrhena, Phellodendron, and Rehmannia Pills (Zhi Bai Di Huang Wan), *Dendrobe Night Lights Pills* (Shi Hu Ye Guang Wan), etc. ② Apply one of the following eye drugs of *Musk and Pearl Eye-Brightening Eye Drop* (She Zhu Ming Mu Di Yan Ye), *Cataract and Nebula Powder* (Zhang Yi San), Pirenoxine Eye Drop, Pirfenoxine Eye Drop, etc.

3.3 其他疗法

（1）手术治疗:超声乳化白内障吸除联合人工晶状体植入术:在手术显微镜下,用超声乳化仪将晶状体核粉碎并吸出,吸净皮质,然后将人工晶状体植入囊袋内。该手术方法切口小,手术时间短,创伤小,可迅速恢复视力,是目前临床最常用的手术方法之一。而人工晶状体也不断地改善其光学特性。

（2）中成药治疗:①根据不同证型可选用杞菊地黄丸、知柏地黄丸及石斛夜光丸等;②麝珠明目滴眼液、障翳散、白内停、卡他林等滴眼液,选用其中之一即可。

4 Speculative map

4 思辨导图

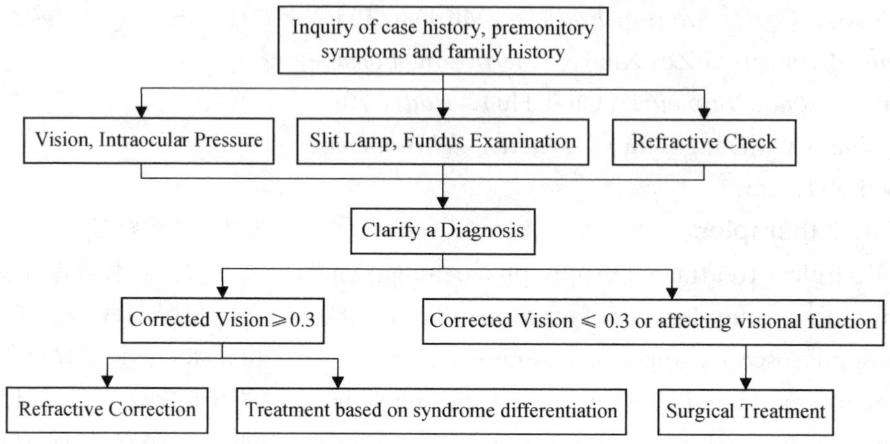

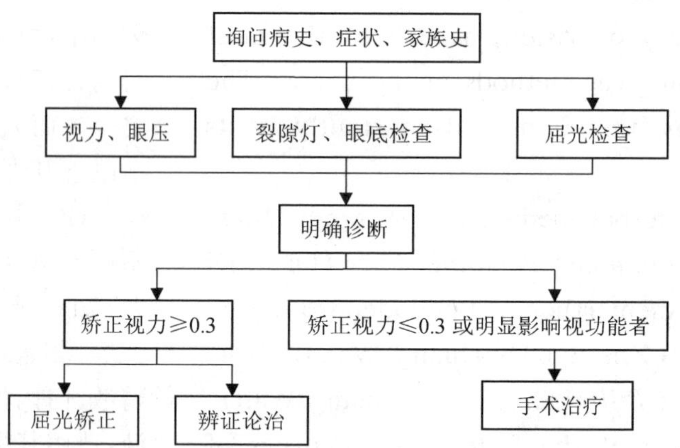

Retinal arterial obstruction

视网膜动脉阻塞

Retinal arterial obstruction is a kind of acute retinal ischemia due to embolism, thrombus or spasm which causes obstruction of retinal central arterial trunk or branches, so as to lead to acute damage or loss of the visual function.

视网膜动脉阻塞是视网膜中央动脉的主干或分支因栓塞、血栓、痉挛而阻塞引起其所供应区域的视网膜发生急性缺血，导致视功能急剧损害或丧失。

In traditional Chinese medicine, the disease is called "sudden blindness due to vessel obstruction" according to its manifestations of normal appearance, sudden decrease of vision of one eye or both eyes, cherry-red spots on fundus and clinical examinations by new technology. Mostly, one eye is affected, often caused by sudden anger which leads to qi activity disturbance, or by indulgence of alcohol and spicy food which leads to internal formation of phlegm-heat obstructing the blood vessels, or by yin and qi deficiency which leads to liver and kidney insufficiency and slow blood circulation, forming stasis to obstruct the vessels.

现代中医依据其外观正常，猝然一眼或双眼视力急剧下降，典型的樱桃红样眼底改变以及临床新技术检查提供的眼底改变命名为“络阻暴盲”。多单眼发病。常因忿怒暴悖，气机逆乱；或恣酒嗜辣，痰热内生，气壅痰阻，血脉闭塞；也有阴亏气弱，肝肾不足，血行滞缓，瘀滞脉络。

1 Etiology and pathogenesis

1 病因病机

1.1 Sudden anger and rage. Qi activity is disturbed, so qi and blood flow upwards to obstruct the blood vessels.

1.1 忿怒暴悖，气机逆乱，气血上壅，血络瘀阻。

1.2 Indulgence of fatty, sweet and greasy food or indulgence of alcohol and spicy food. Phlegm-heat is formed to obstruct the blood vessels.

1.2 偏食肥甘燥腻，或恣酒嗜辣，痰热内生，血脉闭塞。

1.3 Yin deficiency of liver and kidney. Liver yang becomes hyperactive and qi and blood flow upwards, so the stasis is formed to obstruct the blood vessels.

1.3 肝肾阴亏，肝阳上亢，气血并逆，瘀滞脉络。

1.4 Heart qi deficiency. The promoting function decreases, so the blood flows slowly to cause stasis which obstructs the blood vessels.

1.4 心气亏虚，推动乏力，血行滞缓，血脉瘀塞。

2 Diagnostic essentials

2 诊断要点

2.1 Subjective symptoms

2.1 自觉症状

Sudden and severe decrease of vision, even blindness, or partially visual field defect, or transitional premonitory symptoms of blurred vision, headache, dizziness before the onset of the disease in some patients.

突然视力急剧下降，甚至失明，或部分视野缺损。部分患者起病前可有视物模糊、头痛头昏等一过性前驱症状。

2.2 Ocular examinations

At the fundus, the retinal artery is obviously thinned, even in linear shape, the veins are also thinned, and the thrombus is in segmental shape or bead-like shape. There is grey-white colored and turbid edema at the posterior part of retina, and the macular region becomes red due to the visible choroids, the so-called "cherry-red" in the clinic. If the retinal ciliary artery is obstructed, its supplying area becomes red in colour and tongue-shaped. If the branch retinal artery is obstructed, the disease is limited in the area dominated by this branch. Over the years, the retinal turbid edema may be dissolved, but the optic disc becomes light-white.

2.2 眼部检查

眼底可见视网膜动脉显著变细，甚则呈线状；静脉亦变细，血柱呈节段状或串珠状；视网膜后部灰白色混浊水肿，黄斑区因透见脉络膜颜色而呈红色，临床称之为"樱桃红"。如有视网膜睫状动脉存在，则其供血区域呈红色舌状区；分支动脉阻塞时，病变限于该分支支配区域。日久视网膜混浊水肿可消退，但可见视盘色淡白。

2.3 Auxiliary examination, fluorescein fundus angiography

It is difficult to take angiography at the moment of disease onset. Usually this examination is taken several hours, several days even several weeks after the disease onset, so the results vary as follows: ① Non-perfusion in central arterial trunk or non-perfusion in small branches. ② Slow arterial and venous filling, and prolonged retinal circulation. ③ Fluorescein traversing the area of blood flow interruption. ④ Fluorescein leakage at partial blood vessel walls. ⑤ No fluorescein phenomenon of obstruction in patients of late stage.

2.3 辅助检查

荧光素眼底血管造影：但在病变发生时很难及时进行造影检查，多在病变发生后数小时、数日甚至数周后才进行此项检查，因此结果差异较大，其常见的变化有：①中央动脉主干无灌注或动脉小分支无灌注；②动脉及静脉充盈迟缓，视网膜循环时间延长；③检眼镜下所见的血流"中断"部位仍有荧光素通过；④部分血管壁的荧光素渗漏；⑤晚期患者可能见不到阻塞的荧光征象。

3 Therapeutic methods

3.1 Therapeutic principles

It is the acute and severe disease in ophthalmol-

3 治疗方法

3.1 治疗原则

本病为眼科急重症，抢

ogy, so the emergency treatment should be as early as possible. In traditional Chinese medicine, the major therapeutic principles are to move qi and blood so as to unblock the vessels, and to benefit zang-fu organs so as to equilibrate yin and yang.

救应尽早、尽快。行气血以贯络脉，益脏腑以平阴阳是中医临证的基本治则。

3.2 First aid measures

(1) Apply the inhalation of 0.2 ml isoamyl nitrite, another inhalation after 1 to 2 hours, and apply 2 to 3 times in succession. Apply sublingual Trinitroglycerin Tablets, 0.3 to 0.6 mg each time and 2 to 3 times a day.

(2) Apply the retroocular injection of 12.5 mg Tolazoline or 1 mg Atropine.

(3) Apply the intermittently massage of eyeballs, anterior chamber penetration and oral administration of Acetazolamide Tablets, to decrease intraocular pressure.

(4) Apply the inhalation of mixed gas of 95% oxygen and 5% carbon dioxide.

3.2 急救措施

（1）亚硝酸异戊酯 0.2 ml 吸入，每隔 1～2 小时再吸 1 次，连用 2～3 次。舌下含化三硝酸甘油酯片。每次 0.3～0.6 mg，每日 2～3 次。

（2）球后注射妥拉苏林 12.5 mg 或阿托品 1 mg。

（3）间歇性按摩眼球、前房穿刺、口服乙酰唑胺以降低眼压。

（4）吸入 95%氧及 5%二氧化碳混合气体。

3.3 Treatment based on syndrome differentiation

(1) Qi and blood stagnation and obstruction:

Main symptoms: Good appearance of eye, sudden blindness, fundus manifestations matching up with the features of the disease, accompanied by restlessness, anger, distension and fullness at chest and hypochondriac area, headache, distension in eye, purplish spots on tongue, and wiry or choppy pulse.

Therapeutic methods: Move qi, activate blood, dredging aperture and brighten eye.

Herbal formulas and drugs: The major formula is *Aperture-Dredging and Blood-Activating Decoction* (Tong Qiao Huo Xue Tang). The commonly-used

3.3 辨证论治

（1）气血瘀阻

主症：眼外观端好，骤然盲无所见，眼底表现符合本病的特征；伴见急躁易怒，胸胁胀满，头痛眼胀；舌有瘀点，脉弦或涩。

治法：行气活血，通窍明目。

方药：代表方为通窍活血汤，常用药如赤芍、桃仁、红花、川芎等。

herbal drugs are *Radix Paeoniae Rubra* (chi xhao), *Semen Persicae* (Tao Ren), *Flos Carthami* (Hong Hua), *Rhizoma Ligustici Chuanxiong* (Chuan Xiong), etc.

Modification according to symptoms: For insomnia, add *Caulis Polygoni Multiflori* (Shou Wu Teng) and *Semen Zizyphi Spinosae* (Suan Zao Ren) to quiet heart and calm mind. For severe distension and fullness at chest and hypochondriac area, add *Radix Curcumae* (Yu Jin) and *Pericarpium Citri Reticulatae Viride* (Qing Pi) to move qi and relieve depression. For severe retinal edema, add *Succinum* (Hu Po), *Herba Lycopi* (Ze Lan) and *Herba Leonuri* (Yi Mu Cao) to activate blood and dissolve stasis, and to promote water flow and relieve swelling. For severe dizziness, add *Rhizoma Gastrodiae* (Tian Ma) and *Radix Achyranthis Bidentatae* (Niu Xi) to soothe liver and guide the blood flowing downwards.

加减：失眠者，加首乌藤、酸枣仁以宁心安神；胸胁胀满甚者，加郁金、青皮以行气解郁；视网膜水肿甚，加琥珀、泽兰、益母草以活血化瘀、利水消肿；头昏重者，加天麻、牛膝以平肝、引血下行。

(2) **Up-accumulation of phlegm-heat**

(2) **痰热上壅**

Main symptoms: Ocular symptoms and examination matching up to the features of the disease, accompanied by heavy body, dizzy and weighty sensation in head, stuffy chest, restlessness, poor appetite, nausea, bitter taste in mouth, thick sputum, yellow-sticky tongue coating, and wiry-rolling pulse.

主症：眼部症状及检查符合本病的特征；形体多较胖，头眩而重，胸闷烦躁，食少恶心、口苦痰稠；舌苔黄腻，脉弦滑。

Therapeutic methods: Cleanse phlegm, dredge collaterals, activate blood and dredge aperture.

治法：涤痰通络，活血通窍。

Herbal formulas and drugs: The major formula is *Phlegm-Cleansing Decoction* (Di Tan Tang). The commonly-used herbal drugs are *Rhizoma Pinelliae* (Ban Xia), *Exocarpium Citri Grandis* (Ju Hong), *Fructus Aurantii Immaturus* (Zhi Shi), *Sclerotium Poriae* (Fu Ling), *Arisaema cum Bile* (Dan Nan

方药：代表方为涤痰汤，常用药如半夏、橘红、枳实、茯苓、胆南星、竹茹、人参、石菖蒲、生甘草。

Xing), *Caulis Bambusae in Taeniam* (Zhu Ru), *Radix Ginseng* (Ren Shen), *Rhizoma Acori Graminei* (Shi Chang Pu), *Radix Glycyrrhizae Cruda* (Sheng Gan Cao), etc.

Modification according to symptoms: Discretionarily add *Lumbricus* (Di Long), *Rhizoma Ligustici Chuanxiong* (Chuan Xiong), *Radix Curcumae* (Yu Jin), *Radix Achyranthis Bidentatae* (Niu Xi), *Herba Lycopi* (Ze Lan) and *Moschus* (She Xiang) to enhance the action to activate blood, dredge collaterals and open aperture. For severe pathogenic heat, subtract *Radix Ginseng* (Ren Shen), *Rhizoma Zingiberis Recens* (Sheng Jiang) and *Fructus Ziziphi Jujubae* (Da Zao), and add *Rhizoma Coptidis* (Huang Lian) and *Radix Scutellariae* (Huang Qin) to clear heat and cleanse phlegm.

加减:可酌加地龙、川芎、郁金、牛膝、泽兰、麝香,以助活血通络开窍之力;若热邪较甚,方中去人参、生姜、大枣,酌加黄连、黄芩以清热涤痰。

(3) **Liver yang hyperactivity**

Main symptoms: Ocular symptoms and fundus examination matching up to the features of the disease, accompanied by dryness of eyes, headache, distension of eye, dizziness now and then, restlessness, anger, red complexion, feverish sensation, palpitation, poor memory, insomnia, dream-disturbed sleep, bitter taste in mouth, sore throat, and wiry-thready or rapid pulse.

Therapeutic methods: Nourish yin, subdue yang, activate blood and dredge collaterals.

Herbal formulas and drugs: The major formula is *Gastrodia and Cat's Claw Drink* (Tian Ma Gou Teng Yin). The commonly-used herbal drugs are *Rhizoma Gastrodiae* (Tian Ma), *Ramulus Uncariae cum Uncis* (Gou Teng), *Concha Haliotidis Cruda* (Sheng Shi Jue Ming), *Fructus Gardeniae* (Zhi Zi), *Radix Scutellariae* (Huang Qin), *Radix Cyathulae*

(3) **肝阳上亢**

主症:眼部症状及眼底检查符合本病的特征,双目干涩,头痛眼胀,眩晕时作,急躁易怒,面赤烘热,心悸健忘,失眠多梦,口苦咽干,脉弦细或数。

治法:滋阴潜阳,活血通络。

方药:代表方为天麻钩藤饮,常用药如天麻、钩藤、生石决明、栀子、黄芩、川牛膝、杜仲、益母草、桑寄生、夜交藤、茯苓等。

(Chuan Niu Xi), *Cortex Eucommiae* (Du Zhong), *Herba Leonuri* (Yi Mu Cao), *Ramulus Loranthi* (Sang Ji Sheng), *Caulis Polygoni Multiflori* (Ye Jiao Teng), *Sclerotium Poriae* (Fu Ling), etc.

Modification according to symptoms: For dark tongue body and choppy pulse, add *Rhizoma Acori Graminei* (Shi Chang Pu), *Radix Salviae Miltiorrhizae* (Dan Shen), *Lumbricus* (Di Long) and *Rhizoma Ligustici Chuanxiong* (Chuan Xiong) to enhance the action to dredge collaterals and activate blood. For palpitation, poor memory, insomnia and dream-disturbed sleep, add *Concha Margaritifera Usta* (Zhen Zhu Mu) to calm mind. For restlessness and feverish sensation in palms and soles, add *Rhizoma Anemarrhenae* (Zhi Mu), *Cortex Phellodendri* (Huang bai) and *Cortex Lycii Radicis* (Di Gu Pi) to reduce the false fire. For severe retinal edema and opacity, add *Semen Plantaginis* (Che Qian Zi), *Herba Lycopi* (Ze Lan) and *Radix Curcumae* (Yu Jin) to activate blood and promote urination.

加减：舌暗脉涩者，加石菖蒲、丹参、地龙、川芎以助通络活血；心悸健忘、失眠多梦者，加珍珠母镇静安神；五心烦热者，加知母、黄柏、地骨皮降虚火；视网膜水肿混浊明显者，加车前子、泽兰、郁金以活血利尿。

(4) **Qi deficiency and blood stasis**

(4) **气虚血瘀**

Main symptoms: Chronic disease, blurring of vision, thin and light-colored artery, or white-colored and linear artery, retinal edema, light-white colour of optic disc, accompanied by shortness of breath, lassitude, sallow-yellow complexion, fatigue, dislike of speaking, pale tongue body with purple patches, and choppy or irregular pulse.

主症：发病日久，视物昏朦，动脉细而色淡红或呈白色线条状，视网膜水肿，视盘色淡白；或伴短气乏，面色萎黄，倦怠懒言；舌淡有瘀斑，脉涩或结代。

Therapeutic methods: Reinforce qi, nourish blood, dissolve stasis and dredge collaterals.

治法：补气养血，化瘀通脉。

Herbal formulas and drugs: The major formula is *Yang-Invigorating and Recuperating Decoction Modified* (Bu Yang Huan Wu Tang Jia Jian). The commonly-used herbal drugs are *Radix Astragali* (Huang Qi),

方药：补阳还五汤加减，常用药如黄芪、桃仁、红花、当归、赤芍、川芎、地龙等。

Semen Persicae (Tao Ren), *Flos Carthami* (Hong Hua), *Radix Angelicae Sinensis* (Dang Gui), *Radix Paeoniae Rubra* (Chi Shao), *Rhizoma Ligustici Chuanxiong* (Chuan Xiong), *Lumbricus* (Di Long), etc.

Modification according to symptoms: For palpitation, fearful throbbing, insomnia and dream-disturbed sleep, add *Semen Zizyphi Spinosae* (Suan Zao Ren), *Caulis Polygoni Multiflori* (Shou Wu Teng) and *Semen Biotae* (Bai Zi Ren) to nourish heart and calm mind. For light-colored retina, add *Fructus Lycii* (Gou Qi Zi), *Semen Cuscutae* (Tu Si Zi) and *Fructus Ligustri Lucidi* (Nü Zhen Zi) to benefit kidney and brighten eyes. For chronic disease and emotional depression, add *Radix Bupleuri* (Chai Hu), *Radix Paeoniae Alba* (Bai Shao), *Pericarpium Citri Reticulatae Viride* (Qing Pi) and *Radix Curcumae* (Yu Jin) to soothe liver and relieve depression.

加减:心慌心悸、失眠多梦者,加酸枣仁、首乌藤、柏子仁以养心宁神;视衣色淡者,加枸杞子、菟丝子、女贞子等益肾明目;久病情志抑郁者,加柴胡、白芍、青皮、郁金以疏肝解郁。

4 Speculative map

4 思辨导图

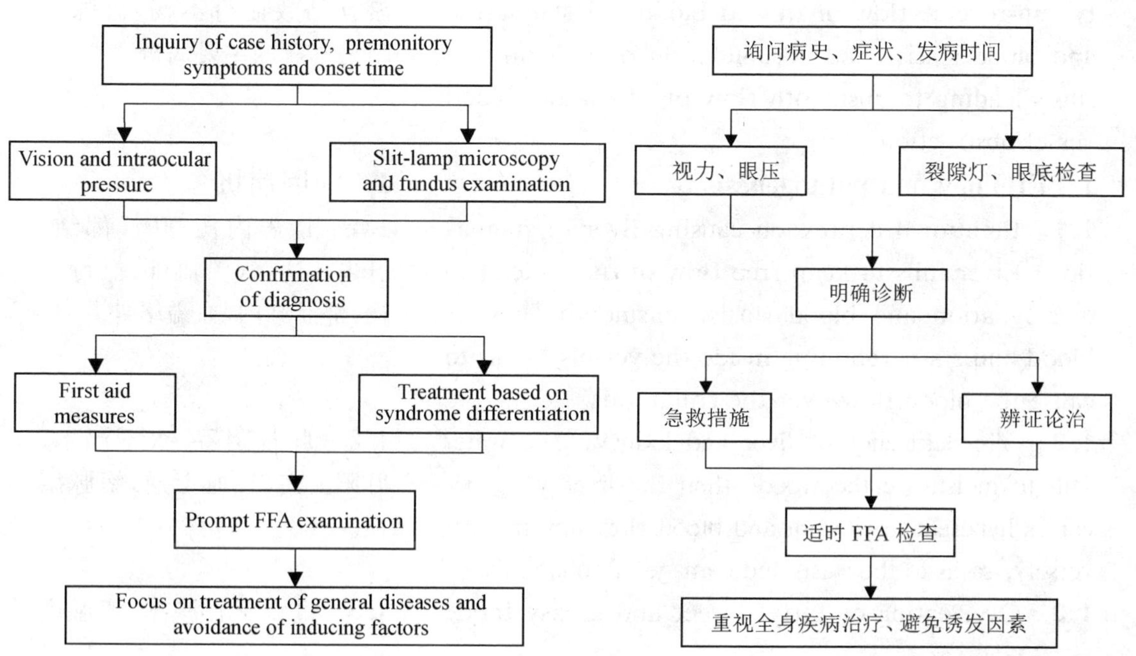

Retinal vein obstruction

视网膜静脉阻塞

Retinal vein obstruction refers to the damages of retinal ischemia, tissue edema, hemorrhage, etc. due to retinal central vein or branch vein obstruction causing reflux obstruction. Clinically, it is divided into central vein obstruction and branch vein obstruction, and divided into ischemic type and non-ischemic type. The condition and visual prognosis are related to the obstruction areas and types.

In traditional Chinese medicine, the disease is called "sudden blindness due to collateral stasis" according to the clinical manifestations of occluded and obstructed veins, overflow of blood and sudden decrease of vision. It is believed that the major pathogenesis of the disease is liver yang hyperactivity, up-reverse flow of qi and blood, qi stagnation and blood stasis, and accumulation of phlegm and stasis leading to unsmooth flow of blood and blood vessel obstruction.

视网膜静脉阻塞是指视网膜中央或分支静脉阻塞回流受阻所导致的视网膜缺血、组织水肿、出血等损害。临床有中央静脉阻塞、分支静脉阻塞；又有缺血型与非缺血型之分；病情与视力预后与阻塞部位及类型相关。

现代中医依据其眼底脉络扭曲瘀阻，血不循经，溢于络外，导致视力突然下降的临床表现命名为“络瘀暴盲”。认为肝阳上亢，气血上逆，气滞血郁，痰凝气滞，痰瘀互结致血行不畅，血脉瘀阻是本病的主要病机。

1 Etiology and pathogenesis

1.1 Emotional depression causing liver qi stagnation: Liver fails to keep free flow of qi, to lead to qi stagnation and blood stasis, unsmooth flow of blood and stasis retaining inside the vessels, so as to cause the blood flow over the collaterals.

1.2 Yin deficiency of liver and kidney: The water fails to moisturize the wood, then the liver yang becomes hyperactive, and qi and blood flow upwards reversely, so as to the stasis and damage of collaterals.

1.3 Over-eating of fatty, sweet and greasy food:

1 病因病机

1.1 情志内伤，肝气郁结，肝失条达，气滞血郁，血行不畅，郁滞脉内，血溢络外。

1.2 肝肾阴亏，水不涵木，肝阳上亢，气血上逆，络脉瘀损。

1.3 过食肥甘厚味，痰湿内

The phlegm-damp is thus formed internally. The phlegm and qi stagnation lead to the unsmooth flow of blood, and accumulation of phlegm and stasis obstructs the blood vessels to cause the disease.

生，痰凝气滞，血行不畅，痰瘀互结，血脉瘀阻而成患。

2 Diagnostic essentials

2 诊断要点

2.1 Subjective symptoms

2.1 自觉症状

Sudden decrease of vision, or black shadow before eye, even hand motion in severe condition.

视力突然减退，或有眼前黑影飘动，严重者可骤降至眼前手动。

2.2 Ocular examinations

2.2 眼部检查

The retinal veins at the affected area become thick-big and twisted, disappearing into the retinal flame hemorrhage and edema. In severe condition, there can be optic disc hemorrhage and edema, accompanied by yellow-white hard exudates or white cotton-wool spots, or cystoid macular edema. There can be sclerotic sign, as reflective enhancement in the retinal artery.

病变区视网膜静脉粗大迂曲，隐没于视网膜火焰状出血及水肿之中，重者可见视盘充血、水肿；或伴有黄白色硬性渗出或棉絮状白斑，或黄斑囊样水肿，视网膜动脉可有反光增强等硬化征象。

2.3 Auxiliary examinations

2.3 辅助检查

In the early stage of fundus fluorescein angiography (FFA), the circulation time of retinal artery and veins is prolonged, the hemorrhagic area covers the fluorescence, and in the obstructing area, the blood capillaries are dilated or microaneurysm can be seen. In the late stage of FFA, there can be fluorescence leakage of blood capillaries, and dying of venous veins. In the chronic condition, there can be the fluorescence forms of non-perfusion area in blood capillaries, macular edema, retinal neovascularization, etc.

眼底荧光血管造影早期可见视网膜动脉—静脉循环时间延长，出血区遮蔽荧光，阻塞区毛细血管扩张或有微动脉瘤；造影后期可见毛细血管荧光素渗漏、静脉管壁着染。病久者可见毛细血管无灌注区、黄斑区水肿、视网膜新生血管等荧光形态。

3 Therapeutic methods

3 治疗方法

3.1 Therapeutic principles

3.1 治疗原则

It is advisable to establish the therapeutic pro-

依据眼底荧光血管造影

gram according to the indications of FFA. It is to apply the comprehensive treatment for non-ischemic type. For ischemic type, it is necessary to apply the retinal laser photocoagulation immediately, so as to decrease retinal edema, promote absorption of hemorrhage, and prevent the occurrence of neovascular glaucoma, and to treat the primary disease positively. In traditional Chinese medicine, the pathogenesis of the disease is vessel and collateral obstruction and overflow of blood from vessels to the eyes. The obstruction is the stasis, and the blood away from meridians is also the stasis, so the blood stasis the most prominent pathogenesis. Therefore, the basic therapeutic principles are to stanch blood, dissolve stasis, move qi and remove phlegm.

提示确定治疗方法，如为非缺血型可综合治疗；缺血型则应立即视网膜激光光凝减少视网膜水肿，促进出血吸收，预防新生血管性青光眼的发生，并积极治疗原发病。因本病的基本病机是脉络瘀阻，血不循经，溢于目内；而阻塞是瘀，离经之血亦是瘀，故血瘀是其最突出的病机，因此，其基本治则是止血逐瘀，行气除痰。

3.2 Treatment based on syndrome differentiation

3.2 辨证论治

(1) Qi stagnation and blood stasis

(1) 气滞血瘀

Main symptoms: Good appearance of eye, sudden decrease of vision, fundus manifestations matching up to the features of the disease, accompanied by distension of eye, headache, distension and pain at chest and hypochondriac area, emotional depression, poor appetite, belching, red tongue body with purple patches and thin-white tongue coating, and wiry or choppy pulse.

主症：眼外观端好，视力急降，眼底表现符合本病特征；可伴见眼胀头痛，胸胁胀痛，或情志抑郁，食少嗳气；舌红有瘀斑，苔薄白，脉弦或涩等。

Therapeutic methods: Regulate qi flow, relieve depression, dissolve stasis and stanch blood.

治法：理气解郁，化瘀止血。

Herbal formulas and drugs: The major formula is *Sanguine Mansion Stasis-Expelling Decoction* (Xue Fu Zhu Yu Tang). The commonly-used herbal drugs are *Semen Persicae* (Tao Ren), *Flos Carthami* (Hong Hua), *Radix Paeoniae Rubra* (Chi Shao), *Radix Achyranthis Bidentatae* (Niu Xi), *Rhizoma*

方药：代表方为血府逐瘀汤，常用药如桃仁、红花、赤芍、牛膝、川芎、枳壳、当归、生地黄、柴胡、桔梗、炙甘草等。

Ligustici Chuanxiong (Chuan Xiong), *Fructus Aurantii* (Zhi Ke), *Radix Angelicae Sinensis* (Dang Gui), *Radix Rehmanniae Cruda* (Sheng Di Huang), *Radix Bupleuri* (Chai Hu), *Radix Platycodi* (Jie Geng), *Radix Glycyrrhizae Praeparata* (Zhi Gan Cao), etc.

Modification according to symptoms: In the early stage, subtract *Rhizoma Ligustici Chuanxiong* (Chuan Xiong) and *Radix Angelicae Sinensis* (Dang Gui), and add *Herba Schizonepetae Carbonisatus* (Jing Jie Tan), *Crinis Carbonisatus* (Xue Yu Tan), *Rhizoma Imperatae* (Bai Mao Gen), *Herba seu Radix Cirsii Japonici* (Da Ji) and *Herba Cephalanoploris* (Xiao Ji) to cool blood and stanch blood. For severe fundus hemorrhage with purple and dark blood, add *Pollen Typhae Cruda* (Sheng Pu Huang), Radix Rubiae (Qian Cao) and *Radix Notoginseng* (San Qi) to dissolve stasis and stanch blood. For severe optic disc hemorrhage and edema and retinal edema, add *Herba Lycopi* (Ze Lan), *Herba Leonuri* (Yi Mu Cao) and *Semen Plantaginis* (Che Qian Zi) to activate blood and promote water flow. For insomnia and dream-disturbed sleep, add *Concha Margaritifera Usta* (Zhen Zhu Mu) and *Caulis Polygoni Multiflori* (Shou Wu Teng) to calm mind.

加减:初期宜去方中川芎、当归,加荆芥炭、血余炭、白茅根、大蓟、小蓟以凉血止血;眼底出血较多,血色紫暗者,加生蒲黄、茜草、三七以化瘀止血;视盘充血水肿,视网膜水肿明显者,宜加泽兰、益母草、车前子以活血利水;失眠多梦者,加珍珠母、首乌藤以镇静安神。

(2) **Yin deficiency and yang hyperactivity**

Main symptoms: Good appearance of eye, sudden decrease of vision, fundus manifestations matching up to the features of the disease, accompanied by dizziness, tinnitus, red complexion, tidal fever, weighty sensation in head and light sensation in feet, insomnia, dream-disturbed sleep, restlessness, anger, aching and weakness at low back and knees, red tongue body with scanty tongue coating, and

(2) **阴虚阳亢**

主症:眼外观端好,视力急降,眼底表现符合本病特征;兼见头晕、耳鸣,面热潮红,头重脚轻,失眠多梦,烦躁易怒,腰膝酸软;舌红少苔,脉弦细。

wiry-thready pulse.

Therapeutic methods: Nourish yin and subdue yang.

治法：滋阴潜阳。

Herbal formulas and drugs: The major formula is *Liver-Sedating and Wind-Eliminating Decoction* (Zhen Gan Xi Feng Tang). The commonly-used herbal drugs are *Radix Achyranthis Bidentatae* (Niu Xi), *Ochra Haematitum* (Dai Zhe Shi), *Os Draconis* (Long Gu), *Concha Ostreae* (Mu Li), *Plastrum Testudinis* (Gui Jia), *Flos Chrysanthemi* (Ju Hua), *Radix Scrophulariae* (Xuan Shen), *Tuber Asparagi* (Tian Men Dong), *Fructus Hordei Germinatus* (Mai Ya), *Herba Artemisiae Scopariae* (Yin Chen Hao), *Radix Glycyrrhizae Praeparata* (Zhi Gan Cao), etc.

方药：代表方为镇肝熄风汤，常用药如牛膝、代赭石、龙骨、牡蛎、龟甲、菊花、玄参、天门冬、麦芽、茵陈蒿、炙甘草等。

Modification according to symptoms: For severe tidal fever and dry mouth, add *Radix Rehmanniae Cruda* (Sheng Di Huang), *Radix Ophiopogonis* (Mai Dong), *Rhizoma Anemarrhenae* (Zhi Mu) and *Cortex Phellodendri* (Huang Bo) to nourish yin and subdue fire. For weighty sensation in head and light sensation in feet, add *Radix Polygoni Multiflori* (He Shou Wu), *Ramulus Uncariae cum Uncis* (Gou Teng) and *Concha Haliotidis* (Shi Jue Ming) to nourish yin and subdue yang.

加减：潮热口干明显者，加生地黄、麦门冬、知母、黄柏以滋阴降火；头重脚轻者，宜加何首乌、钩藤、石决明以滋阴潜阳。

(3) **Mutual accumulation of phlegm-stasis**

(3) **痰瘀互结**

Main symptoms: Same eye symptoms as the above, long course of disease, obvious fundus edema and exudates, or cystoid macular edema, accompanied by heavy body, weighty sensation in head, dizziness, stuffy chest, distension in abdomen, tongue and pulse of those of phlegm-damp.

主症：眼症同前，或病程较长，眼底水肿渗出明显，或有黄斑囊样水肿；形体肥胖，兼见头重眩晕、胸闷脘胀、舌脉等为痰湿之候。

Therapeutic methods: Dissolve phlegm, remove damp, activate blood and dredge collaterals.

治法：化痰除湿，活血通络。

Herbal formulas and drugs: The major formula

方药：代表方为桃红四

is Peach Pit, Safflower and *Four Agents Decoction* (Tao Hong Si Wu Tang) plus *Gallbladder-Warming Decoction* (Wen Dan Tang). The commonly-used herbal drugs are *Radix Rehmanniae Cruda* (Sheng Di Huang), *Radix Paeoniae Rubra* (Chi Shao), *Rhizoma Ligustici Chuanxiong* (Chuan Xiong), *Radix Angelicae Sinensis* (Dang Gui), *Semen Persicae* (Tao Ren), *Flos Carthami* (Hong Hua), *Rhizoma Pinelliae* (Ban Xia), *Pericarpium Citri Tangerinae* (Chen Pi), *Sclerotium Poriae* (Fu Ling), *Radix Glycyrrhizae Praeparata* (Zhi Gan Cao), *Fructus Aurantii Immaturus* (Zhi Shi), *Caulis Bambusae in Taeniam* (Zhu Ru), etc.

物汤合温胆汤,常用药如生地黄、赤芍、川芎、当归、桃仁、红花、半夏、橘皮、茯苓、炙甘草、枳实、竹茹等。

Modification according to symptoms: For severe retinal edema and exudates, add *Semen Plantaginis* (Che Qian Zi), *Herba Leonuri* (Yi Mu Cao) and *Herba Lycopi* (Ze Lan) to activate blood, promote water flow and relieve swelling.

加减:若视网膜水肿、渗出明显者,可加车前子、益母草、泽兰以活血利水消肿。

3.3 Other therapies

(1) Patent herbal medicines: According to the patterns, apply *Compound Thrombosis Relieving Capsule* (Fu Fang Xue Shuan Tong Jiao Nang) for oral administration or *Thrombosis Relieving Injection* (Xue Shuan Tong Zhu She Ye) for intravenous injection.

(2) If the hemorrhagic volume is large to involve the vitreous body, and the accumulated blood has not been absorbed after positive treatment for one month, or the organic hybrid film is formed by B-ultrasonic examination, or retinal detachment occurs, it is advisable to apply vitrectomy.

(3) If OCT indicates macular edema, it is advisable to apply the anti-neovasculatural therapy.

3.3 其他疗法

(1) 中成药治疗:根据临床证型选用复方血栓通胶囊口服或血栓通注射液静脉滴注。

(2) 如出血量多进入玻璃体,腔积血经积极治疗月余仍不能吸收,或经 B 超检查有机化膜形成,甚或有视网膜脱离者,应行玻璃体切除术。

(3) OCT 提示视网膜黄斑水肿,可施行抗新生血管治疗。

4 Speculative map

4 思辨导图

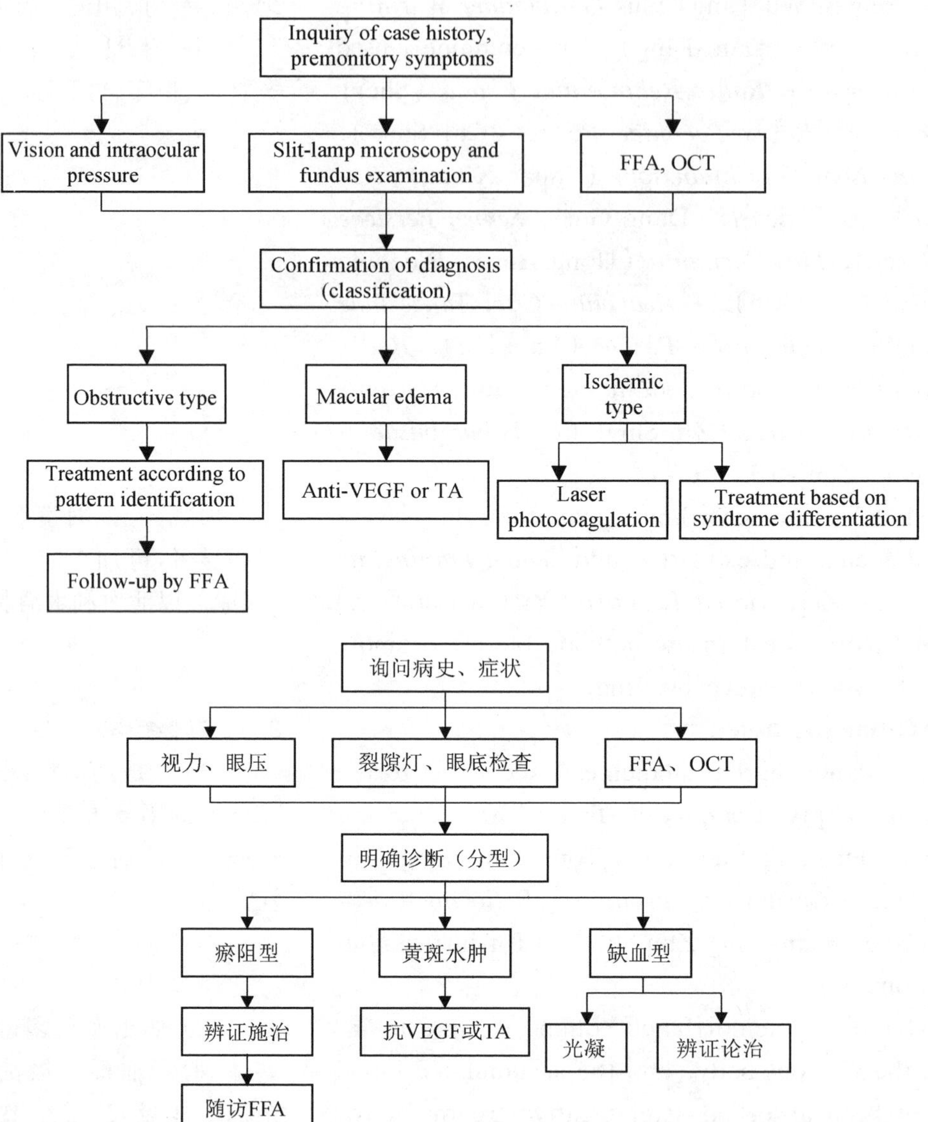

Diabetic retinopathy

Diabetic retinopathy refers to a series of lesions of retinal edema, hemorrhage or exudation, even neoangiogenesis due to retinal microvascular abnormalities, such as retinal ischemia or anoxia, caused by diabetes. The basic essential of the disease is the long-term glucose metabolic disorder, leading to microcirculation disturbance caused by retinal vascular endothelial and pericyte dysfunction.

In traditional Chinese medicine, the disease pertains to the scope of "eye diseases due to diabetes" according to the clinical manifestationsof visual function injury, such as "blurred vision", "vitreous opacity", "sudden visual loss", etc. Xu Ling-tai described the disease as "polydipsia, polyphagia and polyuria, caused by yin deficiency with yang hyperactivity, and body fluid consumption with pathogenic heat". It is believed that the mechanism of microcirculation disturbance in TCM ophthalmology is the loss of equilibrium in lung, spleen and kidney. The chronic disease in the Qi (Energy) Phase involves the Ying (Nutrition) Phase and Xue (Blood) Phase, then the collaterals, so deficiency causes stasis which causes phlegm, as a result, the accumulation of phlegm and stasis. Therefore, the pathogenesis of qi deficiency, blood lesion and collateral damage are applied to guide the clinic practice.

糖尿病性视网膜病变

糖尿病视网膜病变是指因糖尿病引起的视网膜微血管异常导致视网膜缺血、缺氧，进而视网膜水肿、出血、渗出，甚至新生血管形成、增殖等一系列病变，其本质是机体长期糖代谢紊乱导致的眼底血管内皮以及周细胞功能受损引起的微循环障碍。

中医眼科依据其“视瞻昏渺”“云雾移睛”“暴盲”等不同视功能损害的临床表现，可将其归属于“消渴目病”范畴。徐灵胎“三消一证，虽有上、中、下之分，其实不越阴亏阳亢，津枯热淫”的阐述，为现代中医眼科理解其微循环障碍乃肺、脾、肾三焦调理失衡的病机。气分久病伤及营血、络脉，由虚致瘀、由瘀致痰，痰瘀互结，故常以气虚、血病、络损之病机指导临床。

1 Etiology and pathogenesis

1.1 Qi and yin are deficient, so the eyes fail to be nourished, or deficiency causes stasis which leads to unsmooth flow of blood in collaterals.

1.2 Unclean food damages the spleen and stomach, or emotional factors damage the liver, causing liver qi stagnation which attacks the splee. Due to spleen deficiency, its transportation is disturbed, leading to internal formation of phlegm-damp and qi stagnation, as a result, the eyes losing the nourishment.

1.3 Damage of yin due to other chronic diseases, or congenital yin deficiency, causes the endogenous false fire which burns and injures the blood vessels in eyes.

1.4 Due to other chronic diseases, the blood vessels are blocked by stasis, and the false fire burns and injures the blood vessels. The stasis causes phlegm, leading to accumulation of phlegm and stasis. Or in the late stage of chronic diseases, both yin and yang are deficient, so yang deficiency causes phlegm, thus blurred vision occurs.

2 Diagnostic essentials

2.1 Clinical manifestations

Floaters, or blurred vision, or visual decrease, or sudden visual loss.

2.2 Fundus examinations

Hemorrhagic spots on retina, or macular edema, or exudation on area postrema, or grey-colored or brown-colored opacity, hemorrhage and exudative membrane on vitreous body, or limit retinal prominence or proliferation, or failure to detect the

1 病因病机

1.1 气阴两亏，目失所养，或因虚致淤，血络不畅。

1.2 饮食不洁，脾胃受伤，或情志伤肝，肝郁犯脾，致脾虚失运，痰湿内生，气滞湿阻，目失濡养。

1.3 病久伤阴，或素体阴亏，虚火内生，灼伤目中血络。

1.4 久病血络瘀阻，加之虚火灼伤脉络，凝液成痰，瘀滞痰结；或后期阴阳俱损，阳虚痰凝，神光不见。

2 诊断要点

2.1 临床表现

眼前似有飞蚊飘动，或视物模糊，或视力下降，或忽然暴盲不见。

2.2 眼底检查

见视网膜散在出血点，或仅见黄斑部水肿，或见后极区渗出，或见玻璃体内灰色、棕色浑浊，出血、机化，或见局限视网膜隆起、增殖，或

vitreous cavity.

无法窥见玻璃体腔。

2.3 Auxiliary examinations

Fundus fluorescein angiography (FFA) indicating abnormality, OTC indicating macular proliferation or edema, or B-type ultrasonic examination indicating intraocular high-density opacity.

2.3 辅助检查

见荧光血管造影异常、OCT 显示黄斑区组织增厚水肿,或 B 超见球内高密度混浊影。

2.4 Staging criteria

It is divided into the simple type and proliferative type, 6 stages totally.

(1) **Simple type**

Stage Ⅰ: Occurrence of retinal microaneuysm or hemorrhagic spots.

Stage Ⅱ: Occurrence of yellow-white "hard exudates" or combining with hemorrhagic spots.

Stage Ⅲ: Occurrence of "soft exudates" or combined with hemorrhagic spots.

(2) **Proliferative type**

Stage Ⅳ: Occurrence of fundus angiogenesis or combining with vitreous hemorrhage.

Stage Ⅴ: Occurrence of fundus angiogenesis and fibrous proliferation.

Stage Ⅵ: Occurrence of fundus angiogenesis and fibrous proliferation, combining with retinal detachment.

2.4 分期标准

分为单纯型和增殖型,共六期。

单纯期

Ⅰ期:有微动脉瘤或并有小出血点。

Ⅱ期:有黄白色"硬性渗出"或并有出血斑。

Ⅲ期:有白色"软性渗出"或并有出血斑。

(2) **增殖期**

Ⅳ期:眼底有新生血管或并有玻璃体出血。

Ⅴ期:眼底有新生血管和纤维增殖。

Ⅵ期:眼底有新生血管和纤维增殖,并发视网膜脱离。

3 Therapeutic methods

3.1 Therapeutic principles

Control glucose, keep a regular ophthalmic follow-up, and remind the patient to fully understand the hazard of the disease, so as to early detect and timely treat the fundus lesions and protect the vision. In traditional Chinese medicine, the treatment according to pattern identification has a good subsidiary function in all the stages, and the basic ther-

3 治疗方法

3.1 治疗原则

控制血糖,定期眼科随访,提醒患者充分认识疾病的危害性,早期发现及时治疗受损眼底病变,保护视功能。中医辨证论治在各期均有良好的辅助作用,基本治则为除瘀逐痰治其标,益气

apeutic principles are to dissolve stasis and eliminate phlegm to treat the superficial symptoms, and to benefit qi and nourish yin to treat the root causes.

养阴治其本。

3.2 Treatment based on syndrome differentiation

3.2 辨证论治

(1) Deficiency of qi and yin, and stasis blocking the vessels

(1) 气阴亏耗，脉络瘀阻

Main symptoms: Blurred vision or no obvious change of vision, retinal microaneuysm, small amount of spot-like or patch-like hemorrhage or yellow-white exudates in fundus examination, mostly seen in Stage I of retinopathy.

主症：视力模糊或无明显改变。眼底检查可见视网膜微血管瘤，少量点状或者小片状出血或黄白色渗出。多见于视网膜病变Ⅰ期。

Therapeutic methods: Benefit qi, nourish yin, dissolve stasis and dredge collaterals.

治法：益气养阴，化瘀通络。

Herbal formulas and drugs: The major formula is *Pulse-Engendering Powder* (Sheng Mai San) plus *Four Agents Decoction* (Si Wu Tang). The commonly-used herbal drugs are *Radix Ginseng* (Ren Shen), *Radix Ophiopogonis* (Mai Dong), *Fructus Schisandrae* (Wu Wei Zi), *Radix Angelicae Sinensis* (Dang Gui), *Radix Rehmanniae Cruda* (Sheng Di Huang), *Radix Paeoniae Alba* (Bai Shao), *Rhizoma Ligustici Chuanxiong* (Chuan Xiong), etc.

方药：代表方为生脉散合四物汤，常用药如人参、麦门冬、五味子、当归、生地黄、白芍、川芎等。

(2) Qi deficiency with damp blockage, and eyes losing nourishment

(2) 气虚湿阻，目失濡养

Main symptoms: Visual decrease, spot-like and patch-like hemorrhage in four retinal quadrants in fundus examination, yellow-white hard exudates, cotton-wool soft exudates, venous beaded changes at vascular arch or optic nerve, macular star-like exudates, partial edema, mostly seen retinopathy with macular edema.

主症：视力下降。眼底检查可见四个象限中视网膜较多点、片状出血；黄白色硬性渗出；棉绒样软性渗出；血管弓或者视乳头附近静脉串珠样改变；黄斑星芒状渗出，部分水肿。多见于视网膜病变有黄斑水肿者。

Therapeutic methods: Benefit qi, activate

治法：益气活血，健脾利

blood, strengthen spleen and dissolve damp.

Herbal formulas and drugs: The major formula is Center-Supplementing Qi-Boosting Decoction (Bu Zhong Yi Qi Tang). The commonly-used herbal drugs are *Radix Ginseng* (Ren Shen), *Radix Astragali* (Huang Qi), *Rhizoma Atractylodis Macrocephalae* (Bai Zhu), *Radix Angelicae Sinensis* (Dang Gui), *Rhizoma Cimicifugae* (Sheng Ma), *Radix Bupleuri* (Chai Hu), *Pericarpium Citri Tangerinae* (Chen Pi), *Radix Glycyrrhizae Praeparata* (Zhi Gan Cao), etc.

湿。

方药：代表方为补中益气汤，常用药如人参、黄芪、白术、当归、升麻、柴胡、陈皮、炙甘草等。

(3) **False fire burning collaterals to cause frenetic movement of blood**

(3) **虚火灼络，迫血妄行**

Main symptoms: Obviously visual decrease, floaters, large scale of retinal hemorrhage in fundus examination, hemorrhage not covering retinal arteries and veins, or patch-like hemorrhage on retinal surface covering retinal arteries and veins, or large scale of retinal hemorrhage or even air-fluid level, abnormal vascular networks in retina, mostly seen in Stage IV to Stage V of retinopathy with angiogenesis.

主症：视力影响明显，眼前飞蚊遮挡。眼底检查可见视网膜下大片出血，出血不遮盖视网膜动静脉血管，或视网膜平面片状出血，遮盖视网膜动静脉血管，或视网膜前大片出血，甚至有液平；视网膜可见异常血管网。多见于视网膜病变Ⅳ期至Ⅴ期眼底有新生血管者。

Therapeutic methods: Nourish yin, cool blood, stanch blood and dissolve stasis.

治法：滋阴凉血，止血化瘀。

Herbal formulas and drugs: The major formula is *Blood-Quieting Decoction* (Ning Xue Tang) or *Crude Cattail Pollen Decoction* (Sheng Pu Huang Tang). The commonly-used herbal drugs are *Radix Rehmanniae Cruda* (Sheng Di Huang), *Fructus Gardeniae Carbonisatus* (Zhi Zi Tan), *Rhizoma Imperatae* (Bai Mao Gen), *Caumen Biotae* (Ce Bai Ye), *Herba Ecliptae* (Mo Han Lian), *Herba Agrimoniae* (Xian He Cao), *Radix Ampelopsis* (Bai

方药：代表方为宁血汤或生蒲黄汤，常用药如生地黄、栀子炭、白茅根、侧柏叶、墨旱莲、仙鹤草、白蔹、白芍、白及、阿胶、牡丹皮、荆芥炭、蒲黄炭、丹参等。

Lian), *Radix Paeoniae Alba* (Bai Shao), *Rhizoma Bletillae* (Bai Ji), *Colla Corii Asini* (E Jiao), *Cortex Moutan Radicis* (Mu Dan Pi), *Herba Schizonepetae Carbonisatus* (Jing Jie Tan), *Pollen Typhae Carbonisatus* (Pu Huang Tan), *Radix Salviae Miltiorrhizae* (Dan Shen), etc.

(4) Accumulation of stasis and phlegm, and injury of vitreous body

(4) **瘀滞痰结,神膏俱损**

Main symptoms: Severely visual damage, even only light perception or no light perception, large amount of abnormal vascular networks in retina in fundus examination, partially retinal traction detachment, vitreous proliferative change, star-like exudates, severe edema and even cystoid degeneration of macula, large amount of hemorrhage in vitreous body, failure to detect fundus, mostly seen in Stage V to Stage VI of retinopathy.

主症:视力严重受损,甚至光感或者无光感。眼底检查可见视网膜大量异常血管网,甚至部分视网膜牵引性脱离;玻璃体增殖性改变;黄斑部星芒状渗出,高度水肿,甚至囊样变性;玻璃体大量出血,眼底窥不见。多见于视网膜病变Ⅴ期至Ⅵ期者。

Therapeutic methods: Remove stasis, dissolve phlegm, soften the hard and subside swell.

治法:逐瘀化痰,软坚散结。

Herbal formulas and drugs: The major formula is *Vital Gate Drink* (You Gui Yin). The commonly-used herbal drugs are *Radix Rehmanniae Praeparata* (Shu Di Huang), *Rhizoma Dioscoreae* (Shan Yao), *Fructus Lycii* (Gou Qi Zi), *Cortex Eucommiae* (Du Zhong), *Fructus Corni* (Shan Zhu Yu), *Radix Glycyrrhizae Praeparata* (Zhi Gan Cao), *Cortex Cinnamomi* (Rou Gui), *Radix Aconiti Praeparata* (Fu Zi), etc.

方药:代表方为右归饮,常用药如熟地黄、山药、枸杞子、杜仲、山茱萸、炙甘草、肉桂、附子等。

Modification according to symptoms: It is advisable to add the products to soften the hard and subside swell appropriately, such as *Rhizoma Sparganii Stoloniferi* (San Leng), *Rhizoma Zedoariae* (E Zhu), *Bulbus Fritillariae Thumbergii* (Zhe Bei Mu), *Radix Angelicae Dahuricae* (Bai Zhi), *Spina*

加减:可酌加软坚散结之品,如三棱、莪术、浙贝母、白芷、皂角刺等。

Gleditsiae (Zao Jiao Ci), etc.

3.3 Other therapies

(1) Control of primary disease: Stabilize the blood glucose, blood lipid and blood pressure, and control the progression of diabetes. See also the relevant contents in internal medicine as for the detailed medicinal drugs.

(2) Oral administration of medicines: Take Hydroxypropyl sulfonate calcium, pancreatic kallikrein, etc., 3 times a day and 1 to 2 tablets each time.

(3) Fundus photocoagulation: The purpose of photocoagulation therapy is to decrease the retinal oxygen consumption and reduce the angiogenesis. According to the obstructive areas of blood capillaries indicated by FFA, fractionally choose the focal photocoagulation or whole retinal photocoagulation

(4) Anti-VEGF therapy: According to macular edema indicated by OCT, choose antiangiogenic agents or Triamcinolone Acetonide Acetate Injection for intraocular injection. After edema diminishing, apply the continue therapy of macular laser grid photocoagulation (MLGP).

(5) Surgery: For those with non-absorbent vitreous hemorrhage or proliferation for months, apply vitrectomy plus fundus photocoagulation.

(6) Treatment of complications: Apply the symptomatic treatment for neovascular glaucoma.

3.3 其他疗法

(1) 控制原发病：稳定血糖、血脂、血压，控制糖尿病进展。具体药物参见内科相关内容。

(2) 口服药物治疗：口服羟丙磺酸钙、胰激肽释放酶等。每日3次，每次1～2片。

(3) 眼底光凝治疗：光凝治疗的目的是减少视网膜的耗氧量，减少新生血管的生成。依据荧光血管造影提示的毛细血管闭塞部位，分次选择局限性激光或者全视网膜激光。

(4) 抗 VEGF 治疗：依据 OCT 提示的黄斑水肿先选择抗新生血管或曲安耐得给眼内注射，待水肿消退后给与黄斑格栅样激光的续贯疗法。

(5) 手术治疗：玻璃体积血经月不吸收者或增殖选择玻璃体切割术联合眼底激光。

(6) 并发症治疗：新生血管性青光眼的对症处理。

4 Speculative map

4 思辨导图

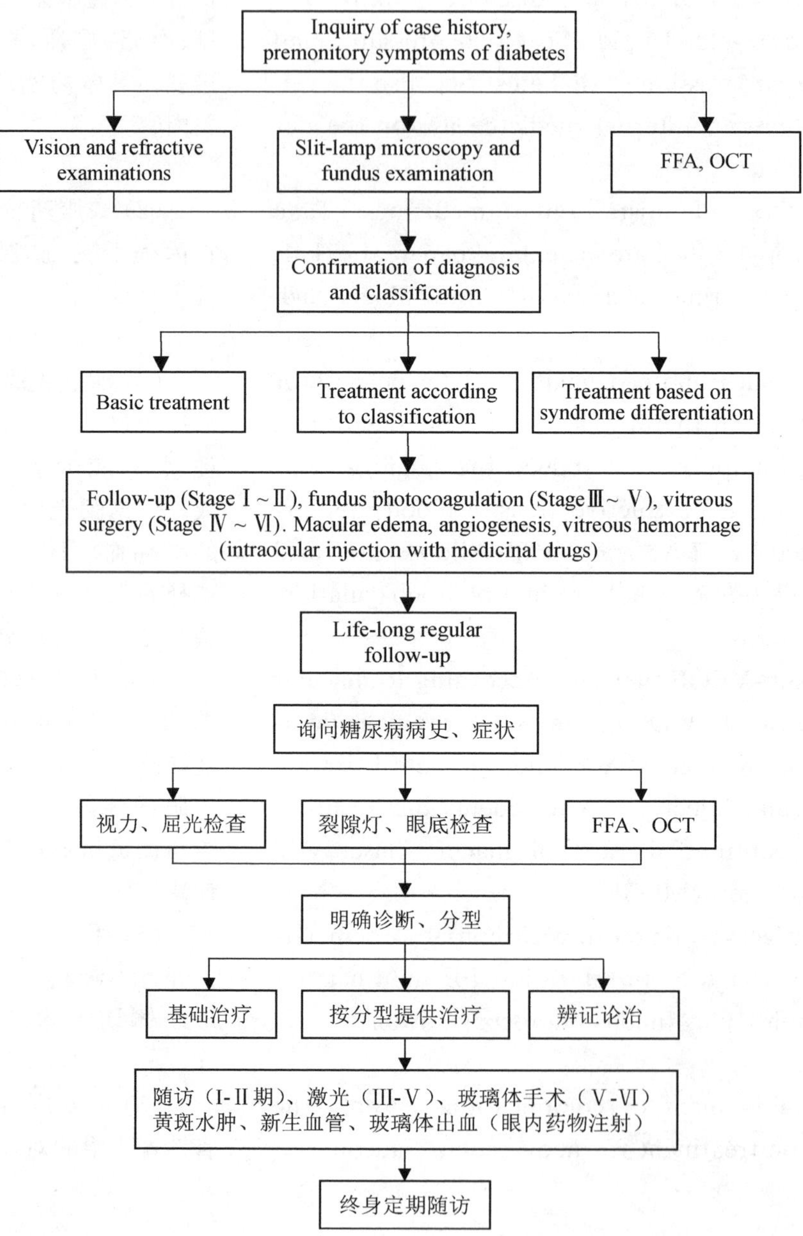

Central serous chorioretinopathy

中心性浆液性脉络膜视网膜病变

Central serous chorioretinopathy (CSC) refers to retinal pigment epithelium defects due to microcirculatory abnormality of choroidal capillary, finally leading to serous defects of retinal neuroepithelium. Its etiology is undetermined. It mostly appears in male adults aged by 20 to 45, as a self-limit disease induced by stress, fatigue, emotional fluctuation and oral administration of steroids.

中心性浆液性脉络膜视网膜病变是指脉络膜毛细血管微循环的异常导致视网膜色素上皮脱离而最终引起视网膜神经上皮层的浆液性脱离。其发病原因不详。好发于20～45岁青壮年男性，通常为自限性疾病，紧张、劳累、情绪波动以及口服激素可诱发。

In traditional Chinese medicine, the disease is regarded as the intraocular diseases, as "colorful vision", "blurred vision", "straight things seen as crooked", "small things seen as large", etc., according to its features of absence of appearance abnormality and subjective feeling of grey or slight-yellow fixed shadow occurring at the central visual field. It is caused by emotional sadness and worry which cause spleen failing to transport normally, or by liver failing to dominate dispersing and dredging which cause upflow of water-damp, or by retention of damp-heat. The principles of treatment are to soothe liver, strengthen spleen, clear heat and dissolve damp.

中医临床依据其外观无异常、自觉视野中心出现灰色或者淡黄色固定阴影；归属于"视瞻有色""视瞻昏渺""视直如曲""视小为大"等内障眼病。认为情志忧思所伤，脾失健运，肝失疏畅致水湿上泛，或湿热滞留为患。治以疏肝健脾，清热化湿为则。

1 Etiology and pathogenesis

1 病因病机

1.1 Over sadness and worry damage the spleen which fails to transport normally, to lead to upflow of water-damp.

1.1 忧思多度，内伤于脾，脾不健运，水湿上泛。

1.2 Emotional depression causes liver qi stagnation which transforms into heat after long-time stagnation, to lead to damp-heat attacking upwards the clear aperture.

1.2 情志不畅，肝气不舒，郁久化热，湿热上犯清窍。

1.3 Insufficiency of liver and kidney causes deficiency of essence and blood, which fail to nourish the eyes.

1.3 肝肾不足，精血亏虚，目失所养。

2 Diagnostic essentials

2 诊断要点

2.1 Clinical manifestations

2.1 临床表现

Subjective feeling of visual decrease or unusual feeling, darkened, discolored, lessened or deformed vision, or sheltered sight by shadow.

自觉视力下降或异样，视物变暗、变色、变小、变形，或暗影遮挡视线。

2.2 Ocular examinations

2.2 眼部检查

(1) Vision: Slight decrease of vision, especially obvious decrease of near vision.

（1）视力：轻度下降，尤以近视力下降明显。

(2) Fundus: A reflected nimbus of circular or oval edema seen at the fundus posterior pole, decrease or disappear of concave reflects in macular center. One week after onset, needle-like grey-white or grey-yellow sub-retinal exudates and deposites seen at the focal region, dome-like retinal detachment seen at the macular area under the binocular indirect ophthalmoscopy or trihedral contact lens examination.

（2）眼底：后极部可见一个圆形或椭圆形水肿反光轮，黄斑中心凹光反射减弱或消失；发病1周后，病灶区可见针尖样灰白或灰黄色视网膜下渗出沉着，在双目间接镜或三面镜下可见黄斑区呈圆顶状视网膜脱离。

2.3 Auxiliary examinations

2.3 辅助检查

(1) Amsler grid table examination: Central scotoma seen, and grid deformation.

（1）Amsler 方格表检查：可见中心暗点，方格变形。

(2) FFA: One or several fluorescein leakage points seen inside the focal area in the venous phase and gradually enlarged in ink-point shape.

（2）荧光素眼底血管造影显示：在静脉期于病灶区内有1个或数个荧光素渗漏点，逐渐呈喷墨样扩大。

(3) OCT: Range and height of serous defects of

（3）OCT 检查：可发现

retinal epithelial layer or pigment layer determined in the focal area.

并测量病灶区视网膜上皮层或色素层浆液性脱离的范围与高度。

3 Therapeutic methods

3 治疗方法

3.1 Therapeutic principles

3.1 治疗原则

The disease is self-limited, usually is cured by itself in 3 to 6 months. If it is not cured for long time or its repeated attacks cause obvious decrease of vision, it is necessary to treat it positively.

本病有一定的自限性，一般3～6个月或能自行痊愈。经久不愈或反复发作者视力下降明显，应积极治疗。

3.2 Treatment based on syndrome differentiation

3.2 辨证论治

(1) **Upflow of damp-turbidity**

(1) **湿浊上泛**

Main symptoms: Blurred vision, colored shadow before eyes, lessened or deformed vision, lessened or deformed fundus, obvious retinal reflects seen at the fundus, macular edema, decrease or disappear of concave reflects in macular center, slippery-sticky tongue coating, and soft or rolling pulse.

主症：视物模糊，眼前出现有色阴影，视物变小或变形，眼底变小或变形，眼底可见视网膜反光晕轮明显，黄斑水肿，中心凹光反射减弱或消失；舌苔滑腻，脉濡或滑。

Therapeutic methods: Promote water flow and dissolve damp.

治法：利水化湿。

Herbal formulas and drugs: The major formula is *Three Seeds Decoction* (San Ren Tang). The commonly-used herbal drugs are *Semen Armeniacae Amarum* (Ku Xing Ren), *Semen Amomi Cardamomi* (Dou Kou Ren), *Semen Coicis* (Yi Yi Ren), *Talcum* (Hua Shi), *Rhizoma Pinelliae* (Ban Xia), *Cortex Magnoliae Officinalis* (Hou Pu), *Medulla Tetrapanacis* (Tong Cao), *Herba Lophatheri* (Dan Zhu Ye), etc.

方药：代表方为三仁汤，常用药如苦杏仁、豆寇仁、薏苡仁、滑石、半夏、厚朴、通草、淡竹叶等。

(2) **Damp-heat in Liver Meridian**

(2) **肝经湿热**

Main symptoms: Blurred vision, brown-yellow shadow before eyes, lessened or deformed vision,

主症：视物模糊，眼前棕黄色阴影，视物变小或变形，

macular edema seen at the fundus, i. e. yellow-white exudates, red tongue body with yellow tongue coating, and thready-rapid pulse.

眼底可见黄斑区水肿即黄白色渗出；舌红苔黄，脉细数。

Therapeutic methods: Soothe liver, relieve depression, clear heat and dissolve damp.

治法：疏肝解郁，清热化湿。

Herbal formulas and drugs: The major formula is *Peony Bark and Capejasmine Free Wanderer Powder* (Dan Zhi Xiao Yao San). The commonly-used herbal drugs are *Radix Bupleuri* (Chai Hu), *Radix Angelicae Sinensis* (Dang Gui), *Radix Paeoniae Alba* (Bai Shao), *Sclerotium Poriae* (Fu Ling), *Rhizoma Atractylodis Macrocephalae* (Bai Zhu), *Cortex Moutan Radicis* (Mu Dan Pi), *Fructus Gardeniae* (Zhi Zi), *Herba Menthae* (Bo He), *Rhizoma Zingiberis Praeparata* (Wei Jiang), etc.

方药：代表方为丹栀逍遥散，常用药如柴胡、当归、白芍、茯苓、白术、牡丹皮、栀子、薄荷、煨姜等。

(3) **Insufficiency of liver and kidney**

(3) **肝肾不足**

Main symptoms: Blurred vision, dark-grey shadow before eyes, lessened or deformed vision, macular pigment disorder seen at the fundus with small amount of white exudates, decrease of concave reflects in macular center, red tongue body with scanty tongue coating, and thready pulse.

主症：视物模糊，眼前可见暗灰色阴影，视物变形或变小，眼底可见黄斑区色素紊乱，少许黄白色渗出，中心凹广反射减弱；舌红少苔，脉细。

Therapeutic methods: Nourish and reinforce liver and kidney, activate blood and brighten eyes.

治法：滋补肝肾，活血明目。

Herbal formulas and drugs: The major formula is *Four Agents and Five Seed Pills* (Si Wu Wu Zi Wan). The commonly-used herbal drugs are *Radix Rehmanniae Praeparata* (Shu Di Huang), *Rhizoma Ligustici Chuanxiong* (Chuan Xiong), *Radix Paeoniae Alba* (Bai Shao), *Fructus Lycii* (Gou Qi Zi), *Fructus Rubi* (Fu Pen Zi), *Fructus Kochiae* (Di Fu Zi), *Semen Plantaginis* (Che Qian Zi), *Semen Cuscutae* (Tu Si Zi), etc.

方药：代表方为四物五子丸，常用药如熟地黄、川芎、白芍、枸杞子、覆盆子、地肤子、车前子、菟丝子等。

3.3 Other therapies

(1) Patent herbal medicines: Take *Lycium, Chrysanthemun and Rehmannia Pills* (Qi Ju Di Huang Wan), *Vintage and Pinellia with Six Nobles Pills* (Chen Xia Liu Jun Zi Wan), *Compound Thrombosis Relieving Capsule* (Fu Fang Xue Sai Tong Jiao Nang), etc. orally according to pattern identification.

(2) Acupuncture: The major points are Tongziliao (GB 1), Cuanzhu (BL 2), Qiuhou (EX-HN 7) and Jingming (BL 1), while the adjunct points are Hegu (LI 4), Zusanli (ST 36), Ganshu (BL 18), Shenshu (BL 23), Pishu (BL 20), Sanyinjiao (SP 6) and Guangming (GB 37). Choose 2 major points and 2—3 adjunct points each time, and choose reinforcing or reducing method according to pattern identification. Apply the treatment once a day and retain the needles for 30 minutes, and 10-day treatments make up a course.

(3) Direct current iontophoresis with herbal drugs in ocular region: Apply Tetramethylpyrazine Injection, Salvia Miltiorrhiza Injection or Panax Notoginseng Injection is applied in iontophoresis, once a day for 15 minutes each time. 10 sessions of treatment make up a course. Start the second course of treatment after a 2 to 5 day break.

(4) Photocoagulation: It is suitable for those with fluorescein leakage after a course of disease for over 3 months and those with continuous serous defects. The obvious fluorescein leakage can be seen, with leakage spot locating outside the visual disk-macular fiber bundles, 250 μm away from the central fovea.

(5) For those with fluorescein leakage locating

3.3 其他疗法

(1) 中成药治疗：根据证型选用杞菊地黄丸、陈夏六君子丸、复方血塞通胶囊等口服。

(2) 针灸治疗：主穴可选瞳子髎、攒竹、球后、睛明；配穴可选合谷、足三里、肝俞、肾俞、脾俞、三阴交、光明。每次选主穴 2 个，配穴2～3个。根据辨证选择补写手法，每日 1 次，留针 30 分钟，10 日为 1 个疗程。

(3) 眼部直流电药物离子导入法：选用川芎秦、丹参或三七注射液作离子导入，每日 1 次，每次 15 分钟，10 次 1 个疗程，间隔 2～5 日再进行第 2 个疗程。

(4) 激光光凝：适用于病程 3 个月以上仍见到荧光渗漏，并有持续存在的浆液性脱离者。有明显荧光渗漏，且渗漏点位于视盘-黄斑纤维束外，离中心凹 250 μm 以外。

(5) 荧光渗漏位于中心

at the contraindicant area of photocoagulation, it is advisable to apply half-dose photodynamic therapy (PDT) or half-dose anti-VEGF for intraocular injection.

凹激光禁忌区，可考虑半剂量光动力（PDT）治疗，或选择抗 VEGF 半剂量眼内注射。

4 Speculative map

4. 思辨导图

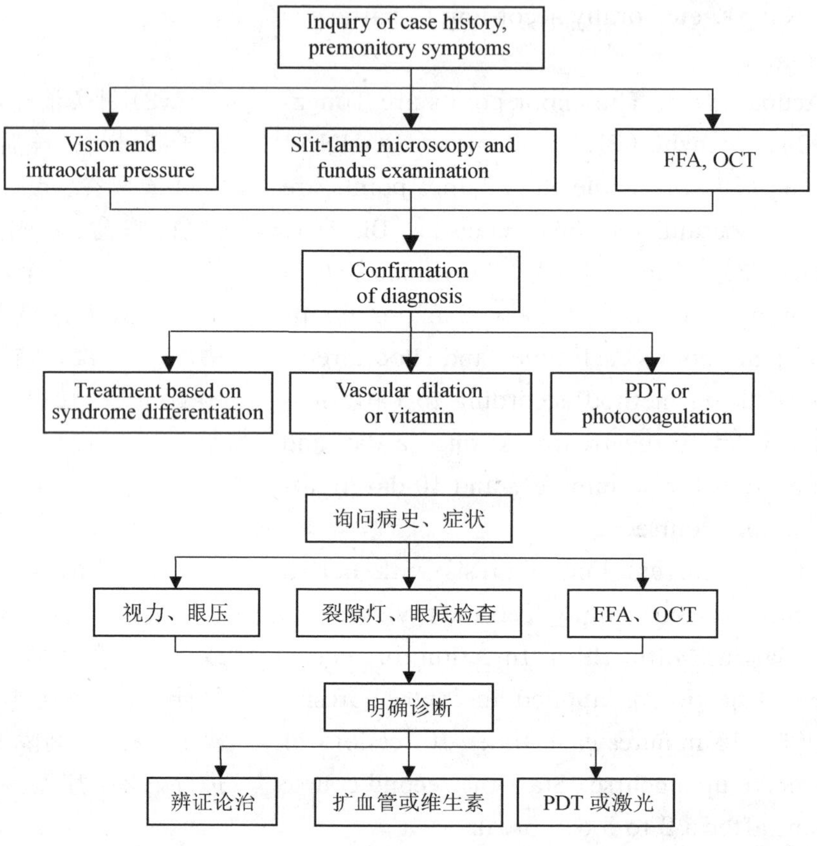

Primary retinal pigment degeneration

原发性视网膜色素变性

Primary retinal pigment degeneration is a genetic disease with progressive functional loss due to retinal photoreceptor cell and retinal pigment epi-

原发性视网膜色素变性是视网膜感光细胞与色素上皮变性导致的功能进行性丧

thelium degeneration. Both eyes are affected, with the onset in the preschoold period and very poor prognosis.

失的遗传性疾病。为双眼患病,学龄期开始发病,预后极差。

In traditional Chinese medicine, the disease is called "sparrow eye due to wind", "intraocular nebula due to wind" or "nebula due to yin wind", according to its clinical features of night blindness and narrowing visual field. Its pathogenesis is deficiency of the central yang which fails to inhibit yin. The principles of treatment are to warm yang, nourish yin, reinforce qi and benefit blood, with the principles of treatment to activate blood and dissolve stasis according to the pathology in western medicine.

中医依据其特有的夜盲和视野渐缩的临床特征名之为"高风雀目",又名"高风内障""阴风障"等;以中阳衰不能抗阴论述其病机,治以温阳、滋阴、补气益血,现代中医遵西医病理而佐以活血化瘀。

1 Etiology and pathogenesis

1 病因病机

1.1 Natural endowment insufficiency: The fire in Ming Men (Vital Gate) is deficient, so yang fails to inhibit yin and sinks into yin, leading to deficiency of yang which fails to warm the eyes to cause the disease.

1.1 禀赋不足,命门火衰,阳虚无以抗阴,阳气陷于阴中,不能自振,目失温煦所致。

1.2 Body constitution of yin deficiency: Yin is deficient and fails to support yang, so the yang qi fails to function normally.

1.2 素体真阴不足,阴虚不能济阳,阳气不能为用所致。

1.3 Spleen qi deficiency: Due to insufficiency of qi and blood, the eyes have no sufficient nutrients to nourish, so as to make them unable to watch things.

1.3 脾气虚弱,气血不足,养目之源匮乏,目不能视物。

2 Diagnostic essentials

2 诊断要点

2.1 Confirmed and short or long phenomenon of night blindness, and visual decrease in the late stage.

2.1 有明确的、长短不一的夜盲现象,晚期视力下降。

2.2 Retinal yellow or white spot-like or irregular-shaped pigmentation at the fundus, diminution of retinal vessels in different degrees and colour change

2.2 眼底视网膜黄色或白色点状或不规则状色素沉着,视网膜血管不同程度变

of optic disc, with progressive development.

细，视盘色泽改变，呈进行性发展。

2. 3 Symmetrical and progressive lessening of visual field, and tubular vision in the late stage.

2. 3 视野呈对称性、进行性缩小，晚期呈管状视野。

2. 4 Characteristic abnormality by visual electrophysiological examination and dark adaptometer examination.

2. 4 视觉电生理检查及暗适应检查特征性异常。

3 Therapeutic methods

3 治疗方法

3. 1 Therapeutic principles

3. 1 治疗原则

The root cause of the disease is deficiency with stasis. On the basis of pattern identification, it is advisable to add the herbal drugs acting to activate blood and dissolve stasis, with supportive nutrition.

本病以虚为本、虚中夹瘀，临床在辨证论治的基础上，均可加活血化瘀药物，辅助支持性营养。

3. 2 Treatment based on syndrome differentiation

3. 2 辨证论治

(1) **Spleen qi deficiency and weakness**

(1) **脾气虚弱**

Main symptoms: Night blindness, narrowing visual field, yellow or white spot-like change at the fundus retina, unobvious change of vessels, slightly pale tongue body with white tongue coating, and weak pulse.

主症：夜盲，视野偏窄，眼底视网膜可见黄、白色斑点样改变，血管改变不显著，舌质偏淡，苔白，脉弱。

Therapeutic methods: Strengthen spleen and benefit qi.

治法：健脾益气。

Herbal formulas and drugs: The major formula is *Center-Supplementing Qi-Boosting Decoction* (Bu Zhong Yi Qi Tang). The commonly-used herbal drugs are *Radix Ginseng* (Ren Shen), *Radix Astragali* (Huang Qi), *Rhizoma Atractylodis Macrocephalae* (Bai Zhu), *Radix Angelicae Sinensis* (Dang Gui), *Rhizoma Cimicifugae* (Sheng Ma), *Radix Bupleuri* (Chai Hu), *Pericarpium Citri Tangerinae* (Chen Pi), *Radix Glycyrrhizae Praeparata* (Zhi Gan Cao), etc.

方药：代表方为补中益气汤，常用药如人参、黄芪、白术、当归、升麻、柴胡、陈皮、炙甘草等。

(2) **Yin deficiency of liver and kidney**

Main symptoms: Night blindness, obvious narrowing visual field, diminution of fundus retinal vessels with irregular pigmentation around, colour change of optic disc, red tongue body with scanty tongue coating, and thready-rapid pulse.

Therapeutic methods: Nourish and reinforce liver and kidney.

Herbal formulas and drugs: The major formula is *Eye-Brightening Rehmannia Pills* (Ming Mu Di Huang Wan). The commonly-used herbal drugs are *Radix Rehmanniae Cruda* (Sheng Di Huang), *Radix Rehmanniae Praeparata* (Shu Di Huang), *Rhizoma Dioscoreae* (Shan Yao), *Fructus Corni* (Shan Zhu Yu), *Cortex Moutan Radicis* (Mu Dan Pi) *Fructus Schisandrae* (Wu Wei Zi), *Radix Angelicae Sinensis* (Dang Gui), *Rhizoma Alismatis* (Ze Xie), *Poria cum Ligno Hospite* (Fu Shen), *Radix Bupleuri* (Chai Hu), etc.

(2) **肝肾阴虚**

主症：夜盲，视野缩窄明显，眼底视网膜血管变细，周边见色素不规则沉着，视盘色泽改变，舌质红，少苔，脉细数。

治法：滋补肝肾。

方药：代表方为明目地黄丸，常用药如生熟地黄、山药、山茱萸、牡丹皮、五味子、当归、泽泻、茯神、柴胡等。

(3) **Insufficiency of kidney yang**

Main symptoms: Night blindness, narrowing and tubular visual field, large amount of osteocyte-like pigmentation at the fundus retina, dark-grey colour of macular area in retina, yellow-colored change of optic disc, accompanied by aching and weakness at low back and knees, chills in body and limbs, pale tongue body with thin tongue coating, and deep-weak pulse.

Therapeutic methods: Warm and reinforce the kidney yang.

Herbal formulas and drugs: The major formula is *Vital Gate Pills* (You Gui Wan). The commonly-used herbal drugs are *Radix Rehmanniae Praeparata* (Shu Di Huang), *Rhizoma Dioscoreae* (Shan Yao),

(3) **肾阳不足**

主症：夜盲，视野呈管状缩窄，眼底视网膜大量色素呈骨细胞样沉着，视网膜黄斑区色泽灰暗，视盘呈蜡黄色改变，或伴腰膝酸软，形寒肢冷，舌质淡，苔薄，脉沉弱。

治法：温补肾阳。

方药：代表方为右归丸，常用药如熟地黄、山药、枸杞子、山茱萸、菟丝子、鹿角胶、杜仲、肉桂、制附子、当归等。

Fructus Lycii (Gou Qi Zi), *Fructus Corni* (Shan Zhu Yu) *Semen Cuscutae* (Tu Si Zi), *Colla Cornus Cervi* (Lu Jiao Jiao), *Cortex Eucommiae* (Du Zhong), *Cortex Cinnamomi* (Rou Gui), *Radix Aconiti Praeparata* (Zhi Fu Zi), *Radix Angelicae Sinensis* (Dang Gui), etc.

3.3 Other therapies

(1) Patent herbal medicines: Apply *Golden Chamber Kidney Qi Pills* (Jin Gui Shen Qi Wan), *Eye-Brightening Rehmannia Pills* (Ming Mu Di Huang Wan), *Center-Supplementing Qi-Boosting Pills* (Bu Zhong Yi Qi Wan), *Compound Red Sage Drop Pills* (Fu Fang Dan Shen Di Wan), *Compound Thrombosis Relieving Capsule* (Fu Fang Xue Sai Tong Jiao Nang), *Compound Codonopsis Injection* (Fu Fang Dang Shen Zhu She Ye), etc., for oral administration or intravenous injection according to pattern identification.

(2) Acupuncture: The major points are Jingming (BL 1), Taiyang (EX-HN 5), Shangjingming (EX-HN), Qiuhou (EX-HN 7), Chengqi (ST 1) and Cuanzhu (BL 2), and the adjunct points are Fengchi (GB 20), Wangu (GB 12), Baihui (GV 20), Hegu (LI 4), Ganshu (BL 18), Shenshu (BL 23), Pishu (BL 20), Zusanli (ST 36), Sanyinjiao (SP 6) and Guanyuan (CV 4). Choose 2 major points and 2 to 4 adjunct points in each treatment and apply reinforcing or reducing method according to pattern identification, once a day.

3.3 其他疗法

（1）中成药治疗：根据证型可选用金匮肾气丸、明目地黄丸、补中益气丸、复方丹参滴丸、复方血塞通胶囊、复方党参注射液等口服或静脉给药。

（2）针灸治疗：主穴选睛明、太阳、上睛明、球后、承泣、攒竹；配穴选风池、完骨、百会、合谷、肝俞、肾俞、脾俞、足三里、三阴交、关元。每次选主穴 2 个，配穴 2～4 个，根据辨证补泻，每日 1 次。

4 Speculative map

4 思辨导图

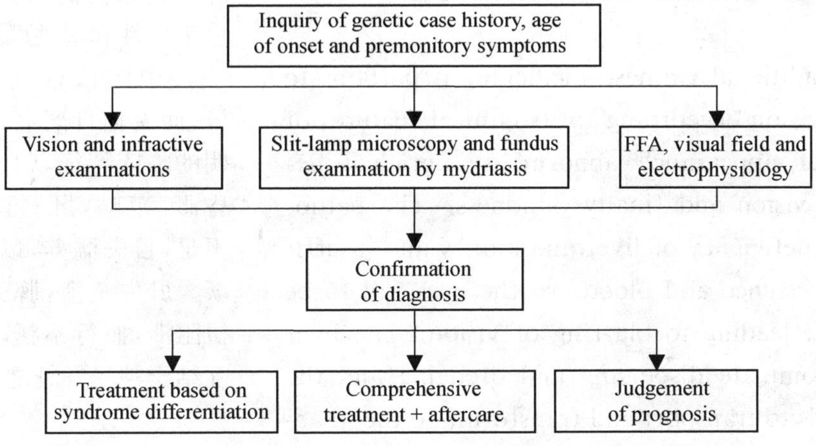

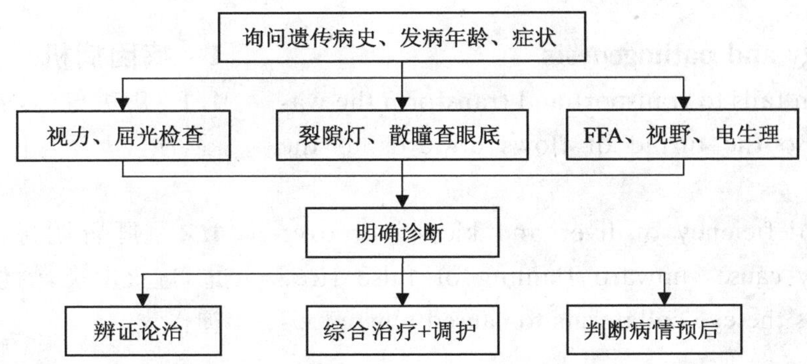

Age-related macular degeneration

老年黄斑变性

Age-related macular degeneration (AMD) is a kind of eye disease, highly age-related, with severe vision damages of hemorrhage, exudates and scars induced by angiogenesis, led by functional degeneration of macular retinal pigment epithelium, Bruch membrane and choroidal vessels. The exact etiology

老年性黄斑变性是指一种与年龄高度相关，黄斑区视网膜色素上皮、Bruch 膜以及脉络膜血管功能退变从而导致新生血管形成引发出血、渗出、瘢痕最终视力严重

is unknown. Clinically it is divided into dry type and damp type according to the fundus lesions.

受损的眼病。确切病因不详。临床上根据眼底的病变分为干性和湿性两种类型。

In traditional Chinese medicine, it pertains to "blurred vision" according to its clinical features of absence of appearance abnormality, gradual decrease of vision and finally blindness. The pathogenesis is deficiency of liver and kidney and insufficiency of essence and blood, so the eyes fail to be nourished, leading to blurring of vision. The liver fails to dominate dispersing and dredging and the spleen fails to transport and transform, so the qi activity is blocked and the blood flow is not smooth, as a result, the phlegm and stasis are accumulated at the eyes.

中医依据其眼外观无异，而视觉日渐衰退，最终失明的临床特征，归属于"视瞻昏渺"范畴，肝肾两虚，精血不足，目失濡养，以致神光暗淡。肝失疏泄，脾失健运，气机阻滞，血行不畅，终致痰瘀互结于神光发越之处。

1 Etiology and pathogenesis

1 病因病机

1.1 Spleen fails to transport and transform the water-damp, so the turbid qi flows upwards to the eyes.

1.1 脾失健运，不能运化水湿，浊气上泛与目。

1.2 Yin deficiency of liver and kidney or over stress-worry causes upward flaming of false fire, which burns the eye collaterals to caused blurred vision.

1.2 肝肾阴虚，或劳思竭虑，虚火上炎，灼伤目络而瞳神昏蒙。

1.3 Emotional change leads to the liver failing to dominate dispersing and dredging, so as to attack the spleen which fails to transport and transform. Qi activity is blocked, the blood flow is not smooth, and the body fluid is accumulated to form up the phlegm. The phlegm and stasis accumulate to cover the eyes and disturb the vision.

1.3 情志内伤，肝失疏泄，肝气犯脾，脾失健运，气机阻滞，血行不畅为瘀，津液凝聚成痰，痰瘀互结，遮蔽瞳神。

1.4 In old age and weak body constitution, both the liver and kidney are deficient, and both the essence and blood are insufficient. The eyes fail to be

1.4 年老体弱，肝肾两虚，精血不足，目失濡养，以致神光暗淡。

nourished, leading to blurred vision.

2 Diagnostic essentials

2.1 Gradual development of blurred vision, deformed vision, or dark shadow covering eyes, and sudden decrease of vision.

2.2 Ocular examination

Decrease of vision which cannot be corrected.

(1) Dry type (also called atrophic type, chronic type or non-angiogenesis type): In the early stage, sporadic and unclear-margin drusens seen at the retinal posterior pole, pigment disturbance at the macular region, and geographic atrophic area of retinal pigment epithelium after pigment disturbance.

(2) Damp type (also called exudative type, acute type and angiogenesis type): In the early stage, sub-retinal angiogenesis of turbid and grey-colored prominence seen at the retinal posterior pole, with dark-red or dark-black hemorrhage in the deep or superficial layer around, and the residual hemorrhagic clots and drusens. 1 optic disc dimeter seen in the small lesion range, while the involvement of whole retineal posterior pole seen in the large lesion range. In severe hemorrhage, preretineal hemorrhage seen, even reaching the inside of vitreous body to form vitreous hemorrhage. In the late stage, hemorrhagic organized thrombosis occurring at the macular region, so as to form up disc-like scar and complete loss of central vision.

2.3 Auxiliary examinations

(1) In FFA and ICGA, the fluorescent focus of drusen, or the blocked fluorescence, or the pigment epithelium damage, or the choroidal neovasculariza-

2 诊断要点

2.1 视物模糊渐重，视物变形，或眼前暗影遮挡，视力骤降。

2.2 眼部检查

视力下降，不能矫正。

（1）干性（也称萎缩性、慢性或非新生血管性）：早期可见后极部视网膜散在、边界欠清楚的玻璃膜疣，黄斑区色素紊乱，呈现色素脱失紊乱后呈地图状色素上皮萎缩区。

（2）湿性（也称渗出性、急性或新生血管性）：初期可见后极部有污秽之灰白色稍微隆起的视网膜下新生血管膜，其周围深层或浅层暗红色或暗黑色出血及残留的出血块和玻璃膜疣。病变范围小者约1个视盘直径，大者波及整个后极部。出血多者可见视网膜前出血，甚至达玻璃体内而成玻璃体积血。晚期黄斑部出血机化，形成盘状瘢痕，中心视力完全丧失。

2.3 辅助检查

（1）荧光素眼底血管造影和脉络膜血管造影检查可显示玻璃膜疣样荧光灶，或

tion, or the fluorescein leakage, or scarred focus indicated.

(2) **OCT examination:** The damp AMD examination clearly shows the choroidal neovascularization, hemorrhage, leakage and the shape, thickness and range of scar.

3 Therapeutic methods

3.1 Therapeutic principles

For those of incipient lesion, intervent the condition with the standardized treatment program guided by evidence-based medicine, by the effective blockage focusing on the angiogenesis, so as to avoid the irreversible damage of vision. In traditional Chinese medicine, the basic principles of treatment are to adjust the zang-fu organs so as to dissolve phlegm-damp, to circulate qi and blood so as to bring back the vision, and to improve the visual quality.

3.2 Treatment based on syndrome differentiation

(1) **Spleen deficiency with damp blockage**

Main symptoms: Blurred vision, deformed vision, macular pigment disturbance, formation of drusen, loss of central fovea reflects, or macular hemorrhage, exudates and edema, accompanied by distension and fullness at chest and hypochondria, dizziness, palpitation, tiredness of body and limbs, pale-white tongue body with teeth-prints on edges and thin-white tongue coating, and deep-thready or thready pulse.

Therapeutic methods: Strengthen spleen and dissolve damp.

荧光遮蔽，或色素上皮损害，或脉络膜新生血管或荧光渗漏或瘢痕病灶等。

（2）OCT 检查：湿性 AMD 检查清晰地显示脉络膜新生血管、出血、渗出及瘢痕的形态、厚度及范围。

3 治疗方法

3.1 治疗原则

初发患者应提供循证医学指导下的规范化治疗方案干预，针对新生血管膜的有效封闭以避免视力的不可逆损害。中医以调脏腑以除痰湿，行气血以复神明，改善其视觉质量为基本治则。

3.2 辨证论治

（1）**脾虚湿困**

主症：视物模糊，视物变形，黄斑色素紊乱，玻璃膜疣形成，中心凹反射消失，或黄斑出血、渗出及水肿；可伴胸膈胀满，眩晕心悸，肢体乏力；舌质淡白，边有齿印，苔薄白，脉沉细或细。

治法：健脾利湿。

Herbal formulas and drugs: The major formula is Ginseng, Poria and Atractylodes Powder (Shen Ling Bai Zhu San). The commonly-used herbal drugs are *Radix Ginseng* (Ren Shen), *Sclerotium Poriae* (Fu Ling), *Rhizoma Atractylodis Macrocephalae* (Bai Zhu), *Rhizoma Dioscoreae* (Shan Yao), *Semen Dolichoris* (Bian Dou), *Semen Nelumbinis* (Lian Zi Rou), *Semen Coicis* (Yi Yi Ren), *Fructus Amomi* (Sha Ren), *Pericarpium Citri Tangerinae* (Chen Pi), *Radix Platycodi* (Jie Geng), *Radix Glycyrrhizae Praeparata* (Zhi Gan Cao), etc.

方药:代表方为参苓白术散,常用药如人参、茯苓、白术、山药、扁豆、莲子肉、薏苡仁、砂仁、陈皮、桔梗、炙甘草等。

(2) **Yin deficiency with fire hyperactivity**

(2) **阴虚火旺**

Main symptoms: Deformed vision, sudden decrease of vision, large amount of fresh hemorrhage, exudates and edema at the macular region, accompanied by dry mouth and thirst, tidal fever, red complexion, feverish sensation in five centers, nocturnal sweats, dream-disturbed sleep, aching and weakness at low back and knees, red tongue body with scanty tongue coating, and thready-rapid pulse.

主症:视物变形,视力突然下降,黄斑部可见大片新鲜出血、渗出和水肿;口干欲饮,潮热面赤,五心烦热,盗汗多梦,腰膝酸软,舌质红,苔少,脉细数。

Therapeutic methods: Nourish yin and reduce fire.

治法:滋阴降火。

Herbal formulas and drugs: The major formula is *Crude Cattail Pollen Decoction* (Sheng Pu Huang Tang) plus *Yin-Nourishing and Fire-Reducing Decoction* (Zi Yin Jiang Huo Tang). The commonly-used herbal drugs are *Radix Rehmanniae Cruda* (Sheng Di Huang), *Pollen Typhae Cruda* (Sheng Pu Huang), *Cortex Moutan Radicis* (Mu Dan Pi), *Herba Ecliptae* (Mo Han Lian), *Herba Schizonepetae Carbonisatus* (Jing Jie Tan), *Radix Curcumae* (Yu Jin), *Radix Salviae Miltiorrhizae* (Dan Shen), *Rhizoma Ligustici Chuanxiong* (Chuan Xiong), *Radix Ophiopogonis* (Mai Men Dong), *Rhizoma Anemarrhenae* (Zhi

方药:代表方为生蒲黄汤合滋阴降火汤,常用药如生地黄、生蒲黄、牡丹皮、墨旱莲、荆芥炭、郁金、丹参、川芎、麦门冬、知母、黄柏、黄芩、柴胡、炙甘草等。

Mu), *Cortex Phellodendri* (Huang Bo), *Radix Scutellariae* (Huang Qin), *Radix Bupleuri* (Chai Hu), *Radix Glycyrrhizae Praeparata* (Zhi Gan Cao), etc.

(3) **Accumulation of phlegm and stasis**

Main symptoms: Deformed vision, visual decrease, prolonged lesion, scar and large amount of pigmentation seen at the fundus, accompanied by fatigue, lassitude, poor appetite, pale tongue body with thin-white-sticky tongue coating, and wiry-rolling pulse.

Therapeutic methods: Dissolve phlegm, soften the hard, activate blood and brighten eyes.

Herbal formulas and drugs: The major formula is *Hard-Softening Double Vintage Decoction* (Hua Jian Er Chen Tang). The commonly-used herbal drugs are *Pericarpium Citri Tangerinae* (Chen Pi), *Rhizoma Pinelliae* (Ban Xia), *Sclerotium Poriae* (Fu Ling), *Radix Glycyrrhizae Praeparata* (Zhi Gan Cao), *Bombyx Batryticatus* (Bai Jiang Can), *Rhizoma Coptidis* (Huang Lian), *Folium Nelumbinis* (He Ye), etc.

(4) **Deficiency of both liver and kidney**

Main symptoms: Blurred vision, deformed vision, old macular exudates seen at fundus, reflective decrease or loss of central fovea, accompanied by dizziness, insomnia, pale complexion, chills in limbs, low spirit, weakness of low back and knees, red tongue body with thin-white tongue coating, and deep-thready-weak pulse.

Therapeutic methods: Reinforce and benefit liver and kidney.

Herbal formulas and drugs: The major formula is *Four Agents and Five Seed Pills* (Si Wu Wu Zi

(3) **痰瘀互结**

主症：视物变形，视力下降，病程日久，眼底可见瘢痕形成及大片色素沉着；伴见倦怠乏力纳食呆顿；舌质淡，苔薄白腻，脉弦滑。

治法：化痰软坚，活血明目。

方药：代表方为化坚二陈丸，常用药如陈皮、半夏、茯苓、炙甘草、白僵蚕、黄连、荷叶等。

(4) **肝肾两虚**

主症：视物模糊，视物变形，眼底可见黄斑陈旧性渗出，中心凹反射减弱或消失；伴有头晕失眠或面白肢冷，精神倦怠，腰膝无力，舌质红苔薄白，脉沉细无力。

治法：补益肝肾。

方药：代表方为四物五子丸或加减驻景丸，常用药

Wan) or *Scenery-Residing Pills Modified* (Jia Jian Zhu Jing Wan). The commonly-used herbal drugs are *Radix Rehmanniae Praeparata* (Shu Di Huang), *Rhizoma Ligustici Chuanxiong* (Chuan Xiong), *Radix Paeoniae Alba* (Bai Shao), *Fructus Lycii* (Gou Qi Zi), *Fructus Rubi* (Fu Pen Zi), *Fructus Kochiae* (Di Fu Zi), *Semen Plantaginis* (Che Qian Zi), *Semen Cuscutae* (Tu Si Zi), *Radix Angelicae Sinensis* (Dang Gui), *Fructus Broussonetiae* (Chu Shi Zi), *Fructus Schisandrae* (Wu Wei Zi), etc.

如熟地黄、川芎、白芍、枸杞子、覆盆子、地肤子、车前子、菟丝子、当归、楮实子、五味子等。

3.3 Definitive therapies

(1) Anti-angiogenesis therapy: It is the effective treatment currently, but the recurrence cannot be controlled, and the continuous treatment costs high.

(2) Laser therapy: The neovascular membranes locate at the sub-retinal membrane 200 μm away from the macular central fovea. The laser therapy blocks the neovascular membranes, so as to avoid the constant development of the lesion, and to extend and influence the central vision. Photodynamic therapy (PDT) is applied to manage the lesion of macular central fovea.

(3) Surgery: For those with severe hemorrhage which causes vitreous hemorrhage which cannot be absorbed in 1 months, it is necessary to apply vitrectomy.

3.3 针对性治疗

(1) 抗新生血管治疗是目前有效的治疗方法,但复发仍无法控制,持续治疗的费用昂贵。

(2) 激光治疗:新生血管膜位于黄斑中心凹200 μm以外的视网膜下,激光封闭新生血管膜,以免病变不断发展、扩大而影响中心视力。光动力疗法可处理黄斑中心凹病变。

(3) 手术:出血量多到进入玻璃体致玻璃体积血者,1月未能吸收,则需行玻璃体切割术。

3.4 Other therapies

(1) Supportive therapy: It is suitable for those of dry type. It is to supplement trace elements and vitamins, as Vitamin C, Vitamin E, etc. for oral administration, so as to protect the optic cells.

(2) Patent herbal medicines: Apply *Ginseng, Poria and Atractylodes Pills* (Shen Ling Bai Zhu

3.4 其他疗法

(1) 支持疗法:适用于本病干性者,补充微量元素及维生素,口服维生素 C、维生素 E 等,以保护视细胞。

(2) 中成药治疗:根据证型选用参苓白术丸、知柏地

Wan), *Anemarrhena, Phellodendron and Rehmannia Pills* (Zhi Bai Di Huang Wan), *Lycium, Chrysanthemun and Rehmannia Pills* (Qi Ju Di Huang Wan), *Pulse-Engendering Drink* (Sheng Mai Yin), *Sanguine Mansion Stasis-Expelling Oral Liquid* (Xue Fu Zhu Yu Kou Fu Ye), *Compound Thrombosis Relieving Capsule* (Fu Fang Xue Sai Tong Jiao Nang), etc. according to pattern identification.

黄丸、杞菊地黄丸、生脉饮、血府逐瘀口服液、复方血塞通胶囊等。

(3) Acupuncture: The major points are Jingming (BL 1), Qiuhou (EX-HN 7), Chengqi (ST 1), Tongziliao (GB 1), Cuanzhu (BL 2) and Fengchi (GB 20), and the adjunct points are Wangu (GB 12), Baihui (GV 20), Hegu (LI 4), Ganshu (BL 18), Shenshu (BL 23), Pishu (BL 20), Zusanli (ST 36), Sanyinjiao (SP 6) and Guangming (GB 37). Choose 2 major points and 2 to 4 adjunct points in each treatment, and apply reinforcing or reducing method according to pattern identification. The treatment once a day with needle retaining for 30 mintues, and 10-day treatments make up a course.

(3) 针灸治疗：主穴选睛明、球后、承泣、瞳子髎、攒竹、风池；配穴选完骨、百会、合谷、肝俞、肾俞、脾俞、足三里、三阴交、光明。每次主穴2个，配穴2～4个，根据辨证补泻，每日1次，留针30分钟，10日1个疗程。

4 Speculative map

4 思辨导图

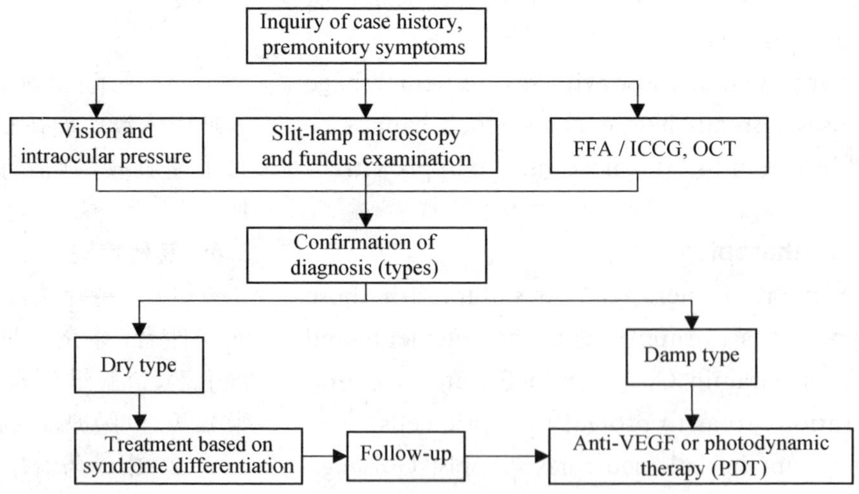

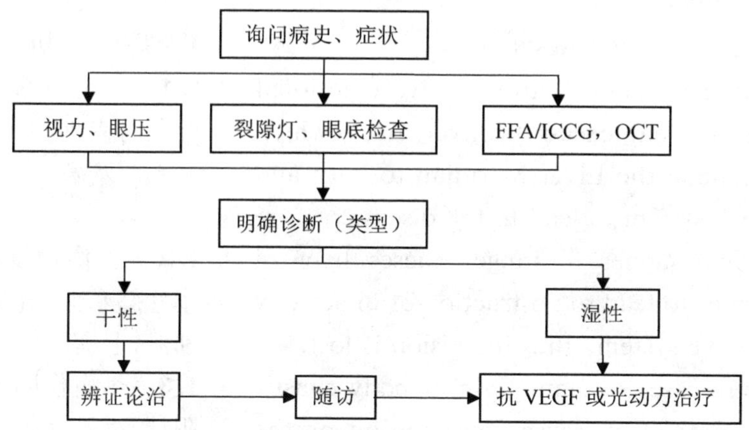

Optic neuropathy

视神经病变

Optic neuropathy is a disease of the optic nerve segment from the optic disc to the optic chiasma, caused by inflammation, edema, ischemia, degeneration, tumor, etc. It is mostly the lesion of inflammation in young people, including optic neuritis and retrobulbar neuritis. It is mostly the lesion of ischemia, including acute ischemia and chronic ischemia. Besides, there are more various pathogenic factors of demyelinating disease, poisoning, hereditary, metabolism, traumatic injury, etc.

In traditional Chinese medicine, the disease is called "sudden visual loss" according to its clinical feature of sudden blindness. In traditional Chinese medicine, it is to treat the disease according to the causes of six exogenous factors, endogenous emotional injuries, febrile disease, chronic disease, etc. According to the theory of five wheels, the liver, kidney, qi and blood are involved, and the therapeutic principles are purifying, dredging, nouris-

视神经病变常因炎症、水肿、缺血、变性、肿瘤等导致的自视盘至视交叉前的视神经段的病变，年轻人以炎性病变多见，有视神经炎与球后视神经炎；老年以缺血为主，有急性缺血和慢性缺血之别；另有脱髓鞘病、中毒、遗传、代谢、外伤等多种致病原因。

根据其患眼倏然盲而不见的临床特征，现代中医命名其为“目系暴盲”，中医依据六淫外感、情志内伤、热病久病等审因论治，以中医轮脏气血学说责之肝、肾、气、血，治以清、疏、滋、补为要。

hing and reinforcing.

1 Etiology and pathogenesis

1.1 The six exogenous factors or five emotional factors cause internal excess of liver fire, which goes upwards along the Liver Meridian to burn and damage the eye system to lead to the disease.

1.2 Emotional sadness or anger causes liver qi stagnation, so as to lead to obstruction of qi activity to disturb the eye system, thus the vision is lost.

1.3 Febrile disease consuming yin or body constitution of yin deficiency cause consumption of the yin essence, so the water fails to moisturize the fire, to lead to the endogenous false fire, which goes upwards to burn the eye system.

1.4 Chronic disease leading to weakness of body or congenital weakness of body, or blood deficiency after delivery causes loss of nourishment of eye system.

2 Diagnostic essentials

2.1 Subjective symptoms

Sudden decrease of vision, even loss of vision, pain in eye movements in some patients, accompanied by headache and vomiting in some patients.

2.2 Ocular examinations

(1) Optic neuritis: Dull light reflect of pupil in those with severe decrease of vision, dilation of pupils and loss of direct or indirect reflect of pupils in those with visual loss of both eyes, relative afferent papillary obstacles (RAPD) showing positive in those with single eye affected or those with both eyes affected but one more severe.

1 病因病机

1.1 六淫外感或五志过极，肝火内盛，循肝经上扰，灼伤目系而发病。

1.2 悲伤过度，情志内伤，或忿怒暴悖，肝失条达，气机郁滞，上壅目系，神光受遏。

1.3 热病伤阴或素体阴亏，阴精亏耗，水不济火，虚火内生，上炎目系。

1.4 久病体虚，或素体虚弱，或产后血亏，目系失养。

2 诊断要点

2.1 自觉症状

突然视力下降，甚或失明。部分患者伴转动眼球时疼痛或眼球深部疼痛，部分患者可伴头痛、呕吐。

2.2 眼部检查

（1）视神经炎：视力下降严重者瞳孔对光反射迟钝；双眼失明者瞳孔散大，瞳孔直接和间接反射均消失；单眼患者患侧或双眼患者受累程度严重的一侧可有相对性传入性瞳孔障碍，即 RAPD 阳性。

Papillitis: Congestion of optic disc withfuzzy boundary, obvious congestion and swelling in severe condition, but usually not more than 3 diopters, filling and circuity of central retinal vein, small amount of hemorrhage, exudates and edema at the optic disc and its nearby, white colour occurring at the temporal side of optic disc in the late stage of the disease.

若为视盘炎，可见视盘充血，边界模糊，严重时视盘充血肿胀明显，但一般不超过3个屈光度，视网膜中央静脉充盈、迂曲，视盘及其周围可见少许出血和渗出、水肿。疾病晚期出现视盘颞侧苍白。

Acute optic neuritis: Medium or severe decrease of vision, even loss of vision, pain in eye movements, edema and hemorrhage at the optic nerve of fundus.

急性视神经炎：视力中、重度下降甚至失明，眼球转动痛。眼底视乳头水肿，出血。

Retrobulbar neuritis: Normal fundus, or slight edema of optic nerve, and pain in eye movements.

球后视神经炎：眼底正常或者视乳头轻度水肿。可有眼球转动痛。

(2) Anterior ischemic optic neuropathy (AION): The circulatory disturbance of posterior ciliary artery which supplies the optic nerve leads to acute ischemia and anoxia of optic nerve, causing edema and linear hemorrhage of optic nerve, and visual function damage. It is an acute eye disease with clinical features of sudden decrease of vision, fan-shaped or side defect of visual field (the upper and lower levels in priority) and edema of optic nerve.

（2）前部缺血性视神经病变：由于供应视乳头的后睫状动脉发生循环障碍引起视乳头的急性缺血、缺氧，以致出现视乳头水肿、线状出血，引起视功能损害。患者以视力突然下降、扇形或半侧（以上下水平为主）视野缺损和视乳头水肿为临床特点的急性眼病。

2.3 Auxiliary examinations

2.3 辅助检查

(1) Visual field examination: Central scotoma, paracentral scotoma or peripheral visual narrowing in those of acute optic neuritis, visual field abnormailities as horizongtal and quadrant defects in those of ischemic optic neuritis.

（1）视野检查：急性视神经炎者中心暗点、旁中心暗点或周边视野缩小；缺血性视神经炎病变者常见水平性、象限性缺损等视野异常。

(2) Visual electrophysiology examination: Visual evoked potential (VEP) showing the prolonged latency and decreased amplitude of P 100 of visible

（2）视觉电生理检测：视觉诱发电位（VEP）检测可见闪光 VEP 和图形 VEP 的

light VEP and graphic VEP.

P100 潜时延长，振幅降低。

(3) Fluorescein fundus angiography (FFA): Capillary dilation and fluorescein leakage seen at the optic disc surface in those of acute neuritis, slow fluorescein filling or uneven fluorescein filling seen at the optic disc in those of ischemic optic neuropathy.

(3) 荧光素眼底血管造影：急性视神经炎者可见视盘表面毛细血管扩张及荧光素渗漏；缺血性视神经病变表现为视盘荧光素充盈迟缓或荧光充盈不均匀。

(4) Head CT、MRI: Exclusion of intracranial space-occupying lesion.

(4) 头部 CT、MRI 检查：排除颅内占位性病变。

3 Therapeutic methods

3 治疗方法

3.1 Therapeutic principles

1.1 治疗原则

The disease is greatly harmful for the vision, as the emergent and critical disease in ophthalmology. It is advisable in the early stage to apply the integrative therapy of both Chinese and western medicines to rescue the vision timely. In traditional Chinese medicine, it is to treat the disease according to its causative factors by applying the purifying, dredging, nourishing and reinforcing methods.

本病对视力危害较大，属眼科急重症，宜早期进行中西医结合治疗，以及时抢救视力。中医以审因论治为原则，临证多用清疏、滋补诸法。

3.2 First-aid measures

3.2 急救措施

(1) Glucocorticoids (GC): Apply Dexamethasone Injection or Triamcinolone Acetonide Acetate Injection for intravenous injection, or apply prednisone for oral administration, or accompanied by Dexamethasone for retrobulbar injection.

(1) 应用糖皮质激素激素：可选用地塞米松或曲安耐得静脉滴注，或口服强的松，也可配合地塞米松球后注射。

(2) Antibiotics: Apply general antibiotics according to the condition if it is caused by inflammation.

(2) 抗生素治疗：如考虑由感染引起者，应根据病情选择抗生素全身应用。

(3) Supportive therapy: Supply Vitamin B and apply vasodilator substances.

(3) 支持疗法：补充 B 类维生素及应用血管扩张剂。

(4) Etiological therapy: Treat the disease by aiming at the pathogenic factors.

(4) 病因治疗：针对病因进行治疗。

3.3 Treatment based on syndrome differentiation

(1) **Excess heat in Liver Meridian**

Main symptoms: Sudden decrease of vision, even loss of vision, accompanied by distending pain at eyeball or pain in eye movements, pupilary dilation, congestion and swelling of optic disc seen at the fundus with fuzzy boundary, peripheral edema, exudates and hemorrhage of optic disc, dilation, circuity and puruple-red colour of central retinal vein, or accompanied by headache, dizziness, red tongue body with yellow tongue coating, and wiry-rapid pulse.

Therapeutic methods: Purify liver, reduce heat, dredge collaterals and dissolve stasis.

Herbal formulas and drugs: The major formula is *Gentian Liver-Draining Decoction* (Long Dan Xie Gan Tang). The commonly-used herbal drugs are *Radix Gentianae* (Long Dan Cao), *Fructus Gardeniae* (Zhi Zi), *Radix Scutellariae* (Huang Qin), *Semen Plantaginis* (Che Qian Zi), *Rhizoma Alismatis* (Ze Xie), *Radix Angelicae Sinensis* (Dang Gui), *Radix Rehmanniae Cruda* (Sheng Di Huang), *Radix Bupleuri* (Chai Hu), *Radix Glycyrrhizae Praeparata* (Zhi Gan Cao), etc.

(2) **Liver qi stagnation**

Main symptoms: Subjective feeling of visual decrease, dull pain at orbit, or distending pain at eyeball, pupilary dilation or invariability, slight congestion of optic disc seen at the fundus with clear boundary, light-colored optic disc over months and years, accompanied by discomforts at chest and hypochondria, deep-red tongue body with thin-yellow tongue coating, and wiry-thready pulse.

3.3 辨证论治

（1）**肝经实热**

主症：视力急降，甚至失明，伴眼球胀痛或转动时痛，瞳神可散大，眼底可见视盘充血肿胀，边界不清，视盘周围水肿、渗出、出血，视网膜静脉扩张迂曲、颜色紫红，或见头痛头晕，舌红，苔黄，脉弦数。

治法：清肝泻热，兼通瘀滞。

方药：代表方为龙胆泻肝汤，常用药如龙胆草、栀子、黄芩、车前子、泽泻、当归、生地黄、柴胡、炙甘草等。

（2）**肝郁气滞**

主症：患眼自觉视力下降，眼眶隐痛或眼球胀痛，瞳神散大或不变，眼底可见视盘轻度充血，边界尚清，日久视盘色淡，或伴胸胁不爽，舌质暗红，苔薄黄，脉弦细。

Therapeutic methods: Soothe liver, relieve depression, move qi and activate blood.

治法:疏肝解郁,行气活血。

Herbal formulas and drugs: The major formula is *Free Wanderer Powder* (Xiao Yao San) plus *Peach Pit, Safflower and Four Agents Decoction* (Tao Hong Si Wu Tang). The commonly-used herbal drugs are *Radix Bupleuri* (Chai Hu), *Radix Angelicae Sinensis* (Dang Gui), *Radix Paeoniae Rubra* (Chi Shao), *Radix Paeoniae Alba* (Bai Shao), *Sclerotium Poriae* (Fu Ling), *Rhizoma Atractylodis Macrocephalae* (Bai Zhu), *Semen Persicae* (Tao Ren), *Flos Carthami* (Hong Hua), *Cortex Moutan Radicis* (Mu Dan Pi), *Rhizoma Ligustici Chuanxiong* (Chuan Xiong), *Radix Rehmanniae Cruda* (Sheng Di Huang), *Herba Menthae* (Bo He), *Rhizoma Zingiberis Recens* (Wei Sheng Jiang) Baked, etc.

方药:代表方为逍遥散合桃红四物汤,常用药如柴胡、当归、赤芍、白芍、茯苓、白术、桃仁、红花、牡丹皮、川芎、生地黄、薄荷、煨生姜等。

(3) **Yin deficiency with fire hyperactivity**

(3) **阴虚火旺**

Main symptoms: Due to old age, subjective feeling of sudden decrease of vision, less obvious eye pain, congestion and swelling of optic disc seen at the fundus with fuzzy boundary, dilation, circuity and puruple-red colour of central retinal vein, linear hemorrhage around the optic disc, or no abnormality seen at the fundus, accompanied by dizziness, blurring of vision, feverish sensation in five centers, red cheeks and lips, dry mouth, red tongue body with scanty tongue coating, and threay-rapid pulse.

主症:患者年高,自觉视力趋降,眼痛不显,眼底可见视盘充血肿胀,边界不清,视网膜静脉扩张迂曲、颜色紫红,视盘周围条状出血,或眼底无异常;伴见头晕目眩,五心烦热,颧赤唇红,口干;舌红,苔少,脉细数。

Therapeutic methods: Nourish yin, subdue fire, activate blood and dissolve stasis.

治法:滋阴降火,活血祛瘀。

Herbal formulas and drugs: The major formula is *Anemarrhena, Phellodendron and Rehmannia Pills* (Zhi Bai Di Huang Wan). The commonly-used

方药:代表方为知柏地黄丸,常用药如知母、黄柏、熟地黄、山茱萸、山药、牡丹

herbal drugs are *Rhizoma Anemarrhenae* (Zhi Mu), *Cortex Phellodendri* (Huang Bo), *Radix Rehmanniae Praeparata* (Shu Di Huang), *Fructus Corni* (Shan Zhu Yu), *Rhizoma Dioscoreae* (Shan Yao), *Cortex Moutan Radicis* (Mu Dan Pi), *Sclerotium Poriae* (Fu Ling), *Rhizoma Alismatis* (Ze Xie), etc.

皮、茯苓、泽泻等。

(4) **Deficiency of both qi and blood**

Main symptoms: Due to chronic disease, or severe hemorrhage, or lactation delivery, weak body constitution, blurred vision, accompanied by pale and lusterless complexion or sallow and yellow complexion, pale-white nails and lips, lack of energy, dislike of speaking, lassitude, low spirit, pale-tender tongue body, and thready-weak pulse.

Therapeutic methods: Reinforce and benefit qi and blood, dredge vessels and open apertures.

Herbal formulas and drugs: The major formula is *Ginseng Nourishing-Flourihing Decoction* (Ren Shen Yang Rong Tang). The commonly-used herbal drugs are *Radix Ginseng* (Ren Shen), *Rhizoma Atractylodis Macrocephalae* (Bai Zhu), *Sclerotium Poriae* (Fu Ling), *Radix Glycyrrhizae Praeparata* (Zhi Gan Cao), *Radix Paeoniae Alba* (Bai Shao), *Radix Angelicae Sinensis* (Dang Gui), *Radix Astragali* (Huang Qi), *Cortex Cinnamomi* (Rou Gui), *Rhizoma Zingiberis Recens* (Sheng Jiang), *Fructus Ziziphi Jujubae* (Da Zao), *Pericarpium Citri Tangerinae* (Chen Pi), *Radix Polygalae* (Yuan Zhi), *Fructus Schisandrae* (Wu Wei Zi), etc.

(4) **气血两虚**

主症：病久体虚，或失血过多，或产后哺乳期发病。症状为视物模糊，兼面白无华或萎黄，爪甲唇色淡白，少气懒言，倦怠神疲；舌淡嫩，脉细弱。

治法：补益气血，通脉开窍。

方药：代表方为人参养荣汤，常用药如人参、白术、茯苓、炙甘草、白芍、当归、黄芪、肉桂、生姜、大枣、陈皮、远志、五味子等。

4 Speculative map

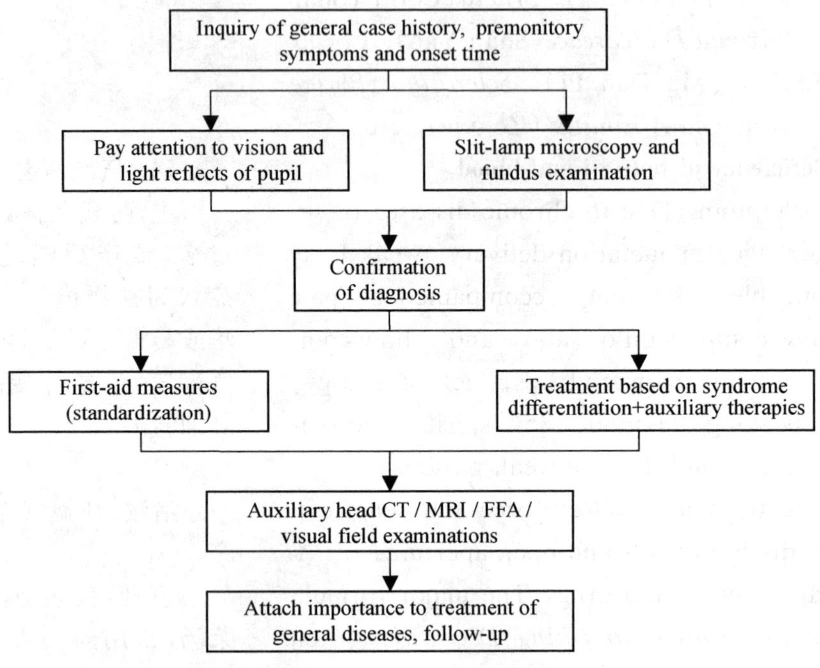

4. 思辨导图

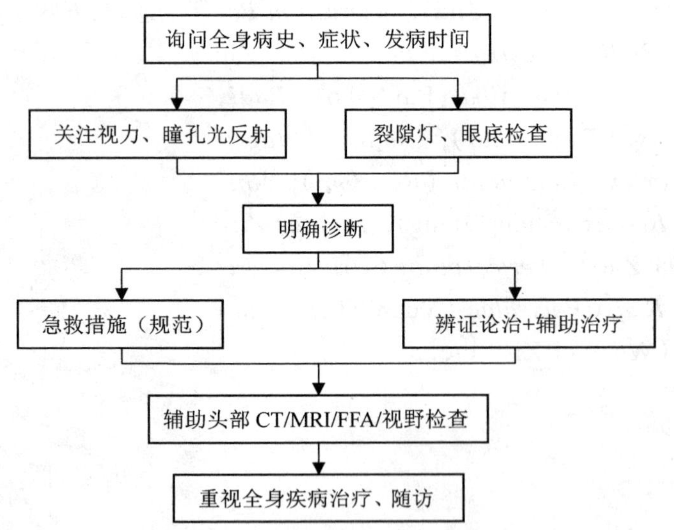

Otorhinolaryngology of Traditional Chinese Medicine

中医耳鼻咽喉科学

Chief Compilers ZHANG Zhijun HUANG Ping

Chief Translator Xu Yao

主编 张治军 黄 平

主译 徐 瑶

Contents

General Introduction

目　　录

总　　论

Specific Introduction

各 论

General Introduction

总 论

Chapter 1 The Relationship between the Ear, Nose and Throat with Zang-fu organs and Meridians

第1章 耳鼻咽喉与脏腑经络的关系

Zang-fu organs are the foundation for the physiological functions and pathological changes of the human body. The meridians are the pathways to circulate qi and blood and communicate with the upper, lower, external and internal parts of the human body. The ear, nose and throat are situated in the head, termed clear aperture, and are linked with Zang-fu organs of the human body via the meridians and are mutually influential, too. Their physiological functions are based upon the normal functions of Zang-fu organs and meridians. Under the pathological situation, the pathological changes of Zang-fu organs can be manifested in the symptoms and signs of the ear, nose and throat. The pathological changes of the clear aperture are often accompanied by the dysfunctions of Zang-fu organs. Although the diseases of the ear, nose and throat are limited, they are closely related to Zang-fu organs and meridians of the whole body.

脏腑是人体生理功能、病理变化的活动基础。经络是人体气血运行，上下表里沟通之脉络。耳鼻咽喉位于头颈，有清窍之称，循经络与人体脏腑相联结，并相互影响，其生理功能的发挥有赖于脏腑经络的正常运行。在病理状态下，脏腑经络病变可反映在耳鼻咽喉的症状与体征上，而清窍病变也常伴有脏腑经络功能的失常。耳、鼻、咽喉疾病虽然局限，但与全身脏腑经络息息相关。

Section 1 The ear and Zang-fu organs and meridians

The ear dominates the auditory sense and governs the balance. It is said in *Spiritual Pivot* (Ling Shu): "the ear is a gathering site of all meridians." The meridians qi of the twelve meridians, three hundred sixty five collaterals of the whole body is linked with the ear. Zang-fu organs closely related to the ear include the kidney, heart, liver, spleen and lung, etc.

1 Ear and kidney

It is said in *Essential Questions* (Su Wen): "The kidney dominates the ear ... opening into the ear." It is also said in *Spiritual Pivot* (Ling Shu): "The ear is an officer of the kidney." It is said in the preface of *Comprehension of Medicine* (Yi Xue Xin Wu): "The kidney can be understood by observing the moistness of the ears." Therefore, the physiological functions of the ear are mainly dominated by the kidney, because the kidney is an organ to store essences and accepts and stores essences from Zang-fu organs. If the essential qi is sufficient and able to flow upward to the ear in its normal nourishing and moistening functions, the hearing ability will be nimble, i. e. the normal auditory sense and balancing functions can be maintained. Exactly as what it is said in *Spiritual Pivot* (Ling Shu): "the kidney qi flows into the ear, if the kidney qi is harmonious, you are able to identify five tones." On contrary, if the kidney essence is deficient and the sea of mar-

第1节 耳与脏腑经络

耳司听觉、主平衡,《灵枢》说:"耳者宗脉之所聚。"全身十二经脉、三百六十五络,其经气皆通于耳。与耳关系较为密切的脏腑有肾、心、肝、胆、脾、肺等。

1 耳与肾

《素问》说:"肾主耳……在窍为耳。"《灵枢》又说:"耳者肾之官也。"《医学心悟》卷首即说:"察耳之枯润,知肾之强弱。"所以耳的生理功能主要由肾主持。因为肾为藏精之脏,受五脏六腑之精而藏之;精气充沛,上通于耳窍,濡养功能正常,则听力聪敏,即正常的听觉与平衡功能得以维系,正如《灵枢》指出:"肾气通于耳,肾和则能闻五音矣。"相反,"肾气不平,则耳为之受病也"(《济生方》);肾精亏损、髓海空虚不能上荣于耳,则出现脑转耳鸣、眩晕等症状。正如《灵枢》所谓:"髓海不足,则脑转耳鸣。"

row is empty, failing to nourish the ear upward, there will be the symptoms of vertigo, tinnitus, and dizziness. Exactly as what it is said in *Spiritual Pivot* (Ling Shu):"if the sea of marrow is insufficient, there will be vertigo and tinnitus."

2 Ear and heart

The heart dominates blood and blood vessels and the heart is a guest of the ear and opens into the ear. The heart manages the ear for the auditory sense under the domination of the heart. The essential qi of the kidney and the meridians and collaterals of the heart are linked with the ear. When the heart and kidney are harmonious, and the water and fire can support each other, the auditory sense will be sensitive. On the contrary, if blood is consumed due to the heart deficiency and the kidney and heart are inharmonious, there will be tinnitus, deafness and vertigo.

2 耳与心

心主血脉，心为耳之客，寄窍于耳，耳司听觉受心主宰。肾之精气与心之脉络通于耳，心肾相交调和、水火既济，则听觉聪敏。反之，心虚血耗、心肾不交，可导致耳鸣、耳聋与眩晕。

3 Ear and liver, gallbladder

The liver and gallbladder are linked in an exterior and interior relationship. The liver qi flows into the ear, and the liver meridian goes along the ear. In the theory of five elements, the liver is a son of the kidney. The liver and kidney share the same resource. The kidney qi flows into the ear and the liver qi does, too. The smooth flow of qi in the liver and gallbladder and nourishment from the liver blood can ensure the normal physiological functions of the ear. If the liver and gallbladder is negligent in their duties, the liver will flow upward reversely or the fire of the liver and gallbladder will flame upward, resulting in tinnitus, deafness, swelling, pain and discharge of pus in the ear.

3 耳与肝、胆

肝与胆互为表里，肝气通于耳，胆脉环绕于耳。五行中肝为肾之子，肝肾同源，肾气既通于耳，肝之气未尝不可。肝胆之气通达与肝血濡养维系耳生理功能的正常发挥。肝胆失职，肝气上逆或肝胆之火上炎可引起耳鸣耳聋、耳部肿痛、流脓等病症。

4 Ear and spleen

The spleen dominates the transportation and transformation and is the source for the production of qi and blood, and its ability to raise the clear yang, which has the effects to nourish the ear. It is related to the normal auditory sense and balance. If the spleen is insufficient, failing to raise the clear yang and to transport water and dampness, and accumulating the turbidity into phlegm and blocking the ear, there will be the symptoms of distending sensation in the ear, discharge of pus, deafness and vertigo, etc.

4 耳与脾

脾主运化，为气血生化之源，其升举清阳之气有荣养耳窍之功，关乎正常听觉与平衡。若脾气不足，清阳不升，水湿失运，聚浊成痰，蒙蔽清窍，可致耳胀、流脓、耳聋及眩晕等症。

5 Ear and lung

The lung is a mother of the kidney and dominates the circulation of qi into the ear, and its meridian also goes around the ear and is related to the auditory sense. If the pathogens attack the lung, the lung will fail to perform its spreading ability, causing distending pain, stuffy sensation and tinnitus. Therefore, there is such a saying: "the lung should be treated for deafness."

5 耳与肺

肺为肾之母，主气贯于耳，其络脉亦循行于耳，关乎听觉。邪气犯肺，肺气不宣可致耳胀痛、闷塞、耳鸣等病，据此有"耳聋治肺"之法。

Section 2 The nose and Zang-fu organs and meridians

The nose is situated in the center of the face, an external aperture of the lung, inhales the clear air and exhales the turbid air, dominates the smell sense and assists the pronunciation, and is a passage for exchange of yin and yang. It is closely related to the twelve meridians and the lung, spleen, heart, kidney and gallbladder.

第2节 鼻与脏腑经络

鼻居面中，为肺之外窍，吸入清气，呼出浊气，司嗅觉，助发音，是阴阳二气交会的通道。与十二经脉，肺、脾、心、肾、胆等脏腑有着密切的关系。

1 Nose and lung

The lung dominates qi and opens into the nose. When the nose is unobstructed, the lung qi will be smooth. The lung qi flows into the nose, and when the lung is harmonious, the nose is able to identify the smells. Two of them coordinate with each other, for displaying the normal physiological functions. Otherwise, the dysfunction of the lung can easily cause nasal problems. The nasal problems can also influence the functions of the lung in the spreading and descending ability. Invasion of exogenous pathogens into the lung, accumulation of heat in the lung meridian or deficiency of the lung qi will cause nasal obstruction, nasal discharge and sneezing, etc.

1 鼻与肺

肺主气，开窍于鼻，鼻窍通畅，则肺气通利；肺气通于鼻，肺和则鼻能知香臭，两者互相协调，才能发挥正常的生理功能。否则，肺的功能失调，易致鼻病发生；鼻病也可影响肺气宣发肃降。外邪犯肺、肺经郁热或肺气虚寒，均可导致鼻塞、流涕、喷嚏等症。

2 Nose and spleen

The spleen contains blood and is a source for the production of qi and blood. The condition of the spleen qi is related to the fullness of blood vessels and normal functions of the nose. The spleen deficiency will cause malnutrition in the nose and retention of the pathogens in the nose, resulting in nasal problems. If the spleen fails to contain blood, there will be nasal bleeding. If dampness and heat are accumulated in the spleen and stomach, there will be red and erosive nose, yellow nasal discharge, and nasal sores, etc.

2 鼻与脾

脾统血，为气血生化之源，脾气的盛衰关系到鼻部血脉盈虚及功能的正常与否。脾虚则鼻失所养，邪毒滞留发鼻病；脾不统血则鼻衄；脾胃湿热则鼻红赤烂、涕黄、生疮。

3 Nose and gallbladder

The Gallbladder Meridian of Foot Shaoyang goes upward to the brain and links with the nose. If heat in the gallbladder is transmitted to the brain or involves the nose directly, there will be running nose, and even nasal hemorrhage due to absurd

3 鼻与胆

足少阳胆经上通于脑，下通頞鼻。胆腑移热于脑，或直犯鼻窍，浊涕下不止也；甚者，迫血妄行而鼻衄。

blood circulation.

4 Nose and heart

The heart dominates the blood and blood vessels. The nose is a gate of the heart and lung. The heart manages the smelling sense, so that the nose is able to identify the smells. If the problem exists in the heart and lung, the nose will be in disorder. If the pathogenic heat damages the heart, nasal hemorrhage will occur.

4 鼻与心

心主血脉，鼻为心肺之门户。心主嗅，故令鼻知香臭。心肺有病，鼻为之不利；邪热伤于心可致鼻衄。

5 Nose and kidney

The kidney dominates water. The kidney meridian intersects with the Governor Vessel through the nose. The inhalation of air is based upon the kidney qi. If the kidney yang is deficient, there will be clear nasal discharge. When the kidney yin is deficient, the nasal cavity will be dry and even its mucous membrane will be atrophic. If the kidney fails to accept qi, there will be panting and flapping of the nasal wings.

5 鼻与肾

肾主水液，肾之经脉交会于循鼻之督脉，气体吸入有赖于肾气。肾阳虚则清涕无摄；肾阴虚则鼻腔干燥，甚至黏膜萎缩；肾不纳气，则喘息鼻煽。

Section 3 The throat and Zang-fu organs and meridians

The pharynx is a tract of water and grain and dominates the input. The larynx links with the mouth and nose upward and connects with the trachea, belongs to a gate for respiration and dominates pronunciation, and manages the output. The throat is a thoroughfare for food ingestion and respiration and is also an important side with the twelve meridians and is closely related to the lung,

第3节 咽喉与脏腑经络

咽为水谷之道，主纳不出；喉上通口鼻，下接气管，为呼吸之门户，司发音，主出不纳。咽喉为饮食呼吸之要道，为十二经脉交会之处，与肺、脾、胃、肝、肾关系较为密切。

spleen, stomach, liver and kidney.

1 Larynx and lung

The larynx links with the airway and communicates with the lung and is connected by the lung. If the lung qi is sufficient, its spreading ability will be smooth and the respiration and pronunciation will be normal. Otherwise, if the lung fails to perform its spreading and descending ability, the pathogens will be accumulated in the throat. If heat is abundant in the lung meridian, it will attack the throat upward. If the lung yin is insufficient, the throat will fail to be nourished by the body fluids. If fire in deficient nature flares upward, it will cause hoarse voice and sore throat, etc.

1 喉与肺

喉接气道与肺相通，为肺之所系。肺气充沛，宣发舒畅，呼吸和发音方能正常。否则，肺失宣降，则邪滞咽喉；肺经热盛，则上攻咽喉；肺阴不足，则咽喉失去津液滋养，甚至虚火上炎，可导致声嘶、喉痛等症。

2 Pharynx and spleen and stomach

The pharynx is the upper mouth of the spleen and stomach, connected by the stomach via the esophagus and dominates the smooth transportation of water and grain. The spleen and stomach jointly decompose water and grain and distribute the essential substances for nourishing the organs and tissues. Therefore, the pharynx is mutually influential to the spleen and stomach. If heat is abundant in the stomach and burns the throat, there can be redness, swelling, heat and pain in the local area. If the spleen qi is deficient, and body fluids are unable to nourish the throat, there will be dry throat and lack of body fluids.

2 咽与脾胃

咽为脾胃之上口，借食道相通，为胃之所系，主司通利水谷；脾胃共主腐熟水谷、输布精微以濡养，故咽与脾胃是相互为用。若胃腑热盛，上灼咽部可致局部红、肿、热、痛；若脾气虚弱，阴津难以滋养，则咽干少津。

3 Throat and kidney

The kidney stores essences. The Kidney Meridian of Foot Shaoyin enters the lung and goes through the throat. When the kidney essence is sufficient and the throat is nourished by the kidney essence,

3 咽喉与肾

肾藏精，足少阴肾经之脉入肺中，循行于咽喉。肾精充沛，咽喉得肾精之濡养而邪毒不易侵犯，则声音洪

the pathogens will not be easy to attack the throat, so the voice will be resonant and the respiration will be forceful. If the kidney yin is deficient, and the fire in deficient nature disturbs the throat upward by the meridians, there will be discomfort in the throat and hoarse voice.

亮,呼吸有力。若肾阴虚,虚火循经上扰咽喉为病,可致咽喉不适,声音嘶哑。

4 Throat and liver

The liver dominates convergence and dispersion. The liver meridian goes along the throat and enters the nasopharynx. The meridian qi of the liver goes upward to the throat. When the liver qi ensures its converging and dispersing ability, the throat will be normal and unobstructed. If the liver qi is stagnant, the liver qi goes abnormally upward or the spleen deficiency due to the liver qi stagnation, resulting in the accumulation of phlegm, or if the liver qi stagnation turns into fire, burning the throat upward, there will be sore throat, and "obstruction of foreign body in the throat", i. e. "globus hysteriocus", etc.

4 咽喉与肝

肝主疏泄,肝之经脉循喉咙入颃颡,肝之经气上于喉咙。肝气疏泄调畅,则咽喉通利。若肝气郁结,肝气上逆,或肝郁脾虚,痰气互结,或肝郁化火,上灼咽喉,则出现咽喉疼痛不利、"喉中介介如梗状"即"梅核气"等症。

Chapter 2 The Commonly Used Examinations of Otorhinolaryngology

第2章 耳鼻咽喉科常用检查方法

Section 1 Basic tools and instruments

第1节 基本检查用具与器械

1 Light source and head mirror

1.1 Light source

Equipped on the one side of the inspector's chair, a little bit above the head, about 25 to 40 cm away from the head mirror of the inspector.

1.2 Head mirror

A concave mirror reflector with the small hole in the center, about 25cm of focal length, connected with the head band by the double ball joint, adjustable and fixable. Precautions in exposure to the light: ① Keep the pupil, mirror hole, reflecting focus and inspected part on a line. ② build up a habit of "single-eye look". ③ the examinee just sits upright and the inspector adjusts the light source for light exposure.

2 Commonly used instruments

There are the commonly used instruments of otoscope (including air blast otoscope, electric otoscope and electric air blast otoscope), atomizer,

1 光源与额镜

1.1 光源

置于受检者座椅一侧，略高出其头部，距检查者所带额镜约25～40厘米。

1.2 额镜

为中央有一小孔的凹面反光镜，焦距约25厘米，以双球关节连于额带，可调节与固定。对光时注意点：①保持瞳孔、镜孔、反光焦点和被检查部位在一直线上；②养成"单眼视"的习惯；③受检者坐姿端正即可，由检查者调整光源对光。

2 常用器械

常用检查器械有耳镜（包括鼓气耳镜、电耳镜或电鼓气耳镜）、喷雾器、压舌板、

tongue depressor, gun-shaped forceps, ear angled forceps, earwax hook, cotton applicator, anterior rhinoscope, indirect nasopharyngoscope, indirect laryngoscope, tuning fork, etc. Alcohol lamp and match should also be ready. Now, alcohol lamp can be replaced by electric heat source in the treatment table of the otorhinolaryngologic clinic.

枪状镊、膝状镊、耵聍钩、卷棉子、前鼻镜、间接鼻咽镜、间接喉镜、音叉等，应备有酒精灯、火柴，现耳鼻咽喉科诊疗台有电热源可取代酒精灯。

Section 2 The commonly used examinations of the ear

第2节 耳部常用检查方法

1 General inspections

It is necessary to inspect the shape, skin colour and activity of the auricle first, mainly observing if there are the deformity, redness and swelling, injury, exudation and preauricular fistula, etc. If the patient complains of ear pain, it is advisable to press the tragus or pull the auricle to see if pain exists, and observe the external auditory canal and tympanic membrane. If lump exists in the auricle or external auditory canal, it is necessary to inspect its size, painful sense, hardness and mobility by the touching method. It is necessary to inspect if pain exists in the mastoid region by the touching method and inspect if there is lymph node enlargement in front of or behind the ear.

1 一般检查法

先观察耳廓的形态、皮肤色泽及活动度，主要看有无畸形、红肿、损伤、渗出及耳前瘘管等。如患者主诉有耳痛，可按压耳屏或牵拉耳廓察有无疼痛，并查看外耳道和鼓膜情况。如遇耳廓或外耳道肿块，以触压法查其大小、痛感、软硬度和活动度。乳突区检查以触压法查有无疼痛，并检查耳前、后有无肿大淋巴结等。

2 Inspection of the external auditory canal and tympanic membrane

After the examinee sits on a chair, facing to one side, the doctor reflects the light on the external auditory meatus. In inspecting the adults, it is advisable to pull the auricle backward, laterally and

2 外耳道和鼓膜检查法

受检者坐椅上，面朝向一侧，医生借额镜反光于外耳道口。检查成人时，可一手将其耳廓向后、外、上方牵

upward with one hand, and press the tragus forward with another hand. In inspecting the babies and infants, it is advisable to pull the auricle backward and downward, in order to straighten the external auditory canal for easy observation. If there is much ear hair, it is advisable to insert the trumpet-shaped otoscope to push away the ear hair. If there is much earwax, it is needed to clean it away. In inspecting the external auditory canal, it is necessary to see clearly if there are blockage, stricture, neoformation, earwax, and foreign body, and to see if there are redness and swelling, erosion, exudation, pus and scab in the skin, etc. In inspecting the tympanic membrane, it is necessary to observe its colour, anatomical landmarks (handle of malleus, tympanic membrane navel, light cone, short process of malleus), mobility and if perforation exists.

拉，另一手食指向前推压耳屏；检查婴幼儿，应将其耳廓向后、下方牵拉，均为使外耳道变直，便于观察。如果耳毛较多，可借助喇叭形耳镜伸入外耳道推开耳毛；如果耵聍较多，需先予清理。查看外耳道应看清有无闭锁、狭窄、新生物、耵聍、异物等，皮肤有无红肿、糜烂、渗液、脓液、结痂等。查看鼓膜时，需注意其色泽、解剖标志（锤骨柄、鼓膜脐部、光锥、锤骨短突等）、活动度及有无穿孔等。

3 Inspection of eustachian tube function

The commonly used methods include the swallowing method, Valsalva manoeuver, Podbielniak ball inflation (mostly for children) and catheterization of eustachian tube. If the eustachian tube is smooth, it is possible to hear light "shh" sound or sound of tympanic vibration from the external auditory canal by the stethoscope and to observe the internal and external activity of the tympanic membrane.

3 咽鼓管功能检查法

常用方法有吞咽法、捏鼻鼓气法、波氏球吹张法（多用于儿童）和导管吹张法。如咽鼓管通畅，用听诊器可从外耳道听到轻柔的"嘘嘘"声或鼓膜振动的声音，也可观察到鼓膜的内外活动。

3.1 Swallowing method

The examinee just does the swallowing action.

3.1 吞咽法

受检者做吞咽动作即可。

3.2 Valsalva manoeuver

The examinee pinches the nose with the fingers (thumb and index finger), closes the mouth and

3.2 捏鼻鼓气法

受检者以手指（大拇指和食指）捏鼻，闭口，用力鼓

blows forcefully.

气。

3.3 Podbielniak ball inflation

After the examinee takes little water in the mouth, the inspector inserts the olive head of the ball into one nostril of the examinee and presses another nostril tightly with the hand, and quickly squeezes the rubber ball in the moment when the examinee swallows.

3.3 波氏球吹张法

受检者口内含水少许，检查者将波氏球橄榄头塞于受检者一侧前鼻孔，同时用手紧压另一侧鼻孔，在受检者吞咽的瞬间迅速捏压橡皮球。

3.4 Catheterization of eustachian tube

A special metal catheter with the curved anterior end is lightly inserted into the nasopharyngeal part from the bottom of the examinee's nasal cavity. The inspector aims at the pharyngeal opening of the auditory tube with the head end of metal catheter by hand feeling, to blow through the tail end of the catheter by the rubber ball (It is necessary to be gentle in operation, not to use the force violently).

3.4 导管吹张法

用特制前端弯曲的金属导管，经受检者鼻腔底部轻轻伸入至鼻咽部，检查者凭手感将金属导管头端对准咽鼓管咽口，用橡皮球经导管尾端吹气(注意操作要轻柔，不可用力过猛)。

4 Inspection of the auditory functions

It is supposed to test if the hearing ability is normal or not, and degree and quality of the hearing loss, in the soundproof room necessarily.

4 听功能检查法

测试听力是否正常，以及听力损失的程度和性质。应在隔音室进行。

4.1 Tuning fork test

The tuning fork of 256 Hz or 512 Hz is most commonly used. By holding the handle of the tuning fork with the hand, the inspector knocks the prong to vibrate it, and then immediately puts the tuning fork 1 cm out of the external auditory meatus with the two prongs in the parallel position for testing air conduction (AC), and puts the handle end of the knocked tuning fork at the skull or tympanic sinus area for testing bone conduction (BC). By the following three tests, the quality of deafness can be judged preliminarily, but the degree of deafness

4.1 音叉试验

最常用的是256赫兹或512赫兹的音叉。检查者手持叉柄，敲击音叉臂使其振动，立即将音叉以两叉臂平行的位置放在耳道口外1厘米处，可查气导；将敲击后的音叉柄底置颅骨或鼓窦区，可查骨导。通过下述三种试验可初步判断耳聋性质，但不能精确判断耳聋程度。

cannot be judged precisely.

In the inspection by the tuning fork, it is necessary to be sure: ① to knock the upper 1/3 of the tuning fork. ② to knock with the same force, without violent force or knocking the hard table surface, for avoiding overtune. ③ to vibrate the surface of the two arms of upper 1/3 of the tuning fork and the vertical axis of the external auditory canal persistently in the inspection of air conduction, at the same level of the external auditory meatus. ④ put the handle bottom at the skull surface in the inspection of bone conduction, and ⑤ not to touch any objects with the vibrating tuning fork.

音叉检测时注意:①应敲击音叉臂的上 1/3 处;②敲击力量应一致,不可用力过猛或敲击台桌硬物,以免产生泛音;③检查气导时应把振动的音叉上 1/3 的双臂平面与外耳道纵轴一致,并同外耳道口同高;④检查骨导时则把柄底置于颅面;⑤振动的音叉不可触及周围任何物体。

(1) Rinne test (RT): To compare the length between the hearing time of air conduction and the hearing time of bone conduction with the tuning fork. If air conduction time is longer than bone conduction time, positive (+) is marked, or negative (−) is marked contrarily, or positive-negative (±) is marked if the two times are equal. If the air conduction time is longer than the bone conduction time, but if the time of the two is shorter than the normal hearing ability, short positive will be marked. Negative or negative-positive results indicate conductive or mixed hearing loss. Positive result is mainly normal. The short positive result is mainly seen in sensorineural deafness.

(1) 气、骨导差比较试验:比较音叉气导听到时间与骨导听到时间的长短。气导时间长于骨导者记为阳性(+),反之记为阴性(−),二者相等者记为阴阳性(±)。若虽气导时间长于骨导,但二者均短于正常听力耳,则记为短阳性。阴性或阴阳性者提示听力损失为传导性或混合性,而阳性者主要为正常;短阳性者主要见于感音神经性聋。

(2) Weber test (WT): The examinee is asked to point out the deviation of the loudness after the tuning fork is put in the middle of the skull. If the deviation inclines to the healthy side or mild side of the hearing loss, the sick ear or serious side of hearing loss is diagnosed as sensorineural deafness, or conductive deafness on contrary. If in the middle,

(2) 骨导偏向试验:音叉置于颅骨正中,令受试者指出响度偏向。如偏向健侧或听力损失较轻一侧,则患耳或听力损失较重侧为感音神经性聋;反之则为传导性聋;如在正中,则或双耳听力正

either the hearing ability is normal in the two ears, or the hearing ability of air conduction, bone conduction in the two ears decreases comparatively.

常,或为双耳气、骨导听力相应减退的综合结果。

(3) Schwabach test (ST): It is used to compare the length of the bone conduction time between the inspecting ear and the normal ear. The time longer than the normal ear is seen in the conductive deafness, and shorter than the normal ear is mostly sensorineural deafness or mixed deafness.

(3) 骨导对比试验:比较受试耳与听力正常耳的骨导时间长短。长于正常耳者见于传导性聋,短于正常者多为感音神经性聋或混合性聋。

Assessment of Tuning Fork Test Results

Methods	Normal Hearing	Conductive Deafness	Sensorineural Deafness
RT	(+)	(-) or (±)	(+)
WT	=	→ Sick ear	→Healthy ear
ST	(±)	(+)	(-)

音叉试验结果评价

试验方法	正常听力	传导性耳聋	感音神经性聋
RT	(+)	(−)或(±)	(+)
WT	=	→患耳	→健耳
ST	(±)	(+)	(−)

4.2 Pure tone test

It is a commonly used method to test the hearing functions of the human ear by the pure tone audiometer in different frequencies and different intensities. The test results are comparatively accurate. Besides the clear definition of the quality in the hearing loss, the nature of the hearing loss can also be defined. The normal hearing thresholds of various frequencies in the audiometer are all in zero (0 dB). Domestically, the hearing threshold means of air conduction at the three different frequencies of 500 Hz, 1 000 Hz and 2 000 Hz are usually used to assess the degree of deafness in the clinic. 25 to

4.2 纯音测听

是借助纯音听力计以不同频率和不同强度的纯音测试人耳听觉功能最常用的方法。测试结果比较准确,除了可以明确听力减退的性质,还可以确定听力减退的程度。听力计各个频率的正常听阈均在零(0 分贝)级。国内临床一般以 500 赫兹,1 000 赫兹和 2 000 赫兹 3 个频率的气导听阈值均数来评价耳聋的程度:25～40 分贝

40 dB is mild, 41 to 55 dB is medium, 56 to 70 dB is severe, and 71 to 90 dB is very severe and >90 dB is complete deafness. The nature of deafness can be judged based upon the feature of the hearing curve line. If bone conduction is normal, the decrease of air conduction is characterized by low frequency. The >10 dB is mostly conductive deafness. The simultaneous decrease of bone conduction and air conduction is mainly characterized by high frequency. No difference between air conduction and bone conduction is sensorineural deafness. If bone conduction and air conduction drop down at the same time, difference between air conduction and bone conduction indicates mixed deafness.

为轻度,41～55 分贝为中度,56～70 为重度,71～90 分贝为严重度,>90 分贝为全聋。根据听力曲线的特点,可以判断耳聋性质。骨导正常,气导下降以低频为主,气骨导间距>10 分贝多为传导性聋;骨气导同时下降以高频为主,无气骨导差为感音神经性聋;骨气导同时下降,有气骨导差为混合性聋。

4.3 Acoustic immittance measurement

A method to objectively test the sound system of the middle ear and auditory pathway function of the brainstem. The curve line of the functions of the tympanic cavity can be achieved by acoustic immittance device. Based upon the shape, peak pressure point, peak height, and gradient and smoothness of the curve line, various tympanic lesions can be objectively reflected, tympanic fluid in particular. By acoustic stapedius reflex, the localization diagnosis of deafness and peripheral facial paralysis can be helpfully made.

4.3 声导抗测试

是客观测试中耳传音系统和脑干听觉通路功能的方法。借助声导抗仪得出鼓室功能曲线,根据曲线形状、峰压点、峰高度以及曲线坡度、光滑度等,可较客观反映各种鼓室病变,尤其是鼓室积液等。通过镫骨肌反射测试,还可以帮助耳聋和周围性面瘫的定位诊断。

4.4 Auditory evoked potential test

The sound wave is converted into nervous impulse by the hair cells in the cochlea, and the biological electricity produced during its transmission through the auditory pathways to the brain is termed auditory evoked potential. Clinically, the cochlear potential, auditory brainstem response, middle latency response and cortex potentials are

4.4 听觉诱发电位测试

声波在耳蜗内由毛细胞转换成神经冲动,沿听觉通路传到大脑的过程中产生的生物电称之为听觉诱发电位。临床应用较多的有耳蜗电位、听性脑干反应测听、中潜伏期反应及皮层电位等,

mostly used as the important means, to objectively test the hearing ability of infants, to diagnose functional deafness and differentiate the location of deafness.

为客观测试婴幼儿听力、诊断功能性聋、鉴别耳聋病位等的重要手段。

4.5 Otoacoustic emission test

4.5 耳声发射检测

Otoacoustic emission refers to sound energy spontaneously produced by the cochlear outer hair cells and transmitted to the middle and external auditory canal, different in spontaneous emission and evoked emission. The evoked otoacoustic emission is objective, simple, time-saving, noninvasive and sensitive, and can be helpful to the early diagnosis of cochlear deafness, beside the extensive application in the hearing screening of the infants.

耳声发射是由耳蜗外毛细胞主动产生，向中耳、外耳道传播的声能，有自发和诱发之分。诱发性耳声发射具有客观、简便、省时、无创和灵敏等优点，除了广泛用于婴幼儿听力筛查，还有助于耳蜗性聋的早期诊断。

5 Inspection of vestibular function

5 前庭功能检查

When the vestibule is irritated, there can be the symptoms of nystagmus, dizziness, topple and fall. The vestibular lesion with the above symptoms is termed spontaneous vestibular symptoms. If the vestibule is irritated artificially, the vestibular symptoms present after induction are termed vestibular function test, used to understand the state of the vestibular functions and help clinical diagnosis. It mainly includes balance function inspection and nystagmus inspection.

当前庭受到刺激时，可发生眼球震颤、眩晕和倾倒等症状。前庭病变出现上述症状，称为自发性前庭症状；若人为方法刺激前庭，诱发出现前庭症状，称为前庭功能试验。用于了解前庭功能状态和帮助临床诊断。主要包括平衡功能检查和眼震检查。

5.1 Balance function inspection

5.1 平衡功能检查

Clinically, there are usually the testing methods of closing the eyes and standing upright, finger to finger, walking, and closing the eyes and writing.

临床常用的有闭目直立、对指、行走和闭眼垂直书写等试验方法。

5.2 nystagmus inspection

5.2 眼震检查

Nystagmus is an involuntary and rhythmic movement of the eyeballs, different in fast phase and slow phase. Slow phase is produced while the

眼震是一种不随意的眼球节律性运动，有快相和慢相之分。慢相为迷路受刺激

labyrinth is irritated, identical in the flowing direction of the endolymph. Fast phase is resulted from the subcortical center in regulating the eyeballs in opposite direction, opposite to the flowing direction of the endolymph. Clinically, the direction of fast phase is defined as the direction of nystagmus, respectively as horizontal, vertical, rotary and diagonal nystagmus. The intensity of nystagmus is divided into three grades: Grade I refers to nystagmus present in looking along the direction of fast phase. Grade II refers to nystagmus present in looking forward. Grade III refers to nystagmus present in looking at any direction. Nystagmus is inspected by naked eyes, Frenzel spectacle and electronystagmography, and the latter can be used to record feeble nystagmus, and provide various parameters of amplitude, frequency and slow-phase velocity, higher in diagnostic value.

所产生，与内淋巴流动方向一致；快相则为皮质下中枢向相反方向调节眼球的结果，与内淋巴流动方向相反。临床将快相指向定为眼震方向，分为水平性、垂直性、旋转性及对角性眼震。眼震强度可分三级：Ⅰ级为向快相方向侧注视时出现眼震；Ⅱ级为向前注视时出现眼震；Ⅲ级为向任意方向注视时均出现眼震。眼震检查有裸眼、Frenzel 眼镜和眼震电图描记等方法，后者可记录到微弱眼震，并提供振幅、频率及慢相角速度等各种参数，诊断价值较高。

(1) A kind of nystagmus detectable without any evoking measure. In the inspection, the patient is told to fix the head and to watch with the two eyes the inspector's fingers 50 cm in the front, and look at the fingers upward, downward, leftward and rightward, with the moving amplitude limited in about 45° from the middle line. The inspector carefully observes the direction, amplitude, intensity, frequency and time of nystagmus. Please refer to the following table for differentiation of three types of nystagmus.

(1) 自发性眼震：是一种无需通过任何诱发措施即可观察到的眼震。检查时患者头部固定，两眼注视前方 50 厘米检查者手指，眼球随手指上下左右移动，移动幅度以距中线约 45°为限。注意观察眼震方向、振幅、强度、频率和时间等。常见 3 种眼震类型鉴别要点见下表：

Differentiation of Three Types of Spontaneous Nystagmus

Types	Peripheral	Central	Ocular
Nature	Horizontal, a little rotary	Vertical, rotary or diagonal	Sowing or tensional
Direction	No change	Changeable	No fast or slow phase
Intensity	Change with disease	Multiple change	Instable
Vegetative nerve symptoms of dizziness, nausea and vomiting	Yes. Severity identical to nystagmus intensity	Nil. If yes, severity identical to nystagmus intensity	Nil

3 种自发性眼震鉴别表

眼震类型	周围性	中枢性	眼病性
性质	水平,略带旋转性	垂直、旋转或对角性	钟摆或张力性
方向	一般不变	可变	无快慢向
强度	随疾病变化	多变	不稳定
眩晕感及恶心、呕吐等植物神经症状	有,严重程度与眼震强度一致	可无;若有,严重程度与眼震强度不一致	无

(2) Positional nystagmus and positioning nystagmus: Positional nystagmus is only present while the head is in certain position. Positioning nystagmus is present by sudden change of the head position or shortly after it.

(2) 位置性眼震和变位性眼震:位置性眼震是头部处于某种位置时才有的眼震;变位性眼震是头位迅速改变过程中或其后短时间内出现的眼震。

(3) A test to evoke the vestibular response by infusing cold and hot water into the external auditory canal. Respectively, 30℃ and 44℃ water (37 ± 7℃) are infused into the external auditory canal to the tympanic membrane, to observe the amplitude, frequency, direction and time of the examinee's nystagmus, for assessing the vestibular functions. There are other methods of optokinetic test, Saccade test, pursuit test, watching test, and fistula test.

(3) 冷热试验:是用冷热水经外耳道诱发前庭反应的试验方法。分别将 30 摄氏度和 44 摄氏度的水(37 ± 7)摄氏度注入外耳道直达鼓膜,观察被检查者眼震的振幅、频率、方向和时间,以评价前庭功能。其他尚有视动性眼震、扫视、跟随、注视和瘘管等试验方法。

6 Imageological inspection

Temporal bone radiography is a traditional inspection for auricular diseases and gradually replaced by temporal bone CT currently. By the showing position, the optional X-ray projection positions include: Lateral oblique position of mastoid process (Runstrome's position), mainly showing the tympanic cavity, aditus ad antrum, tympanic sinus and mastoid air cells. petrous axial position (Mayer's position), mainly showing the upper tympanic cavity, and aditus ad antrum. oblique petrous position (Stenver's position), mainly showing the internal auditory canal, labyrinth, and petrous apex; frontooccipital position of temporal bone (Town's position), mainly showing the petrous apex, internal auditory canal and inner ear.

CT scan of temporal coronal position or axial thin layer (2mm) can clearly show the fine anatomical structure of the temporal bone, such as the external auditory canal, auditory ossicle, facial canal, internal auditory canal, sigmoid sinus, cochlea, vestibule, semicircular canal, vestibular aqueduct and cochlear aqueduct meatus, highly valuable for diagnosis of congenital ear malformation, temporal fracture, various otitis media, and tumors, etc.

Magnetic resonance imaging (MRI) can show the soft tissue structure of the inner ear and internal auditory canal and temporal lesions, beneficial to the diagnosis of tumors, abscess and hemorrhage in the cerebellopontine angle, temporosphenoid lobe and ventricle.

6 影像学检查

颞骨摄片是耳部疾病传统检查方法，目前逐渐被颞骨 CT 取代。依显示部位，可选择的 X 线投照位有：乳突侧斜位（亦称伦氏位），主要显示鼓室、鼓窦入口、鼓窦及乳突气房；岩部轴位（亦称麦氏位），主要显示上鼓室及鼓窦入口；岩部斜位（亦称斯氏位），主要显示内听道、内耳迷路、岩尖部；颞骨额枕位（亦称汤氏位），主要显示岩尖、内听道及内耳。

颞骨冠状位或轴位薄层（2 毫米）CT 扫描可清晰显示颞骨细微解剖结构，如外耳道、听小骨、面神经管、内听道、乙状窦、耳蜗、前庭、半规管、前庭水管和耳蜗导水管开口。对先天性耳畸形、颞骨骨折、各种中耳炎症、肿瘤等具有较高的诊断价值。

磁共振成像（MRI）可显示内耳、内听道软组织结构和颞骨病变，也有利于桥小脑角、颞叶及脑室等部位肿瘤、脓肿及出血等疾病的诊断。

Section 3 The commonly used examinations of the nose

1 Inspection of external nose

It is mainly used to observe if there is any change in the shape and color, and to check by touching the external nose if there are tenderness, thickness and hardness and bone-friction sensation, deformity and migration, etc.

2 Inspection of nasal vestibule

After the examinee uplifts the head, the inspector pushes the nose tip with the thumb to observe if there are redness and swelling, ulcers, scabs, cracks, proliferation and neoformation in the nasal vestibular skin.

3 Anterior rhinoscopy

How to use rhinoscope: Hold the rhinoscope with the left hand, with the handle held by the palm and fingers, and press the joint of the rhinoscope with the thumb, and close the two leaves and insert into the nostrils parallel from the nasal bottom, and then open the two leaves to dilate the nostrils for observing the nasal cavity. The examinee first lowers the head slightly, in order to observe the nasal bottom, inferior nasal passage, inferior nasal concha, and anterioinferior part of the nasal septum. Then, the examinee uplifts the head slightly, in order to observe the middle nasal concha, nasal common meatus, inferior nasal concha and middle part of the nasal septum. The examinee uplifts the head backward in about 30° to 60°, in order to observe the nasal agger, nasal common meatus, middle con-

第3节 鼻部常用检查方法

1 外鼻检查法

主要观察有无形态、色泽改变。触按外鼻有无压痛、增厚、变硬和有无骨摩擦感、畸形及移位等。

2 鼻前庭检查法

受检者头稍后仰，检查者以拇指推起鼻尖即可观察鼻前庭皮肤有无红肿、溃疡、结痂、皲裂、增生及新生物等。

3 前鼻镜检查法

鼻镜使用方法：左手持鼻镜，镜柄置于掌指，拇指按住鼻镜关节，合拢两叶平行于鼻底伸入前鼻孔，张开上下两叶扩大鼻孔，窥视鼻腔。受试者先头微低，以利观察鼻底、下鼻道、下鼻甲和鼻中隔前下部；再头微仰，观察中鼻甲、总鼻道、下鼻甲和鼻中隔中部；头进一步后仰约30°～60°，观察鼻丘、总鼻道、中鼻甲、嗅裂、中鼻道和鼻中隔上部。注意勿将鼻镜伸入过深超过鼻阈，以免损伤鼻黏膜造成疼痛或出血；取出鼻镜时不可两叶完全闭拢以

cha, olfactory cleft, middle nasal meatus, and upper part of the nasal septum. It is necessary not to insert the rhinoscope too deeply over the nasal limen, in order to avoid damaging the nasal membrane and causing pain or hemorrhage. In taking out the rhinoscope, it is necessary not to close the two leaves completely, in order to avoid nipping the nasal hair to cause pain.

免夹住鼻毛造成疼痛。

The rhinoscopy can be processed from the bottom to the top, and from the anterior to the posterior and from the interior to the exterior. If the nasal membrane is swollen, it is advisable to start inspection after using 1% Enpherine spray or cotton slice to contract the nasal membrane, in order to see the lesions in the deep nasal cavity clearly. It is necessary to observe the colour of mucous membrane, and to see if there are congestion, tumefaction, hypertrophy, dryness and atrophy, and ulceration and adhesion in it, and to see if the nasal common meatus is broadened or narrowed, and to see if there are secretions in various nasal meatus and volume, colour and shape of secretions, and to see if there are deviation, bleeding spots, hemangioblastoma, erosion, ulcer or perforation in the nasal septum, and to see if there are foreign body, polyp and tumor in the nasal cavity.

鼻腔检查可按由下向上，由前向后，由内向外的次序进行。如果鼻黏膜肿胀，可用1%麻黄素喷雾或棉片收缩鼻腔黏膜后检查，以便看清鼻腔深处病变。注意黏膜颜色，有无充血、肿胀、肥厚、干燥和萎缩，有无溃疡、粘连；总鼻道有无增宽或狭窄；各鼻道有无分泌物及分泌物的量、色和性状；鼻中隔有无偏曲、出血点、血管扩张、糜烂、溃疡或穿孔；鼻腔有无异物、息肉及肿瘤等。

4 Posterior rhinoscopy

The examinee bends the head slightly to lean on the chair, with the body relaxed, and open the mouth and nose for respiration. After the posterior rhinoscope is slightly heated over the alcohol lamp, the inspector holds the tongue depressor with the left hand to press the anterior 2/3 tongue, and holds

4 后鼻镜检查法

被检者头略前倾靠椅，身体放松，张口用鼻呼吸。将后鼻镜镜面在酒精灯上略为加热后，检查者左手持压舌板，下压舌前2/3，右手持后鼻镜，镜面朝上置于软腭

the posterior rhinoscope with the right hand to put between the soft palate and posterior pharyngeal wall with the mirror upward, and to see the whole picture of the nasopharynx by adjusting the mirror leftward, rightward, anteriorly and posteriorly, including the backside of the soft palate, posterior nostril (including the posterior border of the nasal septum, posterior end of the inferior nasal concha and middle nasal concha), pharyngeal opening of the auditory tube, carina and pharyngeal recess, nasopharyngeal top and adenoid. If pharyngeal reflex is too sensitive, it is advisable to inspect after using 1% tetracaine or surface anesthesia. If the nasopharyn is difficult to expose, it is advisable to pull the soft palate via the mouth and nose by silicone tube. In the inspection, it is necessary to observe if the mucous membrane is congestive, coarse, bleeding, ulcerative, and if there are scabs, purulent fluid and neoformation in its surface.

和咽后壁之间，左右、前后调整镜面以窥清鼻咽全貌，包括软腭背面、后鼻孔（包括鼻中隔后缘、下鼻甲和中鼻甲后端等），咽鼓管咽口、圆枕及咽隐窝，鼻咽顶部和腺样体。如咽反射过于敏感，可用1%丁卡因表面麻醉后施检；如鼻咽显露困难，可用硅胶管经口鼻牵拉软腭。检查时注意黏膜有无充血、粗糙、出血、溃疡，表面有无痂皮、脓液，有无新生物等。

5 Inspection of paranasal sinus

5 鼻窦检查法

5.1 Visual inspection and palpation of nasal sinuses

5.1 鼻窦区视、触诊

It is advisable to observe if there are red tumefaction and tenderness in the buccal region, inner canthus and in the skin of the medial eyebrow, and if there are local hardness or protrusion by pressure, and to observe if there are migration and motor impairment of the eyeballs.

观察面颊部、内眦及眉根处皮肤有无红肿，压痛，按压局部有无硬性或弹性隆起，观察眼球有无移位及运动障碍。

5.2 Rhinoscopy

5.2 鼻镜检查

It is mainly advisable to observe if there are secretions (including purulent fluid, blood, etc) and polyp or neoformation in various nasal meatus, and if there are tumefaction and polyp in the turbinal

主要观察各鼻道有无异常分泌物（包括脓液、血液等）及息肉或新生物，鼻甲黏膜有无肿胀及息变。

mucosa.

5.3 Puncture and flushing of maxillary sinus

Used for diagnosis and treatment of the diseases of the maxillary sinus. It is necessary to pay attention to the quantity and quality of flushing fluid, and to send for cytological examination and bacterial culture if needed. Method: After surface anesthesia of the local mucosa, insert the puncture needle for maxillary sinus from the lateral wall of the inferior nasal meatus of the sick side, about 1.5 cm away from the anterior end of the interior nasal concha, toward the outer canthus into the maxillary sinus cavity to extract purulent fluid, and infuse physiological saline to flush the sinus cavity. Before the withdrawal of the needle, it is necessary to inject medication, such as Houttuynia injection.

5.3 上颌窦穿刺冲洗

用于上颌窦疾病的诊断与治疗。注意冲洗液的量和性质,必要时送细胞学检查和细菌培养等。方法:局部黏膜表面麻醉后,用上颌窦穿刺针,在患侧下鼻道外侧壁距下鼻甲前端约 1.5 厘米处进针,朝外眦方向刺入上颌窦腔,抽吸脓液,灌注生理盐水冲洗窦腔。拔针前可注入药物,如鱼腥草注射等。

6 Inspection of olfactory sensation

The patient is told to smell the different fluids (such as vinegar, soy sauce, sesame oil, alcohol, perfume, gasoline, etc) in the small bottles of different size and same color, for comparing the difference in the two sides. This method is used only to test if there is olfactory sensation. Besides, there are also the olfactory threshold test and olfactory evoked potential test.

6 嗅觉检查

让受检者分别嗅辨多个大小、色泽一致的小瓶内不同液体(如醋、酱油、麻油、酒精、香水、汽油等)的气味,比较两侧异同。此法只能测试有无嗅觉功能。此外还有嗅阈检查及嗅觉诱发电位检查方法。

7 Imageological inspection

Nasomental position (Water's position) mainly shows the maxillary sinus, and also enthmoidal sinus, frontal sinus, nasal cavity and orbit, and nasofrontal position (Caldwell's position) mainly shows the frontal sinus, enthmoidal sinus, and also maxillary sinus, nasal cavity and orbit, for understanding the size and shape of the sinus cavity and observing

7 影像学检查

鼻颏位(亦称华氏位)主要显示上颌窦,也可显示筛窦、额窦、鼻腔和眼眶;鼻额位(亦称柯氏位)主要显示额窦、筛窦,也可显示上颌窦、鼻腔和眼眶。可了解窦腔大小、形状、有无黏膜增厚、占

if there are thickened membrane, occupational lesion and bone destruction, etc.

位性病变和骨质破坏等。

Currently, computed tomography (CT) and magnetic resonance imaging (MRI) extensively used in clinics are used for showing the pathological lesions in the nasal cavity and nasal sinus, more clearly and precisely than the films.

目前临床广泛应用的计算机X线断层摄影术和磁共振成像用于显示鼻腔、鼻窦病变较平片更为清晰、准确。

Section 4 The commonly used examinations of the laryngopharynx

第4节 咽常用检查方法

1 Oropharyngeal inspection

1 口咽检查法

After the examinee takes a frontal sedentary position, in calm respiration, relaxation and opening the mouth, the inspector holds the tongue depressor and presses the tongue at the juncture of anterior 2/3 and posterior 1/3. For those with sensitive pharyngeal reflex, it is advisable to use 1% tetracaine spray for 1 or 2 times for surface anesthesia of mucous membrane.

受检者正坐,安静呼吸,放松,张口。检查者手持压舌板,下压舌前2/3和舌后1/3交界处。对咽反射敏感者,先用1%丁卡因喷雾黏膜表面麻醉1~2次。

It is necessary to observe carefully the shape of the throat, membrane color, size of the tonsil, and see if there are congestion, secretions, pseudomembrane, ulceration, neoformation, and mobility of the soft palate and anterior and posterior palate arch. If the anterior palate arch is pulled with a drawing hook, it is possible to see fine change in the tonsil clearly. By pressing the tongue with a tongue depressor, it is possible to observe if there is caseous stuff or purulent fluid in the tonsillar crypts.

注意观察口咽部形态,黏膜色泽,扁桃体大小,有无充血、分泌物、假膜、溃疡、新生物,软腭和前后腭弓活动情况。若用拉钩牵拉前腭弓,可看清扁桃体细微变化。用压舌板挤压舌腭弓,观察扁桃体隐窝内有无干酪样物或脓液溢出。

2 Inspection of nasopharynx

2.1 Nasopharyngscopy (posterior rhinoscopy).

2.2 Fiberoptic nasopharyngolaryngoscopy

It is an effective tool to check the nasopharyngeal part and throat. Via the nasal cavity, the flexible optical fiber can be inserted to clearly show the condition of the nasal cavity and nasopharynx. If further inserted into the laryngopharynx and laryngeal cavity, it is possible to observe the various parts of laryngopharynx and laryngeal cavity, and to draw material for biopsy, if needed. For those with sensitive pharyngeal reflex, it is advisable to inspect after using 1% tetracaine spray for 1 or 2 times for surface anesthesia of mucous membrane. Electric nasopharyngolaryngoscope is clearer in definition.

2.3 Nasopharyngeal digital inspection

Used for touching and detecting the size of adenoid and lockout of the posterior nostril in children. It is seldom used clinically, because of suffering.

3 Inspection of laryngeopharynx

Please see "indirect laryngoscopy".

4 Imageological inspection

Used for diagnosis of the diseases in the pharyngeal part, retropharyngeal space, cervical vertebras and mandible. Cervical lateral film, skull base film, mandibular film and styloid process film are beneficial to the detection of adenoidal hypertrophy, etc. CT and MRI inspection can clearly show the change in the pharyngeal soft tissues, beneficial to the early diagnosis of nasopharyngeal carcinoma or pterygopalatine fossa lesions, and to the show of tumor scope.

2 鼻咽检查法

2.1 鼻咽镜检查(见“后鼻镜检查”)。

2.2 纤维鼻咽喉镜检查

是检查鼻咽和喉部的有效工具。为可弯曲光导纤维,经鼻腔导入可清晰显示鼻腔和鼻咽情况,继续导入喉咽和喉腔,可观察喉咽各部及喉腔,必要时取材活检或照相。对咽反射敏感者,可用1%丁卡因喷雾黏膜表面麻醉1～2次后施行。电子鼻咽喉镜则清晰度更高。

2.3 鼻咽指诊

用于触探儿童腺样体大小及后鼻孔有无闭锁,有一定痛苦,临床已少用。

3 喉咽检查

见“间接喉镜检查”。

4 影像学检查

用于诊断咽部、咽后间隙、颈椎和下颌骨等处疾病。颈侧位片、颅底片、下颌骨片和茎突片,有助于发现腺样体肥大等。CT和MRI检查可清晰显示咽部软组织变化,有利于鼻咽癌或翼腭窝病变的早期诊断,显示肿瘤范围。

Section 5 The commonly used examinations of the larynx

第 5 节 喉常用检查方法

1 Observation and palpation of laryngeal part

It is supposed to observe the external shape, size, position and symmetry of the throat, and to palpate if there are tumefaction, pain and malformation in the throat, and if there are lymph node enlargement and subcutaneous emphysema in the neck, and to check the mobility and friction of the throat by slightly pressing and moving the laryngeal body with the thumb and index finger.

1 喉部望、触诊

观察喉外形、大小、位置和对称度。触诊喉部有无肿痛、畸形，颈部有无肿大淋巴结、皮下气肿；用拇指和食指轻按喉体并移动，检查喉活动度和摩擦感。

2 Indirect laryngoscopy

It is convenient, simple and mostly commonly used. After the examinee sits upright, uplifting the head slightly, opening the mouth and extending the tongue, the inspector pulls the anterior 1/3 tongue out of the mouth with the gauze-wrapped thumb and middle finger of the left hand, and pushes the upper lip with the index finger, and inserts the heated indirect laryngoscope into the mouth with the right hand, pushes the uvula upward and backward with the back of the scope, with the mirror facing forward and downward, to rotate the mirror leftward and rightward and adjusts the angle forward and backward, for observing the tongue root, epiglottis, epiglottic vallecula, laryngeal inlet, and pyriform sinus successively. If the epiglottis is raised when the patient makes "yee, yee" sound, it is possible to observe the laryngeal surface, aryepiglottic wall, ventricular bands, laryngeal ventricle, vocal

2 间接喉镜检查

简便易行，最常用。受检者正面端坐，头稍后仰，张口伸舌。检查者左手拇指和中指持纱布将舌前 1/3 部轻拉出口外，食指将上唇推开。右手持加温的间接喉镜，伸入口内，用镜背将悬雍垂推向后上方，镜面朝前下方。左右转动镜面、前后调整角度，依次观察舌根、会厌、会厌谷、喉入口、梨状窝等。受检者发“衣……衣……”音时会厌上举，可观察会厌喉面、杓会厌襞、室带、喉室、声带、声门下结构和气管环。咽反射敏感者，可用 1% 丁卡因行咽部黏膜表面麻醉后再检查。注意喉咽及喉部形态、

cords, subglottic structure and tracheal rings. For those with sensitive pharyngeal reflex, it is advisable to inspect after using 1% tetracaine spray for surface anesthesia of mucous membrane. It is necessary to observe the shape of the pharynx and larynx, colour of mucous membrane, and to see if there are secretions, congestion, hypertrophy, ulceration, scars, neoformation and foreign body, and necessary to pay attention to the mobile condition of the vocal cords and aryepiglottic cartilage.

黏膜色泽，有无分泌物、充血、增厚、溃疡、瘢痕、新生物和异物等，特别要留意声带和杓状软骨活动情况。

3 Direct laryngoscopy

The contents to be observed are similar to those in the indirect laryngoscopy. Because the direct laryngoscope is a hard tube, when it is inserted into the laryngeal cavity via the oral cavity, the head needs to be uplifted fully backward, to ensure the vision in a straight line. Therefore, it is very painful and seldom used at present. In addition to the inspection, it can also be used to take out foreign body, polyp and neoformation under the direct laryngoscope.

3 直接喉镜检查

观察内容同间接喉镜检查。由于直接喉镜系硬管，经口腔插入喉腔需头颈部充分后仰，使视觉成一直线，因而痛苦较大，现已少用。除用于检查，还可在直接喉镜下钳取喉部异物、息肉，新生物等。

4 Fiberoptic laryngoscopy

As same as"fiberoptic nasopharyngolaryngoscopy".

4 纤维喉镜检查

同“纤维鼻咽喉镜检查”。

5 Laryngeal electronic endoscopy

The laryngeal electric endoscope image system (including endoscope, tomography system, light source, monitor, video recorder, and printer) is as same as fiberoptic laryngoscopy in the indications and inspecting methods, and can be used to observe, photography and videotape the laryngeal lesions in details.

5 喉电子内镜检查

喉电子内镜影像系统（包括内镜、摄像系统、光源、监视器、录像机及打印机）适应症和检查方法同纤维喉镜，可对喉部病变详细观察、拍照或视频留存。

6 Imageological inspection

There are X-ray inspection, plain films, tomography, radiography, and CT scan, used for diagnosis of tumors and foreign body in the laryngeal part. CT and MRI inspections are more valuable for understanding the scope of tumors in the laryngeal part and lymphatic metastasis and can be selected for clinical use.

6 影像学检查

有透视、平片、体层摄片、造影和 CT 扫描等,用于喉部肿瘤、异物等的诊断。CT 和 MRI 检查对了解喉部肿瘤范围、有无淋巴结转移更有价值,临床可选择应用。

Chapter 3 Pattern Identifications of Otorhinolaryngological Diseases

第3章 耳鼻咽喉科疾病的辨证方法

Section 1 Pattern identifications of otological diseases

第1节 耳科疾病辨证法

The commonly seen clinical symptoms and signs of the otological diseases include ear pain, discharging ear, tinnitus, deafness, vertigo and abnormal tympanic membrane, etc.

耳病常见的临床症状和体征有：耳痛、耳流脓、耳鸣耳聋、眩晕及鼓膜异常等。

1 Identify patterns of ear pain

1 辨耳痛病证

Ear pain is a commonly seen symptom in the otological diseases. Its patterns are usually analyzed based upon the location, degree, time and accompanying symptoms of ear pain. Mild pain with short duration belongs to new disease, mostly caused by invasion of exogenous pathogenic wind, leading to obstruction of the ear. Slow pain tendency, with intermittent pain or alleviation of pain by pressure and long duration, is mostly caused by spleen deficiency or kidney deficiency, resulting in malnutrition in the meridians or obstruction of the ear by blood stasis. Severe pain is mostly caused by fire and heat in the liver and gallbladder, burning the ear

耳痛是耳病常见症状，辨证主要根据耳痛部位、程度、时间和伴随症状来分析。痛轻且病程短属新病，多因风邪外犯，壅滞耳窍；痛势较缓、时痛时止或痛而喜按且病程较长，则多为脾虚或肾虚，经脉失养或瘀血阻滞耳窍所致。痛重者，多因肝胆火热，上灼耳窍所致。

upward.

1.1 Mild ear pain in new disease, possibly accompanied by blockage sensation inside the ear, slight red colour in the tympanic membrane, and decreased hearing ability, is mostly induced by invasion of exogenous pathogenic wind and heat, and the pathogens are still in the exterior region. If the auricular problem lasts for long time, manifested by slight painful, discomfort or distending sensation inside the ear or accompanied by tinnitus and hearing loss, it is mostly identified as pattern of spleen qi deficiency plus accumulation of turbid dampness. The slight red and swelling auricle is mostly due to invasion of pathogens into the auricle, seen in the early stage of ear sores. If the auditory meatus is red and swelling, with pain aggravated by pulling the auricle or pressing the tragus, it is mostly identified as ear furuncle, ear sores. If the tympanic membrane is slightly red, it is mostly the early stage of ear tumefaction or otopyorrhea.

1.1 新病耳痛较轻,可伴有耳内阻塞感,耳膜微红,听力减退,多属风热外袭,邪尚在表。若耳病已久,则耳内微痛不适或有胀闷感,或兼耳鸣重听,多为肝肾不足或脾气虚弱,正不胜邪,邪留耳窍。若耳痛轻,有流脓、耳膜穿孔、听力下降,多为脾气虚兼湿浊停聚证。耳廓微红肿,多为耳廓受邪,见于断耳疮初起;若耳道红肿,牵拉耳廓或按压耳屏痛重,多为耳疖、耳疮;若鼓膜微红,多为耳胀或脓耳初起。

1.2 Serious ear pain, in deep position, manifested by throbbing pain or drilling pain, and accompanied by fever, is mostly caused by flaming of fire in the liver and gallbladder and accumulation and abundance of heat toxin, burning the ear and producing pus. Pain in the auricle is termed sore severing auricle, and in the styloid area behind the ear is termed retroauricular subperiosteal abscess. Pain by pulling the auricle or pressing the tragus is termed sore and furuncle of the auditory meatus, and in the tympanic membrane is termed otopyorrhea.

1.2 耳痛剧烈,部位深在,呈跳痛或钻痛,并有发热,多为肝胆火炽、热毒壅盛,灼耳酿脓之证。在耳廓为断耳疮;在耳后完骨为耳后骨膜下脓肿;牵拉耳廓或压迫耳屏作痛为耳道疮疖;在鼓膜为脓耳。

1.3 Serious ear pain, accompanied by remarkable headache, strong fever, vomiting, or dizziness and delirium, is identified as pattern of internal pene-

1.3 耳痛剧烈,伴有显著头痛、壮热、呕吐或神昏谵语,为火毒内攻、邪犯心包之重

tration of fire toxin and invasion of pathogens into the pericardium, i. e. deteriorated pattern of otopyorrhea.

证,即脓耳变证。

1.4 Traumatic injury, foreign body in the ear and insect bite can also cause ear pain.

1.4 外伤、异物入耳、虫伤亦可致耳疼痛。

2 Identify patterns of discharging ear

2 辨耳流脓病证

The patterns are identified based upon duration of suppuration, colour volume and smell of pus.

从流脓时间长短、脓液颜色及其质地、脓量和气味等方面进行辨证。

2.1 Acute onset with early suppuration is mostly excessive pattern. Slow onset with lingering suppuration is mostly deficient pattern.

2.1 起病急,流脓初起,多为实证;发病缓,流脓日久,多为虚证。

2.2 Ear pus in tenacious nature, yellow colour and large volume in new disease is mostly due to upward steaming of fire and heat from the liver and gallbladder. Pus accompanied by lots of bleeding is related to accumulation and abundance of heat toxin in the liver and gallbladder, damage of the blood phase. Pus in white or blue colour is mostly related to spleen deficiency. Filthy pus is mostly related to kidney deficiency.

2.2 新病耳脓稠黄量多,多为肝胆火热上蒸;脓伴血多为肝胆热毒壅盛,伤及血分;脓色白或色青多为脾虚;脓液污秽,多为肾虚。

2.3 Pus in large volume and tenacious nature is mostly due to excessive body and yang abundance, and upward steaming of dampness and heat. Pus in large volume but in thin and clear nature is mostly related to obstruction of dampness due to spleen deficiency. Stinky and filthy pus with bean dreg-like stuff is mostly regarded as pattern of coexistence of excess and deficiency, due to retention of dampness and heat and deconstruction of bone by deficiency of kidney qi. Pus with sudden decrease in volume, accompanied by headache, aversion to cold, high fever, is mostly a pattern of inward penetration of

2.3 脓量多而质稠,多属体实阳盛,湿热上蒸;脓量多而清稀,多为脾虚湿困;脓液臭秽,有豆渣样物,多为肾元亏虚,湿热滞留,蚀及骨质,属虚实夹杂之证。耳流脓量由多锐减,伴头痛、恶寒高热,多为脓毒内陷之证。

sepsis.

3 Identify patterns of tinnitus and deafness

3.1 Sudden tinnitus, with loud sound, hearing loss, is identified as excessive pattern, heat pattern due to ascension of fire and heat of the liver and gallbladder, or accumulation of phlegm and fire, disturbing the brain upward. Sudden deafness is mostly related to obstruction of the ear by pathogenic wind, heat and dampness.

3.2 Gradual tinnitus, with low sound like cicada, and gradual hearing loss, is mostly identified as deficient pattern of yin deficiency in the liver and kidney and upward flaming of deficient fire, or deficiency and exhaustion of qi and blood and malnutrition in the ear.

3.3 Tinnitus in high tone, with obvious decrease of high-frequency hearing ability, is mostly the pattern of deficiency of the liver and kidney or insufficiency of qi and blood. Tinnitus in low tone, with obvious decrease of low-frequency hearing ability, mostly belongs to heat abundance of the liver and gallbladder or invasion of exogenous pathogenic wind and blockage of ear by pathogens.

3.4 Gradual hearing loss with aging, without history of suppuration, is mostly caused by deficiency of the liver and kidney, insufficiency of qi and blood and malnutrition of the ear.

3.5 Embolism of earwax and foreign body in the ear would also cause tinnitus, deafness, and even sudden deafness.

4 Identify patterns of vertigo

4.1 Vertigo accompanied by unilateral or bilateral tinnitus, accompanied by headache, distending and

3 辨耳鸣耳聋病证

3.1 耳鸣暴发、声大、听力下降,为肝胆火热上逆,或痰火郁结上扰清窍之实证、热证。暴聋多为风、热、湿邪壅塞耳窍。

3.2 耳鸣渐发,鸣声细微如蝉,听力逐渐下降,多为肝肾阴虚、虚火上炎,或气血亏耗、耳失濡养所致的虚证。

3.3 耳鸣呈高音调,高频听力下降明显,多为肝肾虚损或气血不足之证;耳鸣呈低音调,低频听力下降明显,多属肝胆热盛,或风邪外袭,邪气壅滞耳窍之证。

3.4 年老听力渐退,无流脓史,多为肝肾亏损,气血不足,清窍失养所致。

3.5 耵聍栓塞、异物入耳亦可造成耳鸣、耳聋,甚至暴聋。

4 辨眩晕病证

4.1 眩晕伴单侧或双侧耳鸣,伴有头痛、耳胀闷感、面

stuffy sensation in the ear, flushed cheeks, red ears, bitter taste in the mouth, dry mouth, irritability and easy anger, is mostly identified as the pattern of hyperactivity of the liver yang.

红耳赤、口苦咽干、急躁易怒者,多为肝阳上亢之证。

4.2 Vertigo accompanied by heavy sensation in the head, distending sensation in the head, stuffy sensation in the chest, poor appetite, lassitude, serious nausea and vomiting, is mostly regarded as pattern of accumulation of turbid phlegm in the Middle Energizer.

4.2 眩晕伴头重、头胀、胸闷、纳呆倦怠、恶心呕吐较甚者,多属痰浊中阻之证。

4.3 Frequent vertigo, with tinnitus, poor hearing ability, stuffy and distending sensation in the ear, palpitation, shortness of breath, lassitude, occurring or aggravated after fatigue, and body position change, is mostly regarded as the pattern of insufficiency of qi and blood.

4.3 经常眩晕耳鸣,听力差,耳闷胀,心悸,气短,乏力,劳作、体位改变后发生或加重,多属气血不足之证。

4.4 Vertigo, accompanied by discharging ear, is mostly regarded as a deteriorated pattern of otopyorrhea. Vertigo at the beginning of disease, with yellow pus, serious ear pain, is mostly induced by fire and heat in the liver and gallbladder, steaming and burning the ear. Vertigo in long-term illness, with thin and clear pus, is related to retention of dampness due to spleen deficiency. Intermittent vertigo, accompanied by dark spots in vision, and tinnitus, hearing loss, declining memory, and soreness and weakness in the low back and knee, is a pattern of deficiency of kidney essence.

4.4 眩晕伴有耳流脓,多系脓耳变证。初病眩晕,脓黄,耳剧痛,多为肝胆火热蒸灼耳窍;久病眩晕,脓清稀,多为脾虚湿困。时有眩晕,眼前有黑花,并有耳鸣、听力下降、记忆力减退、腰膝酸软,为肾精亏损之证。

5 Identify patterns of abnormal tympanic membrane

5 辨鼓膜异常病证

Abnormal tympanic membrane is mainly manifested by change in the shape and colour and tympanic membrane perforation, etc.

鼓膜异常主要表现为形态、色泽变化及鼓膜穿孔等。

5.1 Slight red tympanic membrane, with clear blood vessel, distension and pain in the ear, is mostly identified as early pattern of ear distension or ear pus due to invasion of exogenous pathogenic wind and heat.

5.2 Fresh red tympanic membrane, with diffuse congestion, and serious ear pain, is mostly ear pus due to fire and heat of the liver and gallbladder, steaming the ear. Convex of tympanic membrane, with small yellow bright spots, is mostly abundance of fire and heat in pus ear, eroding the tympanic membrane and producing the decay into pus. If the tympanic membrane is red in color, with blood blisters, and serious ear pain, it is regarded as bullous myringitis caused by fire and heat of the liver and gallbladder, flaming the ear.

5.3 The tympanic membrane in reddish orange color, with convex, dialysate or air bubble, is diagnosed as tympanic cavity effusion due to accumulation of turbid dampness. The tympanic membrane in blue, with convex, is mostly a pattern of accumulation of blood stasis in the ear.

5.4 Thickened or atrophic tympanic membrane, with calcium plaque, grey, and turbid and lustrousless nature, is mostly blocked ear or long-term ear pus due to insufficiency of qi and blood and malnutrition of the tympanic membrane.

5.5 Tympanic membrane perforation, in round or elliptic shape in the tense part, and smooth perforation border, is mostly induced by invasion of pathogenic wind, heat and dampness into the liver, gallbladder, spleen and lung, attacking the ear. If perforation occurs in the flaccid part or at the border, with cholesteatoma formation, it is mostly caused

5.1 鼓膜微红，血络显露，耳胀痛，多为风热外袭所致的耳胀或脓耳初起之证。

5.2 鼓膜鲜红，弥漫性充血，耳剧痛，多为肝胆火热上蒸耳窍之脓耳；若鼓膜外凸，有小黄亮点，为脓耳火热炽盛，腐蚀鼓膜，化腐酿脓；若鼓膜红赤有血泡，耳痛剧烈，为肝胆火热、燔灼耳窍所致的大疱性鼓膜炎。

5.3 鼓膜呈橘红色、外凸，透出液平或有气泡，为湿浊内聚所致之鼓室积液；鼓膜色蓝、外凸，多为瘀血内聚耳窍之证。

5.4 鼓膜增厚或萎缩，有钙斑，色灰白，浑浊少泽，多为气血不足，鼓膜失养所致的耳闭或脓耳久病者。

5.5 脓耳穿孔，若在紧张部呈圆形、椭圆形，穿孔边缘光滑，常为肝、胆、脾、肺等脏腑受风、热、湿邪侵袭，上犯耳窍所致；若在松弛部或边缘性穿孔，常有胆脂瘤形成，多为肾、脾虚损，邪毒蕴结，腐

by deficiency of kidney and spleen and accumulation of pathogens, eroding the muscles and bones. Acute onset of pus ear, with small perforation of the tympanic membrane, mostly belongs to excessive pattern and heat pattern. Long-term ear pus, with large perforation, mostly belongs to deficient pattern or pattern with coexistence of deficiency and excess.

肌蚀骨而成。脓耳急发，鼓膜穿孔较小，多属实证、热证；脓耳日久，穿孔较大。多属虚证或虚实夹杂之证。

Section 2 Pattern identifications of rhinologic diseases

第2节 鼻科疾病辨证法

The commonly seen clinical symptoms and signs of the rhinologic diseases include nasal obstruction, nasal discharge, sneezing, epistaxis, abnormal nasal concha, olfactory dysfunction and headache, etc.

鼻病常见的临床症状和体征有：鼻塞、流涕、喷嚏、鼻衄、鼻甲异常、嗅觉障碍及头痛等。

1 Identify nasal obstruction and abnormal nasal concha

1 辨鼻塞、鼻甲异常

1.1 Nasal obstruction in the initial stage, red tumefaction in the nasal membrane, aversion to wind, and fever, is mostly caused by invasion of pathogenic wind and heat into the exterior. Nasal membrane in light red tumefaction, with aversion to wind, and fever, is mostly pattern of nasal obstruction due to invasion of exogenous wind and cold.

1.1 鼻塞初起，鼻黏膜红肿，恶风发热，多为风热邪毒犯表；若鼻黏膜淡红肿胀，恶寒发热，为风寒外邪侵袭之伤风鼻塞。

1.2 Severe nasal obstruction, with red tumefaction of the nasal mucous membrane, profuse yellow and tenacious sputum, and serious headache, is mostly regarded as nasal sinusitis due to fire and heat in the lung, gallbladder, spleen and stomach, steaming the nose upward.

1.2 鼻塞重，鼻黏膜色红肿胀，涕黄稠多，头痛较剧，多为肺、胆、脾胃火热上蒸鼻窍之鼻渊。

1.3 Long-term nasal obstruction, mild-to-severe symptoms or in alternation, with slight red nasal mucous membrane, tumefaction, smoothness and softness of the inferior nasal concha (or middle nasal concha), belongs to qi deficiency in the lung and spleen, and retention of pathogens in the nose. Continuous nasal obstruction, with strong nasal breathing, dark red in the nasal mucous membrane, hypertrophic, hard and uneven interior nasal concha, is mostly regarded as chronic rhinitis caused by long-term retention of pathogenic factors and obstruction of qi and blood stasis in the nose.

1.3 鼻塞日久，时轻时重或交替，鼻黏膜淡红，下鼻甲（或伴中鼻甲）肿胀、光滑、柔软，为肺脾气虚，邪滞鼻窍；若鼻塞持续，鼻音重，鼻黏膜暗红，下鼻甲肥大、质硬、凹凸不平，多为邪毒久留，气血瘀阻鼻窍之鼻窒。

1.4 Paroxysmal nasal obstruction, with nasal itching, frequent sneezing, clear nasal discharge, pale and edematous inferior nasal concha (or mmiddle nasal concha), is diagnosed as allergic rhinitis due to deficiency of the lung, spleen and kidney, and accumulation of pathogenic cold.

1.4 阵发性鼻塞、鼻痒、喷嚏频作，涕清稀，下鼻甲（或伴中鼻甲）苍白、水肿，为肺、脾、肾虚，寒邪凝聚之鼻鼽。

1.5 Nasal obstruction, with dry and even atrophic and scabby nasal mucous membrane, is mostly regarded as allergic rhinitis due to invasion of pathogenic dryness into the lung, and malnutrition of the nose, or yin deficiency of the lung and kidney, deficiency of spleen qi, and malnutrition of the nose.

1.5 鼻塞，鼻黏膜干燥甚至萎缩，结痂，多为燥邪犯肺，鼻窍失养，或肺肾阴虚，脾气虚弱，鼻失滋养之鼻槁。

2 Identify nasal discharge

2 辨鼻涕

2.1 Clear and thin nasal discharge is mostly seen in allergic rhinitis due to cold, or deficiency of the lung, spleen and kidney.

2.1 鼻涕清稀者，多见于伤风，或肺、脾、肾虚所致之鼻鼽。

2.2 Thick and tenacious nasal discharge, with white due to dampness, or yellow due to heat, is often seen in chronic rhinitis and nasal sinusitis.

2.2 鼻涕浓稠者，色白属湿，色黄属热，常见于鼻窒、鼻渊。

2.3 Yellow and green nasal discharge in long-term illness, or dryness and scab inside the nose, is most-

2.3 久病涕黄绿，或鼻内干燥结痂，多为肺脾气阴两虚，

ly related to allergic rhinitis due to deficiency of qi and yin in the lung and spleen.

见于鼻槁。

3 Identify olfactory dysfunction

3 辨嗅觉异常

3.1 Anosmia in the beginning of illness, accompanied by nasal obstruction, and red and swelling nasal concha, is caused by accumulation of pathogenic wind and heat in the nose. Pale nasal mucous membrane is induced by invasion of wind and cold.

3.1 初病失嗅，伴鼻塞，鼻甲赤肿，为风热邪毒壅塞鼻窍；鼻膜淡白为受风寒。

3.2 Anosmia in long-term illness, with clear and thin nasal discharge, pale and slight tumefaction in the nasal mucous membrane, is mostly allergic rhinitis.

3.2 久病失嗅，鼻涕清稀，鼻膜淡肿，多为鼻鼽。

3.3 Anosmia, with dry nasal mucous membrane, and atrophic nasal concha, is related to yin deficiency in the lung and kidney or spleen qi deficiency and is seen in atrophic rhinitis.

3.3 失嗅，鼻膜干枯，鼻甲萎缩，为肺肾阴虚或脾气虚弱，见于鼻槁。

3.4 Gradual subsidence of olfactory sensation, with obstruction of lump inside the nose, is mostly related to retention of phlegm and blood stasis in the meridians and is seen in nasal polyp and nasal tumors.

3.4 嗅觉渐退，鼻内肿物堵塞，多为痰凝血瘀，脉络受阻，见于鼻息肉、鼻腔肿瘤等。

4 Identify headache

4 辨头痛

Headache is one of the commonly seen symptoms in the nasal diseases. It is necessary to pay attention to its location, urgency, time and accompanying symptoms.

头痛是鼻病常见症状之一，应注意头痛部位、痛势急缓、时间及其伴随症状。

4.1 Initial headache, accompanied by nasal obstruction, running nose, and sneezing, is mostly related to invasion of pathogenic wind into the nose.

4.1 头痛初起，伴鼻塞、流涕、喷嚏，多为风邪犯鼻。

4.2 Serious headache, in the frontal, occipital or vertex region, in certain time, accompanied by yellow, turbid and purulent nasal discharge in large volume, red and swollen middle and inferior nasal

4.2 头痛剧烈，多在前额、枕后或头顶，有一定时间规律，伴黄浊脓涕，量多，中、下鼻甲肿赤，多为肺、胆、脾胃

concha, is mostly regarded as nasal sinusitis due to upward flaming of abundant heat from the lung, gallbladder, spleen and stomach.

热盛上灼所致之鼻渊。

4.3 Long-term nasal problem, with serious headache and dizziness, tenacious nasal discharge, and pale colour in the nasal mucous membrane, is mostly related to qi deficiency in the lung and spleen, and upward attack of turbid dampness.

4.3 鼻病日久，头痛昏重，涕黏，鼻黏膜色淡，多为肺、脾气虚，湿浊上犯。

4.4 If nasal carbuncle induces red puffiness and pain in the face, high fever and headache, it is regarded as carbuncle complicated by septisemia, due to violence of pathogenic fire toxin.

4.4 若鼻疔引发颜面红肿疼痛、高热头痛，为火毒势猛，为疔疮走黄。

4.5 Headache, accompanied by dryness inside the nose, and broadened nasal cavity, is mostly regarded as atrophic rhinitis by yin deficiency or pathogenic dryness.

4.5 头痛，伴鼻内干燥，鼻腔宽大，多属阴虚或燥邪为患之鼻槁。

Section 3 Pattern identifications of laryngopharyngeal diseases

第3节 咽喉科疾病辨证法

1 Identify red tumefaction

Red tumefaction and pain are the commonly seen clinical manifestations in the laryngopharyngeal diseases, and their severity and urgency are closely related to pattern identification.

1 辨红肿疼痛

红肿疼痛是咽喉疾病常见临床表现，其轻重缓急与辨证密切相关。

1.1 Initial sore and swollen throat is mostly caused by invasion of pathogenic wind and heat, and accumulation of pathogens in the lung. The symptom with slight red, slight swollen and sore throat mostly belongs to exterior pattern of wind and cold.

1.1 初起咽喉红肿疼痛，多为风热外袭，邪在肺卫；若咽喉淡红、微肿而痛，多属风寒表证。

1.2 Serious sore throat, with serious swelling, red

1.2 咽喉疼痛较剧，红肿较

swollen and protruded follicles in the bottom of the throat, or red swollen vocal cords, is mostly related to abundance of heat in the lung and stomach.

甚，喉底滤泡红肿突起，或喉核红肿，或声带红肿，多为肺胃热盛。

1.3 Acute onset, serous sore throat, red swollen mucous membrane of the throat, in deep red color, are related to the abundant accumulation of heat toxin in the lung and stomach, even turning the decay into carbuncle.

1.3 起病急，咽喉疼痛剧烈，咽喉黏膜红肿，色深红，为肺胃热毒壅盛，甚则将化腐成痈。

1.4 Long-term laryngeal problem, with slight red color, slight swelling and slight pain, is mostly deficient pattern. Slight sore throat, dry heat sensation, protrusion of follicles like shade beads in the bottom of the throat, in wet red color, or white dots on the throat nodes, in wet red colour in the front and back, or slight red and swollen vocal cords are mostly due to upward flaming of fire due to yin deficiency.

1.4 咽喉病日久，微红、微肿、微痛，多为虚证；若咽部微痛、干热，喉底滤泡如帘珠状突起，潮红，或喉核有白点、前后潮红；或见声带微红而肿，多为阴虚上火。

2 Identify dry itching and foreign body sensation

2 辨咽干痒、异物感

2.1 Initial dry and sore throat, with burning sensation, itching sensation in the throat, and swollen throat, is mostly due to invasion of exogenous wind and heat.

2.1 初病咽干痛、灼热，咽痒咳嗽，咽部红肿，多为风热外袭。

2.2 Long-term dry throat, with itching sensation, choking sensation, dry cough, scanty sputum, is mostly related to yin deficiency of the lung and kidney, and upward flaming of deficient fire.

2.2 久病咽干、痒感，哽哽不利，干咳少痰，多为肺肾阴虚，虚火上炎。

2.3 Long-term choking sensation in the throat, with gluing sensation of sputum, bland taste in the mouth, no thirst, stuffy sensation in the chest, and nausea, is mostly related to accumulation of dampness due to spleen deficiency. Sensation of foreign body in the throat, tenacious sputum, difficult to

2.3 久病咽喉哽哽，痰黏着感，口淡不渴，胸闷恶心，多为脾虚湿困；若咽喉堵塞异物感，痰粘难咯，喉底颗粒增多暗红，喉核肥大质韧，声带暗红或有小结，多为痰瘀搏

cough up, increased dark red granules in the bottom of the throat, hypertrophic and tough throat nodes, dark red colour or small nodes in the vocal cords are mostly related to the accumulation of phlegm and blood stasis in the throat.

结咽喉。

2.4 Sensation of foreign body in the throat, such as globus hystericus, without problems in food ingestion, accompanied by depression and doubtfulness, vexation and anger, is mostly related to liver qi stagnation and obstruction of phlegm and qi.

2.4 咽喉异物感,如梅核阻塞,饮食无碍,伴抑郁多疑、心烦郁怒者,多为肝郁气滞、痰气交阻。

2.5 Tumors in the throat should be considered while there are obstruction in the throat, difficulties in digestion and respiration.

2.5 咽喉梗阻,饮食难下,影响呼吸,当虑咽喉、食管肿瘤。

3 Identify abnormal voice

3 辨声音异常

3.1 Acute onset, sore and swollen throat, and inarticulate speech, like an object in the mouth, is mostly diagnosed as throat carbuncle due to the accumulation of abundant pathogens and heat in the lung and stomach.

3.1 病急初起,咽喉肿痛,言语不清,口中如含物,多为肺胃邪热壅盛之咽喉痈症。

3.2 Sudden low voice at the beginning of illness, even with hoarse voice, accompanied by sore throat, red and swollen vocal cords, is related to invasion of wind and heat into the lung. Fresh red and swollen vocal cords and yellow sticking sputum are related to the accumulation of phlegm and heat in the lung.

3.2 初病卒然声音不扬,甚则声嘶,伴喉痛,声带红肿,为风热犯肺;若声带鲜红肿胀,上有黏痰泛黄,为痰热壅肺。

3.3 Long-term hoarse voice, dry and slight sore throat, or itching sensation and dry cough, worse in the afternoon, tenacious and scanty sputum are mostly related to yin deficiency in the lung and kidney, and upward flaming of deficient fire. Hoarse and low voice, disability in speaking for long time, hypertrophic vocal cords or with polyp and nodes

3.3 声嘶日久,咽喉干涩微痛,或喉痒干咳,午后尤甚,痰粘而少,多为肺肾阴虚,虚火上炎;若声嘶低沉,讲话不能持久,声带肥厚或有息肉、小结,多为气滞血瘀痰凝;若声嘶音低,讲话费力,伴气短

are mostly due to qi stagnation, blood stasis and accumulation of phlegm. Low and hoarse voice, difficulty in speaking, accompanied by shortness of breath, lassitude, flaccid vocal cords with difficult opening and closure, are mostly deficient pattern, mostly qi deficiency in the lung and spleen.

乏力,声带松弛,闭合欠佳,多为虚证,以肺脾气虚居多。

3.4 Sudden aphasia, normal sound of cough and normal vocal cords are mostly related to internal injury of seven emotional factors, and liver qi stagnation.

3.4 突然失音,咳嗽声如常,声带无异常,多为七情所伤,肝郁气滞。

4 Identify critical conditions of laryngopharyngeal diseases

4 辨咽喉病危候

Inspiratory dyspnea and wheezing present in the laryngopharyngeal diseases, accompanied by red, swollen and sore throat, profuse sputum and saliva, difficult speaking, difficult food intake mostly belong to critical signs and even would lead to death from suffocation in severe condition.

咽喉病证出现吸气性呼吸困难,喘鸣,伴有咽喉红肿疼痛、痰涎壅盛、语言不利、汤水难下等症,多属危候,严重者可窒息死亡。

Chapter 4 Chinese Medical Therapies for otorhinolaryngological diseases

第4章 耳鼻咽喉科疾病中医治法

Section 1 The commonly used internal therapies for otorhinolaryngological diseases

第1节 耳鼻咽喉科疾病常用内治法

The therapeutic principles and therapeutic methods should be drafted from the holistic concept, by following the four diagnostic methods and eight principles, and based upon the integration of local pattern identification and general pattern identification. Additionally, the ear, nose and throat are understood as the clear and hollow apertures, and the pathogens, turbid phlegm, stagnant blood and qi stagnation would usually block those clear and hollow apertures. Therefore, the therapeutic methods to dredge the apertures, dissolve phlegm, expel blood stasis, and soothe the liver and remove stagnation, based upon the routine therapeutic principles.

从整体观出发，遵循四诊八纲，局部辨证与全身辨证相结合，拟定治则与治法。同时耳鼻咽喉为清空之窍，邪毒、痰浊、瘀血、气郁均可闭塞清窍，故在常规治则基础上还需配合通窍、化痰、祛瘀、疏肝解郁等方法。

1 Method to dredge the aperture

The herbal drugs in light and clear nature, in

1 通窍法

运用具有轻清、辛散、芳

spicy and dispersing nature, aromatic nature and migrating effect are used to treat the diseases due to blockage of the clear apertures, for the purpose to expel the pathogens, smoothen qi dynamics, and remove stagnation, so as to dredge and benefit the clear apertures.

香、走窜功效的药物，治疗清窍闭塞性疾病，以透邪外出、舒畅气机、清除壅滞，从而通利清窍。常用的通窍法如下。

1.1 Dredge the aperture by aromatic herbal drugs

The herbal drugs in light and aromatic nature are used to expel the pathogens and disperse the accumulation and reopen the blocked aperture, usually for treating stuffy sensation in the ear, deafness, or nasal obstruction and hyposmia caused by the accumulation of abundant pathogens in the clear aperture. The commonly used herbal drugs include *Fructus Xanthii* (Cang Er Zi), *Flos Magnoliae Liliflorae* (Xin Yi Hua), *Radix Angelicae Dahuricae* (Bai Zhi), *Rhizoma Acori Graminei* (Shi Chang Pu), *Rhizoma Ligustici Chuanxiong* (Chuan Xiong), *Herba Asari* (Xi Xin), and *Herba Menthae* (Bo He), etc.

1.1 芳香通窍

选用轻清芳香之药物祛邪散壅，宣通闭塞之孔窍。常用于邪毒壅滞清窍引起的耳闷塞、耳聋，或鼻塞、嗅觉减退等。常选用苍耳子、辛夷花、白芷、石菖蒲、川芎、细辛、薄荷等。

1.2 Dissolve the turbid and dredge the aperture

The herbal drugs in aromatic nature and dissolving the turbid are selected to disperse and dissolve dampness and turbidity, and normalize qi dynamics and are often used for lingering discharging ear, lingering turbid nasal discharge, vertigo, vomiting and nausea caused by the accumulation of dampness and turbidity in the Middle Energizer, attacking the clear aperture upward. The commonly used herbal drugs include *Herba Agastachis* (Huo Xiang), *Herba Eupatorii* (Pei Lan), *Cortex Magnoliae Officinalis* (Hou Pu), *Fructus Amomi* (Sha Ren), *Pericarpium Citri Tangerinae* (Chen Pi), *Semen Amomi*

1.2 化浊通窍

选用芳香化浊之药物宣化湿浊、舒畅气机。常用于湿浊内阻中焦，上犯清窍引起的耳流脓缠绵难愈、鼻流浊涕不止、眩晕呕恶等。常选用藿香、佩兰、厚朴、砂仁、陈皮、白豆蔻、草豆蔻等。

Cardamomi (Bai Dou Kou), and *Semen Alpiniae Katsumadai* (Cao Dou Kou), etc.

1.3 Remove dampness and dredge the aperture

The herbal drugs to strengthen the spleen, promote diuresis and secrete dampness are selected to remove dampness and dredge the aperture and are often used for exudates in the auditory canal, tympanic cavity effusion, purulent discharge in the ear, lingering nasal discharge, vertigo, vomiting and nausea caused by retention of water and dampness in the clear aperture. The commonly used herbal drugs include *Sclerotium Poria* (Fu Ling), *Rhizoma Alismatis* (Ze Xie), *Semen Coicis* (Yi Yi Ren), *Semen Plantaginis* (Che Qian Zi), *Polyporus Umbellatus* (Zhu Ling), etc.

1.3 利湿通窍

选用健脾利水渗湿之药物利湿通窍。常用于水湿停聚清窍引起的耳道渗液、鼓室积液、耳内流脓、鼻涕长流难止及眩晕呕恶等。常选用茯苓、泽泻、薏苡仁、车前子、猪苓等。

1.4 Raise yang and dredge the aperture

The herbal drugs to raise the clear, dissipate the pathogens and dredge the aperture are selected to raise yang and dissipate the pathogens and are often used for lingering distending and stuffy sensation in the ear, progressive deafness, lingering nasal obstruction, or lingering nasal discharge, and frequent sneezing, caused by retention of exogenous pathogens due to qi deficiency in the lung and spleen, and accumulation of the turbid in the clear aperture. The commonly used herbal drugs include *Radix Bupleuri* (Chai Hu), *Rhizoma Cimicifugae* (Sheng Ma), and *Radix Puerariae* (Ge Gen), etc.

1.4 升阳通窍

选用升清透邪通窍之药物升举阳气、托邪外出。常用于肺脾气虚、清阳不升外邪滞留、浊阴上干清窍引起的耳内胀闷日久不愈、耳聋渐重、鼻窍窒塞日久，或流涕难止、喷嚏频作等。常选用柴胡、升麻、葛根等。

2 Method to expel phlegm

The herbal drugs to dissolve phlegm are selected to treat diseases and patterns due to the accumulation of phlegm and turbidity in the clear aperture, such as auditory vertigo, distending and stuffy sen-

2 祛痰法

选用具有化痰作用的药物，治疗痰浊困结清窍之病证，如耳眩晕、耳胀耳闭、喉痹、喉瘖、痰包及肿瘤等。常

sation in the ear, sore throat, aphonia, phlegmatic nodule and tumor, etc. The commonly used herbal drugs to expel phlegm include *Rhizoma Pinelliae* (Ban Xia), *Rhizoma Arisaematis* (Tian Nan Xing), *Rhizoma Typhonii Gigantei* (Bai Fu Zi), and *Semen Sinapis Albae* (Bai Jie Zi) for warming and dissolving cold phlegm, and *Bulbus Fritillariae Cirrhosae* (Chuan Bei Mu), *Semen Trichosanthis* (Gua Lou Ren), *Radix Peucedani* (Qian Hu), *Caulis Bambusae in Taeniam* (Zhu Ru), *Concretio Siliceae Bambusae* (Tian Zhu Huang), and *Radix Ranunculus Ternati* (Mao Zhua Cao) for clearing away heat and dissolving phlegm, and *Rhizoma Pinelliae* (Ban Xia), *Pericarpium Citri Tangerinae* (Chen Pi), *Sclerotium Poria* (Fu Ling), and *Radix Glycyrrhizae Praeparata* (Zhi Gan Cao) for drying up dampness and dissolving phlegm, and *Herba Siegesbeckiae* (Xi Xian Cao), and *Bombyx Batryticatus* (Bai Jiang Can) for expelling wind and dissolving phlegm, etc.

用祛痰药有温化寒痰的半夏、天南星、白附子、白芥子等；清热化痰的贝母、瓜蒌仁、前胡、竹茹、天竺黄、猫爪草等；燥湿化痰的半夏、陈皮、茯苓、炙甘草等；祛风化痰的豨莶草、白僵蚕等。

3　Method to expel blood stasis

The herbal drugs to dredge the blood vessels and expel blood stasis are selected to treat diseases and patterns caused by poor blood circulation, qi stagnation and blood stasis or retention of phlegm and blood stasis in the clear aperture, such as traumatic injury, tumor, tinnitus, deafness, chronic rhinitis, acute tonsillitis, pharyngitis, aphonia, etc. The commonly used herbal drugs include *Rhizoma Ligustici Chuanxiong* (Chuan Xiong), *Radix Salviae Miltiorrhizae* (Dan Shen), *Herba Lycopi* (Ze Lan), *Semen Vaccariae* (Wang Bu Liu Xing), *Radix Ilex pubescens* (Mao Dong Qing), *Semen Persicae* (Tao Ren), *Flos Carthami* (Hong Hua), *Radix Curcumae* (Yu

3　祛瘀法

选用具有通血脉、祛瘀滞作用的药物，治疗血行不畅、气滞血瘀或痰瘀互结清窍之病证，如外伤、肿瘤、耳鸣耳聋、鼻窒、乳蛾、喉痹、喉瘖等。常选用川芎、丹参、泽兰、王不留行、毛冬青、桃仁、红花、郁金、五灵脂等。

Jin), and *Faeces Trogopterorum* (Wu Ling Zhi), etc.

4 Method to ease up the voice

The herbal drugs to benefit the throat and ease up the voice are selected to treat hoarse voice. The commonly used herbal drugs include *Herba Menthae* (Bo He), *Periostracum Cicadae* (Chan Tui), *Radix Platycodi* (Jie Geng), *Rhizoma Belamecandae* (She Gan), *Lasiosphaera Seu Calvatia* (Ma Bo), *Semen Sterculiae Lychnophorae* (Pang Da Hai), *Semen Oroxyli* (Mu Hu Die), *Radix Curcumae* (Yu Jin), and *Fructus Terminaliae Chebulae* (He Zi), etc.

4 开音法

选用具有利喉开音作用的药物治疗声嘶之证。常选用薄荷、蝉蜕、桔梗、射干、马勃、胖大海、木蝴蝶、郁金、诃子等。

5 Method to eliminate carbuncle and discharge pus

It is used to treat carbuncle, sores, and furuncles.

5 消痈排脓法

用于治疗痈疮疖肿。

5.1 Clear away heat, resolve toxin and eliminate carbuncle

The herbal drugs to clear away the internal heat are selected to treat diseases and patterns caused by the abundant accumulation of pathogenic fire and heat, steaming the clear aperture upward, such as red tumefaction in the auditory canal, congestion in the tympanic membrane, red tumefaction and pain in the nose and throat. The commonly used herbal formulas include *Five Ingredients Detoxifying Drink* (Wu Wei Xiao Du Yin), *Coptis Detoxifying Decoction* (Huang Lian Jie Du Tang), etc.

5.1 清热解毒消痈

选用具有清解里热作用的药物,治疗火热邪毒壅盛、上蒸清窍之病证,如耳道红肿、鼓膜充血、鼻窍与咽喉红肿疼痛等。常用方如五味消毒饮、黄连解毒汤等。

5.2 Disperse blood stasis and discharge pus

The herbal drugs to clear away heat, resolve toxin, activate blood, disperse blood stasis, discharge pus and erupt the hardness are selected to treat diseases and patterns caused by the accumula-

5.2 散瘀排脓

选用具有清热解毒、活血祛瘀、透脓溃坚作用的药物,治疗热毒壅聚、气滞血瘀之病证,如鼻疔、耳疖、咽喉

tion of heat toxin, qi stagnation and blood stasis, such as nasal furuncle, auricular furuncle, and carbuncle in the throat, etc. The commonly used herbal formulas include *Fairy Formula Life-Saving Decoction* (Xian Fang Huo Ming Yin), and *Four-Agents Brave and Peaceful Decoction* (Si Miao Yong An Tang), etc.

痈等。常用方如仙方活命饮、四妙勇安汤等。

5.3 Expel toxin and discharge pus

The herbal drugs to expel the pathogens, resolve toxin, nourish blood and reinforce qi are selected to treat diseases and pattern caused by insufficiency of qi and blood, retention of pathogenic toxin, and lingering suppuration, such as pus ear, nasal sinusitis, etc.

5.3 托毒排脓

选用具有祛邪解毒、养血补气作用的药物，治疗气血不足、邪毒滞留、流脓经久不愈之病证，如脓耳、鼻渊等。

6 Method to soothe the liver and remove stagnation

The herbal drugs to circulate qi, dissolve phlegm, soothe the liver and remove stagnation are selected to treat diseases and patterns caused by liver qi stagnation, coagulation of phlegm by qi stagnation, such as obstructive sensation in the throat, difficult to throw up and swallow down, stuffy sensation in the chest, etc. The commonly used herbal drugs include *Rhizoma Pinelliae* (Ban Xia), *Cortex Magnoliae Officinalis* (Hou Pu), and *Radix Curcumae* (Yu Jin), etc.

6 疏肝解郁法

选用具有行气、化痰、疏肝解郁作用的药物，治疗肝气郁结、气滞痰凝之病证，如咽喉哽哽不利，吐之不出，咽之不下，胸中痞闷等。常选用半夏、厚朴、郁金等。

Section 2 The commonly used external therapies for otorhinolaryngological diseases

第2节 耳鼻咽喉科疾病常用外治法

1 The commonly used external therapies in the otology

1 耳科常用外治法

1.1 Cleaning method

Physiological saline, 3% hydrogen peroxide solution or herbal decoction are used to rinse pus and scabs inside and outside the external auditory canal, in order for convenient observation, mostly used for pus ear, ear sores, ear eczema, auricular fistula, etc.

1.1 清洁法

用生理盐水、3%双氧水或中药煎水清洗外耳道内外脓液、结痂等，以利清洁后便于观察。多用于脓耳、耳疮、旋耳疮、耳瘘等。

1.2 Ear dropping method

After the ear faces upward and is pulled lightly, ear drops (3 to 5 drops) are dripped into the external auditory canal, mostly used for ear pain, and pus ear.

1.2 滴耳法

患耳朝上，轻拉耳廓，将滴耳液(3～5滴)滴入外耳道内，多用于耳痛、脓耳者。

1.3 Insufflating method

Some herbal powder with the effects to clear away heat, resolve toxin, promote astringency, stop pain, dissipate the decay and promote granulation is blown to the sick area of the external ear or into the auditory canal. The dose should be proper, in order to avoid accumulating herbal powder and hindering pus drainage.

1.3 吹药法

将少许具有清热解毒、收敛止痛、祛腐生肌作用的药粉吹入外耳患处或耳道内。用量不宜过多，以免药粉积聚，妨碍脓液引流。

1.4 Smearing method

The herbal ointment or paste with the effects to clear away heat, resolve toxin, stop inflammation and alleviate pain is smeared on the auricle or sick area of the auditory canal. *Coptis Detoxifying*

1.4 涂敷法

将具有清热解毒、消炎止痛的中药膏或糊剂涂敷于耳廓或耳道患处。常选用黄连解毒膏、青黛散或紫金锭

Ointment (Huang Lian Jie Du Gao), *Indigo Powder* (Qing Dai San) or *Purple Gold Ingot* (Zi Jin Ding) are often used for ear eczema, ear furuncle, and ear sores, etc.

等,用于旋耳疮、耳疖、耳疮等病证。

1.5 Inflating method

It can be used to dredge the eustachian tube directly or indirectly, to eliminate the pressure of the tympanic cavity and remove tympanic cavity effusion. There are Valsalva maneuver, Podbielniak ball inflation, and catheterization of eustachian tube, etc.

1.5 吹张法

可直接或间接疏通咽鼓管,消除鼓室负压,利于鼓室积液排除。有捏鼻鼓气自行吹张法、波氏球吹张法、金属管吹张法等。

2 The commonly used external therapies in the rhinology

2 鼻科常用外治法

2.1 Nose-dripping method

Nose drops are dripped into the nasal cavity to display the direct therapeutic effect in the local area. The commonly used medications include 1% Ephedrine Nasal Drops, 1% Furaclin and Ephedrine Nasal Drops, Compound Camphor Peppermint Oil Nasal Drops, Fish Liver Oil Nasal Drops, Magnolia and Small Centipeda Nasal Drops, etc, mainly for nasal sinusitis, allergic rhinitis, rhinitis sicca, and nasal hemorrhage, etc.

2.1 滴鼻法

将滴鼻药滴入鼻腔以发挥局部直接的治疗作用。常用药物有1%麻黄素滴鼻剂、1%呋喃西林麻黄素滴鼻剂、复方樟脑薄荷油滴鼻剂、鱼肝油滴鼻剂、辛夷鹅不食草滴鼻液等。主要治疗鼻-鼻窦炎、过敏性鼻炎、干燥性鼻炎、鼻出血等。

2.2 Nose-insufflating method

The herbal powder with the effects to diminish swelling, dredge the aperture, moisten the mucous membrane and arrest bleeding is inhaled or blown into the nasal cavity. Borneol and Coptis Powder (Bing Lian San) can be used for excessive patterns. *Blue Clouds Powder* (Bi Yun San) can be used for deficient patterns.

2.2 吹鼻法

将具有消肿通窍、滋润黏膜、止血作用的药粉吸入或吹入鼻腔。实证可选冰连散等,虚证可选碧云散等。

2.3 Nose-smearing method

The herbal paste with the effects to clear away

2.3 涂鼻法

将具有清热解毒、润燥

heat, resolve toxin, moisten dryness and promote granulation is smeared on the sick area. *Four Yellowness Powder* (Si Huang San) and *Purple Gold Ingot* (Zi Jin Ding) can be selected for red nose tip or erosive nostril. *Coptis Ointment* (Huang Lian Gao) and *Golden Yellow Ointment* (Jin Huang Gao) can be selected for erosion, cracks and bleeding of the nasal mucous membrane.

生肌作用的药膏涂敷患处。治疗鼻头红赤或鼻孔糜烂可选用四黄散、紫金锭等;鼻黏膜糜烂、干裂渗血可选用黄连膏、金黄膏等。

2.4 Nose-flushing method

Around 37℃ physiological saline, or warm water or herbal decoction (filtered liquid) with the effects to clear away heat, resolve toxin and discharge pus is used to flush the nasal cavity, in order to eliminate purulent nasal discharge or dry scabs inside the nose, for atrophic rhinitis, nasal sinusitis, etc.

2.4 洗鼻法

用 37 摄氏度左右的生理盐水、温开水或具有清热解毒排脓作用的中药煎剂(滤清液)冲洗鼻腔,以清除鼻内脓涕或干痂。可用于鼻槁、鼻渊等病证。

2.5 Aerosolization inhaling method

The herbal decoction (filtered clear liquid) with the effects to clear away heat, resolve toxin, diminish swelling and dredge the aperture is inhaled into the nasal cavity by ultrasonic atomizer or steam inhaler. *Radix Angelicae Dahuricae* (Bai Zhi), *Rhizoma Atractylodis* (Cang Zhu) and *Pericarpium Punicae Granati* (Shi Liu Pi) can be used for nasal polyp.

2.5 雾化吸入法

将具有清热解毒、消肿通窍的中药煎剂(滤清液)通过超声雾化器或蒸汽吸入器吸入鼻腔。鼻息肉可用白芷、苍术、石榴皮等。

2.6 Nose-plugging method

Ribbon gauze soaked with medication or Vaseline gauze is plugged into the nasal cavity, mainly for epistaxis.

2.6 塞鼻法

用浸药纱条或凡士林纱条,塞入鼻腔内,主要治疗鼻衄。

3 The commonly used external therapies for the pharyngolaryngeal diseases

3 咽喉病常用外治法

3.1 Insufflating method

The herbal powder with the effects to clear a-

3.1 吹药法

将具有清热解毒、消肿

way heat, resolve toxin, diminish swelling, stop pain, dissipate the decay and promote granulation is blown to the sick area of the throat. The commonly used herbal powders include *Swelling-Diminishing Powder* (Xiao Zhong San), *Yin-Nourishing and Granulation-Promoting Powder* (Yang Yin Sheng Ji San), and *Borneol and Borax Powder* (Bing Peng San), etc.

止痛、祛腐生肌作用的药粉吹布于咽喉患处。常用的有消肿散、养阴生肌散、冰硼散等。

3.2 Sublingual administrating method

The herbal pills and herbal tablets with the effects to clear away heat, resolve toxin, diminish swelling, stop pain, produce body fluid, moisten dryness, benefit qi and ease up voice are taken into the mouth and melted slowly, often used for tonsillitis, pharyngitis, hoarse voice, and oral ulcers. Optionally, there are *Throat-Easing Dripping Pills* (Qing Yan Di Wan), *Honeysuckle and Scutellaria Oral Tablets* (Yin Huang Han Pian), and *Throat-Clarifying Oral Pills* (Yan Li Shuang Kou Han Di Wan), etc.

3.2 噙化法

将具有清热解毒、消肿止痛、生津润燥、益气开音等作用的药丸、药片含于口内慢慢噙化咽下。常用于乳蛾、喉痹、喉瘖、口疮等病证。可选用清咽滴丸、银黄含片、咽立爽口含滴丸等。

3.3 Mouth-rinsing method

The herbal liquid or solution with the effects to clear away heat, resolve toxin, diminish swelling, stop pain, dissipate the decay and promote granulation is used to rinse the throat and oral cavity, often used for pharyngitis, tonsillitis, and paradentitis, etc. *Honeysuckle Gargle* (Yin Hua Han Shu Ji) is optional.

3.3 含漱法

将具有清热解毒、消肿止痛、祛腐生肌作用的药水或溶液漱洗咽喉口腔。常用于喉痹、乳蛾、牙周炎等病证,可选用银花含漱液等。

3.4 Aerosolization inhaling method

The herbal decoction (filtered clear liquid) with the effects to clear away heat, resolve toxin, diminish swelling and dredge the aperture is inhaled into the throat by ultrasonic atomizer or steam inhaler, often used for pharyngitis, tonsillitis, retro-

3.4 雾化吸入法

将具有清热解毒、消肿止痛、滋润咽喉的中药煎剂(滤清液)通过超声雾化器或蒸汽吸入器吸入咽喉。常用于治疗喉痹、乳蛾、喉痈、口

pharyngeal abscess, oral ulcers, etc.

疮等。

3.5 Application method

The herbal stuffs are applied topically on the sick area or acupoints along the meridians. For instance, *Four Yellowness Powder* (Si Huang San) or *Lucky Golden Yellow Powder* (Ru Yi Jin Huang San) can be used for red swelling and pain in the neck. For yang deficient pattern of pharyngeal problems, *Fructus Evodiae* (Wu Zhu Yu) can be powdered or *Radix Aconiti Praeparata* (Fu Zi) can be pounded and apply on the sole.

3.5 敷贴法

将药物敷贴于患处或循经所取之穴位处。如颈部红肿疼痛,用四黄散或如意金黄散;如咽喉病之阳虚证,用吴茱萸研粉或附子捣烂敷贴于足心。

3.6 Ironing method

A specially-made iron (about 20 cm in the handle, 0.5 to 1 cm in diameter at the head, different in size, round, or lengthwise, crosstrail round shape) is burnt red in its head over an alcohol lamp and then dipped in sesame oil to iron quickly the sick area, for 10 to 20 times per session. The treatment is given once every other day, till sick area is cured. It is often used for tonsillitis, and pharyngitis,

3.6 烙治法

用特制烙铁(柄长约20厘米,头端直径为0.5~1厘米,大小不等,圆形或纵长、横长圆形)头端在酒精灯上烧红,蘸香油后迅速烙于患处,每次10~20下,隔日1次至患处平复。常用于治疗乳蛾、喉痹。

Specific Introduction

各论

Chapter 1 Otological Diseases

第1章 耳科疾病

External otitis

外耳道炎

External otitis is an inflammatory disease characterized by red tumefaction and pain in the external auditory canal. It belongs to the scope of "ear sores" in Chinese medicine and often occurs in the summer and autumn and is caused by bacterial or viral infection. Its inducing factors include traumatic injury (pick ear, flush the external auditory canal), eczema, and diabetes. It is divided into acute and chronic type.

外耳道炎是以外耳道红肿疼痛为特征的炎症性疾病。属中医学"耳疮"范畴，好发于夏秋季，为细菌或病毒感染。可有诱发因素，如外伤(挖耳、外耳道冲洗等)、湿疹和糖尿病等。分为急性和慢性两类。

1 Diagnostic essentials

1 诊断要点

1.1 Acute external otitis

1.1 急性外耳道炎

① Ear pain in different severity, pain present in opening the mouth and chewing food or pulling the auricle. ② diffuse red tumefaction in the external auditory canal, with secretions on the surface, possible stenosis or blockage of the external auditory canal by serious tumefaction. ③ and needed to be differentiated from furuncle of the external auditory canal, eczema of the external ear, and necrotizing external otitis.

①耳痛轻重不等，可有张口咀嚼及牵拉耳廓痛；②外耳道弥漫性红肿，表面可有分泌物，肿胀剧烈可致外耳道狭窄及闭塞；③须与外耳道疖、外耳道湿疹，坏死性外耳道炎鉴别。

1.2 Chronic external otitis

1.2 慢性外耳道炎

① Ear itching or discomfort, pain in the skin

①耳痒或不适，若挖耳

lesion present after picking the ear, and ② thickened and narrowed skin in the external ear, with squamous crust, or stinky secretions, lustrousless, thickened and granulomatous tympanic membrane in long-term illness, and even hearing loss.

后皮损可有疼痛；②外耳皮肤增厚、狭窄，可有鳞屑状痂皮，或臭味分泌物，久病者鼓膜光泽消失、增厚、有肉芽，甚者听力可下降。

2 Therapeutic methods

2 治疗方法

2.1 Therapeutic principles

2.1 治疗原则

In Chinese medicine, external otitis is identified into pattern of invasion of pathogenic wind, heat and dampness, pattern of dampness and heat in the liver and gallbladder, and pattern of yin deficiency and fire hyperactivity. Acute stage is mainly treated to clear away fire and heat from the liver and gallbladder, and to expel wind as well. The chronic stage is mainly treated to nourish yin and clear away heat.

外耳道炎中医分为风热湿毒外侵证、肝胆湿热证和阴虚火旺证。急性期治疗以清泻肝胆火热为主，兼以疏风；慢性期则以养阴清热为主。

2.2 Treatment based on syndrome differentiation

2.2 辨证论治

(1) **Pattern of invasion of pathogenic wind, heat and dampness**

(1) **风热湿毒外侵**

Main symptoms: Redness, swelling and pain in the external auditory canal, pain aggravated in chewing food or pressing the auricle, or with little effusion, possibly accompanied by fever, headache, white or thin and yellow tongue coating, superficial and rapid pulse.

主症：外耳道红肿疼痛，咀嚼或压迫耳屏时疼痛加重，或有少许渗液。可伴发热、头痛。舌苔白或薄黄，脉浮数。

Therapeutic methods: To expel wind, clear away heat, resolve toxin and diminish swelling.

治法：疏风清热，解毒消肿。

Herbal formulas and drugs: ① *Lonicera and Forsythia Powder* (Yin Qiao San) (modified). *Flos Lonicerae* (Jin Yin Hua) 10g, *Fructus Forsythiae* (Lian Qiao) 10g, *Rhizoma Phragmitis* (Lu Gen) 30g, *Herba Menthae* (Bo He) (decoct later) 6g, *Herba Schizonepetae* (Jing Jie) 10g, *Radix Platycodi* (Jie

方药：①银翘散加减。金银花 10 克，连翘 10 克，芦根 30 克，薄荷(后下)6 克，荆芥 10 克，桔梗 6 克，蒲公英 10 克，甘草 3 克。若疼痛甚，加夏枯草 10 克、黄芩 10 克；

Geng) 6g, *Herba Taraxaci* (Pu Gong Ying) 10g, and *Radix Glycyrrhizae* (Gan Cao) 3g. For serious pain, add *Spica Prunellae* (Xia Ku Cao) 10g, and *Radix Scutellariae* (Huang Qin) 10g. ② *Five Ingredients Detoxifying Drink* (Wu Wei Xiao Du Yin) (modified). *Flos Lonicerae* (Jin Yin Hua) 15g, *Flos Chrysanthemi Indici* (Ye Ju Hua) 6g, *Herba Taraxaci* (Pu Gong Ying) 6g, *Herba Violae* (Zi Hua Di Ding) 6g, and *Radix Semiaquilegiae* (Tian Kui Zi) 6g.

有渗液,加苦参10克。②五味消毒饮加减。金银花15克,野菊花6克,蒲公英6克,紫花地丁6克,天葵子6克。

(2) **Pattern of dampness and heat in the liver and gallbladder:**

(2) **肝胆湿热**

Main symptoms: Diffusive red tumefaction, serious pain, or with pus discharge, hearing loss, lymph node enlargement in front of and behind the ear, accompanied by fever, bitter taste in the mouth, dry throat, irritability, brown urine, constipation, red tongue, yellow and greasy tongue coating, wiry and rapid pulse.

主症:外耳道弥漫性红肿、疼痛剧烈,或有流脓,听力减退,耳前或耳后淋巴结肿大,伴发热,口苦咽干,烦躁,溲黄便结。舌红苔黄腻,脉弦数。

Therapeutic methods: To clarify the liver and gallbladder, discharge fire and eliminate tumefaction.

治法:清泄肝胆,泻火消肿。

Herbal formulas and drugs: ① *Gentian Liver-Draining Decoction* (Long Dan Xie Gan Tang) (modified). *Radix Gentianae* (Long Dan Cao) 3g, *Radix Scutellariae* (Huang Qin) 10g, *Fructus Gardeniae* (Zhi Zi) 10g, *Rhizoma Alismatis* (Ze Xie) 10g, *Radix Rehmanniae Cruda* (Sheng Di Huang) 15g, *Radix Angelicae Sinensis* (Dang Gui) 10g, *Spica Prunellae* (Xia Ku Cao) 10g, and *Radix Glycyrrhizae* (Gan Cao) 3g. For profuse pus, add *Squama Manitis* (Chuan Shan Jia) 10g, and *Spina Gleditsiae* (Zao Jiao Ci) 10g. For serious thirst, add *Radix Adenophorae* (Nan Sha Shen) 10g, and *Radix*

方药:①龙胆泻肝汤加减。龙胆草3克,黄芩10克,栀子10克,泽泻10克,生地黄15克,当归10克,夏枯草10克,甘草3克。若脓多,加穿山甲10克、皂角刺10克;口渴甚,加南沙参10克、麦门冬10克。②银花解毒汤加减。金银花25克,地丁25克,赤茯苓10克,连翘10克,牡丹皮10克,黄连10克,夏枯草6克,犀角2.5克。③仙

Ophiopogonis (Mai Dong) 10g. ② *Honeysuckle Toxin-Resolving Decoction* (Yin Hua Jie Du Tang) (modified). *Flos Lonicerae* (Jin Yin Hua) 25g, *Herba Violae* (Zi Hua Di Ding) 25g, *Rubra Poria* (Chi Fu Ling) 10g, *Fructus Forsythiae* (Lian Qiao) 10g, *Cortex Moutan Radicis* (Mu Dan Pi) 10g, *Rhizoma Coptidis* (Huang Lian) 10g, *Spica Prunellae* (Xia Ku Cao) 6g, and *Cornu Rhinoceri Asiatici* (Xi Jiao) 2.5g. ③ *Fairy Formula Life-Saving Decoction* (Xian Fang Huo Ming Yin) (modified). *Squama Manitis* (Chuan Shan Jia) 5g, *Radix Angelicae Dahuricae* (Bai Zhi) 5g, *Radix Trichosanthis* (Tian Hua Fen) 5g, *Spina Gleditsiae* (Zao Jiao Ci) 5g, *Radix Angelicae Sinensis* (tail) (Dang Gui Wei) 5g, *Radix Glycyrrhizae* (Gan Cao) 5g, *Radix Paeoniae Rubra* (Chi Shao) 5g, *Resina Olibani* (Ru Xiang) 5g, *Myrrha* (Mo Yao) 5g, *Radix Ledebouriellae* (Fang Feng) 5g, *Bulbus Fritillariae Cirrhosae* (Chuan Bei Mu) 5g, *Pericarpium Citri Tangerinae* (Chen Pi) 15g, and *Flos Lonicerae* (Jin Yin Hua) 15g.

方活命饮加减。炙穿山甲5克，白芷5克，天花粉5克，皂角刺5克，当归尾5克，甘草5克，赤芍药5克，乳香5克，没药5克，防风5克，贝母5克，陈皮15克，金银花15克。

(3) **Pattern of yin deficiency and fire hyperactivity**

Main symptoms: Itching and discomfort in the external auditory canal, with a little volume of secretions, coarse and thickened skin in the external auditory canal, or with crusts and scales, lustrousless complexion, dry skin, red tongue, scanty body fluid, thin tongue coating, thready and rapid pulse.

Therapeutic methods: To nourish yin, moisten dryness, resolve toxin and expel pathogens.

Herbal formulas and drugs: ① *Anemarrhena, Phellodendron, and Rehmannia Pills* (Zhi Bai Di Huang Wan) (modified). *Rhizoma Anemarrhenae* (Zhi Mu) 10g, *Cortex Phellodendri* (Huang Bo)

(3) **阴虚火旺**

主症：外耳道发痒不适，可有少量分泌物，外耳道皮肤粗糙、增厚，或有痂皮、鳞屑。面色无华，皮肤干涩。舌红少津，苔薄，脉细数。

治法：滋阴润燥，解毒祛邪。

方药：①知柏地黄丸加减。知母10克，黄柏10克，生地黄10克，牡丹皮6克，茱萸肉10克，茯苓10克，泽泻

10g, *Radix Rehmanniae Cruda* (Sheng Di Huang) 10g, *Cortex Moutan Radicis* (Mu Dan Pi) 6g, *Fructus Corni* (Shan Zhu Yu) 10g, *Sclerotium Poria* (Fu Ling) 10g, *Rhizoma Alismatis* (Ze Xie) 10g, *Rhizoma Dioscoreae* (Shan Yao) 10g, *Flos Lonicerae* (Jin Yin Hua) 10g, and *Spica Prunellae* (Xia Ku Cao) 10g. For serious itching sensation in the external auditory canal, add *Flos Chrysanthemi* (Ju Hua) 10g, and *Periostracum Cicadae* (Chan Tui) 3g. For chapped skin, add *Radix Rubiae* (Qian Cao) 10g, and *Radix Arnebiae seu Lithospermi* (Zi Cao) 10g. ② *Angelica, White Paeonia and Rehmannia Decoction* (Gui Shao Di Huang Tang) (modified). *Radix Angelicae Sinensis* (Dang Gui) 15g, *Radix Paeoniae Albae* (Bai Shao) 15g, *Radix Rehmanniae Cruda* (Sheng Di Huang) 15g, *Rhizoma Dioscoreae* (Shan Yao) 20g, *Fructus Corni* (Shan Zhu Yu) 15g, *Sclerotium Poria* (Fu Ling) 15g, *Rhizoma Alismatis* (Ze Xie) 15g, and *Cortex Moutan Radicis* (Mu Dan Pi) 15g.

10 克,山药 10 克,金银花 10 克,夏枯草 10 克。若外耳道痒甚,加菊花 10 克、蝉蜕 3 克,皮肤皲裂,加茜草 10 克、紫草 10 克。②归芍地黄汤加减。当归 15 克,白芍 15 克,生地 15 克,山药 20 克,山茱萸 15 克,茯苓 15 克,泽泻 15 克,丹皮 15 克。

2.3 Other therapies

(1) Simple and proved formula: ① *Spica Prunellae* (Xia Ku Cao) 30g, decoct with water for oral administration. ② *Flos Chrysanthemi* (Ju Hua) 20g. and *Herba Lobeliae Chinensis* (Ban Zhi Lian) 20g, decoct with water for oral administration, one dose per day, for pattern of invasion of pathogenic wind and heat into the ear, and pattern of fire abundance of the liver and gallbladder.

(2) External therapies: ① For exudates in the auditory canal, after cleaning with 3% hydrogen peroxide solution, blow *Corktree Bark Powder* (Huang Bo Fen) or *Indigo Powder* (Qing Dai San) to the sick area, for once per day. ② Apply *Lucky*

2.3 其他疗法

(1) 单验方:①夏枯草 30 克,水煎服;②菊花 20 克,半枝莲 20 克,水煎服,每日 1 剂。用于风热犯耳证和肝胆火盛证。

(2) 外治法:①耳道有渗液者,用 3%双氧水清洗干净后,用黄柏粉或青黛散吹撒于患处,每日 1 次。②如意金黄膏、或黄连膏、或青黛散

Golden Yellow Ointment (Ru Yi Jin Huang Gao), or *Coptis Ointment* (Huang Lian Gao), or *Indigo Powder* (Qing Dai San) on the sick area, for once per day. ③ For profuse exudates in the auditory canal, after cleaning with 3% hydrogen peroxide solution, blow and sprinkle a little *Corktree Bark Powder* (Huang Bo Fen) into the external auditory canal, for once per day, or drip 20% *Corktree Bark Ear Drops* (Huang Bo Di Er Ye) every 3 to 4 hours, or insert the small gauze dipped with *Coptis and Safflower Oil* (Huang Lian Hong Hua You) into the external auditory canal, for once per day.

涂患处，每日 1 次。③外耳道渗液较多者，3%双氧水清洗后，用少许黄柏粉吹撒于外耳道，每日 1 次。或每隔 3～4 小时滴入 20%黄柏滴耳液；或用蘸有黄连红花油的小纱布填塞外耳道，每日 1 次。

Eczema of external ear

外耳湿疹

It refers to the polymorphous skin rash, part of eczema on the face and scalp, and belongs to the scope of "eczema around the ear" in Chinese medicine. It is commonly seen in the infants. Generally, it is divided into acute, subacute and chronic types.

外耳湿疹是指发生在耳廓、外耳道及其周围皮肤的多形性皮疹，可为面部和头皮湿疹的一部分。属中医学"旋耳疮"范畴。小儿多见，一般分为急性、亚急性、慢性三类。

It may be related to allergic reaction, mental factors, nerve dysfunction, endocrine disorder, metabolic disturbance, and indigestion. Among them, allergic reaction is a major factor.

湿疹可能与变态反应、精神因素、神经功能障碍、内分泌失调、代谢障碍、消化不良等有关，其中过敏反应是主因。

1 Diagnostic essentials

1.1 Acute eczema

Serious itching sensation in the local area, accompanied by burning sensation, pain, elevated body temperature, involving the deep part of the external auditory canal and tympanic membrane,

1 诊断要点

1.1 急性湿疹

局部剧痒，伴有烧灼感。继发感染，则有疼痛、体温升高。累及外耳道深部及鼓膜，则有耳鸣和轻度传导性

and tinnitus and mild conductive deafness, and including red swelling, red spots, papule, blisters, slight yellow watery secretions and scabs seen in the inspection.

耳聋。检查见外耳道皮肤红肿、红斑、丘疹、水疱、淡黄色水样分泌物和结痂。

1.2 Subacute eczema

Developed from lingering acute eczema, itching sensation, red swelling, mild exudates, but with scales and crusts.

1.2 亚急性湿疹

急性湿疹迁延所致。瘙痒、红肿和渗液较轻,但有鳞屑、结痂。

1.3 Chronic eczema

Caused by long-term eczema, manifested by serious itching, thickened, coarse and cracked skin in the external auditory canal, with lichenification and scales.

1.3 慢性湿疹

湿疹病久所致。表现为剧痒、外耳道皮肤增厚、粗糙、表皮龟裂、苔癣样变、脱屑等。

1.4 It is necessary to differentiate it from contact dermatitis and seborrheic dermatitis.

1.4 注意与接触性皮炎和脂溢性皮炎鉴别。

2 Therapeutic methods

2 治疗方法

2.1 Therapeutic principles

Clinically in Chinese medicine, it is divided into pattern of pathogenic wind, dampness and heat toxin, pattern of dampness and heat in the liver and gallbladder, and pattern of blood deficiency turning into dryness. Acute stage is mainly treated to discharge dampness and heat from the liver and gallbladder, and to expel wind and clear away heat as well. Chronic stage is mainly treated to nourish blood and activate blood.

2.1 治疗原则

中医临床分为风湿热毒证、肝胆湿热证和血虚化燥证。急性期以清泄肝胆湿热为主,兼以疏风清热;慢性期则以养血活血为主。

2.2 Treatment based on syndrome differentiation

(1) **Pattern of pathogenic wind, dampness and heat toxin**

Main symptoms: Red swelling in the skin of the ear, burning sensation, itching sensation, blisters, and yellow exudates, yellow and greasy tongue coating, wiry and rapid pulse.

2.2 辨证论治

(1) **风湿热毒**

主症:耳部皮肤红肿、灼热、瘙痒、水疱、糜烂和黄色渗液。舌苔黄腻,脉弦数。

Therapeutic methods: To clear away heat, dissipate dampness, expel wind and stop itching.

Herbal formulas and drugs: ① *Wind-Expelling Powder* (Xiao Feng San) plus *Sevenlobed Yam and Dampness-Eliminating Decoction* (Bi Xie Shen Shi Tang) (modified). *Radix Ledebouriellae* (Fang Feng) 10g, *Herba Schizonepetae* (Jing Jie) 10g, *Flos Chrysanthemi* (Ju Hua) 10g, *Rhizoma Dioscorea Septemlobae* (Bi Xie) 10g, *Cortex Phellodendri* (Huang Bo) 10g, *Cortex Dictamni* (Bai Xian Pi) 10g, *Radix Sophorae flavescentis* (Ku Shen) 10g, and *Rhizoma Alismatis* (Ze Xie) 10g. For serious pain, add *Radix Paeoniae Rubra* (Chi Shao) 6g, and *Radix Angelicae Sinensis* (tail) (Dang Gui Wei) 10g. For profuse exudates, add *Semen Plantaginis* (Che Qian Zi) 10g, and *Rubra Poria* (Chi Fu Ling) 10g. ② *Lonicera and Forsythia Powder* (Yin Qiao San) or *Five Ingredients Detoxifying Drink* (Wu Wei Xiao Du Yin) (modified), Please see “External otitis”.

治法：清热祛湿，疏风止痒。

方药：①消风散合萆薢渗湿汤加减。防风10克，荆芥10克，菊花10克，萆薢10克，黄柏10克，白鲜皮10克，苦参10克，泽泻10克。若疼痛甚，加赤芍药6克、当归尾10克；渗液多，加车前子10克、赤茯苓10克。②银翘散或五味消毒饮加减，参见“外耳道炎”。

(2) **Pattern of blood deficiency turning into dryness**

(2) **血虚化燥**

Main symptoms: Itching in the ear, coarse, thickened, dry, cracked, scabbed and scaled skin in the external auditory canal, slight red tongue, thin and white tongue coating, thready and feeble pulse.

Therapeutic methods: To nourish blood, moisten dryness, extinguish wind and stop itching.

Herbal formulas and drugs: *Four Ingredients Wind-Eliminating Drink* (Si Wu Xiao Feng Yin) (modified). *Flos Carthami* (Hong Hua) 10g, *Radix Rehmanniae Praeparata* (Shu Di Huang) 10g, *Rhizoma Ligustici Chuanxiong* (Chuan Xiong) 6g, *Radix Angelicae Sinensis* (Dang Gui) 10g, *Radix*

主症：耳部瘙痒，外耳道皮肤粗糙、增厚、干燥、皲裂、结痂和鳞屑。舌淡红，苔薄白，脉细弱。

治法：养血润燥，息风止痒。

方药：四物消风饮加减。红花10克，熟地黄10克，川芎6克，当归10克，赤芍药6克，郁金10克，蝉蜕3克，白芷10克，甘草3克。若局部红肿而痒，加牡丹皮6克、泽

Paeoniae Rubra (Chi Shao) 6g, *Radix Curcumae* (Yu Jin) 10g, *Periostracum Cicadae* (Chan Tui) 3g, *Radix Angelicae Dahuricae* (Bai Zhi) 10g, and *Radix Glycyrrhizae* (Gan Cao) 3g. For local red swelling and itching, add *Cortex Moutan Radicis* (Mu Dan Pi) 6g, and *Herba Lycopi* (Ze Lan) 10g. For scratch and bleeding, add *Radix Rubiae* (Qian Cao) 10g, and *Radix Arnebiae seu Lithospermi* (Zi Cao) 10g.

兰 10 克；有抓痕出血，加茜草 10 克、紫草 10 克。

2.3 Other therapies

(1) Simple and proved formula: ① *Flos Lonicerae* (Jin Yin Hua) 20g, *Spica Prunellae* (Xia Ku Cao) 30g, decoct with water for oral administration, for pattern of pathogenic wind, dampness and heat toxin. ② *Semen Coicis* (Yi Yi Ren) 30g, *Semen Oryza Sativae* (Jing Mi) 30g. for cooking congee, take twice per day, for pattern of pathogenic wind, dampness and heat toxin, and pattern of blood deficiency turning into dryness.

(2) External therapies: ① *Corktree Bark Powder* (Huang Bo Fen) or *Indigo Powder* (Qing Dai San): After cleaning with 3% hydrogen peroxide solution, blow herbal powder to the local area, for three times per day, for pattern of pathogenic wind, dampness and heat toxin, and pattern of dampness and heat of the liver and gallbladder. ② *Coptis Ointment* (Huang Lian Gao): Smear on the local area, for three times per day, for pattern of blood deficiency turning into dryness. ③ Smoking therapy: *Ignite Folium Artemistae Argyi* (Ai Ye) and smoke skin lesions of eczema, for pattern of blood deficiency turning into dryness.

2.3 其他疗法

（1）单验方：①金银花 20 克，夏枯草 30 克。水煎服。用于风湿热毒证。②薏苡仁 30 克，粳米 30 克，煮粥，每日分 2 次服食。用于风湿热毒证，血虚化燥证。

（2）外治法：①黄柏粉或青黛散：先用 3%双氧水清洗耳道，再局部吹撒药粉，每日 3 次。用于风湿热毒证和肝胆湿热证。②黄连膏：涂搽局部，每日 3 次。用于血虚化燥证。③烟熏疗法：用艾叶点燃后以烟气薰及湿疹皮损之处，用于血虚化燥证。

Secretory otitis media

分泌性中耳炎

It refers to a disease of otitis media mainly characterized by tympanic cavity effusion and hearing loss. It is termed in many ways, such as exudative otitis media, serous otitis media, mucinous otitis media, catarrhal otitis media, non-suppurative otitis media, glue ear, and it belongs to the scope of "ear distention" and "ear blockage" in Chinese medicine. It mainly occurs in winter and spring.

分泌性中耳炎是以鼓室积液及听力下降为主要特征的中耳炎性疾病。称谓甚多,有渗出性中耳炎、浆液性中耳炎、黏液性中耳炎、卡他性中耳炎、非化脓性中耳炎、胶耳等,属中医"耳胀""耳闭"范畴。好发于冬春季。

1 Diagnostic essentials

1 诊断要点

1.1 The main symptoms include stuffy sensation in the ear, ear pain, tinnitus and hearing loss.

1.1 主要症状包括耳闷塞、耳痛、耳鸣和听力下降。

1.2 In the inspection, invagination can be seen in the tympanic membrane, and fluid levels and bubbles in fluid can be seen through the tympanic membrane. In profuse effusion, the tympanic membrane protrudes outward, with limited motion. Tuning fork test shows negative in Rinne test negative and deviation to the sick side in Weber test.

1.2 检查见鼓膜内陷,透过鼓膜可见液平面和液中气泡。积液多时鼓膜向外隆凸,活动受限,音叉检查Rinne 试验阴性,Weber 试验偏向患侧。

1.3 Tympanic cavity effusion can be extracted in the diagnostic puncture.

1.3 诊断性穿刺可抽出鼓室积液。

1.4 Audiological inspection

1.4 听力学检查

Pure tone test shows mild conductive deafness. Acoustic immitance test shows flat type (B type), and high pressure type (C type). Acoustic reflex disappears.

纯音测听为轻度传导性聋;声导抗测试为平坦型(B型)、高负压型(C型);声反射消失。

1.5 In CT scan of the skull, dense and even shadow can be seen in the tympanic cavity, and fluid levels can be seen in the mastoid air cells.

1.5 颞骨 CT 扫描可见鼓室内有密度均匀一致的阴影,乳突气房中可见液气面。

1.6 If sensorineural deafness is complicated with this problem, the diagnosis will be easily missed.

1.6 患感音神经性聋小儿合并本病时易漏诊。

1.7 The diagnosis should be differentiated from nasopharyngeal cancer, cerebrospinal fluid otorrhea, perilymph fistula, and cholesterol granuloma.

1.7 鉴别诊断包括鼻咽癌、脑脊液耳漏、外淋巴漏和胆固醇肉芽肿。

2 Therapeutic methods

2 治疗方法

2.1 Therapeutic principles

2.1 治疗原则

The commonly seen patterns of secretory otitis media include four types: pattern of invasion of pathogenic wind into the lung, pattern of dampness and heat in the liver and gallbladder, pattern of accumulation of dampness due to spleen deficiency, and pattern of qi stagnation and blood stasis. The initial problem accompanied by exterior pattern is treated to expel wind and promote the lung in its spreading ability. The long-term problem is mainly treated to regulate qi, disperse blood stasis, clarify the liver, strengthen the spleen, dissipate dampness and dredge the aperture.

分泌性中耳炎常见证型有风邪犯肺、肝胆湿热、脾虚湿困、气滞血瘀四类。病初兼有表证,治宜疏风宣肺,日久以理气化瘀、清肝健脾、祛湿通窍为主。

2.2 Treatment based on syndrome differentiation

2.2 辨证论治

(1) **Pattern of invasion of pathogenic wind into the lung**

(1) 风邪犯肺

Main symptoms: Mostly distending sensation in the ear after cold, nasal obstruction, and nasal discharge, or slight pain, hearing loss, loud self-listening, tinnitus like wind, feeling comfortable by pressing Ermen (TE 21), possibly accompanied by headache, fever, and aversion to cold, slight red, invagination and fluid levels of the tympanic membrane seen in the inspection, red tongue, white tongue coating, superficial and rapid pulse.

主症:多在伤风、鼻塞、流涕后耳内作胀,或微痛,听力减退,自听过响,耳鸣如闻风声。轻按耳门常感舒适。可伴有头痛、发热恶寒等症。检查见鼓膜微红、内陷或有液平,呈传导性聋。舌红苔白,脉浮数。

Therapeutic methods: To expel wind, promote the lung in its spreading ability, disperse the pathogens and dredge the aperture.

治法:疏风宣肺,散邪通窍。

Herbal formulas and drugs: ① *Three Disobedience*

方药:① 三拗汤加减。

Decoction (San Ao Tang) (modified). *Herba Ephedrae* (Ma Huang) 5g, *Semen Armeniacae Amarum* (Ku Xing Ren) 10g, *Fructus Arctii* (Niu Bang Zi) 10g, *Herba Spirodelae* (Fu Ping Cao) 10g, *Herba Menthae* (Bo He) (decoct later) 6g, *Fructus Aristolochiae* (Ma Dou Ling) 10g, *Fructus Liquidambaris* (Lu Lu Tong) 10g, *Periostracum Cicadae* (Chan Tui) 3g, and *Radix Glycyrrhizae* (Gan Cao) 3g. For bitter taste in the mouth and dry throat, add *Spica Prunellae* (Xia Ku Cao) 10g, and *Flos Chrysanthemi* (Ju Hua) 10g. For profuse effusion in the tympanic cavity, add *Semen Plantaginis* (Che Qian Zi) (decoct in bag) 10g, and *Cortex Mori Radicis* (Sang Bai Pi) 10g. ②*Lonicera and Forsythia Powder* (Yin Qiao San). *Flos Lonicerae* (Jin Yin Hua) 12g, *Fructus Forsythiae* (Lian Qiao) 12g, *Radix Ledebouriellae* (Fang Feng) 10g, *Periostracum Cicadae* (Chan Tui) 6g, *Lumbricus* (Di Long) 9g, *Herba Schizonepetae* (Jing Jie) 10g, *Radix Peucedani* (Qian Hu) 10g, *Rhizoma Phragmitis* (Lu Gen) 15g, *Radix Platycodi* (Jie Geng) 10g, *Radix Glycyrrhizae* (Gan Cao) 3g, and *Rhizoma Acori Graminei* (Shi Chang Pu) 9g. For cough and yellow sputum, add *Cortex Mori Radicis* (Sang Bai Pi) 12g, *Bulbus Fritillariae Thumbergii* (Zhe Bei Mu) 12g, and *Herba Houttuyniae* (Yu Xing Cao) 15g. For nasal obstruction and tenacious nasal discharge, add *Flos Magnoliae Liliflorae* (Xin Yi Hua) 10g, and *Radix Angelicae Dahuricae* (Bai Zhi) 9g. ③ *Schizonepeta and Ledebouriella Detoxifying Powder* (Jing Fang Bai Du San). *Herba Schizonepetae* (Jing Jie)(decoct later) 10g, *Radix Ledebouriellae* (Fang Feng) 10g, *Rhizoma seu Radix Notopterygii* (Qiang Huo) 6g, *Fructus Aurantii* (Zhi Qiao) 10g, *Radix Angelicae*

麻黄5克,杏仁10克,牛蒡子10克,浮萍10克,薄荷(后下)6克,马兜铃10克,路路通10克,蝉蜕3克,甘草3克。若有口苦、咽干,加夏枯草10克、菊花10克;鼓室积液较多,加车前子(包煎)10克、泽泻10克、桑白皮10克。②银翘散。金银花12克,连翘12克,防风10克,蝉蜕6克,地龙9克,荆芥(后下)10克,前胡10克,芦根15克,桔梗10克,甘草3克,石菖蒲9克。若咳嗽、痰黄,加桑白皮12克、浙贝母12克、鱼腥草15克;鼻塞,涕稠,加辛夷花10克、白芷9克。③荆防败毒散。荆芥10克,防风10克,羌活6克,枳壳10克,独活10克,柴胡10克,桔梗10克,茯苓12克,川芎5克,甘草5克。若中耳积液,加车前子15克、泽泻15克;鼻塞、流涕,加辛夷10克、白芷10克、苍耳子10克。

Pubescentis (Du Huo) 10g, *Radix Bupleuri* (Chai Hu) 10g, *Radix Platycodi* (Jie Geng) 10g, *Sclerotium Poria* (Fu Ling) 12g, *Rhizoma Ligustici Chuanxiong* (Chuan Xiong) 5g, *Radix Glycyrrhizae* (Gan Cao) 5g. For effusion in the ear, add *Semen Plantaginis* (Che Qian Zi) 15g, and *Rhizoma Alismatis* (Ze Xie) 15g. For nasal obstruction and nasal discharge, add *Flos Magnoliae Liliflorae* (Xin Yi Hua) 10g, and *Radix Angelicae Dahuricae* (Bai Zhi) 10g, and *Fructus Xanthii* (Cang Er Zi) 10g.

(2) **Pattern of dampness and heat in the liver and gallbladder**

(2) **肝胆湿热**

Main symptoms: Stuffy and blocking sensation in the ear, or slight pain, autophonai, tinnitus, possible irritability and easy anger, bitter taste in the mouth, dry mouth, stuffy sensation in the chest, and congestion and invagination of the tympanic cavity, with fluid levels, conductive deafness, red tongue, yellow and greasy tongue coating, wiry and rapid pulse.

主症:耳胀闷堵塞,或微痛,自听过响,耳鸣。可有烦躁易怒,口苦口干,胸胁苦闷等症。检查见鼓膜充血、内陷或有液平,呈传导性聋。舌红苔黄腻,脉弦数。

Therapeutic methods: To clarify the liver and gallbladder, remove dampness and dredge the aperture.

治法:清泻肝胆,利湿通窍。

Herbal formulas and drugs: *Gentian Liver-Draining Decoction* (Long Dan Xie Gan Tang) (modified). *Radix Bupleuri* (Chai Hu) 10g, *Radix Gentianae* (Long Dan Cao) 8g, *Radix Scutellariae* (Huang Qin) 12g, *Fructus Gardeniae* (Zhi Zi) 10g, *Rhizoma Alismatis* (Ze Xie) 12g, *Semen Plantaginis* (Che Qian Zi) 10g, *Radix Rehmanniae Cruda* (Sheng Di Huang) 10g, *Caulis Akebiae* (Mu Tong) 6g, and *Radix Glycyrrhizae* (Gan Cao) 5g. For serious stuffy sensation in the ear, add *Fructus Xanthii* (Cang Er Zi) 3g, and *Rhizoma Acori Graminei* (Shi

方药:龙胆泻肝汤加减。柴胡10克,龙胆草8克,黄芩12克,栀子10克,泽泻12克,车前子10克,生地10克,木通6克,甘草5克。若耳闷塞甚,加苍耳子3克、石菖蒲10克;大便秘结,加大黄10克。

Chang Pu) 10g. For constipation, add *Rhizoma Rhei* (Da Huang) 10g.

(3) **Pattern of accumulation of dampness due to spleen deficiency**

Main symptoms: Long-term stuffy sensation in the ear, gradual hearing loss, loud self-listening, noise tinnitus, feeling comfortable by pressing Ermen (TE 21), possibly accompanied by stuffy sensation in the chest, poor appetite, abdominal distension, loose stool, tiredness in the limbs, lassitude, lustrousless complexion, invaginated, turbid and thickened tympanic cavity in the inspection, possible effusion by puncture, conductive deafness, pale and swollen tongue with teeth marks on the margin, thready and rolling or thready and slow pulse.

Therapeutic methods: To strengthen the spleen, remove dampness, dissolve the turbid and dredge the aperture.

Herbal formulas and drugs: *Ginseng, Poria and Atractylodes Powder* (Shen Ling Bai Zhu San) (modified). *Semen Nelumbinis* (Lian Zi) 9g, *Semen Coicis* (Yi Yi Ren) 9g, *Fructus Amomi* (Sha Ren) 6g, *Radix Platycodi* (Jie Geng) 6g, *Semen Dolichoris Album* (Bai Bian Dou) 12g, *Sclerotium Poria* (Fu Ling) 15g, *Radix Ginseng* (Ren Shen) 15g, *Radix Glycyrrhizae* (Gan Cao) 9g, *Rhizoma Atractylodis Macrocephalae* (Bai Zhu) 15g, and *Rhizoma Dioscoreae* (Shan Yao) 15g. For tenacious and profuse effusion, add *Herba Agastachis* (Huo Xiang) 10g, and *Herba Eupatorii* (Pei Lan) 10g. For thin effusion, add *Rhizoma Alismatis* (Ze Xie) 10g, and *Ramulus Cinnamomi* (Gui Zhi) 6g. For liver qi stagnation, vexation and stuffy sensation in the chest, add *Radix Bupleuri* (Chai Hu) 10g,

(3) **脾虚湿困**

主症:耳内闷塞日久,听力渐降,自听过响,耳鸣声嘈杂。轻按耳门常感舒适。可伴有胸闷纳呆,腹胀便溏,肢倦乏力,面色不华等症。检查见鼓膜内陷、混浊、增厚,穿刺可有积液,呈传导性聋。舌淡体胖,边有齿印,脉细滑或细缓。

治法:健脾利湿,化浊通窍。

方药:参苓白术散加减。莲子肉9克,薏苡仁9克,砂仁6克,桔梗6克,白扁豆12克,白茯苓15克,人参15克,甘草9克,白术15克,山药15克。若积液黏稠量多,加藿香10克、佩兰10克;若积液稀薄,加泽泻10克、桂枝6克;肝气不舒,心烦胸闷,加柴胡10克、白芍10克、香附6克;脾虚甚,加黄芪15克。

Radix Paeoniae Albae (Bai Shao) 10g, and *Rhizoma Cyperi* (Xiang Fu) 6g. For severe spleen deficiency, add *Radix Astragali* (Huang Qi) 15g.

(4) **Pattern of qi stagnation and blood stasis**

Main symptoms: Lingering stuffy and blocking sensation in the ear, gradual hearing loss, tinnitus like cicada, or noisy sound, obvious invagination and decreased mobility in the tympanic cavity, with grey white plague, conductive deafness in the audiological inspection, purple and dark tongue, wiry and choppy pulse.

Therapeutic methods: To circulate qi, activate blood and dredge the aperture and break up blockage.

Herbal formulas and drugs: *Aperture-Opening and Blood-Activating Decoction* (Tong Qiao Huo Xue Tang) (modified). *Rhizoma Ligustici Chuanxiong* (Chuan Xiong) 5g, *Radix Bupleuri* (Chai Hu) 10g, *Rhizoma Cyperi* (Xiang Fu) 10g, *Flos Carthami* (Hong Hua) 5g, *Semen Persicae* (Tao Ren) 10g, *Cortex Moutan Radicis* (Mu Dan Pi) 12g, *Sclerotium Poria* (Fu Ling) 15g, *Radix Curcumae* (Yu Jin) 10g, *Lumbricus* (Di Long) 10g, *Rhizoma Acori Graminei* (Shi Chang Pu) 10g, *Radix Glycyrrhizae* (Gan Cao) 5g. For accompanying qi deficiency in the lung and spleen, add *Radix Codonopsis Pilosulae* (Dang Shen) 15g, and *Radix Astragali* (Huang Qi) 15g. For accompanying kidney yang deficiency, add *Cortex Eucommiae* (Du Zhong) 15g, *Semen Cuscutae* (Tu Si Zi) 15g, and *Radix Morindae Officinalis* (Ba Ji Tian) 15g. For aversion to cold, and cold sensation in the four limbs, add *Radix Aconiti Praeparata* (Fu Zi) 5g, and *Cortex Cinnamomi* (Rou Gui) 5g.

(4) **气滞血瘀**

主症：耳胀闷闭塞，日久不愈，听力渐退，耳鸣如蝉，或声音嘈杂。检查见鼓膜内陷较明显，活动度减低，有灰白色斑块。听力检查呈传导性聋。舌质紫暗，脉弦涩。

治法：行气活血，通窍开闭。

方药：通窍活血汤加减。川芎 5 克，柴胡 10 克，香附 10 克，红花 5 克，桃仁 10 克，牡丹皮 12 克，茯苓 15 克，郁金 10 克，地龙 10 克，石菖蒲 10 克，甘草 5 克。若兼肺脾气虚，加党参 15 克、黄芪 15 克；兼肾阳虚，加杜仲 15 克、菟丝子 15 克、巴戟天 15 克；畏寒、四肢不温加附子 5 克、肉桂 5 克。

2.3 Other therapies

(1) Massage the tympanic membrane: It is advisable to insert the middle finger into the external auditory canal, and press slightly, again and again, and press for 15 to 30 times on the two sides respectively, for three sessions per day, or to shake lightly inside the external auditory canal for dozen times for massaging the tympanic membrane, in order to initiate the circulation of qi and blood. It is certainly effective for the restoration of the hearing ability.

(2) Pinch the nose and puff out the cheeks: It is advisable to pinch the nostrils tightly with the thumb and index finger of the right hand, in an action to blow the nose, in order to blow the air current into the auditory tube, for three times per day, for alleviating the distending and blocking sensation in the ear.

(3) Strike the heavenly drum: After regulating the respiration, press the occipital part with the index, middle, ring and small fingers of the two hands in opposition, with the two middle fingers touched, and cover the auricles with the two palms, and then put the two index fingers on the middle fingers and slide forcefully from the middle fingers to knock the occipital part, with a resonant and clear sound like striking a drum. It is advisable to do for 24 times with the left hand and right hand respectively, and then to do for 48 times with the two hands at the same time. This method is supposed to dredge the meridians and circulate qi and blood.

(4) Chinese patent medicine: ① *Gentian Liver-Draining Pills* (Long Dan Xie Gan Wan) Take 6g each time, for three times per day, for secretory o-

2.3 其他疗法

(1) 鼓膜按摩法:用中指指尖插入外耳道口,轻轻按压,一按一放,两侧各捺按15～30下,每日3次;或在外耳道内轻轻摇动数十次,以按摩鼓膜,引动气血流通,对恢复听力有一定的作用。

(2) 捏鼻鼓气法:以右手拇指和食指捏紧鼻孔,做擤鼻涕动作,使气流冲入咽鼓管,每日3次,可缓解耳胀、耳闭。

(3) 鸣天鼓法:调整好呼吸,两手食指、中指、无名指、小指对称地横按在枕部,两中指相接触,手掌捂住耳廓,后将两食指翘起叠放并从中指上用力弹向枕骨,叩击脑后枕部,有宏亮清晰之声响如击鼓。可左手、右手各做24次,再两手同时做48次。本法亦可疏通经络、运行气血。

(4) 中成药:①龙胆泻肝丸 每次6克,每日3次。治疗肝胆湿热型分泌性中耳

titis media in pattern of dampness and heat in the liver and gallbladder. ② *Deafness Pills* (Er Long Wan) Take two pills each time, for twice per day, appropriate for ear distension and ear blockage in excessive pattern of the liver and gallbladder. ③ *Center-Supplementing Qi-Boosting Pills* (Bu Zhong Yi Qi Wan) Take 8 pills each time, for three times per day, appropriate for pattern of accumulation of dampness due to spleen deficiency.

炎。②耳聋丸 每次 2 丸，每日 2 次。适用于肝胆实证之耳胀耳闭。③补中益气丸 每次 8 丸，每日 3 次。适用于脾虚湿困之证。

Acute suppurative otitis media

急性化脓性中耳炎

It refers to an acute suppurative inflammation in the mucous membrane of the middle ear. The main pathogenic bacteria are pneumococcus, Haemophilus influenzae, beta hemolytic streptocossus, staphylococcus and Pseudomonas aeruginosa, ect. The infective channels include: ① auditory tube. ② external auditory canal-tympanic membrane, and ③ hematogenous infection. It is termed "pus ear" in Chinese medicine, and often occurs in children.

急性化脓性中耳炎是中耳黏膜的急性化脓性炎症。主要致病菌为肺炎球菌、流感嗜血杆菌、乙型溶血性链球菌、葡萄球菌及绿脓杆菌等，感染途径包括：①咽鼓管；②外耳道—鼓膜；③血行感染。中医学称为"脓耳"，好发于儿童。

1 Diagnostic essentials

1 诊断要点

1.1 General symptoms

1.1 全身症状

Obvious perforation of the tympanic membrane than before, possible fever, aversion to cold, tiredness, poor appetite, often high fever in children.

鼓膜穿孔前较明显，可有发热、恶寒、倦怠、食欲减退，小儿常高热。

1.2 Ear pain

1.2 耳痛

Sharp pain or fluctuating throbbing pain in the deep part of the ear, possible radiating to the forehead, temple and vertex of the same side. Ear pain is decreased immediately after perforation of the tympanic membrane.

耳深部锐痛或波动性跳痛，可向同侧额、颞、顶部放射。鼓膜穿孔后，耳痛顿减。

1.3 Tinnitus and hearing loss

Tinnitus can be fluctuating. Hearing loss will be worse after perforation of the tympanic membrane

1.4 Otorrhea

After perforation of the tympanic membrane, fluid will flow from the ear, serous-hemic initially, and mucous or purulent later.

1.5 Otoscopy

Congestion in the tympanic membrane in the early stage, fluctuation seen in the outward protrusion of the tympanic membrane, perforation mostly in the tense part, tenderness possible in the mastoid apex and tympanic antrum.

1.6 Conductive deafness is present in the hearing test. The total white blood cells and neutrophil are elevated in routine blood test.

1.7 It is necessary to differentiate it from acute furuncle of external auditory canal.

2 Therapeutic methods

2.1 Therapeutic principles

The commonly seen patterns of acute suppurative otitis media include two types: pattern of invasion of pathogenic wind and heat, and pattern of fire abundance in the liver and gallbladder. The treatment is mainly given to expel wind, clear away heat, discharge fire and resolve toxin.

2.2

(1) **Pattern of invasion of pathogenic wind and heat**

Main symptoms: Distending pain in the ear, hearing loss, tinnitus like wind sound, accompanied by fever, aversion to cold, body ache, nasal obstruction, and nasal discharge.

1.3 耳鸣及听力减退

耳鸣可为波动性，听力减退在鼓膜穿孔后有所提高。

1.4 耳漏

鼓膜穿孔后耳内有液体流出，初为浆液—血性，以后变为黏液脓性或脓性。

1.5 耳镜检查

早期鼓膜充血，鼓膜外凸并可见搏动。穿孔多位于紧张部，乳突尖及鼓窦区可有压痛。

1.6 听力检查呈传导性聋。血常规检查白细胞总数及中性粒细胞增高。

1.7 应与急性外耳道疖鉴别。

2 治疗方法

2.1 治疗原则

急性化脓性中耳炎常见证型有风热外袭、肝胆火盛两类。治疗以疏风清热、泻火解毒为主。

2.2 辨证论治

(1) 风热外袭

主症：耳胀痛，听力减退，耳鸣如闻风声。伴有发热、恶寒、身疼、鼻塞、流涕等症。鼓膜色红，听力检查呈传导性聋。舌边尖红，脉浮数。

Therapeutic method: To expel wind, clear away heat, promote the lung in its spreading ability and dredge the aperture.

治法：疏风清热，宜肺通窍。

Herbal formulas and drugs: ① *Chastetree Fruit Powde* (Man Jing Zi San) (modified). *Fructus Viticis* (Man Jing Zi) 10g, *Flos Chrysanthemi* (Ju Hua) 10g, *Rhizoma Cimicifugae* (Sheng Ma) 10g, *Fructus Arctii* (Niu Bang Zi) 10g, *Herba Menthae* (Bo He) (decoct later) 6g, *Folium Llicis Latifoliae* (Ku Ding Cha) 10g, *Flos Lonicerae* (Jin Yin Hua) 10g, *Radix Scutellariae* (Huang Qin) 6g, and *Radix Glycyrrhizae* (Gan Cao) 3g. For bitter taste in the mouth and dry throat, add *Spica Prunellae* (Xia Ku Cao) 15g, and *Radix Bupleuri* (Chai Hu) 10g. For cough and expectoration, add *Cortex Mori Radicis* (Sang Bai Pi) 15g, and *Semen Armeniacae Amarum* (Ku Xing Ren) 10g. ② *Five Ingredients Detoxifying Drink* (Wu Wei Xiao Du Yin) (modified). Please see "External otitis".

方药：①蔓荆子散加减。蔓荆子 10 克，菊花 10 克，升麻 10 克，牛蒡子 10 克，薄荷（后下）6 克，苦丁茶 10 克，金银花 10 克，黄芩 6 克，甘草 3 克。若口苦、咽干，加夏枯草 15 克、柴胡 10 克；咳嗽、咯痰，加桑白皮 15 克、杏仁 10 克。②五味消毒饮加减。见"外耳道炎"。

(2) **Pattern of fire abundance in the liver and gallbladder**

(2) **肝胆火盛**

Main symptoms: Serious ear pain, sharp like needle pricking, manifested crying and screaming in infants, more obvious hearing loss; deep red colour in the tympanic membrane, bulged or with small yellow spots, premonitory sign of tympanic membrane perforation, or small perforation in the tympanic membrane, still lots of purulent fluid, red tongue, yellow tongue coating, wiry and rapid pulse.

主症：耳痛剧烈，如锥如刺，小儿表现为哭闹不安；听力减退更为明显；检查见鼓膜呈深红色，向外膨出，或可见小黄点，为鼓膜穿孔先兆；或鼓膜有小穿孔，但大量脓液仍未流出。舌红，苔黄，脉弦数。

Therapeutic principles: To clarify the liver and gallbladder, reduce fire and dredge the aperture.

治法：清泻肝胆，降火通窍。

Herbal formulas and drugs: *Gentian Liver-Draining Decoction* (Long Dan Xie Gan Tang) (modified) (Please see "External otitis"). For constipation, add *Rhizoma Rhei Cruda* (Sheng Da Huang) 10g. For thirst with preference of drinks, add *Herba Dendrobii* (Shi Hu) 10g and *Radix Trichosanthis* (Tian Hua Fen) 10g.

方药：龙胆泻肝汤（见"外耳道炎"）加减。若大便秘结，加生大黄 10 克；口渴多饮，加石斛 10 克、天花粉 10 克。

2.3 Other therapies

Simple and proved formula: ① Pound the fresh *Herba Saxifragae Stoniferae* (Hu Er Cao) and extract its liquid to drip the ear, three drop each time, for three times per day. ② *Coptis (or Corktree Bark) Ear Drops [Huang Lian (Huang Bo) Di Er Ye]*, in concentration of 20% to 30%, drip the ear, for three drops per session, for three times per day. ③ *Decoct Rhizoma Coptidis* (Huang Lian) 15g, and *Herba Taraxaci* (Pu Gong Ying) 30g. with water for oral administration.

2.3 其他疗法

单验方：①新鲜虎耳草捣烂取汁，滴耳，每次 3 滴，每日 3 次。②黄连（或黄柏）滴耳液，浓度为 20%～30%，滴耳，每次 3 滴，每日 3 次。③黄连 15 克，蒲公英 30 克，水煎服。

Chronic suppurative otitis media

慢性化脓性中耳炎

It refers to suppurative inflammation in the mucous membrane of the middle ear, periosteum or deep to the bone substance. It often exists together with chronic mastoiditis. The commonly seen pathogenic bacteria are mostly staphylococcus aureus, and Pseudomonas aeruginosa. It belongs to the scope of "pus ear" in Chinese medicine.

慢性化脓性中耳炎是中耳黏膜、骨膜或深达骨质的化脓性炎症，常与慢性乳突炎合并存在。常见致病菌以金黄色葡萄球菌最多，绿脓杆菌次之。属中医"脓耳"范畴。

1 Diagnostic essentials

1.1 Long-term continuous or intermittent discharge of pus inside the ear, perforation of the tympanic membrane and hearing loss in varying degree.

1.2 Imageological inspection includes X-ray or CT

1 诊断要点

1.1 耳内长期持续或间断流脓，鼓膜穿孔和不同程度的听力下降。

1.2 影像学检查包括颞骨

scan of the temporal bone, beneficial to the pattern identification.

X线或CT,有助于明确病变分型。

1.3 It is necessary to differentiate it from chronic granular myringitis, carcinoma of the middle ear and tuberculous otitis media.

1.3 注意与慢性肉芽性鼓膜炎、中耳癌和结核性中耳炎鉴别。

Differential Essentials for Three Types of Chronic Suppurative Otitis Media

Types	Pus Discharge	Perforation in Tympanic Membrane	Tympanum and Contents	Deafness	Imageology
Simple	Intermittent mucous pus	Central in the tense part	Red swelling	Mild, acoustic	Sclerosing mastoid
Carious (or granular)	Persistent mucous and stinky pus	Large or marginal	Polyp or granular	Severe, acoustic	Lump shadow & bone destruction
Epidermoid tumor	Persistent ill-stinky pus	In flaccid part, posterior & superior marginal	Grey white scales or white bean dreg-like substance	Mixed type	Regular margin of bone destruction

三型慢性化脓性中耳炎鉴别要点

分型	流脓	鼓膜穿孔	鼓室及内容	耳聋	影像学
单纯型	间歇黏液脓	紧张部中央性	红肿	轻,传音性	硬化型乳突
骨疡(或肉芽)型	持续黏臭脓	大或边缘性	息肉或肉芽	重,传音性	软组织影及骨破坏
表皮样瘤型	持续奇臭脓	松弛部、后上边缘性	灰白色鳞片或白色豆渣样物	混合性	骨破坏边缘整齐

2 Therapeutic methods

2 治疗方法

2.1 Therapeutic principles

2.1 治疗原则

The commonly seen patterns of chronic suppurative otitis media include pattern of dampness accumulation due to spleen deficiency, pattern of kidney qi deficiency, and pattern of kidney deficiency and liver hyperactivity. The treatment is mainly given to strengthen the spleen, benefit the kidney, and expel toxic substance and discharge pus by reinforcement.

慢性化脓性中耳炎的常见证型有脾虚挟湿、肾元亏虚和肾虚肝旺等证。治疗以健脾益肾、补托排脓为主。

2.2 Treatment based on syndrome differentiation

(1) Pattern of dampness accumulation due to spleen deficiency

Main symptoms: Long-term discharging ear, in intermittent nature, in large volume and thin quality, without smell, hearing loss or tinnitus, possible dizziness, lassitude, lustrousless complexion, poor appetite, tiredness, loose stool, central perforation, in turbid, thickened and calcium-spotted nature, in the tense part of the tympanic membrane, slight red or pale colour in the mucous membrane of the tympanum, conductive deafness by auditory test, pale tongue, white and greasy tongue coating, slow and feeble pulse.

Therapeutic methods: To strengthen the spleen, secrete dampness, expel toxin and discharge pus.

Herbal formulas and drugs: ① *Ginseng, Poria and Atractylodes Powder* (Shen Ling Bai Zhu San) plus *Two Wonderful Ingredients Pills* (Er Miao Wan) (modified). *Radix Codonopsis Pilosulae* (Dang Shen) 10g, *Sclerotium Poria* (Fu Ling) 10g, *Radix Astragali* (Huang Qi) 15g, *Rhizoma Atractylodis* (Cang Zhu) 6g, *Rhizoma Atractylodis Macrocephalae* (Bai Zhu) 6g, *Rhizoma Dioscoreae* (Shan Yao) 10g, *Cortex Phellodendri* (Huang Bo) 10g, and *Radix Glycyrrhizae* (Gan Cao) 3g. For loose stool, add *Rhizoma Cimicifugae* (Sheng Ma) 10g, and *Radix Bupleuri* (Chai Hu) 10g. For profuse pus, add *Semen Coicis* (Yi Yi Ren) 15g, and *Radix Platycodi* (Jie Geng) 6g. ② *Sevenlobed Yam and Dampness-Eliminating Decoction* (Bi Xie Shen Shi Tang)(modified). *Rhizoma Dioscorea Septemlobae* (Bi Xie) 15g, *Semen Coicis* (Yi Yi Ren) 30g, *Rhizoma Smilacis Glabrae* (Tu Fu Ling) 30g,

2.2 辨证论治

(1) 脾虚湿困

主症：耳流脓日久，多呈间歇性，量较多，质稀，无臭味，听力下降或有耳鸣。可有头晕乏力，面色少华，纳差，倦怠乏力，大便溏薄。鼓膜呈紧张部中央性穿孔、浑浊、增厚及钙斑，鼓室黏膜淡红或苍白，听力检查呈传导性聋。舌淡，苔白腻，脉缓弱。

治法：健脾渗湿，托毒排脓。

方药：①参苓白术散合二妙丸加减。党参 10 克，茯苓 10 克，黄芪 15 克，苍术 6 克，白术 6 克，山药 10 克，黄柏 10 克，甘草 3 克。若大便溏薄，加升麻 10 克、柴胡 10 克；流脓量多，加薏苡仁 15 克、桔梗 6 克。②萆薢渗湿汤加减。萆薢 15 克，薏苡仁 30 克，土茯苓 30 克，滑石 30 克，牡丹皮 12 克，泽泻 12 克，通草 12 克，黄柏 12 克。若便秘，加大黄 12 克；湿热较盛者，加龙胆草 12 克、栀子 12 克；剧痒者，加浮萍 9 克、白蒺藜 15 克。

Talcum (Hua Shi) 30g, *Cortex Moutan Radicis* (Mu Dan Pi) 12g, *Rhizoma Alismatis* (Ze Xie) 12g, *Medulla Tetrapanacis* (Tong Cao) 12g, and *Cortex Phellodendri* (Huang Bo) 12g. For constipation, add *Rhizoma Rhei* (Da Huang) 12g. For abundant dampness and heat, add *Radix Gentianae* (Long Dan) 12g, and *Fructus Gardeniae* (Zhi Zi) 12g. For serious itching, add *Herba Spirodelae* (Fu Ping) 9g, and *Fructus Tribuli* (Bai Ji Li) 15g.

(2) **Pattern of kidney qi deficiency**

(2) **肾元亏虚**

Main symptoms: Long-term discharging ear, in a little volume, with pus in filthy or bean-dreg nature and stinky smell, obvious hearing loss, possible accompanied by dizziness, slow spirit, lassitude, soreness and weakness in the low back and knee, perforation of the tympanic membrane in the flaccid part or in the margin, with grey-white or bean-dreg pus, granulation or polyp in the tympanum, conductive deafness or mixed deafness, bone destruction or soft tissue shadow present in CT or X-ray film of the mastoid, red tongue, scanty tongue coating, thready and feeble pulse.

主症：耳内流脓，日久不愈，量不多，脓液污秽或呈豆渣样，有恶臭味，听力明显减退。可有头晕，神疲乏力，腰膝酸软。鼓膜呈松弛部或边缘性穿孔，有灰白色或豆渣样脓，鼓室内有肉芽或息肉，传导性聋或混合性脓。乳突CT或X线片可显示骨质破坏或软组织影。舌红，苔少，脉细弱。

Therapeutic methods: To reinforce the kidney, build up primary qi, dissipate the decay and dissolve dampness.

治法：补肾培元，祛腐化湿。

Herbal formulas and drugs: *Anemarrhena, Phellodendron, and Rehmannia Pills* (Zhi Bai Di Huang Wan) (modified). Please see “External otitis”.

方药：知柏地黄丸加减。见“外耳道炎”。

2.3 Other therapies

2.3 其他疗法

Simple and proved formulas: ①*Coptis (or Corktree Bark) Ear Drops [Huang Lian (Huang Bo) Di Er Ye]*, in concentration of 20% to 30%, drip the ear, for three drops per session, for three times per

单验方：①黄连（或黄柏）滴耳液，浓度为20%～30%，滴耳，每次3滴，每日3次。②枯矾10克，冰片3克，

day. ②Alumen (Ku Fan) 10g, *Borneolum Syntheticum* (Bing Pian) 3g, *Aloe* (Lu Hui) 4g, *Halloysitum Rubrum* (Chi Shi Zhi) 10g, *Moschus* (She Xiang) 0. 3g (now man-made), and *Margarita* (Zhen Zhu) 4g. *Except Moschus* (She Xiang), the ingredients are grinded into power and mixed, for topical application, once per day.

芦荟4克,赤石脂10克,麝香0.3克(现用人工麝香),珍珠4克。除麝香外研细末,混合外用,每日1次。

Patency of Patulous Eustachian tube

咽鼓管异常开放症

It refers to the pathological change of uncomfortable sensation caused by ventilation higher than the normal state in the auditory tube, or in the persistent opening state. Clinically, it is mainly manifested by breezing-like respiration in the patient's ear. In the inspection, the internal and external flapping motion can be seen in the tympanic membrane with respiration. The pathogenic factors are numerous and can be divided into two types of organic reason and functional reason. The organic problem is seen in the diseases near the auditory tube, such as atrophic rhinitis, pharyngitis, catarrhal otitis media, or local tissue atrophy after nasopharyngeal surgery or after large-dose radiotherapy, or scar contracture and nerve paralysis, resulting in the loss of the normal closing and opening function of the auditory tube and hence persistent opening of the auditory tube. The functional problem is induced by excessive nervous tension, causing the opening muscles of the auditory tube in a state of high tension. This situation can gradually disappear naturally, while the spiritual state gets better. It be-

咽鼓管异常开放症是指咽鼓管通气高于常态,或总是处于开放状态而引起患者不适感觉的病变。临床主要表现为患者自己听到耳中吹风样呼吸声,检查时可见鼓膜随着呼吸而内外扇动。发病原因较多,分为器质性和功能性两类。器质性见于咽鼓管邻近部位的疾病,如萎缩性鼻炎、咽炎,或卡他性中耳炎,或鼻咽部手术后和接受大剂量放疗后局部组织萎缩,或瘢痕挛缩、神经麻痹,使咽鼓管失去正常的闭合功能,造成咽鼓管的持久开放。功能性如神经过度紧张,司咽鼓管开放的肌群处于高张力状态,这种情况随着精神状态转好,可逐渐自行恢复。该症属中医学“耳鸣”“耳痛”范畴。

longs to the scope of "tinnitus" and "ear pain" in Chinese medicine.

1 Diagnostic essentials

1.1 Self-listening of breezing-like tinnitus in low tone, identical to the rhythm of spontaneous respiration, with sound of tinnitus related the depth and velocity of respiration, tinnitus decreased or faded away in lying down or lowering the head, and tinnitus occurring or aggravated in speaking, swallowing, opening the mouth and yawning.

1.2 Autophony (self voice transmitted via the auditory tube, amplifying the voice), the patient feels uncomfortable and annoyed and unwilling to speak.

1.3 Stuffy sensation, ear pain, or flapping sensation inside the nose, also possible stuffy sensation in the ear, distending pain in the sick ear in deep breathing or blowing the nose, or an opening and closing sensation of the flapper in the nasopharynx during the respiration.

1.4 Internal and external flapping motion of the tympanic membrane with the respiration, present in the inspection, inward depression of the tympanic membrane during inhalation, and slight outward bulge during exhalation. In mild condition, flapping motion in the tympanic membrane can only be seen in the patient in pinching the nose and exhaling by closed mouth. In the nasopharyngeal inspection, scar adhesion can be seen in the pharyngeal recess, and the torus of the auditory tube becomes thin or its pharyngeal opening becomes larger.

1.5 In acoustic immittance inspection, abnormal pressure can be seen in the tympanum.

1 诊断要点

1.1 可闻及低音调的吹风样耳鸣，与自主呼吸节律一致，耳鸣声大小亦与呼吸深度、速度相关。平卧或低头时常可减轻或消失。说话、吞咽、张口、打哈欠时，耳鸣即可发生或加重。

1.2 自听过响(自己的说话声音经咽鼓管传入，致使声音放大)，患者感觉不适甚至十分烦恼而不愿说话。

1.3 耳闷、耳痛，或鼻内有活瓣感。亦可有耳中闷气的感觉。在深呼吸或擤涕时患耳有胀痛感，或在呼吸时感觉鼻咽部有活瓣开闭感。

1.4 检查时可见鼓膜随呼吸内外扇动。吸气时鼓膜向内凹陷，呼气时向外微凸。轻者在患者捏鼻闭口呼气时才可见到鼓膜扇动。鼻咽部检查见咽隐窝有瘢痕粘连，咽鼓管圆枕变薄或其咽口扩大。

1.5 声阻抗检查，可见鼓室内压力异常。

2 Therapeutic methods

2.1 Therapeutic principles

The commonly seen patterns of abnormal patency of Eustachian tube include pattern of spleen qi deficiency, and pattern of qi stagnation and blood stasis. The treatment is mainly given to benefit qi, strengthen the spleen, regulate qi, activate blood and dredge the aperture.

2.2 Treatment based on syndrome differentiation

(1) **Pattern of spleen qi deficiency**

Main symptoms: Long duration, flapping sensation inside the nose during respiration, loud self-listening, incommunicative, pale and lustrousless complexion, dizziness, lassitude, poor appetite, pale and swollen tongue, white or greasy tongue coating, thready and feeble pulse.

Therapeutic method: To reinforce qi, nourish blood, raise the clear and dredge the aperture.

Herbal formulas and drugs: *Center-Supplementing Qi-Boosting Decoction* (Bu Zhong Yi Qi Tang) (modified). *Radix Codonopsis Pilosulae* (Dang Shen) 10g, *Rhizoma Atractylodis Macrocephalae* (Bai Zhu) 10g, *Sclerotium Poria* (Fu Ling) 10g, *Radix Astragali* (Huang Qi) 15g, *Radix Puerariae* (Ge Gen) 10g, *Rhizoma Cimicifugae* (Sheng Ma) 10g, *Radix Angelicae Sinensis* (Dang Gui) 10g, *Flos Carthami* (Hong Hua) 6g, *Cortex Moutan Radicis* (Mu Dan Pi) 6g, and *Radix Glycyrrhizae* (Gan Cao) 3g.

(2) **Pattern of qi stagnation and blood stasis**

Main symptoms: Breezing-like tinnitus inside the ear, present with the respiration, sometimes

2 治疗方法

2.1 治疗原则

咽鼓管异常开放症常见证型有脾气虚弱、气滞血瘀等证。治疗以益气健脾、理气活血通窍为主。

2.2 辨证论治

(1) **脾气虚弱**

主症：病程较长，呼吸时鼻内有活瓣感，自听过响。患者沉默寡言，面白无华，头晕乏力，饮食量少。舌质淡胖，苔白或腻，脉细弱。

治法：补气养血，升清通窍。

方药：补中益气汤加减。党参 10 克，白术 6 克，茯苓 10 克，黄芪 15 克，葛根 10 克，升麻 10 克，当归 10 克，红花 6 克，牡丹皮 6 克，甘草 3 克。

(2) **气滞血瘀**

主症：耳内吹风样耳鸣，随自身呼吸产生。有时耳内

distending pain inside the ear, more obvious in blowing the nose, internal and external flapping motion in the tympanic membrane during the respiration, purple dark tongue, white tongue coating, choppy pulse.

胀痛，擤涕时尤为明显。检查见鼓膜随呼吸内外扇动。舌质紫暗，苔白，脉涩。

Therapeutic methods: To circulate qi, activate blood, disperse blood stasis and dredge the aperture.

治法：行气活血，化瘀通窍。

Herbal formulas and drugs: *Aperture-Opening and Blood-Activating Decoction* (Tong Qiao Huo Xue Tang) (modified). Please see "secretory otitis media".

方药：通窍活血汤加减。见"分泌性中耳炎"。

Sudden sensorineural hearing loss

突发性聋

It refers to sudden hearing loss of unknown reason, mostly in one ear. The incidence rate is in increasing tendency, but is not different in the males and females, and in the left side or right side. It belongs to the scope of "sudden deafness" in Chinese medicine.

突发性聋是指突然发生的原因不明的听力损失。多单耳发病，发病率有增加趋势，但男女及左右侧无差别。属中医学"暴聋"范畴。

1 Diagnostic essentials

1 诊断要点

1.1 Deafness can occur instantly, within several hours or several days, from mild to complete deafness, mostly in one ear, occasionally in the two ears in succession or at the same time. Some patients can be accompanied by the blocking sensation in the ear.

1.1 耳聋可在瞬间、几小时或几天内发生。其程度从轻度至全聋，多为单耳，偶有双耳先后或同时发生。部分患者可伴有耳内堵塞感。

1.2 Tinnitus is mostly manifested by bumming sound or cicada sound, as the primary symptom.

1.2 耳鸣多数为嗡嗡声或蝉鸣音，可为首发症状。

1.3 Vertigo is often rotatory, mostly accompanied by nausea, vomiting, cold sweating, and even rota-

1.3 眩晕常为旋转性，多伴有恶心、呕吐、出冷汗，甚至

tion of objects, and reluctance in opening the eyes.

视物旋转，不欲睁眼。

1.4 Conductive deafness is often present in the hearing test. The hearing loss of high frequency is more obvious. The loudness recruitment test is negative at the beginning and becomes positive afterward.

1.4 听力检查多呈感音神经性聋，高频段听力损失更明显。响度重振试验，初起阴性，后转为阳性。

1.5 No obvious abnormality is seen in CT scan of the middle ear and internal auditory canal.

1.5 中耳及内听道 CT 检查未见明显异常。

2 Therapeutic methods

2 治疗方法

2.1 Therapeutic principles

2.1 治疗原则

The commonly seen patterns of sudden deafness include pattern of invasion of pathogenic wind and heat, pattern of upward disturbance of liver fire, pattern of accumulation of phlegm and fire, pattern of qi stagnation and blood stasis. The treatment is mainly given to expel wind, clear away heat, sedate the liver, dissipate phlegm, regulate qi and disperse blood stasis.

突发性聋常见证型有风热侵袭、肝火上扰、痰火郁结、气滞血瘀等证。治疗以疏风清热、泻肝祛痰、理气化瘀为主。

2.2 Treatment based on syndrome differentiation

2.2 辨证论证

(1) Pattern of invasion of pathogenic wind and heat

(1) 风热侵袭

Main symptoms: Sudden tinnitus like breeze, hearing loss, or accompanied by distending and stuffy sensation in the ear, possibly accompanied by nasal obstruction, nasal discharging, cough, pain, fever, aversion to cold, and normal external auditory canal and tympanic membrane, red tongue, thin and yellow tongue coating, superficial and rapid pulse.

主症：突起耳鸣如吹风，听力下降，或伴有耳胀闷感。可伴有鼻塞、流涕、咳嗽、疼痛、发热恶寒等。外耳道、鼓膜如常。舌红，苔薄黄，脉浮数。

Therapeutic method: To expel wind, clear away heat, promote the lung in its spreading ability and dredge the aperture.

治法：疏风清热，宣肺通窍。

Herbal formulas and drugs: ① *Mulberry and*

方药：①桑菊饮加减。

Chrysanthemum Drink (Sang Ju Yin) (modified). *Folium Mori* (Sang Ye) 6g, *Flos Chrysanthemi* (Ju Hua) 10g, *Semen Armeniacae Amarum* (Ku Xing Ren) 10g, *Fructus Arctii* (Niu Bang Zi) 10g, *Herba Spirodelae* (Fu Ping) 10g, *Herba Menthae* (Bo He) (decoct later) 6g, *Fructus Aristolochiae* (Ma Dou Ling) 10g, *Fructus Liquidambaris* (Lu Lu Tong) 10g, *Periostracum Cicadae* (Chan Tui) 3g, and *Radix Glycyrrhizae* (Gan Cao) 3g. For bitter taste in the mouth and dry throat, add *Spica Prunellae* (Xia Ku Cao) 10g, and *Flos Chrysanthemi* (Ju Hua) 10g. ② *Lonicera and Forsythia Powder* (Yin Qiao San) (modified). Please see "External otitis".

桑叶6克，菊花10克，杏仁10克，牛蒡子10克，浮萍10克，薄荷(后下)6克，马兜铃10克，路路通10克，蝉蜕3克，甘草3克。若口苦、咽干，加夏枯草15克、菊花10克；②银翘散加减。见"外耳道炎"。

(2) **Pattern of upward disturbance of liver fire**

(2) **肝火上扰**

Main symptoms: Sudden anger, or emotional depression, sudden hearing loss, distending and stuffy sensation in the ear, loud tinnitus, complete tympanic membrane with clear landmarks, sensorineural deafness in the hearing test, possible dizziness, red tongue, thin and white tongue coating, wiry and rapid pulse.

主症：暴怒，或情志抑郁，听力突然减退，耳内胀闷不舒，耳鸣轰轰。检查见鼓膜完整标志清楚，听力呈感音神经性聋。可有头晕，面目红赤。舌质红，苔薄黄，脉弦数。

Therapeutic principles: To clarify the liver, discharge fire, circulate qi and dredge the aperture.

治法：清肝泻火，行气通窍。

Herbal formulas and drugs: *Gentian Liver-Draining Decoction* (Long Dan Xie Gan Tang) (modified). Please see "External otitis".

方药：龙胆泻肝汤加减。见"外耳道炎"。

(3) **Pattern of accumulation of phlegm and fire**

(3) **痰火郁结**

Main symptoms: Sudden hearing loss, or accompanied by tinnitus, possible dizziness, blurring vision, stuffy sensation in the chest, nausea, expectoration in yellow color, bitter taste or bland taste in the mouth, sensorineural deafness in the hearing test, red tongue, yellow and greasy tongue coating, rolling and rapid pulse.

主症：听力突然下降，或伴耳鸣。可有头晕目眩，胸闷，泛恶，咳痰色黄，口苦或淡而无味。听力呈感音神经性聋。舌红，苔黄腻，脉滑数。

Therapeutic principles: To dissolve phlegm, clear away heat, regulate qi and dredge the aperture.

治法：化痰清热，理气通窍。

Herbal formulas and drugs: *Ingredient-Added Double Vintage Decoction* (Jia Wei Er Chen Tang) (modified). *Pericarpium Citri Tangerinae* (Chen Pi) 6g, *Rhizoma Pinelliae* (Ban Xia) 10g, *Radix Scutellariae* (Huang Qin) 6g, *Rhizoma Coptidis* (Huang Lian) 3g, *Semen Trichosanthis* (Gua Lou Zi) 10g, *Rhizoma Arisaematis cum Bile* (Dan Nan Xing) 10g, *Fructus Aurantii Immaturus* (Zhi Shi) 6g, *Rhizoma Acori Graminei* (Shi Chang Pu) 3g, *Sclerotium Poria* (Fu Ling) 10g, and *Radix Glycyrrhizae* (Gan Cao) 3g.

方药：加味二陈汤加减。陈皮6克，半夏10克，黄芩6克，黄连3克，瓜蒌仁10克，胆南星10克，枳实6克，石菖蒲3克，茯苓10克，甘草3克。

(4) **Pattern of qi stagnation and blood stasis**

(4) **气滞血瘀**

Main symptoms: Sudden deafness, accompanied by tinnitus like cicada, not obvious general symptoms, sensorineural deafness in the hearing test, purple dark tongue or with speckle, thready and choppy pulse.

主症：突发耳聋，或伴耳鸣如蝉。全身症状可不明显。听力呈感音神经性聋。舌质紫暗或有瘀斑，脉细涩。

Therapeutic principles: To circulate qi, activate blood, dissolve blood stasis and dredge the aperture.

治法：行气活血，化瘀通窍。

Herbal formulas and drugs: ① *Aperture-Opening and Blood-Activating Decoction* (Tong Qiao Huo Xue Tang) (modified). Please see "secretory otitis media". ② *Peach Pit, Safflower and Four Agents Decoction* (Tao Hong Si Wu Tang) (modified). *Radix Angelicae Sinensis* (Dang Gui) 9g, *Rhizoma Ligustici Chuanxiong* (Chuan Xiong) 9g, *Radix Paeoniae Rubra* (Chi Shao) 9g, *Radix Rehmanniae Cruda* (Sheng Di Huang) 9g, *Semen Persicae* (Tao Ren) 9g, *Flos Carthami* (Hong Hua) 6g, *Sclerotium Poria* (Fu Ling) 15g, *Polyporus Umbellatus* (Zhu Ling) 9g, *Rhizoma Alismatis* (Ze Xie) 9g, *Rhizoma Atractylodis Macrocephalae* (Bai Zhu) 9g,

方药：①通窍活血汤加减。参见"分泌性中耳炎"。②桃红四物汤加减。当归、川芎、赤芍、生地、桃仁各9克，红花6克，茯苓15克，猪苓、泽泻、白术、桂枝、川贝母各9克。

Ramulus Cinnamomi (Gui Zhi) 9g, and *Bulbus Fritillariae Cirrhosae* (Chuan Bei Mu) 9g,

Meniere's disease

Meniere's disease is characterized by repeated rotatory vertigo, fluctuating sensorineural deafness, tinnitus and distending and full sensation in the ear. The pathological factor is unknown and may be related to autoimmunity, infection, traumatic injury, autonomic dysfunction, and congenital hypoplasia of the vestibular aqueduct and endolymphatic sac. The basic pathological change is labyrinthine hydrops. Mostly single-earorset, involving about 10% to 15% both ears. It often occurs in the young and middle-aged adults, with significant difference between the genders. It belongs to the scope of "vertigo" in Chinese medicine.

1 Diagnostic essentials

1.1 Sudden and serious rotatory vertigo lasts from several minutes to several hours, and fades away several hours later, accompanied by autonomic nerve reflex symptoms, such as nausea, vomiting, pale complexion, etc. It is often accompanied by tinnitus, deafness, and distending and full sensation in the ear. The symptoms are aggravated by opening the eyes or turning the head. The patient is conscious during vertigo. Vertigo can occur repeatedly but there is no vertigo in the intervals. Usually, it will fade away naturally. The interval usually will last from several days, to several months and to several years. The repeated seizure will shorten the in-

梅尼埃病

梅尼埃病的特点为反复发作旋转性眩晕、波动性感音神经性聋、耳鸣和耳内胀满感。病因不明，可能与自身免疫、感染、外伤、自主神经功能紊乱及先天性前庭水管与内淋巴囊发育不全有关。基本病理改变为膜迷路积水。多为单耳发病，累及双耳者约10%～15%。好发于青、中年，性别差异不显著。属中医学“眩晕”范畴。

1 诊断要点

1.1 突发剧烈旋转性眩晕，持续数十分钟至数小时，几小时后缓解。伴自主神经反射症状，如恶心、呕吐、面色苍白等。常伴有耳鸣、耳聋、耳内胀满感。睁眼或转头时，症状加重。眩晕时神志清醒，眩晕常反复发作，但间歇期无眩晕。一般能自行缓解。间歇期少则数日，多则数月，甚至数年。反复发作则间歇期缩短。发作时眩晕程度较剧烈，但患者神志清

tervals. During the seizure, vertigo is comparatively serious but the patient is conscious.

楚。

1.2 Tinnitus sounds like breeze at the beginning and like cicada after long time. There is distending and full sensation in the ear.

1.2 耳鸣初如吹风,久呈蝉鸣;耳内有胀满感。

1.3 The auditory function test shows mostly sensorineural deafness. The auditory curve in the early stage is present with hearing loss of low frequency, flat type or descending type in the later stage. The recruitment test is positive. The electrocochleogram shows enlargement in - SP, and - SP/AP larger than 40%. The otoacoustic emission chart shows early cochlear dysfunction. The auditory brain stem response (ABR) excludes retrocochlear lesions.

1.3 听功能检查多为感音神经性聋,听力曲线早期多呈低频听力受损,晚期呈平坦型或下降型。重振试验阳性。耳蜗电图示 - SP 增大,- SP/AP 大于 40%。耳声发射提示早期耳蜗功能受损。听性脑干反应(ABR)排除蜗后病变。

1.4 In the vestibular inspection, disturbance of balance function, spontaneous horizontal rotatory nystagmus and positional nystagmus are present during the seizure. In ENG check, spontaneous nystagmus can last for several days. Various types of vestibular ocular reflex show peripheral lesions. The caloric test shows weakness in the sick ear.

1.4 前庭功能检查见发作时有平衡功能障碍,自发水平旋转性眼震和位置性眼震。ENG 检查,自发性眼震可持续数日。各项前庭眼动反射示外周病变。变温试验,患耳反应减退。

1.5 Hennerbert sign is positive. In about 1/3 patients, in the active stage of labyrinthine hydrops, adhesion is formed between the membranous labyrinth (saccule) and pedal palate of the stapes. Vertigo and nystagmus are present in the decompression of the auditory canal.

1.5 Hennerbert 征阳性,约 1/3 患者,膜迷路积水活动期或膜迷路(球囊)与镫骨足板间有粘连形成,外耳道减压时出现眩晕和眼震。

1.6 The glycerol test is positive

After 50% glycerol saline is administrated, about 2.4 to 3 ml/kg. The hearing ability is tested again at the first hour, second hour and third hour after the administration. The hearing threshold decreasing over 10 to 15 dB in the three frequencies is positive.

1.6 甘油试验阳性

方法是服 50% 甘油盐水,2.4～3 ml/kg。服后第 1、第 2 及第 3 小时复测听力。三个频率听阈下降 10～15 dB 以上为阳性。

1.7 CT and MRI inspection of the temporal bone exclude the relevant vertigo problems caused by inflammation, traumatic injury, tumor and developing malformation, such as retarded endolymphatic hydrops, large vestibular aqueduct syndrome, and retrocochlear lesion, like acoustic neuroma.

1.7 颞骨 CT 及 MRI 检查排除有炎症、外伤、肿瘤、发育畸形等所致的相关眩晕疾病，如迟发性内淋巴积水、大前庭水管综合征及蜗后病变如听神经瘤等。

2 Therapeutic mehtods

2 治疗方法

2.1 Therapeutic principles

2.1 治疗原则

The commonly seen patterns of Meniere's disease include pattern of invasion of pathogenic wind, pattern of insufficiency of marrow sea, pattern of insufficiency of central qi, pattern of upward overflow of cold water, pattern of upward disturbance of liver yang, and pattern of central obstruction of phlegm and dampness. The treatment is given to expel wind, balance the liver, warm up yang, promote diuresis, regulate qi and dissolve phlegm, and to benefit the kidney and fill up essence, reinforce qi and raise yang.

梅尼埃病常见证型有风邪外袭、髓海不足、上气不足、寒水上犯、肝阳上扰和痰浊中阻等证。治疗以祛风平肝、温阳利水、理气化痰，配合益肾填精、补气升阳。

2.2 Treatment based on syndrome differentiation

2.2 辨证论治

(1) **Pattern of invasion of pathogenic wind and heat**

(1) **风热侵袭**

Main symptoms: Sudden vertigo, like motion sickness, nausea, vomiting, possibly accompanied by tinnitus like breeze, hearing loss, or distending and stuffy sensation in the ear, and simultaneously by nasal obstruction, nasal discharge, cough, pain, fever, and aversion to cold, but normal tympanic membrane, red tongue, thin and yellow tongue coating, superficial and rapid pulse.

主症：突发眩晕，如坐舟车，恶心呕吐，可伴耳鸣如吹风，听力下降，或伴耳胀闷感。同时伴有鼻塞、流涕、咳嗽、疼痛、发热恶寒等。外耳道、鼓膜如常。舌红，苔薄黄，脉浮数。

Therapeutic methods: To expel wind, clear away heat, promote the lung for its spreading ability and dredge the aperture.

治法：疏风清热，宣肺通窍。

Herbal formulas and drugs: ① *Mulberry and Chrysanthemum Drink* (Sang Ju Yin)(modified). *Folium Mori* (Sang Ye) 6g, *Flos Chrysanthemi* (Ju Hua) 10g, *Semen Armeniacae Amarum* (Ku Xing Ren) 10g, *Fructus Arctii* (Niu Bang Zi) 10g, *Herba Spirodelae* (Fu Ping Cao) 10g, *Herba Menthae* (Bo He) (decoct later) 6g, *Fructus Aristolochiae* (Ma Dou Ling) 10g, *Fructus Liquidambaris* (Lu Lu Tong) 10g, *Periostracum Cicadae* (Chan Tui) 3g, and *Radix Glycyrrhizae* (Gan Cao) 3g. For serious vertigo, add *Rhizoma Gastrodiae* (Tian Ma), *Ramulus Uncariae cum Uncis* (Gou Teng) and *Fructus Tribuli* (Bai Ji Li). For serious vomiting, add *Rhizoma Pinelliae* (Ban Xia), and *Caulis Bambusae in Taeniam* (Zhu Ru).

方药:①桑菊饮加减。桑叶 6 克,菊花 10 克,杏仁 10 克,牛蒡子 10 克,浮萍 10 克,薄荷(后下)6 克,马兜铃 10 克,路路通 10 克,蝉蜕 3 克,甘草 3 克,眩晕甚者,加天麻、钩藤、白蒺藜,呕吐甚者,加半夏、竹茹。

(2) **Pattern of insufficiency of marrow sea**

(2) **髓海不足**

Main symptoms: Repeated seizure of vertigo, tinnitus, deafness, low spirit, soreness and weakness of the low back and knee, insomnia, dreamfulness, vexation, poor memory, seminal emission, feverish sensation in the palms and soles, red tongue, scanty tongue coating, thready and rapid pulse.

主症:眩晕频发、耳鸣耳聋。精神萎靡,腰膝酸软,失眠多梦,心烦,记忆力差,遗精,手足心热。舌红苔少,脉细数。

Therapeutic methods: To nourish yin, replenish the kidney, fill up essence and benefit marrow.

治法:滋阴补肾,填精益髓。

Herbal formulas and drugs: *Lycium, Chrysanthemun and Rehmannia Pills* (Qi Ju Di Huang Wan) (modified). *Fructus Lycii* (Gou Qi Zi) 10g, *Flos Chrysanthemi* (Ju Hua) 10g, *Radix Rehmanniae Praeparata* (Shu Di Huang) 10g, *Fructus Corni* (Shan Zhu Yu) 10g, *Rhizoma Dioscoreae* (Shan Yao) 10g, *Cortex Moutan Radicis* (Mu Dan Pi) 6g, *Rhizoma Alismatis* (Ze Xie) 10g, and *Sclerotium Poria* (Fu Ling) 10g. For seizure of vertigo, add *Concha Haliotidis* (Shi Jue Ming), and *Concha*

方药:杞菊地黄丸加减。枸杞子 10 克,菊花 10 克,熟地黄 10 克,山茱萸 10 克,山药 10 克,牡丹皮 6 克,泽泻 10 克,茯苓 10 克。眩晕发作时加石决明、牡蛎;髓海不足甚者,加鹿角胶或龟甲胶。

Ostreae (Mu Li), For serious insufficiency of marrow sea, add *Colla Cornus Cervi* (Lu Jiao Jiao) or *Colla Plastri Testudinis* (Gui Jia Jiao).

(3) **Pattern of insufficiency of central qi**

Main symptoms: Intermittent vertigo, tinnitus, deafness, possibly accompanied by lustrousless complexion, tiredness, lassitude, shortness of breathing, reluctance in speaking, low voice, panting with exertion, poor appetite, loose stool, pale tongue, thready and feeble pulse.

Therapeutic methods: To reinforce and benefit qi and blood, strengthen the spleen and calm down the mind.

Herbal formulas and drugs: ① *Angelica Splenic Decoction* (Gui Pi Tang) (modified). *Radix Codonopsis Pilosulae* (Dang Shen) 10g, *Radix Astragali* (Huang Qi) 10g, *Rhizoma Atractylodis Macrocephalae* (Bai Zhu) 10g, *Sclerotium Poria* (Fu Ling) 10g, *Radix Angelicae Sinensis* (Dang Gui) 10g, *Arillus Longan* (Long Yan Rou) 10g, *Semen Zizyphi Spinosae* (Suan Zao Ren) 10g, *Fructus Tribuli* (Bai Ji Li) 10g, and *Radix Glycyrrhizae* (Gan Cao) 3g. ② *Eight Jewel Decoction* (Ba Zhen Tang)(modified). *Radix Angelicae Sinensis* (Dang Gui) 10g, *Rhizoma Ligustici Chuanxiong* (Chuan Xiong) 10g, *Radix Rehmanniae Praeparata* (Shu Di Huang) 15g, *Radix Paeoniae Albae* (Bai Shao) 12g, *Radix Codonopsis Pilosulae* (Dang Shen) 10g, *Rhizoma Atractylodis Macrocephalae* (Bai Zhu) 15g, *Sclerotium Poria* (Fu Ling)(peeled) 12g, *Radix Glycyrrhizae Praeparata* (Zhi Gan Cao) 10g, *Rhizoma Zingiberis Recens* (Sheng Jiang) 3 pieces, and *Fructus Ziziphi Jujubae* (Da Zao) 10 pieces. ③ *Center-Supplementing Qi-Boosting Pills* (Bu Zhong Yi Qi Wan). Please see

(3) **中气不足**

主症：眩晕时发，耳鸣耳聋。可伴面色不华，倦怠乏力，少气懒言，语声低微，动则喘促，食少便溏。舌淡，脉细弱。

治法：补益气血，健脾安神。

方药：①归脾汤加减。党参10克，黄芪10克，白术10克，茯苓10克，当归10克，龙眼肉10克，酸枣仁10克，白蒺藜10克，甘草3克。②八珍汤加减。当归10克，川芎10克，熟地黄15克，白芍药12克，党参10克，白术15克，茯苓（去皮）12克，炙甘草10克，生姜3片，大枣10枚；③补中益气汤。见“咽鼓管异常开放症”。

"Abnormal patency of Eustachian tube".

(4) **Pattern of upward overflow of cold water**

Main symptoms: Frequent vertigo, tinnitus, deafness, palpitation, cough with white sputum, nausea, clod sensation in the low back and back, cold sensation in the four limbs, low spirit, frequent nocturnal urination with profuse urine, pale and swollen tongue, white tongue coating, deep, thready and feeble pulse.

Therapeutic principles: To warm up the kidney, strengthen yang, promote diuresis and stop vertigo.

Herbal formulas and drugs: *True Warrior Decoction* (Zhen Wu Tang)(modified). *Radix Aconiti Praeparata* (Fu Zi) 6g, *Rhizoma Zingiberis Recens* (Sheng Jiang) 10g, *Rhizoma Atractylodis Macrocephalae* (Bai Zhu) 10g, *Sclerotium Poria* (Fu Ling) 10g, *Pericarpium Zanthoxyli* (Hua Jiao) 10g, *Herba Asari* (Xi Xin) 3g, *Ramulus Cinnamomi* (Gui Zhi) 6g, and *Radix Glycyrrhizae* (Gan Cao) 3g. For serious cold, use *Ramulus Cinnamomi* (Gui Zhi) in 12g and add *Radix Morindae Officinalis* (Ba Ji Tian) 10g.

(4) **寒水上泛**

主症:眩晕常作,耳鸣耳聋,心下悸动。咳嗽痰白,恶心欲呕,腰痛背冷,四肢不温,精神萎靡,夜尿频而清长。舌淡胖,苔白,脉沉细弱。

治法:温肾壮阳,利水止眩。

方药:真武汤加减。制附子 6 克,生姜 10 克,白术 10 克,茯苓 10 克,川椒 10 克,细辛 3 克,桂枝 6 克,甘草 3 克。若寒甚者,桂枝可用至 12 克,加巴戟天 10 克。

(5) **Pattern of upward disturbance of liver yang**

Main symptoms: Serious vertigo, occurring with emotional fluctuation, bad mood and vexation, loud tinnitus, bitter taste in the mouth, red eyes, flushed cheeks, irritability, easy anger, poor and dreamful sleep, red tongue, thin and yellow tongue coating, wiry and rapid pulse.

Therapeutic principles: To nourish yin, suppress yang, balance the liver and extinguish wind.

Herbal formulas and drugs: ① *Gastrodia and Uncaria Cool Decoction* (Tian Ma Gou Teng Yin) (modified). *Rhizoma Gastrodiae* (Tian Ma) 9g,

(5) **肝阳上扰**

主症:眩晕较剧,多发于情绪波动、心情不舒及烦恼之时。耳鸣轰轰,口苦咽干,目赤面红,烦躁易怒,少寐多梦。舌红苔薄黄,脉弦数。

治法:滋阴潜阳,平肝息风。

方药:①天麻钩藤饮加减。天麻 9 克,栀子 9 克,黄芩 9 克,桑寄生 9 克,杜仲 9

Fructus Gardeniae (Zhi Zi) 9g, *Radix Scutellariae* (Huang Qin) 9g, *Ramulus Loranthi* (Sang Ji Sheng) 9g, *Cortex Eucommiae* (Du Zhong) 9g, *Herba Leonuri* (Yi Mu Cao) 9g, *Caulis Polygoni Multiflori* (Ye Jiao Teng) 9g, *Poria cum Ligno Hospite* (Zhu Fu Shen) (processed with Cinnabar) 9g, *Ramulus Uncariae cum Uncis* (Gou Teng) (Decoct later) 12g, and *Radix Cyathulae* (Chuan Niu Xi) 12g. ② *Gentian Liver-Draining Decoction* (Long Dan Xie Gan Tang) (modified). Please see "External otitis". ③*Lycium, Chrysanthemun and Rehmannia Pills* (Qi Ju Di Huang Wan)(modified). Please see "pattern of insufficiency of marrow sea". ④*Free Wanderer Powder* (Xiao Yao San) (modified). *Radix Bupleuri* (Chai Hu) 15g, *Radix Angelicae Sinensis* (Chao Dang Gui) 15g, *Radix Paeoniae Albae* (Bai Shao) 15g, *Rhizoma Atractylodis Macrocephalae* (Bai Zhu) 15g, *Sclerotium Poria* (Fu Ling) 15g, *Radix Glycyrrhizae Praeparata* (Zhi Gan Cao) 6g, *Rhizoma Zingiberis Recens* (Sheng Jiang) 15g, and *Herba Menthae* (Bo He) 6g.

克，益母草9克，夜交藤9克，朱茯神9克，钩藤（后下）12克，川牛膝12克。②龙胆泻肝汤加减。参见“外耳道炎”。③杞菊地黄汤加减。见“髓海不足型”。④逍遥散加减。柴胡15克，炒当归15克，白芍药15克，白术15克，茯苓15克，炙甘草6克，生姜15克，薄荷6克。

(6) **Pattern of central obstruction of phlegm and dampness**

（6）**痰浊中阻**

Main symptoms: Vertigo, tinnitus, deafness, heavy sensation in the head, stuffy sensation in the chest, palpitation, serious nausea, profuse phlegm and saliva, poor appetite, tiredness, white and greasy tongue coating, soft and rolling or wiry and rolling pulse.

主症：眩晕，耳鸣耳聋。头重如蒙，胸闷不舒，心悸，呕恶甚，痰涎多，纳呆倦怠。舌苔白腻，脉濡滑或弦滑。

Therapeutic methods: To strengthen the spleen, dry up dampness, dissipate phlegm and stop vertigo.

治法：健脾燥湿，涤痰止眩。

Herbal formulas and drugs: ①*Pinellia, Atractylodes and Gastrodia Decoction* (Ban Xia Bai Zhu Tian Ma Tang) (modified). *Rhizoma Pinelliae*

方药：①半夏白术天麻汤加减。半夏10克，白术6克，天麻10克，陈皮6克，党

(Ban Xia) 10g, *Rhizoma Atractylodis Macrocephalae* (Bai Zhu) 6g, *Rhizoma Gastrodiae* (Tian Ma) 10g, *Pericarpium Citri Tangerinae* (Chen Pi) 6g, *Radix Codonopsis Pilosulae* (Dang Shen) 10g, and *Radix Astragali* (Huang Qi) 10g, *Radix Puerariae* (Ge Gen) 10g, *Fructus Tribuli* (Bai Ji Li) 10g, and *Radix Glycyrrhizae* (Gan Cao) 3g. For serious dampness, double the dose of *Rhizoma Pinelliae* (Ban Xia) and add *Rhizoma Alismatis* (Ze Xie) 10g. For fire hyperactivity, add *Radix Scutellariae* (Huang Qin) 6g, and *Radix Scrophulariae* (Xuan Shen) 10g. For qi deficiency, add *Radix Astragali* (Huang Qi) 15g, and *Radix Ginseng* (Ren Shen) 9g. ② Tangerine Peel and Pinellia with *Six Nobles Decoction* (Chen Xia Liu Jun Zi Tang)(modified). *Pericarpium Citri Tangerinae* (Chen Pi) 3g, *Rhizoma Pinelliae* (Ban Xia) 4.5g, *Radix Codonopsis Pilosulae* (Dang Shen) 10g, *Sclerotium Poria* (Fu Ling) 10g, *Rhizoma Atractylodis Macrocephalae* (Bai Zhu) 10g, and *Radix Glycyrrhizae Praeparata* (Zhi Gan Cao) 6g.

参10克，黄芪10克，葛根10克，白蒺藜10克，甘草3克。若湿重，倍半夏，加泽泻10克；上火者，加黄芩6克，玄参10克；气虚者加黄芪15克，人参9克。②陈夏六君子汤。陈皮3克，半夏4.5克，党参10克，茯苓10克，白术10克，炙甘草6克。

Chapter 2 Rhinologic Diseases

第2章 鼻科疾病

Nasal vestibulitis

鼻 前 庭 炎

It refers to the diffuse inflammation in the skin of the nasal vestibule. It is divided into the acute and chronic type and easily occurs in the patients with diabetes. The commonly seen pathogenic factors include acute and chronic rhinitis, nasosinusitis, foreign body in the nasal cavity or secondary infection caused by long-term harmful dust irritation and picking the nose. It belongs to the scope of "nose sores" in Chinese medicine.

鼻前庭炎是鼻前庭皮肤的弥漫性炎症。分急、慢性，糖尿病患者易发。常见病因有急慢性鼻炎，鼻窦炎，鼻腔异物或长期有害粉尘刺激，挖鼻等继发细菌感染所致。属中医学"鼻疮"范畴。

1 Diagnostic essentials

1.1 Acute condition is manifested by serious pain in the nasal vestibule, diffusive red swelling and erosion in the local and nearby skin.

1.2 Chronic condition is manifested by itching, burning hot, dry and foreign body sensation in the nasal vestibule, sparse nasal hair, thickened local skin, even with scabs or cracks, and possible bleeding after removal of scabs.

1.3 It is necessary to differentiate it from eczema of the nasal vestibule.

1 诊断要点

1.1 急性者，鼻前庭剧痛，局部及附近皮肤弥漫红肿、糜烂。

1.2 慢性者，鼻前庭痒、灼热、干和异物感，鼻毛稀疏脱落，局部皮肤增厚，甚或结痂或皲裂，揭痂后可有出血。

1.3 应与鼻前庭湿疹鉴别。

2 Therapeutic methods

2.1 Therapeutic principles

The commonly seen patterns of nasal vestibulitis include pattern of accumulation of heat in the lung meridian, pattern of accumulation of dampness and heat in the spleen and stomach, and pattern of dryness produced by blood deficiency. The treatment is mainly given to clear away heat from the lung and stomach, expel dampness and replenish blood.

2.2 Treatment based on syndrome differentiation

(1) **Pattern of accumulation of heat in the lung meridian**

Main symptoms: Local burning hot sensation, swelling, pain, erosion and yellow fluid discharge in the nasal vestibule, no obvious general symptoms, by accompanied possibly by headache, fever, cough, shortness of breath, constipation, red tongue, yellow tongue coating, and rapid pulse.

Therapeutic method: To expel wind, disperse the pathogens, clear away and discharge heat from the lung.

Herbal formulas and drugs: ① *Large-Flowered Skullcap Decoction* (Huang Qin Tang) combined with *Lung-Draining Powder* (Xie Bai San) (modified). *Cortex Mori Radicis* (Sang Bai Pi) 10g, *Radix Scutellariae* (Huang Qin) 6g, *Cortex Lycii Radicis* (Di Gu Pi) 10g, *Flos Lonicerae* (Jin Yin Hua) 10g, *Fructus Forsythiae* (Lian Qiao) 10g, *Flos Chrysanthemi* (Ju Hua) 10g, *Cortex Moutan Radicis* (Mu Dan Pi) 6g, and *Radix Glycyrrhizae* (Gan Cao) 3g. For serious itching, accompanied by aversion to cold, add *Herba Schizonepetae* (Jing Jie)

2 治疗方法

2.1 治疗原则

鼻前庭炎常见证型有肺经郁热、脾胃湿热、血虚化燥等。治疗以清肺胃之热、祛湿补血为法。

2.2 辨证论治

(1) **肺经郁热**

主症：鼻前庭局部灼热肿痛，糜烂，流黄水。无明显全身症状，但可有头痛发热，咳嗽气促，便秘。舌质红，苔黄，脉数。

治法：疏风散邪，清泄肺热。

方药：①黄芩汤合泻白散加减。桑白皮10克，黄芩6克，地骨皮10克，金银花10克，连翘10克，菊花10克，牡丹皮6克，甘草3克。若痒甚，伴有恶风，加荆芥10克、薄荷（后下）6克、蝉蜕3克；头痛，加川芎6克、蔓荆子10克；皮肤皲裂出血，加牡丹皮6克、赤芍药6克；大便干结，加生大黄6克、全瓜蒌10克。

10g, *Herba Menthae* (Bo He) (decoct later) 6g, and *Periostracum Cicadae* (Chan Tui) 3g. For headache, add *Rhizoma Ligustici Chuanxiong* (Chuan Xiong) 6g, and *Fructus Viticis* (Man Jing Zi) 10g. For cracks and bleeding of the skin, add *Cortex Moutan Radicis* (Mu Dan Pi) 6g, and *Radix Paeoniae Rubra* (Chi Shao) 6g. For constipation, add *Rhizoma Rhei Cruda* (Sheng Da Huang) 6g, and *Fructus Trichosanthis* (Gua Lou) 10g. ② *Lonicera and Forsythia Powder* (Yin Qiao San) (modified). (Please refer to "External otitis").

②银翘散加减。见"外耳道炎"。

(2) **Pattern of accumulation of dampness and heat in the spleen and stomach**

(2) **脾胃湿热**

Main symptoms: Local itching and erosion of the nasal vestibule, yellow exudation, lingering condition, possibly accompanied by abdominal distention, loose stool, red tongue, yellow and greasy tongue coating, rolling and rapid pulse.

主症：鼻前庭局部瘙痒，糜烂，黄色渗液，经久不愈。可有腹胀，大便溏薄。舌红，苔黄腻，脉滑数。

Therapeutic method: To clear away heat, remove dampness, resolve toxin and harmonize the center.

治法：清热利湿，解毒和中。

Herbal formulas and drugs: ① *Dampness-Removing and Stomach Scutellaria Decoction* (Chu Shi Wei Qin Tang) (modified). *Rhizoma Atractylodis* (Cang Zhu) 6g, *Cortex Magnoliae Officinalis* (Hou Pu) 3g, *Polyporus Umbellatus* (Zhu Ling) 10g, *Sclerotium Poria* (Fu Ling) 10g, *Rhizoma Alismatis* (Ze Xie) 10g, *Radix Scutellariae* (Huang Qin) 6g, *Talcum* (Hua Shi) 10g, *Pericarpium Citri Tangerinae* (Chen Pi) 6g, and *Radix Glycyrrhizae* (Gan Cao) 3g. For sticky condition in the mouth, add *Herba Agastachis* (Huo Xiang) 10g, and *Herba Eupatorii* (Pei Lan) 10g. For local itching, add *Radix Sophorae flavescentis* (Ku Shen) 10g, *Cortex*

方药：①除湿胃苓汤加减。苍术6克，厚朴3克，猪苓10克，茯苓10克，泽泻10克，黄芩6克，滑石10克，陈皮6克，甘草3克。若口中黏腻，加藿香10克、佩兰10克；局部瘙痒，加苦参10克、白鲜皮10克、地肤子10克。②萆薢渗湿汤加减。黄柏10克，木通10克，萆薢25克，薏苡仁25克，滑石15克，茯苓15克，丹皮12克。③参苓白术散。见"分泌性中耳炎"。

Dictamni (Bai Xian Pi) 10g and *Fructus Kochiae* (Di Fu Zi) 10g. ② *Wind-Expelling Powder* (Xiao Feng San) plus *Sevenlobed Yam and Dampness-Eliminating Decoction* (Bi Xie Shen Shi Tang)(modified). *Cortex Phellodendri* (Huang Bo) 10g, *Caulis Akebiae* (Mu Tong) 10g, *Semen Coicis* (Yi Yi Ren) 25g, *Talcum* (Hua Shi) 15g, *Sclerotium Poria* (Fu Ling) 15g, and *Cortex Moutan Radicis* (Mu Dan Pi) 12g. ③ *Ginseng, Poria and Atractylodes Powder* (Shen Ling Bai Zhu San) (modified). Please refer to "Secretory otitis media".

(3) **Pattern of dryness produced by blood deficiency**

Main symptoms: Itching, burning hot and dry pain in the nose, possibly accompanied by dry mouth and throat, sallow complexion, constipation, coarse, thickened and cracked skin in the nasal vestibule, with many crusts and scales, red tongue, scanty tongue coating, thready and rapid pulse.

Therapeutic method: To nourish yin, nourish blood, moisten dryness and extinguish wind.

Herbal formulas and drugs: *Rehmannia Decoction* (Di Huang Yin Zi) (modified). *Radix Rehmanniae Cruda* (Sheng Di Huang) 10g, *Radix Angelicae Sinensis* (Dang Gui) 10g, *Radix Paeoniae Albae* (Bai Shao) 10g, *Radix Adenophorae* (Nan Sha Shen) 15g, *Radix Ophiopogonis* (Mai Dong) 10g, *Rhizoma Polygonati* (Huang Jing) 10g, *Rhizoma Polygonati Odorati* (Yu Zhu) 10g, and *Radix Glycyrrhizae* (Gan Cao) 3g. For cracks and bleeding, add *Radix Paeoniae Rubra* (Chi Shao) 6g, and *Caumen Biotae* (Ce Bai Ye) 10g. For serious itching, add *Radix Salviae Miltiorrhizae* (Dan Shen) 10g, and Seedcoat Glycine max 10g.

(3) **血虚化燥**

主症:鼻部瘙痒,灼热干痛。可伴口干咽燥,面色萎黄,大便干结。鼻前庭皮肤粗糙、增厚或皲裂,有较多痂皮、鳞屑。舌红苔少,脉细数。

治法:滋阴养血,润燥熄风。

方药:地黄饮子加减。生地黄10克,当归10克,白芍药10克,南沙参15克,麦门冬10克,黄精10克,玉竹10克,甘草3克。若皲裂出血,加赤芍药6克、侧柏叶10克;痒甚,加丹参10克、穞豆衣10克。

2.3 Other therapies

(1) **Simple and proved formula** *Radix Scutellariae* (Huang Qin) 10g, and *Cortex Phellodendri* (Huang Bo) 10g: Decoct with water for oral administration, one dose per day, and take for two times, appropriate for acute stage of nasal vestibulitis.

(2) **External therapies** ① *Coptis Ointment* (Huang Lian Gao): Apply a little on the sick area, for three times per day, appropriate for local dryness and cracks of the nasal vestibule. ② *Cortex Phellodendri* (Huang Bo): Grind into powder and mix with a little sesame oil and smear on the sick area, appropriate for acute stage of nasal vestibulitis.

2.3 其他疗法

(1) **单验方**:黄芩10克,黄柏10克,水煎服,每日1剂,分2次服,适用于鼻前庭炎急性期。

(2) **外治法**:①黄连膏,取少许,涂于患处,每日3次,适用于鼻前庭炎局部干燥,皲裂者。②黄柏,研细末,少量麻油调和,敷于患处,适用于鼻前庭炎急性期。

Nasal vestibular eczema

It refers to allergic inflammation in the nasal vestibular and nearby skin, clinically manifested by polymorphous skin lesions of burning hot, itching and painful sensation, flushing, erosion, effusion and scabs in the skin of nasal vestibule, nasal wings, nasal tip and upper lip. It can be divided into acute type and chronic type and often occurs in children, and may be related to allergic reaction, endocrine disorder, metabolic dysfunction, and indigestion. It belongs to the scope of "nose sores" in Chinese medicine.

1 Diagnostic essentials

1.1 Acute stage is manifested by flushing, blisters, erosion, effusion and scabs in the skin of the nasal vestibule, around the nose and upper limb. Chronic

鼻前庭湿疹

鼻前庭湿疹是指发于鼻前庭及其周围皮肤的变态反应性炎症。临床主要表现为鼻前庭、鼻翼、鼻尖及上唇皮肤灼热痒痛、潮红、糜烂、渗液及结痂等多形性皮损。分为急性和慢性两型,多发于儿童,可能与变态反应、内分泌失调、代谢障碍、消化不良等有关。属中医学"鼻疮"范畴。

1 诊断要点

1.1 急性发作者,表现为鼻前庭、鼻孔周围、上唇皮肤痒痛潮红、水疱、糜烂、渗液、结

stage is manifested by itching, thickeness, coarseness, scales, cracks and ichenification in the skin of the sick area.

痂等；慢性期表现为患处皮肤发痒、增厚、粗糙、鳞屑、皲裂、苔藓化等。

1.2 The pathological condition is sometimes mild and sometimes severe and is easy to reoccur.

1.2 病情时轻时重，易于反复发作。

1.3 It showld be differentiated from nasal vestibulitis.

1.3 应与鼻前庭炎相鉴别。

2 Therapeutic methods

2 治疗方法

2.1 Therapeutic principles

2.1 治疗原则

Nasal vestibular eczema includes the commonly seen pattern of accumulation of heat in the lung meridian, pattern of dampness and heat in the spleen and stomach, and pattern of dryness produced by blood deficiency. The treatment is mainly given to clear away heat from the lung and stomach, and expel dampness and replenish blood.

鼻前庭湿疹多为肺经郁热、脾胃湿热、血虚化燥等常见证型。治疗以清肺胃之热、祛湿补血为法。

2.2 Treatment based on syndrome differentiation

2.2 辨证论治

(1) **Pattern of accumulation of heat in the lung meridian**

(1) **肺经郁热**

Main symptoms: Local itching, burning hot sensation, red swelling in the nasal vestibule, possible pain, erosion and effusion after scratch, possible without general symptoms, or possible headache, nasal obstruction, nasal discharge, fever, dry mouth, brown urine, dry stool, red tongue, yellow tongue coating, superficial and rapid pulse.

主症：鼻前庭局部瘙痒、灼热、红肿，若搔抓破溃后可疼痛、糜烂，有渗液。可无全身症状，或可有头痛，鼻塞，流涕，发热，口干，溲黄便干。舌质红，苔黄，脉浮数。

Therapeutic method: To clear away and discharge heat from the lung, expel wind and remove dampness.

治法：清泻肺热，疏风利湿。

Herbal formulas and drugs: *Large-Flowered Skullcap Decoction* (Huang Qin Tang) combined with *Lung-Draining Powder* (Xie Bai San) (modified). *Cortex Mori Radicis* (Sang Bai Pi) 10g,

方药：黄芩汤合泻白散加减。桑白皮 10 克，黄芩 6 克，地骨皮 10 克，金银花 10 克，连翘 10 克，菊花 10 克，甘

Radix Scutellariae (Huang Qin) 6g, *Cortex Lycii Radicis* (Di Gu Pi) 10g, *Flos Lonicerae* (Jin Yin Hua) 10g, *Fructus Forsythiae* (Lian Qiao) 10g, *Flos Chrysanthemi* (Ju Hua) 10g, and *Radix Glycyrrhizae* (Gan Cao) 3g. For serious itching, accompanied by aversion to wind, add *Herba Schizonepetae* (Jing Jie) 10g, *Herba Menthae* (Bo He) (decoct later) 6g, and *Periostracum Cicadae* (Chan Tui) 3g. For headache, add *Rhizoma Ligustici Chuanxiong* (Chuan Xiong) 6g, and *Fructus Viticis* (Man Jing Zi) 10g. For cracks and bleeding of the skin, add *Cortex Moutan Radicis* (Mu Dan Pi) 6g, and *Radix Paeoniae Rubra* (Chi Shao Yao) 6g. For constipation, add *Rhizoma Rhei Cruda* (Sheng Da Huang) 6g, and *Fructus Trichosanthis* (Gua Lou) 10g.

草3克。若痒甚,伴有恶风,加荆芥10克、薄荷(后下)6克、蝉蜕3克;头痛,加川芎6克、蔓荆子10克;皮肤皲裂出血,加牡丹皮6克、赤芍药6克;大便干结,加生大黄6克、全瓜蒌10克。

(2) **Pattern of dampness and heat in the spleen and stomach**

(2) **脾胃湿热**

Main symptoms: Serious itching, profuse blisters, effusion and wetness, and mild pain in the skin of the nasal vestibule, slight red tongue, yellow and greasy tongue coating, thready and feeble pulse.

主症:鼻前庭皮肤瘙痒较甚,水泡较多,渗液而潮湿不干,疼痛较轻。舌质偏红,苔黄腻,脉细弱。

Therapeutic method: To strengthen the spleen, remove dampness, clear away heat and resolve toxin.

治法:健脾利湿,清热解毒。

Herbal formulas and drugs: *Scutellaria and* Talcum *Decoction* (Huang Qin Hua Shi Tang)(modified). *Radix Scutellariae* 6g, *Talcum* (Hua Shi) 15g, *Polyporus Umbellatus* (Zhu Ling) 10g, *Sclerotium Poria* (Fu Ling) 10g, *Rhizoma Alismatis* (Ze Xie) 10g, *Medulla Tetrapanacis* (Tong Cao) 5g, and *Radix Glycyrrhizae* (Gan Cao) 3g. For local yellowish fluid, add *Rhizoma Coptidis* (Huang Lian) 3g. For sticky sensation in the mouth, add *Herba Agastachis* (Huo Xiang) 10g, and *Herba*

方药:黄芩滑石汤加减。黄芩6克,滑石15克,猪苓10克,茯苓10克,泽泻10克,通草5克,甘草3克。若局部黄水淋漓,加黄连3克;口中黏腻,加藿香10克、佩兰10克。

Eupatorii (Pei Lan) 10g.

(3) **Pattern of dryness produced by blood deficiency**

Main symptoms: Long duration, itching, uncomfortable, coarse, thickened, dry or lichenoid skin of the nasal vestibule, slight red tongue, thin and white tongue coating, thready and feeble pulse.

Therapeutic method: To nourish yin, nourish blood, moisten dryness and eliminate wind.

Herbal formulas and drugs: *Four Ingredients Wind-Eliminating Drink* (Si Wu Xiao Feng Yin) (modified). *Flos Carthami* (Hong Hua) 10g, *Radix Rehmanniae Praeparata* (Shu Di Huang) 10g, *Rhizoma Ligustici Chuanxiong* (Chuan Xiong) 6g, *Radix Angelicae Sinensis* (Dang Gui) 10g, *Radix Paeoniae Rubra* (Chi Shao) 6g, *Radix Ledebouriellae* (Fang Feng) 10g, *Radix Angelicae Dahuricae* (Bai Zhi) 10g, and *Radix Glycyrrhizae* (Gan Cao) 3g. For local red swelling and itching, add *Cortex Moutan Radicis* (Mu Dan Pi) 6g, and *Herba Lycopi* (Ze Lan) 10g. For dryness and cracks, add *Radix Adenophorae* (Nan Sha Shen) 10g, and *Radix Ophiopogonis* (Mai Dong) 10g.

(3) **血虚化燥**

主症：病程较长，鼻前庭皮肤瘙痒不适、粗糙、增厚、干燥，或呈苔藓化。舌淡红，苔薄白，脉细弱。

治法：滋阴养血，润燥消风。

方药：四物消风饮加减。红花10克，熟地黄10克，川芎6克，当归10克，赤芍药6克，防风10克，白芷10克，甘草3克。若局部红肿而痒，加牡丹皮6克、泽兰10克；干燥皲裂，加沙参10克、麦门冬10克。

2.3 Other therapies

(1) Simple and proved formula: ① *Caulis Lonicerae* (Ren Dong Teng) 20g, and *Radix Sophorae flavescentis* (Ku Shen) 20g: Decoct with water for oral administration, used for acute stage of nasal vestibular eczema in pattern of accumulation of heat in the lung meridian, and pattern of dampness and heat in the spleen and stomach. ② *Semen Coicis* (Yi Yi Ren) 30g, *Semen Oryza Sativae* (Jing Mi) 30g. for cooking congee, take twice per day, for pattern of acute and chronic nasal vestibular eczema.

2.3 其他疗法

(1) 单验方：①忍冬藤20克，苦参20克，水煎服。用于肺经郁热证和脾胃湿热证之鼻前庭湿疹急性期。②薏苡仁30克，粳米30克。煮粥，每日分2次食用。急、慢性鼻前庭湿疹均适合。

(2) External therapies: ① *Corktree Bark Powder* (Huang Bo Fen) or *Indigo Powder* (Qing Dai San). Blow herbal powder to the local area, for three times per day, used for pattern of accumulation of heat in the lung meridian, and pattern of dampness and heat in the spleen and stomach. ② *Coptis Ointment* (Huang Lian Gao). Smear on the local area, for three times per day, for pattern of dryness produced by blood deficiency.

(2) 外治法:①黄柏粉或青黛散。吹撒局部,每日 3 次。用于肺经郁热证和脾胃湿热证。②黄连膏。涂搽局部,每日 3 次,用于血虚化燥证。

Acute rhinitis

急性鼻炎

It refers to acute infectious inflammation of the mucous membrane of the nasal cavity, mainly caused by viral infection, combined with bacterial infection in the later stage. Many infectious diseases are manifested by rhinitis as the premonitory symptom. It can occur in four seasons, more frequently in the winter. It belongs to the scope of "cold and nasal obstruction" in Chinese medicine.

急性鼻炎系鼻腔黏膜的急性感染性炎症,主要为病毒感染,后期可合并细菌感染。许多急性传染病常以鼻炎为其前驱症状。四季均可发病,冬季更见。属中医"伤风鼻塞"范畴。

1 Diagnostic essentials

1 诊断要点

1.1 In the initial stage, there are dry and itching sensation and frequent sneezing in the nose and nasopharynx.

1.1 初期有鼻内和鼻咽部干燥、瘙痒感,频发喷嚏。

1.2 Nasal obstruction can be aggravated, frequently accompanied by wet red and dry nasal membrane. 1 to 2 days after the onset, there are nasal obstruction, profuse nasal discharge, congestion in the mucous membrane of the nose, and tenacious nasal discharge inside the nasal cavity, and sore throat, fever, and distending and stuffy sensation in the head for 1 to 2 days continuously. In the later

1.2 鼻塞,可逐渐加重。常伴有,鼻黏膜潮红、干燥。起病1～2 日后即有鼻塞、大量流清涕,鼻黏膜充血,鼻腔内有黏涕。常有咽痛、发热,头闷胀,持续 1～2 日。后期鼻塞,鼻涕为脓性,下鼻甲肿胀,鼻道多量脓涕,持续 3～5 日。

stage, there are purulent nasal discharge, tumefaction of the inferior nasal concha, and profuse purulent nasal discharge in the nasal passage, lasting for 3 to 5 days.

1.3 Nasal discharge is watery in the beginning, and becomes tenacious in 1 to 2 days, and becomes purulent in the later stage.

1.3 流涕，始为清水样涕，1～2日后转为黏涕，后期多量脓涕。

1.4 There can be general symptoms of fever, aversion to cold, fatigue, headache, uncomfortable sensation in the whole body, aching pain in the four limbs, and poor appetite, etc.

1.4 全身可有发热、恶寒、疲乏、头痛、周身不适、四肢酸痛、食欲下降等。

1.5 Local inspection shows flushing and dryness in the nasal membrane, swollen inferior nasal concha, tenacious or purulent nasal discharge in the nasal passage, etc.

1.5 局部检查：鼻黏膜潮红、干燥、下鼻甲肿大、鼻道黏涕或脓涕等。

1.6 White blood cell count is usually lower than normal level.

1.6 白细胞计数常偏低。

1.7 It should be differentiated from allergic rhinitis, acute infectious diseases (measles, scarlet fever, etc).

1.7 应与过敏性鼻炎，急性传染病（如麻疹、猩红热等）鉴别。

2 Therapeutic methods

2 治疗方法

2.1 Therapeutic methods

2.1 治疗原则

The commonly seen patterns of acute rhinitis include pattern of invasion of wind and cold into the lung, and pattern of invasion of wind and heat into the lung. The treatment is given to expel wind, and disperse cold and clear away heat in combination.

急性鼻炎的常见证型有风寒犯肺和风热犯肺证。治疗以疏风结合散寒和清热为法。

2.2 Therapeutic principles

2.2 辨证论治

(1) **Pattern of invasion of wind and cold into the lung**

(1) **风寒犯肺**

Main symptoms: Nasal obstruction, aggravated by exposure to cold, relieved by warmth, thin and

主症：鼻塞，遇寒加重，得热减轻，鼻涕清稀，量多，

clear nasal discharge, in profuse volume and white color, heavy and deep voice, headache, distending sensation in the head, or accompanied by aversion to cold, fever, swollen inferior nasal concha, edema in the mucous membrane, in light color, a little clear nasal discharge, slight red tongue, thin and white tongue coating, and superficial pulse.

色白。语声重浊,头痛头胀,或伴恶寒、发热。检查见下鼻甲肿大,黏膜水肿,色淡,少量清涕。舌质淡红,苔薄白,脉浮。

Therapeutic method: To expel wind, disperse cold, promote the lung for its spreading ability and dredge the aperture.

治法:疏风散寒,宣肺通窍。

Herbal formulas and drugs: ① *Schizonepeta and Ledebouriella Detoxifying Powder* (Jing Fang Bai Du San). *Herba Schizonepetae* (Jing Jie) 10g, *Radix Ledebouriellae* (Fang Feng) 10g, *Radix Angelicae Dahuricae* (Bai Zhi) 10g, *Flos Magnoliae Liliflorae* (Xin Yi Hua) 6g, *Fructus Xanthii* (Cang Er Zi) 10g, *Rhizoma Ligustici Chuanxiong* (Chuan Xiong) 6g, *Radix Glycyrrhizae* (Gan Cao) 3g. For aversion to cold, and no sweating, add *Herba Ephedrae* (Ma Huang) 10g. For headache, add *Fructus Viticis* (Man Jing Zi) 10g. For cough and profuse sputum, add *Semen Armeniacae Amarum* (Ku Xing Ren) 10g, and *Radix Peucedani* (Qian Hu) 10g. ② *Aperture-Dredging Decoction* (Tong Qiao Tang). *Herba Ephedrae* (Ma Huang) 12g, *Radix Ledebouriellae* (Fang Feng) 12g, *Rhizoma seu Radix Notopterygii* (Qiang Huo) 12g, *Rhizoma Ligustici* (Gao Ben) 12g, *Rhizoma Ligustici Chuanxiong* (Chuan Xiong) 10g, *Radix Angelicae Dahuricae* (Bai Zhi) 10g, *Radix Puerariae* (Ge Gen) 10g, *Herba Asari* (Xi Xin) 3g, *Rhizoma Cimicifugae* (Sheng Ma) 5g, *Pericarpium Zanthoxyli* (Hua Jiao) 5g, *Rhizoma Atractylodis* (Cang Zhu) 10g, and *Radix Glycyrrhizae* (Gan Cao) 10g.

方药:①荆防败毒散加减。荆芥 10 克,防风 10 克,白芷 10 克,辛夷 6 克,苍耳子 10 克,川芎 6 克,甘草 3 克。若恶寒、无汗,加麻黄 10 克;头痛,加蔓荆子 10 克;咳嗽痰多,加杏仁 10 克、前胡 10 克。②通窍汤。麻黄 12 克,防风 12 克,羌活 12 克,藁本 12 克,川芎 10 克,白芷 10 克,葛根 10 克,细辛 3 克,升麻 5 克,川椒 5 克,苍术 10 克,甘草 10 克。

(2) **Pattern of invasion of wind and heat into the lung**

Main symptoms: Intermittent severity of nasal obstruction, profuse nasal discharge, in tenacious nature and yellow or white color, headache, dry throat, cough, scanty and tenacious sputum difficult to cough up, or accompanied by fever, aversion to cold, swollen inferior nasal concha, endematous mucous membrane in red color, red tongue, thin and white or thin and yellow tongue coating, superficial and rapid pulse.

Therapeutic method: To expel wind, promote the lung for its spreading ability, clear away heat and dredge the aperture.

Herbal formulas and drugs: ① *Xanthium Powder* (Cang Er Zi San) (modified). *Fructus Xanthii* (Cang Er Zi) 10g, *Flos Magnoliae Liliflorae* (Xin Yi Hua) 6g, *Radix Angelicae Dahuricae* (Bai Zhi) 10g, *Radix Ledebouriellae* (Fang Feng) 10g, *Herba Menthae* (Bo He) (decoct later) 6g, *Flos Chrysanthemi* (Ju Hua) 10g, *Flos Lonicerae* (Jin Yin Hua) 10g, *Radix Scutellariae* (Huang Qin) 6g, *Fructus Aristolochiae* (Ma Dou Ling) 10g, and *Radix Glycyrrhizae* (Gan Cao) 3g. For profuse yellow nasal discharge, add *Herba Houttuyniae* (Yu Xing Cao) 10g, and *Folium Isatidis* (Da Qing Ye) 15g. For headache, add *Rhizoma Ligustici Chuanxiong* (Chuan Xiong) 6g, and *Fructus Viticis* (Man Jing Zi) 10g. For cough and profuse sputum, add powder of *Bulbus Fritillariae Cirrhosae* (Chuan Bei Mu) (drink after infused) 3g, and *Concretio Siliceae Bambusae* (Tian Zhu Huang) 6g. ② *Lonicera and Forsythia Powder* (Yin Qiao San) (modified). Please refer to "External otitis". ③ *Mulberry and*

(2) **风热犯肺**

主症：鼻塞时轻时重，鼻涕量多，质黏稠，色黄或白。头痛、咽干、咳嗽、痰少而黏，不易咳出，或伴发热、恶寒；检查见下鼻甲肿大，黏膜水肿，色红。舌红，苔薄白或薄黄，脉浮数。

治法：疏风宣肺，清热通窍。

方药：①苍耳子散加减。苍耳子10克，辛夷6克，白芷10克，防风10克，薄荷（后下）6克，菊花10克，金银花10克，黄芩6克，马兜铃10克，甘草3克。若涕黄量多，加鱼腥草10克、大青叶15克；头痛甚，加川芎6克、蔓荆子10克；咳嗽痰多，加川贝粉（另冲服）3克、天竺黄6克。②银翘散。见“外耳道炎”。③桑菊饮。见“突发性聋”。

Chrysanthemum Drink (Sang Ju Yin). Please refer to "sudden deafness".

2.3 Other therapies

(1) Chinese patent medicines: ① *Climbing Groundsel and Selaginella Rhinitis Tablets* (Qian Bai Bi Yan Pian): Take three tablets each time, for three times per day, used for pattern of invasion of wind and heat into the lung. ② *Sinusitis Oral Liquid* (Bi Yuan Shu Kou Fu Ye) or *Nasosinusitis Oral Liquid* (Bi Dou Yan Kou Fu Ye): Take 10 mL each time, for 2 to 3 times per day, used for cold and nasal obstruction in pattern of pathogenic wind and heat.

(2) Simple and proved formula: *Flos Magnoliae Liliflorae* (Xin Yi Hua) 10g. and *Flos Chrysanthemi* (Ju Hua) 15g: Decoct with water for oral administration, one dose per day, and take in two times.

(3) External therapies: Nose-teaming method: Use 30 grams of vinegar and add a little water, and heat it hot and steam the nose, for three sessions per day, and ten minutes for each time.

2.3 其他疗法

（1）中成药：①千柏鼻炎片，每次3片，每日3次，用于风热犯肺证；②鼻渊舒口服液或鼻窦炎口服液：每次10毫升，每日2～3次，用于风热型伤风鼻塞。

（2）单验方：辛夷10克，菊花15克。水煎，每日1剂，分2次服。

（3）外治法：薰鼻法，用食醋30克，加水少许，烧热，用热气薰鼻，每日3次，每次10分钟。

Chronic rhinitis

It refers to chronic inflammation in the nasal mucous membrane and lower layer of the mucous membrane, characterized by nasal obstruction, tumefaction of the mucous membrane, and increased secretions. Generally, it is divided into chronic simple rhinitis and chronic hypertrophic rhinitis. It belongs to the scope of "chronic rhinitis" in Chinese medicine.

慢 性 鼻 炎

慢性鼻炎是鼻黏膜和黏膜下层的慢性炎症，以鼻塞、黏膜肿胀、分泌物增多为特点。一般分为慢性单纯性鼻炎和慢性肥厚性鼻炎两类。属中医学"鼻窒"范畴。

1 Diagnostic essentials

1.1 Chronic simple rhinitis

① typical symptoms of intermittent or alternative nasal obstruction, nasal discharge, hyposmia; ② tumefaction in the inferior nasal concha, without obvious hypertrophy, and sensitive to vasoconstrictor, ③ and it is needed to check the abnormal structure of the nasal cavity and have CT scan of the nasal sinus if necessary.

1.2 Chronic hypertrophic rhinitis

① serious nasal obstruction, mostly persistent, hyposmia, heavy nasal voice, and tenacious nasal discharge difficult to blow out, ② hypertrophic, pale and uneven inferior nasal concha, and like mulberry fluid in severe condition, poor contractive effect by reducing decongestant, and ③ it is needed to exclude sinusitis, nasal polyp, and tumor in the nasal cavity, etc.

1.3 Chronic simple rhinitis should be differentiated from chronic hypertrophic rhinitis

Please see the following table.

1 诊断要点

1.1 慢性单纯性鼻炎

①有间歇性或交替性鼻塞、流涕、嗅觉减退等典型临床症状;②下鼻甲肿胀,不伴明显增生,对血管收缩剂反应敏感;③注意鼻腔结构异常,必要时行鼻窦 CT 检查。

1.2 慢性肥厚性鼻炎

①鼻塞较重,多为持续性,嗅觉减退,鼻音重,黏涕不易擤出。②下鼻甲肥大、苍白,表面不光滑,严重者呈桑葚状。减充血剂收缩效果差。③需排除鼻窦炎、鼻息肉、鼻腔肿瘤等。

1.3 慢性单纯性鼻炎和慢性肥厚性鼻炎鉴别

见下表。

Differentiation betweenchronic simple rhinitis and chronic hypertrophic rhinitis

Types	Chronic simple rhinitis	chronic hypertrophic rhinitis
Nasal obstruction	Intermittent or alternative	Persistent
Nasal discharge	Mucous	Mucous or sticky purulent, difficult to blow out
Hyposmia	Not obvious	Possible
Obstructive nasal voice	Nil	Yes
Headache, dizziness	Possible	Often yes
Dry throat, sore throat	Possible	Often yes
Tinnitus, ear obstruction	Possible	Possible
Inferior nasal concha	Tumefaction, smooth surface, dark red color, soft, and elastic in membrane	Hypertrophic membrane, in dark red color, smooth or uneven surface, or in nodes, mulberry fruit or lobular shape, and hard sense
Reaction to 1% ephedrine	Obvious contractive in membrane, shrunken inferior nasal concha	No contraction or slight contraction in mucous membrane, no obvious change in its size.

慢性单纯性鼻炎和慢性肥厚性鼻炎鉴别要点

分型	慢性单纯性鼻炎	慢性肥厚性鼻炎
鼻塞	间歇性或交替性	持续性
鼻涕	黏液性	黏液性或黏脓性,不易擤出
嗅觉减退	不明显	可有
闭塞性鼻音	无	有
头痛,头昏	可有	常有
咽干,咽痛	可有	常有
耳鸣,耳闭塞感	可有	可有
下鼻甲	黏膜肿胀,表面光滑,暗红色,柔软,有弹性	黏膜肥厚,暗红色,表面光滑或不平,或呈结节状、桑葚状或分叶状,有硬实感
对1%麻黄素的反应	黏膜收缩明显,下鼻甲缩小	黏膜不收缩或轻微收缩,下鼻甲大小无明显改善

2 Therapeutic methods

2.1 Therapeutic principles

The commonly seen patterns of chronic rhinitis include pattern of accumulation of heat in the lung meridian, pattern of deficiency and cold of lung qi, pattern of abundant dampness due to spleen deficiency, and pattern of qi stagnation and blood stasis. The treatment is mainly given to clear away heat from the lung, regulate qi, dissolve dampness, and correct deficiency for benefiting the lung and strengthen the spleen.

2.2 Treatment based on syndrome differentiation

(1) Pattern of accumulation of heat in the lung meridian

Main symptoms: Intermittent nasal obstruction, heavy voice, scanty nasal discharge, in tenacious nature and yellow color, headache, distention in the head, dry throat, cough, scanty, yellow and tenacious sputum, difficult to cough up, even respiration by opening the mouth, irritability, poor sleep, tu-

2 治疗方法

2.1 治疗原则

慢性鼻炎的常见证型有肺经郁热、肺气虚寒、脾虚湿盛,气滞血瘀等。治疗驱邪以清热泻肺、理气化湿,补虚以益肺健脾为主。

2.2 辨证论治

(1)肺经郁热

主症:间歇性鼻塞,语声重浊,涕不多,质黏稠,色黄。头痛头胀,咽干,咳嗽,痰少而黄稠不易咳出,甚则张口呼吸,烦躁,影响睡眠。检查见下鼻甲肿大,黏膜水肿,色

mefaction in the inferior nasal concha, edematous mucous membrane, good contraction by 1% ephedrine, red tongue, yellow tongue coating, rapid or wiry and rapid pulse.

红，用1%麻黄素收缩良好。舌质红，苔黄，脉数或弦数。

Therapeutic method: To expel wind, promote the lung for its spreading ability, clear away heat and dredge the aperture.

治法：疏风宣肺，清热通窍。

Herbal formulas and drugs: *Xanthium Powder* (Cang Er Zi San) (modified). *Fructus Xanthii* (Cang Er Zi) 10g, *Flos Magnoliae Liliflorae* (Xin Yi Hua) 6g, *Radix Angelicae Dahuricae* (Bai Zhi) 10g, *Herba Menthae* (Bo He) (decoct later) 6g, *Herba Agastachis* (Huo Xiang) 10g, *Flos Chrysanthemi alba* (Bai Ju Hua) 10g, *Cortex Mori Radicis* (Sang Bai Pi) 10g, *Radix Scutellariae* (Huang Qin) 6g, *Cortex Moutan Radicis* (Mu Dan Pi) 6g, *Fructus Aristolochiae* (Ma Dou Ling) 10g, and *Radix Glycyrrhizae* (Gan Cao) 3g. For severe heat and yellow nasal discharge, add *Flos Lonicerae* (Jin Yin Hua) 10g, *Herba Taraxaci* (Pu Gong Ying) 10g, and *Folium Isatidis* (Da Qing Ye) 15g. For headache, add *Rhizoma Ligustici Chuanxiong* (Chuan Xiong) 6g, and *Fructus Viticis* (Man Jing Zi) 10g. For cough and profuse sputum, add powder of *Bulbus Fritillariae Cirrhosae* (Chuan Bei Mu) (drink after infused) 3g, *Radix Peucedani* (Qian Hu) 10g. and *Concretio Siliceae Bambusae* (Tian Zhu Huang) 6g.

方药：苍耳子加减。苍耳子10克，辛夷6克，白芷10克，薄荷（后下）6克，藿香10克，白菊花10克，桑白皮10克，黄芩6克，牡丹皮6克，马兜铃10克，甘草3克。若热重、涕黄，加金银花10克、蒲公英10克、大青叶15克；头痛，加川芎6克、蔓荆子10克；咳嗽痰多，加川贝粉（冲服）3克、前胡10克、天竺黄6克。

(2) **Pattern of deficiency and cold of lung qi**

（2）**肺气虚寒**

Main symptoms: Alternative nasal obstruction, aggravated by exposure to cold, or relieved sometimes or worsen sometimes, pale tumefaction of the mucous membrane inside the nose, accompanied by cough with thin sputum, shortness of breathing,

主症：交替性鼻塞，遇寒加重；或时轻时重，鼻涕黏稀。检查见鼻内黏膜肿胀色淡，伴有咳嗽痰稀，气短，面白。舌质淡红，苔薄白，脉缓

pale complexion, slight red tongue, thin and white tongue coating, slow or thready and feeble pulse.

或细弱。

Therapeutic method: To replenish the lung, benefit qi, disperse cold and dredge the aperture.

治法：补肺益气，散寒通窍。

Herbal formulas and drugs: *Lung-Warming and Nose-Drying Elixi* (Wen Fei Zhi Liu Dan)(modified). *Radix Codonopsis Pilosulae* (Dang Shen) 10g, *Herba Schizonepetae* (Jing Jie) 10g, *Radix Astragali* (Huang Qi) 10g, *Herba Asari* (Xi Xin) 3g, *Fructus Terminaliae Chebulae* (He Zi) 10g, *Fructus Schisandrae* (Wu Wei Zi) 10g, *Rhizoma Atractylodis Macrocephalae* (Bai Zhu) 6g, *Radix Platycodi* (Jie Geng) 6g, *Flos Magnoliae Liliflorae* (Xin Yi Hua) 6g, *Rhizoma Acori Graminei* (Shi Chang Pu) 6g, and *Radix Glycyrrhizae* (Gan Cao) 3g. For pale and swelling nasal mucous membrane, add *Ramulus Cinnamomi* (Gui Zhi) 6g.

方药：温肺止流丹加减。党参10克，荆芥10克，黄芪10克，细辛3克，诃子10克，五味子10克，白术6克，桔梗6克，辛夷6克，石菖蒲6克，甘草3克。若鼻黏膜苍白肿胀，加桂枝6克。

(3) **Pattern of abundant dampness due to spleen deficiency**

(3) **脾虚湿盛**

Main symptoms: Long-term nasal obstruction and loud voice, tenacious and profuse nasal discharge, hyposmia, poor appetite, loose stool, stuffy sensation in the chest and epigastric region, pale and lustrousless complexion, figure, lassitude, pale tongue, white and greasy tongue coating, slow and feeble pulse.

主症：病久鼻塞声重，鼻涕稠而量多，嗅觉减退；纳差、便溏、胸脘闷胀，面白无华，体倦乏力，舌淡，苔白腻，脉缓弱。

Therapeutic method: To strengthen the spleen, secrete dampness, dissolve the turbid and dredge the aperture.

治法：健脾渗湿，化浊通窍。

Herbal formulas and drugs: *Ginseng, Poria and Atractylodes Powder* (Shen Ling Bai Zhu San)(modified). *Radix Codonopsis Pilosulae* (Dang Shen) 10g, *Rhizoma Dioscoreae* (Shan Yao) 10g, *Rhizoma Atractylodis Macrocephalae* (Bai Zhu) 6g,

方药：参苓白术散加减。党参10克，山药10克，白术6克，茯苓10克，薏苡仁15克，扁豆10克，石菖蒲6克，路路通10克，辛夷6克，苍术

Sclerotium Poria (Fu Ling) 10g, *Semen Coicis* (Yi Yi Ren) 15g, *Semen Dolichoris* (Bian Dou) 10g, *Rhizoma Acori Graminei* (Shi Chang Pu) 6g, *Fructus Liquidambaris* (Lu Lu Tong) 10g, *Flos Magnoliae Liliflorae* (Xin Yi Hua) 6g, *Rhizoma Atractylodis* (Cang Zhu) 6g, and *Radix Glycyrrhizae* (Gan Cao) 3g. In summer, add *Herba Agastachis* (Huo Xiang) 10g, and *Herba Eupatorii* (Pei Lan) 10g, and *Herba Elsholtziae* (Xiang Ru) 10g. For afraid of cold, add *Ramulus Cinnamomi* (Gui Zhi) 6g, and *Herba Asari* (Xi Xin) 3g.

6克,甘草3克。若逢暑季,加藿香10克、佩兰10克、香薷10克;畏寒者,加桂枝10克、细辛3克。

(4) **Pattern of qi stagnation and blood stasis**

Main symptoms: Persistent nasal obstruction, profuse nasal discharge, hyposmia, or headache, dry mouth, tumefaction in the nasal mucous membrane, firm nasal concha, in mulberry fruit shape or uneven surface, insensitive to 1% ephedrine, dark red tongue or with purple spot, thin and white tongue coating, choppy pulse.

Therapeutic method: To regulate and harmonize qi and blood, remove stagnation and dissolve blood stasis.

Herbal formulas and drugs: ① Angelica and Peony Decoction (Dang Gui Shao Yao Tang)(modified). *Radix Angelicae Sinensis* (Dang Gui) 10g, *Rhizoma Atractylodis Macrocephalae* (Bai Zhu) 6g, *Radix Paeoniae Rubra* (Chi Shao) 6g, *Rhizoma Ligustici Chuanxiong* (Chuan Xiong) 6g, *Rhizoma Alismatis* (Ze Xie) 10g, *Sclerotium Poria* (Fu Ling) 10g, *Semen Persicae* (Tao Ren) 10g, *Flos Carthami* (Hong Hua) 10g, *Lumbricus* (Di Long) 10g, and *Radix Glycyrrhizae* (Gan Cao) 3g. For headache and dizziness, add *Radix Angelicae Dahuricae* (Bai Zhi) 10g, *Fructus Tribuli* (Bai Ji Li) 10g, and

(4) **气滞血瘀**

主症:持续性鼻塞,较多黏涕,嗅觉迟钝。或有头痛,口干。检查见鼻黏膜肿胀,鼻甲硬实,呈桑椹样或表面不平,1%麻黄素收缩不敏感。舌质暗红或有紫斑,苔薄白,脉涩。

治法:调和气血,行滞化瘀。

方药:①当归芍药汤加减。当归10克,白术6克,赤芍6克,川芎6克,泽泻10克,茯苓10克,桃仁10克,红花10克,地龙10克,甘草3克。若头痛头昏,加白芷10克、白蒺藜10克、蔓荆子10克;咳嗽痰多,加桔梗6克、瓜蒌仁10克、杏仁10克。②通窍活血汤。见“分泌性中耳炎”。

Fructus Viticis (Man Jing Zi) 10g. For cough and profuse sputum, add *Radix Platycodi* (Jie Geng) 6g, *Semen Trichosanthis* (Gua Lou Zi) 10g, and *Semen Armeniacae Amarum* (Ku Xing Ren) 10g. ② *Aperture-Opening and Blood-Activating Decoction* (Tong Qiao Huo Xue Tang). Please refer to "Secretory otitis media".

2.3 Other therapies

(1) Chinese patent medicines: ① *Climbing Groundsel and Selaginella Rhinitis Tablets* (Qian Bai Bi Yan Pian). Take three tablets each time, for three times per day. ② *Sinusitis Oral Liquid* (Bi Yuan Shu Kou Fu Ye) or *Nasosinusitis Oral Liquid* (Bi Dou Yan Kou Fu Ye). Take 10 mL each time, for 2 to 3 times per day, used for pattern of wind and head in the lung meridian, and pattern of accumulation of heat in the liver and gallbladder. ③ *Magnolia Granules* (Xin Yi Ke Li). Take 5 grams each time, for three times per day, used for pattern of insufficiency of lung qi, and pattern of infection of exogenous wind.

(2) Simple and proved formula: *Magnolia Powder* (Xin Yi San). *Grind Rhizoma Ligustici Chuanxiong* (Chuan Xiong), *Caulis Akebiae* (Mu Tong), *Radix Ledebouriellae* (Fang Feng), *Radix Glycyrrhizae* (Gan Cao), *Flos Magnoliae Liliflorae* (Xin Yi Hua), *Herba Asari* (Xi Xin), *Rhizoma Ligustici* (Gao Ben), *Rhizoma Cimicifugae* (Sheng Ma), *Radix Angelicae Dahuricae* (Bai Zhi), in equal portion, into fine powder, and take 5 grams each time, after infused with tea water.

(3) External therapies: ① *Green Jade Powder* (Bi Yu San). *Grind Herba Centipedae* (E Bu Shi Cao), *Rhizoma Ligustici Chuanxiong* (Chuan

2.3 其他疗法

(1) 中成药:①千柏鼻炎片,每服3片,每日3次;②鼻渊舒口服液或鼻窦炎口服液:每次10毫升,每日2～3次,用于肺经风热及肝胆郁热证;③辛芩颗粒,每次5克,每日3次,用于肺气不足,风邪外感证。

(2) 单验方:辛夷散。川芎、木通、防风、甘草、辛夷、细辛、藁本、升麻、白芷,上药各等分共研细末,每服5克,清茶调服。

(3) 外治法:①碧玉散。鹅不食草、川芎、细辛、辛夷、青黛,上药各等分,共研细

Xiong), *Herba Asari* (Xi Xin), *Flos Magnoliae Liliflorae* (Xin Yi Hua), and *Indigo Naturalis* (Qing Dai), in equal portion, into the fine powder, and take a little to blow into the nose each time. ② *Yellow Croaker Earstone Powder* (Yu Nao Shi San). Inhale into the nose the fine powder made of *Asteriscus Pseudosciaenae* (Yu Nao Shi) 9g, *Borneolum Syntheticum* (Bing Pian) 6g, *Flos Magnoliae Liliflorae* (Xin Yi Hua) 6g, and *Herba Asari* (Xi Xin) 3g.

末,和匀,每取少许,吹鼻。②鱼脑石散。鱼脑石粉9克,冰片1克,辛夷6克,细辛3克,共为细末,吸鼻中。

Atrophic rhinitis

萎缩性鼻炎

It refers to gradual atrophic process of the nasal membrane. Its pathogenic factors are unknown and may be related to nutrition, heredity and environmental pollution. It belongs to the scope of "atrophic rhinitis" in Chinese medicine.

萎缩性鼻炎是鼻腔黏膜逐渐萎缩的过程,病因不甚明确。与营养、遗传和环境污染有关。属中医"鼻槁"范畴。

1 Diagnostic essentials

1 诊断要点

1.1 There are typical clinical symptoms of dry sensation in the nasal cavity and throat, nasal obstruction, hyposmia or loss of smelling sense, nasal bleeding, dizziness, headache and stink, etc.

1.1 具有典型临床症状,如鼻腔和咽部干燥感、鼻塞、嗅觉减退或消失、鼻出血、头昏、头痛及鼻恶臭等。

1.2 There are dilated nasal cavity, dry mucosa, atrophy of nasal concha, large volume of gray green purulent dry scabs, etc.

1.2 鼻腔宽大,黏膜干燥,鼻甲萎缩,大量灰绿色脓性干痂等。

2 Therapeutic methods

2 治疗方法

2.1 Therapeutic principles

2.1 治疗原则

The commonly seen patterns of atrophic rhinitis include pattern of lung dryness due to yin deficiency, and pattern of qi and blood deficiency. The treatment is mainly given to nourish blood, benefit

萎缩性鼻炎常见症型有阴虚肺燥症和气血虚弱证。治疗以养血益阴润燥为主。

yin and moisten dryness.

2.2 Treatment based on syndrome differentiation

(1) Pattern of lung dryness due to yin deficiency

Main symptoms: Dry, burning hot and painful sensation in the nose, atrophy of nasal muscular membrane, hyposmia, profuse nasal scabs, yellow and green and turbid nasal discharge, mixed with blood streak, aggravated in dry weather, possibly accompanied by dry and sore throat, cough, lassitude, and reluctance in speaking, feverish sensation in the chest, palms and soles, red tongue, scanty tongue coating, thready and rapid pulse.

Therapeutic method: To nourish yin, moisten dryness, promote the lung for its spreading ability and disperse the pathogens.

Herbal formulas and drugs: ① Dryness-Eliminating and Lung-Rescuing Decoction (Qing Zao Jiu Fei Tang)(modified). *Folium Mori* (Sang Ye) 10g, *Gypsum Fibrosum* (Shi Gao) (Decoct first) 30g, *Colla Corii Asini* (E Jiao) (Melt first) 10g, *Radix Ophiopogonis* (Mai Dong) 10g, *Semen Sesami* (Hu Ma Ren) 10g, *Radix Codonopsis Pilosulae* (Dang Shen) 10g, *Radix Glycyrrhizae* (Gan Cao) 3g, *Semen Armeniacae Amarum* (Ku Xing Ren) 10g, and *Folium Eriobotryae* (Pi Pa Ye) 10g. For serious dry nose, add *Rhizoma Glehniae* (Bei Sha Shen) 10g, *Herba Dendrobii* (Shi Hu) 10g, and *Cortex Mori Radicis* (Sang Bai Pi) 10g. For epistaxis, add *Caumen Biotae* (Ce Bai Ye) 10g, *Radix Rubiae* (Qian Cao) 10g, and *Cortex Moutan Radicis* (Mu Dan Pi) 6g. For soreness and pain of low back and knee due to kidney yin deficiency, add *Fructus Ligustri Lucidi* (Nü Zhen Zi) 10g, *Herba Ecliptae* (Han Lian Cao) 10g, *Tuber Asparagi* (Tian Men Dong) 10g,

2.2 辨证论治

(1) 阴虚肺燥

主症：鼻内干燥，灼热疼痛，鼻内肌膜萎缩，嗅觉减退，鼻痂多，有黄绿色浊涕，间有血丝，每于气候干燥之时症状加重；可伴咽喉干痛，咳嗽，乏力懒言，五心烦热。舌红少苔，脉细数。

治法：养阴润燥，宣肺散邪。

方药：①清燥救肺汤加减。桑叶10克，石膏（先煎）30克，阿胶（烊化）10克，麦门冬10克，胡麻仁10克，党参10克，甘草3克，杏仁10克，枇杷叶10克。若鼻干燥较甚，加沙参10克、石斛10克、桑白皮10克；鼻衄者，加侧柏叶10克、茜草10克、牡丹皮6克；肾阴虚而腰膝酸痛，加女贞子10克、旱莲草10克、天门冬10克、干地黄10克。②百合固金汤。熟地15克，生地10克，麦门冬7.5克，贝母5克，百合5克，当归5克，炒芍药5克，甘草5克，玄参4克，桔梗4克。

and *Radix Rehmanniae* (Di Huang) 10g. ② *Lily Metal-Consolidating Decoction* (Bai He Gu Jin Tang): *Radix Rehmanniae Praeparata* (Shu Di Huang) 15g, *Radix Rehmanniae Cruda* (Sheng Di Huang) 10g, *Radix Ophiopogonis* (Mai Dong) 7.5g, *Bulbus Fritillariae Cirrhosae* (Chuan Bei Mu) 5g, *Bulbus Lilii* (Bai He) 5g, *Radix Angelicae Sinensis* (Dang Gui) 5g, *Radix Paeoniae* (Shao Yao) 5g, *Radix Glycyrrhizae* (Gan Cao) 5g, *Radix Scrophulariae* (Xuan Shen) 4g, and *Radix Platycodi* (Jie Geng) 4g.

(2) **Pattern of qi and blood deficiency**

Main symptoms: Comparatively serious atrophy of the nasal muscular membrane, stinky nasal discharge like thick liquid and like crease, or with yellow green purulent scabs, poor appetite, abdominal distension, fatigue, loose stool, pale tongue, white tongue coating, thready and feeble pulse.

Therapeutic method: To replenish middle-Jiao, benefit qi, nourish blood and moisten dryness.

Herbal formulas and drugs: *Center-Supplementing Qi-Boosting Decoction* (Bu Zhong Yi Qi Tang) (modified). *Radix Codonopsis Pilosulae* (Dang Shen) 10g, *Radix Astragali* (Huang Qi) 10g, *Rhizoma Atractylodis Macrocephalae* (Bai Zhu) 6g, *Sclerotium Poria* (Fu Ling) 10g, *Radix Ophiopogonis* (Mai Dong) 10g, *Rhizoma Dioscoreae* (Shan Yao) 10g, *Radix Glycyrrhizae* (Gan Cao) 3g, and *Fructus Ziziphi Jujubae* (Hong Zao) 10g. For ulcerative nasal membrane, stinky breath, add *Cortex Phellodendri* (Huang Bo) 10g, *Radix Sophorae flavescentis* (Ku Shen) 10g, and *Rhizoma Atractylodis* (Cang Zhu) 6g. For hyposmia, add *Fructus Xanthii* (Cang Er Zi) 10g, *Flos Magnoliae Liliflorae* (Xin

(2) **气血虚弱**

主症：鼻窍肌膜萎缩较甚，鼻涕腥臭如浆如酪或有黄绿色脓痂，纳差腹胀，倦怠疲乏，大便溏薄。舌质淡，苔白，脉细弱。

治法：补中益气，养血润燥。

方药：补中益气汤加减。党参10克，黄芪10克，白术6克，茯苓10克，麦门冬10克，山药10克，百合10克，甘草3克，红枣10克。若鼻黏膜溃烂，鼻气腥臭，加黄柏10克、苦参10克、苍术6克；嗅觉失灵，加苍耳子10克、辛夷6克、白芷10克；鼻黏膜萎缩较甚，加红花10克、桃仁10克、丹参10克。

Yi Hua) 6g, and *Radix Angelicae Dahuricae* (Bai Zhi) 10g. For serious atrophy of the nasal membrane, add *Flos Carthami* (Hong Hua) 10g, *Semen Persicae* (Tao Ren) 10g, and *Radix Salviae Miltiorrhizae* (Dan Shen) 10g.

2.3 Other therapies

(1) Chinese patent medicines: ① Rehmannia Pills with Six Ingredients (Liu Wei Di Huang Wan). Take 6 grams each time, for three times per day, appropriate for pattern of lung dryness due to yin deficiency. ② Center-Supplementing Qi-Boosting Pills (Bu Zhong Yi Qi Wan). Take 9 grams each time, for 2 to 3 times per day, appropriate for pattern of qi and blood deficiency.

(2) Simple and proved formula: Reed Rhizome Decoction (Lu Gen Tang). Decoct *Rhizoma Phragmitis* (Lu Gen) 30g, and *Flos Magnoliae Liliflorae* (Xin Yi Hua) 10g. with water for oral administration, one dose per day, and take in two times, used for various patterns of atrophic rhinitis.

(3) External therapies: *Coptis Ointment* (Huang Lian Gao): Smear a little inside the nasal cavity, for three times per day.

2.3 其他疗法

（1）中成药：①六味地黄丸。每服 6 克，每日 3 次，适用于阴虚肺燥证。②补中益气丸。每服 9 克，每日 2～3 次，适用于气血虚弱证。

（2）单验方：芦根汤。芦根 30 克，辛夷 10 克。水煎，每日 1 剂，分 2 次服。用于萎缩性鼻炎各症型。

（3）外治法：黄连油膏，取少许涂擦鼻腔内，每日 3 次。

Allergic rhinitis

It refers to chronic inflammatory reaction of the nasal membrane, due to the release of media (mainly histamine) by IgE mediated mast cells, after the specific individuals contact with allergens, together with participation of many inflammatory cells and histocytes. It is seasonal and perennial. It belongs to the scope of "allergic rhinitis" in Chinese

变应性鼻炎

变应性鼻炎是特应性个体接触致敏原后 IgE 介导肥大细胞释放介质（主要是组胺）和多种炎性细胞、组织细胞等参与的鼻黏膜慢性炎症反应，分季节性和常年性。属中医学“鼻鼽”范畴。

medicine.

1 Diagnostic essentials

1.1 Typical symptoms

Nasal itching, sneezing, clear nasal discharge and nasal obstruction, possibly accompanied by itching in the throat and eye, conjunctival congestion and edema, swelling of eyelids, also hyposmia,

1.2 Inspection

Pale color, edema or congestion in the mucous membrane of the interior nasal concha, clear, thin and profuse secretions in the nasal cavity.

1.3 In the initial stage, the eosinophil granulocytes are positive by nasal secretion smear.

1.4 Allergic skin test presents positive reaction and elevation of serum IgE.

2 Therapeutic methods

2.1 Therapeutic principles

The commonly seen patterns of allergic rhinitis include pattern of invasion of wind and cold into the lung, pattern of accumulation of heat in the lung meridian, pattern of qi deficiency in the lung and spleen, and pattern of kidney yang deficiency. In the seizure stage, the treatment is mainly given to expel wind, cut off allergen, and to clarify the lung and benefit qi as well. In the remission stage, the treatment is mainly given to replenish and benefit the lung, spleen and kidney.

2.2 Treatment based on syndrome differentiation

(1) **Pattern of invasion of wind and cold into the lung**

Main symptoms: Paroxysmal nasal itching, sneezing, and clear nasal discharge, accompanied by nasal obstruction, or cough with white sputum,

1 诊断要点

1.1 典型症状

鼻痒、喷嚏、清涕和鼻塞。可伴咽痒、眼痒、结膜充血、水肿和眼睑肿胀等。也可有嗅觉减退。

1.2 检查

下鼻甲黏膜苍白、水肿或充血、肿胀。鼻腔内分泌物清稀量多。

1.3 鼻分泌物涂片在发病期嗜酸性粒细胞阳性。

1.4 变应性皮肤试验呈阳性反应，血清 IgE 升高。

2 治疗方法

2.1 治疗原则

变应性鼻炎常见证型有风寒犯肺、肺经郁热、肺脾气虚和肾阳虚弱等证。发作期治疗以祛风截敏为主，佐以清肺、益气等法。缓解期以补益肺脾肾三脏为主。

2.2 辨证论治

(1) 风寒犯肺

主症：发作性鼻痒、喷嚏、清涕，伴鼻塞，或有咳嗽痰白，恶风，鼻黏膜色淡白，水肿。舌

aversion to wind, pale and edematous nasal membrane, slight red tongue, thin and white tongue coating, superficial and tense pulse.

淡红，苔薄白，脉浮紧。

Therapeutic method: To expel wind, promote the lung for its spreading ability, dissipate cold and dredge the aperture.

治法：疏风宣肺，祛寒通窍。

Herbal formulas and drugs: Cinnamon-Twig Decoction (Gui Zhi Tang) (modified). *Ramulus Cinnamomi* (Gui Zhi) 5g, *Radix Paeoniae Albae* (Bai Shao) 10g, *Rhizoma Zingiberis Recens* (Sheng Jiang) 2 pieces, *Fructus Ziziphi Jujubae* (Da Zao) 5g, *Radix Ledebouriellae* (Fang Feng) 10g, *Flos Magnoliae Liliflorae* (Xin Yi Hua) 6g, and *Radix Glycyrrhizae* (Gan Cao) 3g. For serious nasal obstruction, add *Fructus Aristolochiae* (Ma Dou Ling) 10g, and *Fructus Liquidambaris* (Lu Lu Tong) 10g.

方药：桂枝汤加减。桂枝 5 克，白芍药 10 克，生姜 2 片，大枣 5 克，防风 10 克，辛夷 6 克，甘草 3 克。若鼻塞重，加马铃兜 10 克、路路通 10 克。

(2) **Pattern of accumulation of heat in the lung meridian**

(2) **肺经郁热**

Main symptoms: Repeated paroxysmal nasal itching, sneezing, and clear nasal discharge, in scanty volume, nasal obstruction, intermittent dryness in the nasal cavity, thirst with preference of drinks, red and swelling nasal membrane, red tongue, white or yellow tongue coating, and rapid pulse.

主症：反复发作鼻痒，喷嚏，鼻流清涕，量不多，鼻塞，间歇性鼻腔干燥，口渴喜饮。鼻黏膜色红，肿胀。舌红，苔白或黄，脉数。

Therapeutic method: To clear away heat, promote the lung for its descending ability, cool blood and induce desensitization.

治法：清热肃肺，凉血脱敏。

Herbal formulas and drugs: Desensitization-Inducing Decoction (Tuo Ming Tang)(modified). *Radix Arnebiae seu Lithospermi* (Zi Cao) 10g, *Radix Rubiae* (Qian Cao) 10g, *Herba Ecliptae* (Han Lian Cao) 10g, *Radix Cynanchi Paniculati* (Xu Chang Qing) 10g, *Periostracum Cicadae* (Chan Tui) 3g,

方药：脱敏汤加减。紫草 10 克，茜草 10 克，旱莲草 10 克，徐长卿 10 克，蝉蜕 3 克，辛夷 10 克，鹅不食草 10 克，甘草 3 克。若嗅觉差，加苍耳子 10 克、白芷 10 克。

Flos Magnoliae Liliflorae (Xin Yi Hua) 10g, *Herba Centipedae* (E Bu Shi Cao) 10g, and *Radix Glycyrrhizae* (Gan Cao) 3g. For poor smelling sense, add *Fructus Xanthii* (Cang Er Zi) 10g, and *Radix Angelicae Dahuricae* (Bai Zhi) 10g.

(3) **Pattern of qi deficiency in the lung and spleen**

Main symptoms: Long duration, repeated nasal itching, sneezing, profuse clear nasal discharge, nasal obstruction, seizure or aggravation after fatigue, or cough, expectoration, poor appetite, loose stool, and weakness in the limbs, pale nasal membrane, serious edema, slight red tongue, thin and white or white and greasy tongue coating, thready and feeble pulse.

Therapeutic method: To replenish and benefit the lung and spleen, raise yang and consolidate Wei-defensive qi.

Herbal formulas and drugs: *Jade Wind-Barrier Powder* (Yu Ping Feng San) plus *Center-Supplementing Qi-Boosting Decoction* (Bu Zhong Yi Qi Tang) (modified). *Radix Astragali* (Huang Qi) 15g, *Radix Codonopsis Pilosulae* (Dang Shen) 10g, *Radix Ledebouriellae* (Fang Feng) 10g, *Rhizoma Atractylodis Macrocephalae* (Bai Zhu) 6g, *Sclerotium Poria* (Fu Ling) 10g, *Rhizoma Cimicifugae* (Sheng Ma) 10g, *Radix Puerariae* (Ge Gen) 10g, and *Radix Glycyrrhizae* (Gan Cao) 3g. For serious nasal obstruction, add Rhizoma Zingiberis (Gan Jiang) 10g, and *Herba Asari* (Xi Xin) 3g.

（3）**肺脾气虚**

主症：病程长，反复鼻痒、喷嚏，鼻流清涕量多，鼻塞，每在疲劳后发作或症状加重。或有咳嗽咯痰、食少、大便溏薄、肢体乏力等证。鼻黏膜苍白、水肿较甚。舌淡红，苔薄白或白腻，脉细弱。

治法：补益肺脾，升阳固卫。

方药：玉屏风散合补中益气汤加减。黄芪 15 克，党参 10 克，防风 10 克，白术 6 克，茯苓 10 克，升麻 10 克，葛根 10 克，甘草 3 克。若鼻塞甚，加干姜 10 克、细辛 3 克。

(4) **Pattern of kidney yang deficiency**

Main symptoms: Long duration, paroxysmal nasal itching, sneezing, clear nasal discharge, nasal obstruction, hyposmia, aversion to cold, cold limbs, loose stool, frequent nocturnal urination,

（4）**肾阳虚弱**

主症：病程长，发作性鼻痒、喷嚏，鼻流清涕，鼻塞失嗅。畏寒、肢冷，大便溏薄，夜尿频多。鼻黏膜苍白，或

pale or green grey nasal membrane, swollen nasal concha, pale tongue, white tongue coating, deep and thready pulse.

呈青灰色,鼻甲肿大。舌淡,苔白,脉沉细。

Therapeutic method: To warm and replenish the kidney, consolidate Wei-defensive qi and dredge the aperture.

治法:温补肾阳,固卫通窍。

Herbal formulas and drugs: *Golden Chamber Kidney Qi Pills* (Jin Kui Shen Qi Wan) (modified). *Radix Aconiti Praeparata* (Fu Zi) 5g, *Cortex Cinnamomi* (Rou Gui) 5g, *Radix Rehmanniae Praeparata* (Shu Di Huang) 15g, *Fructus Corni* (Shan Zhu Yu) 10g, *Rhizoma Dioscoreae* (Shan Yao) 10g, *Cortex Moutan Radicis* (Mu Dan Pi) 6g, *Rhizoma Alismatis* (Ze Xie) 10g, *Sclerotium Poria* (Fu Ling) 10g, and *Radix Glycyrrhizae* (Gan Cao) 3g. For aversion to wind, and perspiration, add *Radix Astragali* (Huang Qi) 15g.

方药:金匮肾气丸加减。制附子5克,肉桂5克,熟地黄15克,山萸肉10克,山药10克,牡丹皮6克,泽泻10克,茯苓10克,甘草3克。若恶风、汗出,加黄芪15克。

2.3 Other therapies

2.3 其他疗法

(1) Simple and proved formula: Decoct *Flos Magnoliae Liliflorae* (Xin Yi Hua) 15g, Herba Centipedae (E Bu Shi Cao) 10g. with water for oral administration, one dose each day, used for various patterns of allergic rhinitis.

(1) 单验:辛夷15克,鹅不食草10克。水煎服,每日1剂。用于变应性鼻炎各型。

(2) Chinese patent medicines: ① *Center-Supplementing Qi-Boosting Pills* (Bu Zhong Yi Qi Wan): Take 9 grams each time, for 2 to 3 times per day, appropriate for pattern of qi and blood deficiency. ② *Asarum and Scutellaria Granules* (Xin Qin Ke Li) or *Jade Wind-Barrier Granules* (Yu Ping Feng Ke Li): Take 5 grams each time, for 3 times per day, appropriate for pattern of qi deficiency in the lung and spleen. ③ *Golden Chamber Kidney Qi Pills* (Jin Kui Shen Qi Wan): Take 5 grams each time, twice per day, appropriate for pattern of kid-

(2) 中成药:①补中益气丸,每服9克,每日2~3次,适用于气血虚弱证;②辛芩颗粒或玉屏风颗粒,每服5克,每日3次,适用于肺脾气虚证;③金匮肾气丸,每服5克,每日2次,适用于肾阳虚证。

ney qi deficiency.

(3) External therapies ① *Magnolia and Centipeda Nasal Drops* (Xin Yi E Bu Shi Cao Di Bi Ye): Drip the nose, twice per day. ② Please refer to the herbal products for external therapies in "chronic rhinitis".

(3) 外治法:①辛夷鹅不食草滴鼻液,滴鼻,每日 2 次。②可参考"慢性鼻炎"的药物外治方法。

Nasal polyp

鼻 息 肉

It refers to high edematous neoplasm in the nasal cavity and sinus mucosa, mostly in the ethmoidal sinus, mainly characterized by nasal obstruction, hyposmia clinically, polyp presents in the nasal inspection, mostly in the middle nasal passage. It is related to the allergic reaction and chronic irritating stimulation. It belongs to the scope of "nasal polyp" in Chinese medicine.

鼻息肉是鼻腔及鼻窦黏膜高度水肿性赘生物,以筛窦为多见。主要临床表现为鼻塞、失嗅,鼻腔检查可见息肉,以中鼻道为多见。与变态反应及慢性炎症刺激有关。属中医学"鼻痔"范畴。

1 Diagnostic essentials

1 诊断要点

1.1 Unilateral or bilateral nasal obstruction, possibly accompanied by hyposmia.

1.1 单侧或双侧鼻塞,可伴嗅觉减退。

1.2 Accompanied by nasosinusitis, often disturbed by symptoms of distending pain in the head, and yellow and turbid nasal discharge.

1.2 伴有鼻窦炎者,常有头胀痛、流涕黄浊等症状。

1.3 When bilateral nasal polyp grows big, there will be an appearance of "frog nose".

1.3 双侧性鼻息肉生长过大时,可有"蛙鼻"外观。

1.4 In inspection, single or multiple gray white or light gray, in even surface, semi-transparent swollen stuffs are present, in shape of fresh lyche pulp, with pedicle, soft and uneasy to bleed by touching.

1.4 检查可见鼻腔单个或多个灰白或淡灰色,表面光滑、半透明肿物,形同新鲜荔枝肉状,可带蒂,质软,触之不易出血。

1.5 The sinus lesions and resource of polyp can be confirmed by nasal endoscopy, X-ray radiography or CT scan.

1.5 鼻内镜、X 线摄片或 CT 扫描可明确鼻窦病变情况和息肉来源。

2 Therapeutic methods

2.1 Therapeutic principles

Nasal polyp is usually caused by accumulation of dampness and heat and accumulation of cold and dampness in the nose. The treatment is mainly given to expel dampness and dredge the aperture, and clear away heat or disperse cold as well.

2.2 Treatment Based on Syndrome Differentiation

(1) **Pattern of accumulation of dampness and heat in the nose**

Main symptoms: Progressive or continuous nasal obstruction, hyposmia, profuse nasal discharge, often accompanied by dizziness and headache, single or multiple neoplasm inside the nose, in smooth surface, grey white or slight red or dark red color, in shape of semi-transparent lyche pulp, soft and not painful, mobile, not easy to bleed, possible widened and bulged nasal bridge due to numerous and big polyps, red tongue, yellow and greasy tongue coating, rolling and rapid pulse.

Therapeutic method: To clear away heat, remove dampness, disperse accumulation and dredge the aperture.

Herbal formulas and drugs: *Magnolia Lung-Cleaning Decoction* (Xin Yi Qing Fei Tang) (modified). *Radix Scutellariae* (Huang Qin) 10g, *Fructus Gardeniae* (Zhi Zi) 10g, *Gypsum Fibrosum* (Shi Gao) (Decoct first) 30g, *Rhizoma Anemarrhenae* (Zhi Mu) 10g, *Cortex Mori Radicis* (Sang Bai Pi) 10g, *Flos Magnoliae Liliflorae* (Xin Yi Hua) 6g, *Folium Eriobotryae* (Pi Pa Ye) 10g, *Semen Plantaginis* (Che Qian Zi) (Decocted after packed) 10g, *Rhizoma Alismatis* (Ze Xie) 10g, *Bombyx Batryticatus* (Bai Jiang Can) 10g, *Rhizoma*

2 治疗方法

2.1 治疗原则

鼻息肉主要由湿热壅结鼻窍和寒湿凝聚鼻窍所致。治疗以祛湿通窍佐以清热或散寒。

2.2 辨证论治

（1）**湿热壅结鼻窍**

主症：渐进性或持续性鼻塞，嗅觉减退，鼻涕多，常有头昏、头痛，可见鼻腔内单个或多个赘生物，表面光滑，色灰白或淡红或暗红，半透明荔枝样，触之柔软不痛，可移动，不易出血。若息肉较多较大，鼻梁可变宽而膨大。舌红苔黄腻，脉滑数。

治法：清热利湿，散结通窍。

方药：辛夷清肺饮加减。黄芩10克，栀子10克，石膏（先煎）30克，知母10克，桑白皮10克，辛夷6克，枇杷叶10克，车前子（包煎）10克，泽泻10克，白僵蚕10克，川芎6克，白芷10克。若涕痰较多，加贝母10克、枳实10克、丝瓜络5克。

Ligustici Chuanxiong (Chuan Xiong) 6g, and *Radix Angelicae Dahuricae* (Bai Zhi) 10g. For profuse nasal discharge and sputum, add *Bulbus Fritillariae Cirrhosae* (Chuan Bei Mu) 10g, *Fructus Aurantii Immaturus* (Zhi Shi) 10g, and *Retinervus Luffae Fructus* (Si Gua Luo) 5g.

(2) **Pattern of accumulation of cold and dampness in the nose**

Main symptoms: Progressive or continuous nasal obstruction, hyposmia, clear and thin or white and sticky nasal discharge, susceptible to cold, aversion to wind and cold, frequent dizziness, and headache, single or multiple neoplasm inside the nose, in smooth surface, grey white or white transparency, soft and not painful, mobile, not easy to bleed, possible widened and bulged nasal bridge due to numerous and big polyps, pale tongue, white and greasy tongue coating, slow and feeble pulse.

Therapeutic method: To warm and dissolve cold and dampness, disperse accumulation and dredge the aperture.

Herbal formulas and drugs: *Lung-Warming and Nose-Drying Elixi* (Wen Fei Zhi Liu Dan) (modified). *Herba Schizonepetae* (Jing Jie) 10g, *Herba Asari* (Xi Xin) 3g, *Radix Codonopsis Pilosulae* (Dang Shen) 10g, *Fructus Terminaliae Chebulae* (He Zi) 10g, *Radix Platycodi* (Jie Geng) 6g, *Asteriscus Pseudosciaenae* (Yu Nao Shi) 10g, *Fructus Xanthii* (Cang Er Zi) 10g, *Flos Magnoliae Liliflorae* (Xin Yi Hua) 6g, *Radix Angelicae Dahuricae* (Bai Zhi) 10g, *Rhizoma Atractylodis Macrocephalae* (Bai Zhu) 6g, and *Radix Glycyrrhizae* (Gan Cao) 3g. For cold and painful forehead, add *Rhizoma Ligustici Chuanxiong* (Chuan Xiong) 6g, and *Rhizoma*

(2) **寒湿凝聚鼻窍**

主症：渐进性或持续性鼻塞，嗅觉减退，鼻涕清稀或白粘，易感冒、畏风寒，常有头昏、头痛，可见鼻腔内单个或多个赘生物，表面光滑，色灰白或白而透明，触之柔软不痛，可移动，不易出血。若息肉较多较大，鼻梁可变宽而膨大。舌淡苔白腻，脉缓弱。

治法：温化寒湿，散结通窍。

方药：温肺止流丹加减。荆芥 10 克，细辛 3 克，党参 10 克，诃子 10 克，桔梗 6 克，鱼脑石 10 克，苍耳子 10 克，辛夷 6 克，白芷 10 克，白术 6 克，甘草 3 克。若额头冷痛，加川芎 6 克、藁本 10 克。

Ligustici (Gao Ben) 10g.

2.3 Other therapies

(1) Chinese patent medicine: *Rhinitis Tablets* (Bi Yan Kang): Take 3 to 4 tablets each time, for 3 times per day, used for pattern of accumulation of dampness and heat in the lung meridian.

(2) Simple and proved formula: Decoct *Cortex Mori Radicis* (Sang Bai Pi) 10g, *Flos Magnoliae Liliflorae* (Xin Yi Hua) 6g, and *Radix Scutellariae* (Huang Qin) 10g. with water for oral administration, one dose per day.

(3) External therapies: Steaming inhalation. Boil *Rhizoma Atractylodis* (Cang Zhu), *Radix Angelicae Dahuricae* (Bai Zhi) and *Pericarpium Punicae Granati* (Shi Liu Pi), each 10g, and inhale the herbal steaming, for twice per day, for 30 minutes each time. Each dose can be used for 3 times. This method should be applied continuously for 1 to 2 months.

2.3 其他疗法

（1）中成药：鼻炎康，每服3～4片，每日3次。用于肺经湿热证。

（2）单验方：桑白皮10克，辛夷6克，黄芩5克，水煎服。每日一剂。

（3）外治法：蒸汽吸入法，苍术、白芷、石榴皮各10克，煎沸后，乘热吸入药物蒸汽，每日2次，每次30分钟。每剂药3次，连薰1～2个月。

Acute nasosinusitis

It refers to acute suppurative inflammation in the sinus mucosa, involving the bone substance and complications in the peripheral tissues and nearby organs in severe condition, and often leading to acute rhinitis. The pathogenic bacteria include Streptococcus pneumoniae, streptococcus, staphylococcus, bacillus coli, bacillus proteus, bacillus influenza, and anaerobe, etc. The incidence rate is high in the children and teenagers. Nasosinusitis occurs frequently in the maxillary sinus, ethmoidal sinus next, frontal sinus and sphenoid sinus less. It be-

急性鼻窦炎

急性鼻窦炎是指鼻窦黏膜的急性化脓性炎症，严重者可累及骨质，可引起周围组织和邻近器官的并发症。常继发于急性鼻炎，致病菌有肺炎双球菌、链球菌、葡萄球菌、大肠杆菌、变形杆菌、流感杆菌及厌氧菌等。儿童和青少年发病率较高，鼻窦炎发于上颌窦最多，筛窦次之、额窦和蝶窦最少。属中

longs to the scope of "nasal sinusitis" in Chinese medicine.

医学"鼻渊"范畴。

1 Diagnostic essentials

1 诊断要点

1.1 Purulent nasal discharge, accompanied by nasal obstruction, headache, and hyposmia, mostly fever, discomfort in the whole body, possible high fever, vomiting and diarrhea in children.

1.1 鼻流脓涕,伴鼻塞,头痛,嗅觉减退等症状。多有发热、全身不适、周身不适,小儿可有高热、呕吐、腹泻等。

1.2 Inspection

Congestion and edema in the nasal mucosa, large volume of sticky or purulent nasal discharge, flowing down from the middle nasal passage or olfactory cleft, possible tenderness in the glabella, and cheeks, etc.

1.2 检查

鼻黏膜充血、水肿,鼻腔大量黏脓或脓涕,自中鼻道或嗅裂处流下。眉间、面颊部可有压痛等。

1.3 White blood cell count and neutrophil count are elevated.

1.3 白细胞及中性粒细胞计数可升高。

1.4 Thickened mucosa and fluid levels of the sinus cavity are present in X-ray radiography of the sinus. The elevated density of the sinus cavity can be present more clearly in CT scan.

1.4 鼻窦X线片可显示窦腔黏膜增厚及液平。CT扫描可见窦腔密度增高,显示更清晰。

2 Therapeutic methods

2 治疗方法

2.1 Therapeutic principle

The commonly seen patterns of acute nasosinusitis include pattern of accumulation of wind and heat in the meridian, pattern of accumulation of heat in the gallbladder, and pattern of accumulation of heat in the spleen and stomach. The treatment is mainly applied to clear away heat from the lung and stomach.

2.1 治疗原则

急性鼻窦炎的常见证型有肺经风热、胆经郁热和脾胃温热等证。治疗以清肺、泻胃为主。

2.2 Treatment based on syndrome differentiation

(1) **Pattern of accumulation of wind and heat in the meridian**

Main symptoms: Intermittent or continuous na-

2.2 辨证论治

(1) **肺经风热**

主症:间歇或持续鼻塞,

sal obstruction, yellow or sticky and white nasal discharge, in profuse volume, hyposmia, congestion in the nasal mucosa, swelling in the two conchas, purulent fluid in the nasal passage, possible tenderness in the glabella and cheeks, and general symptoms of fever, aversion to cold, headache, stuffy sensation in the chest, cough, profuse sputum, red tongue, slight yellow tongue coating, superficial and rapid pulse.

鼻涕色黄或黏白,量多,嗅觉减退。检查见鼻黏膜充血,双下甲肿大,鼻道有脓液,眉间或颧部可有压痛。全身有发热,恶寒,头痛,胸闷,咳嗽,痰多。舌质红,苔微黄,脉浮数。

Therapeutic method: To expel wind, clear away heat, promote the lung for its spreading ability and dredge the aperture.

治法:疏风清热,宣肺通窍。

Herbal formulas and drugs: *Xanthium Powder* (Cang Er Zi San) (modified). *Fructus Xanthii* (Cang Er Zi) 10g, *Flos Magnoliae Liliflorae* (Xin Yi Hua) 6g, *Herba Menthae* (Bo He) (decoct later) 6g, *Radix Angelicae Dahuricae* (Bai Zhi) 10g, *Folium Mori* (Sang Ye) 10g, *Flos Chrysanthemi* (Ju Hua) 10g, *Radix Scutellariae* (Huang Qin) 10g, *Herba Taraxaci* (Pu Gong Ying) 15g, *Fructus Forsythiae* (Lian Qiao) 10g, and *Radix Glycyrrhizae* (Gan Cao) 3g.

方药:苍耳子散加味。苍耳子10克,辛夷6克,薄荷(后下)6克,白芷10克,桑叶10克,菊花10克,黄芩10克,蒲公英15克,连翘10克,甘草3克。

(2) **Pattern of accumulation of heat in the gallbladder**

(2) **胆经郁热**

Main symptoms: Yellow, turbid and tenacious nasal discharge, in profuse volume and stinky smell, poor smelling sense, tumefaction and redness in the nasal mucosa, serious headache, obvious tenderness in the glabella and cheeks, possibly accompanied by fever, bitter taste in the mouth, dry throat, dizziness, tinnitus, deafness, poor sleep, dreamful sleep, irritability, easy anger, red tongue, thin and yellow tongue coating, wiry and rapid pulse.

主症:鼻涕黄浊黏稠,量多有臭味,嗅觉差,鼻黏膜肿胀、红赤。头痛剧烈,眉间及颧部叩压痛明显。可伴发热、口苦、咽干、目眩、耳鸣、耳聋、少寐、多梦,急躁易怒。舌质红,苔薄黄,脉弦数。

Therapeutic method: To clear away heat from

治法:清泄胆热,利湿通

the gallbladder, remove dampness and dredge the aperture.

窍。

Herbal formulas and drugs: ① *Gentian Liver-Draining Decoction* (Long Dan Xie Gan Tang) (modified). *Radix Gentianae* (Long Dan) 3g, *Radix Scutellariae* (Huang Qin) 10g, *Radix Bupleuri* (Chai Hu) 10g, *Fructus Gardeniae* (Zhi Zi) 10g, *Spica Prunellae* (Xia Ku Cao) 15g, *Flos Chrysanthemi* (Ju Hua) 10g, *Herba Houttuyniae* (Yu Xing Cao) 10g, *Radix Trichosanthis* (Tian Hua Fen) 10g, *Rhizoma Alismatis* (Ze Xie) 10g, *Semen Plantaginis* (Che Qian Zi)(Decoct after wrapped) 10g, *Herba Taraxaci* (Pu Gong Ying) 15g, *Flos Magnoliae Liliflorae* (Xin Yi Hua) 6g, *Fructus Xanthii* (Cang Er Zi) 10g, and *Radix Glycyrrhizae* (Gan Cao) 3g. For constipation, add *Rhizoma Rhei Cruda* (Sheng Da Huang) 10g. ② Specially Instructed Agastache Pills (Qi Shou Huo Xiang Wan). 50 grams of *Herba Agastachis* (Huo Xiang) are prepared with boar's bile into pills. Take 10g each time, for twice per day.

方药:①龙胆泻肝汤加减。龙胆草3克,黄芩10克,柴胡10克,山栀子10克,夏枯草15克,菊花10克,鱼腥草10克,天花粉10克,泽泻10克,车前子(包煎)10克,蒲公英15克,辛夷6克,苍耳子10克,甘草3克。若大便干结,加生大黄10克。②奇授藿香丸。藿香末50克,公猪胆汁熬稠膏为丸,每服10克,每日2次。

(3) **Pattern of accumulation of heat in the spleen and stomach**

(3) **脾胃湿热**

Main symptoms: Distending pain in the nose, yellow, turbid and profuse nasal discharge, persistent nasal obstruction, no smelling sense, red swelling of nasal mucosa, and general symptoms of dizziness, headache, fatigue in the body, lassitude, distending and stuffy sensation in the chest and hypochondriac region, poor appetite, brown urine, red tongue, yellow and greasy tongue coating, soft or rolling and rapid pulse.

主症:鼻内胀痛,鼻涕黄浊量多,鼻塞持续,嗅觉消失,鼻腔内黏膜红肿。全身可有头晕、头痛,体倦乏力,脘胁胀闷,食欲不振,小便黄,舌质红,苔黄腻,脉濡或滑数。

Therapeutic method: To clear away heat, remove dampness, expel the turbid and dredge the ap-

治法:清热利湿,祛浊通窍。

erture.

Herbal formulas and drugs: ① *Scutellaria and* Talcum *Decoction* (Huang Qin Hua Shi Tang)(modified). *Radix Scutellariae* (Huang Qin) 10g, *Talcum* (Hua Shi) 10g, *Caulis Akebiae* (Mu Tong) 10g, *Herba Agastachis* (Huo Xiang) 10g, *Herba Eupatorii* (Pei Lan) 10g, *Sclerotium Poria* (Fu Ling) 10g, *Polyporus Umbellatus* (Zhu Ling) 10g, *Flos Magnoliae Liliflorae* (Xin Yi Hua) 6g, *Fructus Xanthii* (Cang Er Zi) 10g, *Rhizoma Acori Graminei* (Shi Chang Pu) 3g, and *Radix Glycyrrhizae* (Gan Cao) 3g. For severe heat, add *Rhizoma Coptidis* (Huang Lian) 3g, *Rhizoma Rhei* (Da Huang) 10g, and *Talcum* (Hua Shi)(Decoct first) 30g. For serious nasal obstruction, add *Radix Angelicae Dahuricae* (Bai Zhi) 10g, and *Fructus Liquidambaris* (Lu Lu Tong) 10g. ② *Ingredient-Added Four Funguses Powder* (Jia Wei Si Ling San). *Sclerotium Poria* (Fu Ling) 15g, *Polyporus Umbellatus* (Zhu Ling) 15g, *Rhizoma Alismatis* (Ze Xie) 15g, *Rhizoma Atractylodis Macrocephalae* (Bai Zhu) 15g, *Cortex Magnoliae Officinalis* (Hou Pu) 10g, and *Pericarpium Citri Tangerinae* (Chen Pi) 10g. ③ Sweet Dew Toxin-Dispersing Drinks (Gan Lu Xiao Du Yin). *Talcum* (Hua Shi) 15g, *Radix Scutellariae* 10g, Herba Artemisiae Scopariae (Yin Chen) 10g, *Herba Agastachis* (Huo Xiang) 4g, *Fructus Forsythiae* (Lian Qiao) 4g, *Semen Amomi Cardamomi* (Bai Dou Kou) 4g, *Herba Menthae* (Bo He) 4g, *Caulis Akebiae* (Mu Tong) 5g, *Rhizoma Belamecandae* (She Gan) 5g, and *Bulbus Fritillariae Cirrhosae* (Chuan Bei Mu) 5g.

方药:①黄芩滑石汤加减。黄芩 10 克,滑石 10 克,木通 10 克,藿香 10 克,佩兰 10 克,茯苓 10 克,猪苓 10 克,辛夷 6 克,苍耳子 10 克,石菖蒲 3 克,甘草 3 克。若热重,加黄连 3 克、大黄 10 克、石膏(先煎)30 克;鼻塞甚,加白芷 10 克、路路通 10 克。②加味四苓散。茯苓 15 克,猪苓 15 克,泽泻 15 克,白术 15 克,厚朴 10 克,陈皮 10 克。③甘露消毒饮。飞滑石 15 克,黄芩 10 克,茵陈 10 克,藿香 4 克,连翘 4 克,石菖蒲 6 克,白豆蔻 4 克,薄荷 4 克,木通 5 克,射干 4 克,川贝母 5 克。

2.3 Other therapies

(1) Chinese patent medicine: ① *Agastache and*

2.3 其他疗法

(1) 中成药:①藿胆丸,

Boar's Bile Pills (Huo Dan Wan), Take 6g each time, for twice per day. ② *Sinusitis Oral Liquid* (Bi Yuan Shu Kou Fu Ye) or *Nasosinusitis Oral Liquid* (Bi Dou Yan Kou Fu Ye), Take 10 ml each time, for 2 to 3 times per day, used for various patterns of acute nasosinusitis.

每次6克,每日2次。②鼻渊舒口服液或鼻窦炎口服液,每次10 ml,每日2～3次,用于急性鼻窦炎各证型。

(2) Simple and proved formula: *Magnolia, Peucedanum, Platycodon and Liquorice Decoction* (Xin Qian Gan Ju Tang): *Flos Magnoliae Liliflorae* (Xin Yi Hua) 6g, *Radix Ledebouriellae* (Fang Feng) 6g, *Radix Peucedani* (Qian Hu) 10g, *Radix Trichosanthis* (Tian Hua Fen) 10g, *Semen Coicis* (Yi Yi Ren) 12g, *Radix Platycodi* (Jie Geng) 5g, and *Radix Glycyrrhizae* (Gan Cao) 3g. Take one dose in two times per day, used for various patterns of nasosinusitis.

(2)单验方:辛前甘桔汤,辛夷,防风各6克,前胡、天花粉各10克,薏苡仁12克,桔梗5克,生甘草3克,水煎,每日1剂分2次服。用于鼻窦炎各证型。

(3) External therapies: *Green Jade Powder* (Bi Yu San): Please refer to "other therapies for chronic rhinitis".

(3)外治法:碧玉散吹鼻,参考"慢性鼻炎的其他疗法"。

Chronic nasosinusitis

慢性鼻窦炎

It refers to chronic suppurative inflammation of the sinus mucosa, mostly caused by repeated seizure and lingering situation of acute nasosinustitis. It can occur in single sinus, multiple sinuses or whole nasal sinuses. It belongs to the scope of "nasosinusitis" in Chinese medicine.

慢性鼻窦炎是鼻窦黏膜的慢性化脓性炎症。多因急性鼻窦炎反复发作,未彻底治愈迁延而致。可单窦、多窦或全鼻窦发病,属中医学"鼻渊"范畴。

1 Diagnostic essentials

1 诊断要点

1.1 Profuse purulent nasal discharge, nasal obstruction with intermittent aggravation, possible with the symptoms of hyposmia, dizziness, head-

1.1 多脓涕、鼻塞时轻时重,可有嗅觉减退、头昏、头痛、精神不振、倦怠、记忆力

ache, low spirit, fatigue, and poor memory.

减退等症状。

1.2 Inspection

Congestion in the nasal mucosa, swollen inferior nasal concha, polypoid change in the middle nasal concha, or nasal polyp, and purulent secretions in the middle nasal passage or auditory cleft.

1.2 检查

鼻黏膜充血,下鼻甲肿大,中鼻甲息肉样变,或鼻腔息肉,中鼻道或嗅裂有脓性分泌物等。

1.3 Purulent fluid in puncture of the maxillary sinus, possibly diagnosed as maxillary sinusitis.

1.3 上颌窦穿刺有脓液,可诊断为上颌窦炎。

1.4 Obscure sinus cavity or elevated density is present in X-ray or CT scan of the nasal sinus.

1.4 鼻窦 X 线或 CT 检查见窦腔模糊或密度增高等。

2 Therapeutic methods

2 治疗方法

2.1 Therapeutic principles

The commonly seen patterns of chronic nasosinustitis include pattern of deficiency and cold of the lung qi, and pattern of spleen qi deficiency. The treatment is mainly given to warm up the lung and strengthen the spleen

2.1 治疗原则

慢性鼻窦炎的常见证型有肺气虚寒和脾气虚弱两种。治疗以温肺健脾为主。

2.2 Treatment based on syndrome differentiation

(1) Pattern of deficiency and cold of the lung qi

Main symptoms: Nasal obstruction in intermittent severity, tenacious and white nasal discharge, hyposmia, slight red swelling of the muscular membrane inside the nose, swollen nasal concha, nasal obstruction and nasal discharge aggravated by cold, and general symptoms of dizziness, cold sensation in the body and limbs, shortness of breath, lassitude, cough with sputum, pale tongue, thin and white tongue coating, thready and feeble pulse.

Therapeutic method: To warm and replenish the lung qi, disperse wind and cold.

Herbal formulas and drugs: *Lung-Warming and Nose-Drying Elixi* (Wen Fei Zhi Liu Dan) (modified). Please refer to “nasal polyp”

2.2 辨证论治

(1) 肺气虚寒

主症:鼻塞或重或轻,鼻涕黏白,嗅觉减退,鼻内肌膜淡红肿胀,鼻甲肿大,遇冷鼻塞、流涕加重。全身可有头昏脑胀,形寒肢冷,气短乏力,咳嗽有痰。舌质淡,苔薄白,脉细弱。

治法:温补肺气,疏散风寒。

方药:温肺止流丹加减,见“鼻息肉”。

(2) **Pattern of spleen qi deficiency**

Main symptoms: White and tenacious nasal discharge, in large volume, nasal obstruction, hyposmia, slight red or deep red muscular membrane inside the nose, serious tumefaction, and general symptoms of lassitude in the limbs, poor appetite, abdominal distension, loose stool, sallow complexion, pale tongue, thin and white tongue coating, slow and feeble pulse.

Therapeutic method: To strengthen the spleen, benefit qi, and remove warm turbidity.

Herbal formulas and drugs: *Ginseng, Poria and Atractylodes Powder* (Shen Ling Bai Zhu San) (modified). *Radix Astragali* (Huang Qi) 10g, *Radix Codonopsis Pilosulae* (Dang Shen) 10g, *Rhizoma Atractylodis Macrocephalae* (Bai Zhu) 6g, *Rhizoma Dioscoreae* (Shan Yao) 10g, *Semen Dolichoris* (Bian Dou) 10g, *Sclerotium Poria* (Fu Ling) 10g, *Semen Coicis* (Yi Yi Ren) 15g, *Flos Magnoliae Liliflorae* (Xin Yi Hua) 6g, *Fructus Xanthii* (Cang Er Zi) 10g, *Rhizoma Acori Graminei* (Shi Chang Pu) 3g, *Herba Houttuyniae* (Yu Xing Cao) 10g, and *Radix Glycyrrhizae* (Gan Cao) 3g.

(2) **脾气虚弱**

主症：鼻涕色白黏稠，量较多，鼻塞，嗅觉减退，鼻内肌膜淡红或深红，肿胀较甚。全身可有肢体乏力，食少腹胀，便溏，面色萎黄。舌质淡，苔薄白，脉缓弱。

治法：健脾益气，清利温浊。

方药：参苓白术散加减。黄芪10克，党参10克，白术6克，山药10克，扁豆10克，茯苓10克，薏苡仁15克，辛夷6克，苍耳子10克，石菖蒲3克，鱼腥草10克，甘草3克。

2.3 Other therapies

(1) Chinese patent medicine: Asarum and Scutellaria Granules (Xin Qin Ke Li), Take 5g each time, for three times per day, used for various patterns of chronic nasosinusitis.

(2) Simple and proved formula: Decoct *Flos Magnoliae Liliflorae* (Xin Yi Hua) 10g, and *Radix Astragali* (Huang Qi) 20g. with water for oral administration, take one dose in two times per day, used for various patterns of chronic naslsinusitis.

(3) Puncture and flush: Used for chronic max-

2.3 其他疗法

(1) 中成药：辛芩颗粒，每服5克，每日3次。用于慢性鼻窦炎各证型。

(2) 单验方：辛夷10克，黄芪20克。水煎，每日1剂分2次服。用于慢性鼻窦炎各证型。

(3) 穿刺冲洗：用于慢性

illary sinusitis. Please refer to "Commonly used inspections of the nose".

上颌窦炎。见"鼻部常用检查法"。

Nasal hemorrhage

鼻 出 血

It refers to the symptom of nasal bleeding caused by various reasons due to rupture of blood vessels or peripheral blood vessels in the nasal cavity and sinus mucosa, with blood flowing through the anterior and posterior nostrils. The local pathogenic factors include traumatic injury, inflammation, malformation and tumor of the nasal cavity and sinus. The general pathogenic factors include systematical vascular and coagulating dysfunctions. It can occur in any age, mostly in children and middle-aged and old people. It is termed "epistaxis" in Chinese medicine.

鼻出血系各种原因引起的鼻腔、鼻窦黏膜血管或周围血管破裂，血液经前后鼻孔流出的症状。局部病因为鼻腔、鼻窦外伤，炎症，畸形和肿瘤等，全身病因可为系统性血管和凝血功能障碍等。可发生于任何年龄，儿童和中老年人多见。中医称之为"鼻衄"。

1 Diagnostic essentials

1 诊断要点

1.1 Nasal hemorrhage, dripping down in mild condition, flowing down in severe condition, often accompanied by dizziness, lassitude and palpitation, hemorrhagic shock present in severe condition. Anemia can be caused due to repeated hemorrhage in fewer cases.

1.1 鼻出血，轻者点滴而下，重者血流汹涌，常伴头昏、乏力、心慌等症状。严重者可出现失血性休克，少量反复出血可导致贫血。

1.2 To define the bleeding location is the key for diagnosis and treatment. If necessary, nasal endoscopy is needed. Hemorrhage often occurs in the Litter's zone anterior and interior to the middle nasal septum in teenagers, and mostly in the nose-nasopharyngeal venous plexus in the posterior part of the nasal cavity in the middle-aged and old people.

1.2 明确出血部位是诊断和治疗的关键，必要时行鼻内镜检查。青少年出血多发生在鼻中隔前下方 litter's 区，中老年出血以鼻腔后部的鼻—鼻咽静脉丛为多见。

1.3 Blood routine and coagulation function may be

1.3 血常规及凝血功能可

abnormal.

1.4 It is necessary to exclude hemoptysis, hematemesis, and exclude the general diseases, such as hypertension and hematological diseases.

2 Therapeutic methods

2.1 Therapeutic principles

The commonly seen patterns of nasal hemorrhage include pattern of abundant heat in the lung meridian, pattern of abundance of stomach fire, pattern of upward disturbance of liver fire, and pattern of yin deficiency in the liver and kidney and failure of qi in containing blood. The treatment is mainly applied to clear away the fire from the lung, liver and stomach for heat patterns and to benefit qi and nourish yin for deficient patterns.

2.2 Treatment based on syndrome differentiation

(1) **Pattern of abundant heat in the lung meridian**

Main symptoms: Dripping nasal bleeding, in fresh red colour and scanty volume, dry and burning sensation in the nasal cavity, accompanied by cough scanty sputum, dry mouth, feverish sensation in the body, red tongue margin nd tip, thin, white and dry tongue coating, rapid or superficial and rapid pulse.

Therapeutic method: To expel wind, clear away heat, cool blood and stop bleeding.

Herbal formulas and drugs: *Mulberry and Chrysanthemum Drink* (Sang Ju Yin) plus *Lung-Draining Powder* (Xie Bai San) (modified). *Folium Mori* (Sang Ye) 10g, *Flos Chrysanthemi* (Ju Hua) 10g, *Cortex Mori Radicis* (Sang Bai Pi) 10g, *Cortex Lycii Radicis* (Di Gu Pi) 10g, *Caumen Biotae* (Ce Bai Ye) 10g, *Radix Rubiae* (Qian Cao) 10g, *Cortex*

异常。

1.4 排除咯血和呕血，排查全身性疾病如高血压、血液病等。

2 治疗方法

2.1 治疗原则

鼻出血的常见证型有肺经热盛、胃火炽盛、肝火上扰、肝肾阴虚和气不摄血证等。热证以清肺、肝、胃之火为主，虚证以益气养阴为法。

2.2 辨证论治

（1）**肺经热盛**

主症：点滴鼻出血，色鲜红，量不多，鼻腔干燥、灼热感，兼有咳嗽、痰少、口干、身热。舌边尖红，苔薄白而干，脉数或浮数。

治法：疏风清热，凉血止血。

方药：桑菊饮合泻白散加减。桑叶10克，菊花10克，桑白皮10克，地骨皮10克，侧柏叶10克，茜草10克，牡丹皮6克，白茅根10克。

Moutan Radicis (Mu Dan Pi) 6g, and *Rhizoma Imperatae* (Bai Mao Gen) 10g.

(2) **Pattern of abundance of stomach fire**

(2) **胃火炽盛**

Main symptoms: Nasal bleeding in large volume, fresh red or deep red color, dry mouth and dry nose, foul breath, frequent thirst with preference of drinks, constipation, scanty and brown urine, red tongue, yellow, thick and dry tongue coating, floody and rapid pulse.

主症：鼻出血，量多，色鲜红或深红，口鼻干燥，口臭，烦渴引饮，大便燥结，小便短赤。舌质红，苔黄厚而干，脉洪大而数。

Therapeutic method: To clarify the stomach, discharge fire, cool blood and stop bleeding.

治法：清胃泻火，凉血止血。

Herbal formulas and drugs: *Rhinoceros Horn and Rehmannia Decoction* (Xi Jiao Di Huang Tang) (modified). *Cornu Bubali* (Shui Niu Jiao) (Decoct first) 30g, *Radix Rehmanniae Cruda* (Sheng Di Huang) (fresh) 15g, *Gypsum Fibrosum* (Shi Gao) (Decoct first) 30g, *Rhizoma Anemarrhenae* (Zhi Mu) 10g, *Cortex Moutan Radicis* (Mu Dan Pi) 6g, *Radix Paeoniae Rubra* (Chi Shao) 6g, *Caumen Biotae* (Ce Bai Ye) 10g, *Rhizoma Coptidis* (Huang Lian) 3g, *Radix Scrophulariae* (Xuan Shen) 10g, *Herba seu Radix Cirsii Japonici* (Da Ji) 10g, and *Radix Glycyrrhizae* (Gan Cao) 3g. For constipation, add *Rhizoma Rhei* (Da Huang) 10g, and *Semen Trichosanthis* (Gua Lou Zi) 10g.

方药：犀角地黄汤加减。水牛角(先煎)30克，鲜生地黄15克，生石膏(先煎)30克，知母10克，牡丹皮6克，赤芍药6克，侧柏叶10克，黄连3克，玄参10克，大蓟10克，生甘草3克。若大便燥结，加大黄10克、瓜蒌仁10克。

(3) **Pattern of upward disturbance of liver fire**

(3) **肝火上扰**

Main symptoms: Epistaxis in profuse volume and deep red color, headache, dizziness, bitter taste in the mouth, dry throat, full sensation in the chest, flushed complexion, red eyes, irritability, easy anger, red tongue, yellow tongue coating, wiry and rapid pulse.

主症：鼻衄量多，色深红，头痛头晕，口苦咽干，胸胁苦满，面红目赤，急躁易怒。舌质红，苔黄，脉弦数。

Therapeutic method: To clarify the liver, discharge fire, cool blood and stop bleeding.

治法：清肝泻火，凉血止血。

Herbal formulas and drugs: *Gentian Liver-Draining Decoction* (Long Dan Xie Gan Tang) (modified). *Radix Gentianae* (Long Dan) 5g, *Fructus Gardeniae* (Zhi Zi) 10g, *Radix Scutellariae* Carbonisatus (Huang Qin Tan) 10g, *Spica Prunellae* (Xia Ku Cao) 15g, *Cortex Moutan Radicis* (Mu Dan Pi) 6g, *Radix Paeoniae Rubra* (Chi Shao) 10g, *Caumen Biotae* (Ce Bai Ye) 10g, *Radix Achyranthis Bidentatae* (Niu Xi) 10g, *Radix Rehmanniae Cruda* (Sheng Di Huang) 10g, *Radix Glycyrrhizae* (Gan Cao) 3g. For severe dizziness and headache, add Magnetitum (Ci Shi) (Decoct first) 30g, and *Concha Margaritifera Usta* (Zhen Zhu Mu) (Decoct first) 30g.

方药:龙胆泻肝汤加减。龙胆草5克,山栀子10克,黄芩炭10克,夏枯草15克,牡丹皮6克,赤芍药10克,侧柏叶10克,盐水炒牛膝10克,生地黄10克,生甘草3克。若头晕头痛较甚,加磁石(先煎)30克、珍珠母(先煎)30克。

(4) **Pattern of yin deficiency in the liver and kidney**

(4) **肝肾阴虚**

Main symptoms: Fresh red epistaxis, intermittent occurrence, not big in volume, dry mouth with less body fluid, dizziness, blurred vision, tinnitus, palpitation, insomnia, feverish sensation in the chest, palms and soles, tender red or crimson tongue with scanty body fluid, scanty tongue coating, thready and rapid pulse.

主症:鼻衄色红,时作时止,量不多,口干少津,头晕眼花,耳鸣,心悸,失眠,五心烦热。舌质嫩红或绛而少津,舌苔少,脉细数。

Therapeutic method: To nourish the liver and kidney, reduce fire and stop bleeding.

治法:滋养肝肾,降火止血。

Herbal formulas and drugs: *Anemarrhena, Phellodendron, and Rehmannia Pills* (Zhi Bai Di Huang Wan) (modified). *Rhizoma Anemarrhenae* (Zhi Mu) 10g, *Radix Rehmanniae Cruda* (Sheng Di Huang) 10g, *Cortex Phellodendri* (Huang Bo) 10g, *Radix Rehmanniae Praeparata* (Shu Di Huang) 10g, *Cortex Moutan Radicis* (Mu Dan Pi) 6g, *Fructus Corni* (Shan Zhu Yu) 10g, *Radix Paeoniae Rubra* (Chi Shao) 60g, *Fructus Ligustri Lucidi* (Nü Zhen

方药:知柏地黄丸加减。知母10克,黄柏10克,生地黄10克,熟地黄10克,牡丹皮6克,山萸肉10克,赤芍药60克,女贞子10克,旱莲草10克,生甘草3克。

Zi) 10g, *Herba Ecliptae* (Han Lian Cao) 10g, and *Radix Glycyrrhizae* (Gan Cao) 3g.

(5) **Pattern of spleen qi deficiency**

Main symptoms: Oozing epistaxis, in light red color, and in profuse or scanty volume, lustrousless complexion, poor appetite, low spirit, reluctance in speaking, pale tongue, thin and white tongue coating, thready and feeble pulse.

Therapeutic method: To strengthen the spleen, benefit qi, contain blood and stop bleeding.

Herbal formulas and drugs: *Angelica Splenic Decoction* (Gui Pi Tang) (modified): *Radix Astragali* (Huang Qi) 15g, *Radix Codonopsis Pilosulae* (Dang Shen) 10g, *Rhizoma Atractylodis Macrocephalae* (Bai Zhu) 6g, *Radix Paeoniae Albae* (Bai Shao) 6g, *Radix Angelicae Sinensis* (Dang Gui) 10g, *Semen Zizyphi Spinosae* (Suan Zao Ren) 10g, Colla Corii Asini (E Jiao) processed with Pollen Typhae (Pu Huang) 10g, Herba Agrimoniae (Xian He Cao) 10g, Radix Polygalae (Yuan Zhi) 10g, and *Radix Glycyrrhizae* (Gan Cao) 3g.

(5) **脾气虚弱**

主症：鼻衄渗渗而出，色淡红，量或多或少，面色不华，饮食减少，神疲懒言。舌淡，苔薄白，脉细弱。

治法：健脾益气，摄血止血。

方药：归脾汤加减。炙黄芪 15 克，炒党参 10 克，炒白术 6 克，白芍药 6 克，当归 10 克，酸枣仁 10 克，蒲黄炒阿胶 10 克，仙鹤草 10 克，炙远志 10 克，生甘草 3 克。

2.3 Other therapies

(1) Chinese patent medicine: ① *Ten Ashes Pills* (Shi Hui Wan), Take 6 grams each time, for twice per day, appropriate for pattern of lung heat, stomach fire and liver fire. ② *Anemarrhena, Phellodendron, and Rehmannia Pills* (Zhi Bai Di Huang Wan): Take 6g each time, for twice per day, appropriate for pattern of yin deficiency in the liver and kidney.

(2) Simple and proved formulas: ① *Decoct Rhizoma Imperatae* (Bai Mao Gen) 20g. with water for oral administration, one dose per day and take in twice, or take 3g of powder of *Herba Bletillae*

2.3 其他疗法

(1) 中成药：①十灰丸，每次 6 克，每日 2 次。适用于肺热、胃火及肝火证。②知柏地黄丸，每次 6 克，每日 2 次。适用于肝肾阴虚证。

(2) 单验方：①白茅根 20 克，水煎，每日 1 剂分 2 次服。或白及粉 3 克，每日 2 次，饭后服。用于少量鼻出

(Bai Ji), for twice per day, after meal, used for scanty nasal bleeding. ② *Decoct Herba Agrimoniae* (Xian He Cao) 15g, and *Herba Ecliptae* (Han Lian Cao) 10g. with water for oral administration, one dose per day and take in twice, used for nasal bleeding in pattern of lung heat, stomach fire and liver fire.

血。②仙鹤草 15 克,旱莲草 10 克,水煎,每日 1 剂分 2 次服。用于鼻出血之肺热、胃火及肝火证。

(3) External therapies

(3) 外治法

1) Herbal powder-blowing method: ① *Grind Crinis Carbonisatus* (Xue Yu Tan) 3g, and *Notoginseng Powder* (San Qi Fen) 3g. into very fine powder and slow a little into the nose each time. ② Grind *Herba Bletillae* (Bai Ji) and *Lasiosphaera Seu Calvatia* (Ma Bo), in equal portion, into very fine powder, and blow a little into the nose each time.

1) 吹药法:①血余炭 3 克,三七粉 3 克,研极细末,每次少许吹鼻孔中。②白及、马勃各等分,研极细末,每取少许,吹鼻孔中。

2) Finger-pressing method: Appropriate for a little bleeding in the Litter's zone anterior to the nasal septum, pinch the bilateral nasal wings tightly with the fingers, breathe through the mouth, and usually press with the fingers for about 10 minutes, and at the same time give cold compress on the forehead and neck.

2) 指压止血法:适用于鼻中隔前部 litter's 区少量出血,用手指捏紧两侧鼻翼,用口呼吸,指压时间一般 10 分钟左右,同时可在前额部及颈部给予冷敷。

3) Burning method: Burn the bleeding spots with a specially-made iron, or with silver nitrate crystals, or electric burner.

3) 烧灼法:烙法,用特制的小烙铁,或用硝酸银结晶、电灼烧器,烧灼出血点。

4) Nasal cavity-stuffing method: Mostly stuff the nose to stop bleeding by using the sterile gauze soaked with *Coptis Ointment* (Huang Lian Gao) Vaseline ointment, also stuff the nose with gelatin sponge and prothrombin. After 48 hours, it is necessary to take away the gauze, in order to avoid causing infection. If bleeding still exist, it is advisable to repeat this method.

4) 鼻腔填塞止血法:多用浸有黄连油膏或凡士林油膏的消毒纱条堵塞止血。亦可用明胶海绵加凝血酶原填塞止血,简便快捷。填塞 48 小时后应抽出纱条,以免引起感染。若仍有出血,再行填塞。

Nose injury

鼻外伤

It refers to swelling pain, hemorrhage and bone fracture of the nose by the external forces and is one of the clinically common emergent symptoms. The nose injuries include injury of soft tissues in the nose and fracture of the nasal bone commonly, and sinus fracture, orbital fracture, skull fracture and cerebrospinal fluid rhinorrhea. If not managed properly, severe nose injury will endanger the life in the early and middle stage and will result in the negative effects of cicatricial stenosis, malformation and dysfunctions in the later stage. It is termed "nose injury" in Chinese medicine.

鼻外伤是鼻部遭受外力作用而致肿痛，出血，骨折等，是临床常见急症之一。常见的有鼻部软组织损伤、鼻骨骨折等，少见的有鼻窦骨折、眼眶骨折、颅底骨折、脑脊液鼻漏等。鼻外伤严重，或处理不当，早中期可危及生命，后期有瘢痕狭窄、畸形或功能障碍等不良后果。中医学称之为"鼻损伤"。

1 Diagnostic essentials

1 诊断要点

1.1 The most common symptoms include local pain, bleeding, or tumefaction of the external nose, deviation of the nasal bridge or concave of nose dorsum, subcutaneous bruises, and sensation of bone friction.

1.1 最常见的症状是局部疼痛、出血，或有外鼻肿胀、鼻梁偏斜或鼻背塌陷，皮下淤血，触及骨擦感等。

1.2 If injured by sharp device, there can be skin lesions, exposure and defect of bone or cartilage, etc.

1.2 若锐器所伤，则可有皮肤破损、骨或软骨暴露及缺损等。

1.3 Fever, red swelling and suppuration can be present in local infection after injury.

1.3 外伤后局部感染，可出现发热、红肿及化脓等。

1.4 By X-ray radiography or CT scan of the nasal bone, bone fracture of the nose and dislocation of bone fracture can be confirmed. The latter is more significant for multiple fractures of the sinus and craniofacial region.

1.4 鼻骨X线侧位片或CT扫描，可以确定有无鼻骨骨折及骨折有无错位。后者对鼻窦、颅面多发骨折意义更大。

2 Therapeutic methods

2 治疗方法

2.1 Therapeutic principles

2.1 治疗原则

The commonly seen patterns of the nose injury

鼻损伤的常见证型有瘀

include pain caused by ecchymoma, skin lesions, nose fracture, and nose injury and epistaxis. The treatment is mainly given to diminish swelling and disperse blood stasis.

肿疼痛、皮肉受损、鼻梁骨折和鼻伤衄血等。治疗以消肿散瘀为主。

2.2 Treatment based on syndrome differentiation

2.2 辨证论治

(1) **Pain caused by ecchymoma**

(1) **瘀肿疼痛**

Main symptoms: Tumefaction in the nose, subcutaneous bruises, pain and obvious tenderness, also subcutaneous bruises in the eyehole and eyelid in severe condition, dark red tongue or with purple spots, thin and white tongue coating, wiry and tense pulse.

主症:鼻部肿胀,皮下青紫,疼痛和压痛明显,重者眼窝、眼睑也见皮下青紫肿胀。舌暗红或有紫斑,苔薄白,脉弦紧。

Therapeutic method: To circulate qi, activate blood, diminish swelling and stop pain.

治法:行气活血,消肿止痛。

Herbal formulas and drugs: *Peach Pit, Safflower and Four Agents Decoction* (Tao Hong Si Wu Tang) (modified). *Semen Persicae* (Tao Ren) 10g, *Flos Carthami* (Hong Hua) 10g, *Radix Angelicae Sinensis* (Dang Gui) 10g, *Rhizoma Ligustici Chuanxiong* (Chuan Xiong) 10g, *Radix Paeoniae Rubra* (Chi Shao) 6g, *Radix Rehmanniae Cruda* (Sheng Di Huang) (fresh) 10g, *Rhizoma Cyperi* (Xiang Fu) 10g, *Rhizoma Corydalis* (Yan Hu Suo) 10g, and *Radix Glycyrrhizae* (Gan Cao) 3g.

方药:桃红四物汤加味。桃仁 10 克,红花 10 克,当归 10 克,川芎 10 克,赤芍药 6 克,生地黄 10 克,香附 10 克,延胡索 10 克,甘草 3 克。

(2) **Skin lesions**

(2) **皮肉破损**

Main symptoms: Epidermal abrasion and blood oozing, breakage and rupture of skin and flesh in severe condition, exposure of bone and cartilage, and even tissue defect, bleeding and pain in the wound, local red swelling, pain and suppuration several days after secondary infection, red tongue, yellow tongue coating, rapid pulse.

主症:轻者表皮擦破渗血,重者皮肉破损裂开,骨与软骨暴露,甚至组织缺损。伤口可有出血、疼痛。继发感染数日后局部红肿疼痛,化脓。舌红,苔黄,脉数。

Therapeutic method: To clear away heat, resolve toxin, activate blood and diminish swelling.

治法:清热解毒,活血消肿。

Herbal formulas and drugs: ① *Coptis Detoxifying Decoction* (Huang Lian Jie Du Tang) plus *Five Ingredients Detoxifying Drink* (Wu Wei Xiao Du Yin) (modified). *Rhizoma Coptidis* (Huang Lian) 3g, *Radix Scutellariae* (Huang Qin) 6g, *Cortex Phellodendri* (Huang Bo) 10g, *Flos Lonicerae* (Jin Yin Hua) 10g, *Herba Taraxaci* (Pu Gong Ying) 10g, *Flos Chrysanthemi Indici* (Ye Ju Hua) 10g, *Radix Rubiae* (Qian Cao) 10g, *Radix Notoginseng* (San Qi) 10g, and *Pollen Typhae* (Pu Huang) 10g. ② *Eight Jewel Decoction* (Ba Zhen Tang): *Radix Angelicae Sinensis* (Dang Gui) 10g, *Rhizoma Ligustici Chuanxiong* (Chuan Xiong) 10g, *Radix Rehmanniae Praeparata* (Shu Di Huang) 20g, *Radix Codonopsis Pilosulae* (Dang Shen) 20g, *Radix Paeoniae Albae* (Bai Shao) 15g, *Sclerotium Poria* (Fu Ling) 15g, *Rhizoma Atractylodis Macrocephalae* (Bai Zhu) 10g, *Radix Glycyrrhizae* (Gan Cao) 10g, *Rhizoma Zingiberis Recens* (Sheng Jiang) 3 pieces, *Fructus Ziziphi Jujubae* (Da Zao) 5 pieces.

方药：①黄连解毒汤合五味消毒饮加减。黄连3克，黄芩6克，黄柏10克，金银花10克，蒲公英10克，野菊花10克，茜草10克，三七10克，蒲黄10克。②八珍汤。当归10克，川芎10克，熟地黄20克，党参20克，白芍15克，茯苓15克，白术10克，甘草10克，生姜3片，大枣5枚。

(3) **Nose fracture**

(3) **鼻骨骨折**

Main symptoms: Nose pain, tumefaction several hours later, green purple skin, obvious swelling and pain in the bridge of the nose, or convex, deviation, nose fracture present in X-ray radiography, dark red tongue, thin and white tongue coating, wiry or choppy pulse.

主症：鼻部疼痛，数小时后肿胀，皮色青紫，鼻梁肿痛明显，或有凹陷、歪曲。X线片可见鼻骨骨折。舌质暗红，苔薄白，脉弦或涩。

Therapeutic method: To stop pain, diminish swelling, expel blood stasis and promote granulation.

治法：止痛消肿，祛瘀生新。

Herbal formulas and drugs: *Blood-Activating and Pain-Alleviating Decoction* (Huo Xue Zhi Tong Tang) in the initial stage. *Resina Olibani* (Ru Xiang) 3g, *Myrrha* (Mo Yao) 3g, *Lignum Sappan*

方药：初期用活血止痛汤。乳香3克，没药3克，苏木10克，红木10克，三七10克，当归10克，川芎10克，赤

(Su Mu) 10g, *Cortex Bixa orellanae* (Hong Mu) 10g, *Radix Notoginseng* (San Qi) 10g, *Radix Angelicae Sinensis* (Dang Gui) 10g, *Rhizoma Ligustici Chuanxiong* (Chuan Xiong) 10g, *Radix Paeoniae Rubra* (Chi Shao) 6g, *Herba Centellae Asiaticae* (Luo De Da) 10g, and *Pericarpium Citri Tangerinae* (Chen Pi). *Bone-Setting Purple Gold Elixir* (Zheng Gu Zi Jin Dan) in the middle stage. *Flos Carthami* (Hong Hua) 10g, *Radix Angelicae Sinensis* (Dang Gui) 10g, *Cortex Moutan Radicis* (Mu Dan Pi) 6g, *Rhizoma Rhei* (Da Huang) 10g, Resina Draconis (Xue Jie) 10g, Catechu (Er Cha) 10g, *Flos Caryophylli* (Ding Xiang) 6g, *Radix Aucklandiae* (Mu Xiang) 10g, *Radix Paeoniae Rubra* (Chi Shao) 6g, and *Sclerotium Poria* (Fu Ling) 10g. *Ginseng and Purple Gold Elixir* (Ren Shen Zi Jin Dan) in the later stage. *Radix Ginseng* (Ren Shen) 10g, *Sclerotium Poria* (Fu Ling) 10g, *Radix Angelicae Sinensis* (Dang Gui) 10g, *Cortex Acanthopanacis Radicis* (Wu Jia Pi) 10g, *Resina Draconis* (Xue Jie) 10g, *Myrrha* (Mo Yao) 3g, Flos Caryophylli (Ding Xiang) 6g, *Rhizoma Drynariae* (Gu Sui Bu) 10g, *Fructus Schisandrae* (Wu Wei Zi) 10g, and *Radix Glycyrrhizae* (Gan Cao) 3g.

芍药6克,落得打10克,陈皮6克。中期用正骨紫金丹。红花10克,当归10克,牡丹皮6克,大黄10克,血竭10克,儿茶10克,丁香6克,木香10克,赤芍药6克,茯苓10克。后期用人参紫金丹。人参10克,茯苓10克,当归10克,五加皮10克,血竭10克,没药3克,丁香6克,骨碎补10克,五味子10克,甘草3克。

(4) **Nose injury and epistaxis**

Main symptoms: Traumatic injury in the nose, rupture of skin and flesh, or fracture, possible bleeding due to rupture of the blood vessels inside the nose, in large volume and fresh red color, red tongue, thin and white tongue coating, wiry pulse.

Therapeutic method: To activate blood, disperse blood stasis, cool blood and stop bleeding.

Herbal formulas and drugs: ① *Ten Ashes Pills* (Shi Hui Wan) (modified). *Cortex Moutan Radicis*

(4) **鼻伤衄血**

主症:鼻部外伤,皮肉破损或有骨折,可有鼻内血脉破裂出血,量多,色鲜红。舌红,苔薄白,脉弦。

治法:活血化瘀,凉血止血。

方药:①十灰丸加减。牡丹皮6克,赤芍药6克,制

(Mu Dan Pi) 6g, *Radix Paeoniae Rubra* (Chi Shao) 6g, *Rhizoma Rhei* (Da Huang) 10g, *Pollen Typhae* (Pu Huang) 10g, *Herba Agrimoniae* (Xian He Cao) 10g, *Fructus Gardeniae Carbonisatus* (Zhi Zi Tan) 10g, *Caumen Biotae* (Ce Bai Ye) 10g, *Radix Rubiae* (Qian Cao) 10g, *Rhizoma Imperatae* (Bai Mao Gen) 10g. and *Nodus Nelumbinis Rhizomatis* (Ou Jie) 10g. For severe ecchymoma and pain, add *Flos Carthami* (Hong Hua) 10g, *Rhizoma Cyperi* (Xiang Fu) 10g, and *Rhizoma Corydalis* (Yan Hu Suo) 10g. For scanty bleeding but long duration, add *Radix Polygoni Multiflori* (He Shou Wu) 10g, *Radix Rehmanniae* (Di Huang) 10g, *Fructus Mori* (Sang Shen Zi) 10g, and *Radix Angelicae Sinensis* (Dang Gui) 10g. ② *Trauma Five-Ingredient Decoction* (Chuang Shang Wu Wei Tang). *Herba Lagotis Brachystachydis* (Tu Er Cao) 200g, *Rhizoma Drynariae* (Gu Sui Bu) 100g, *Radix Gentianae* Macrophyllae (Qin Jiao) 100g, *Fel Ursi* (Xiong Dan) 50g, and *Radix Arnebiae seu Lithospermi* (Zi Cao) 100g.

大黄10克，蒲黄10克，仙鹤草10克，栀子炭10克，侧柏叶10克，茜草10克，白茅根10克，藕节10克。若瘀肿疼痛甚，加红花10克、香附10克、延胡索10克；出血量少，但病程较长，加何首乌10克、干地黄10克、桑椹子10克、当归10克。②创伤五味汤。兔耳草200克，骨碎补(去毛)100克，秦艽100克，熊胆50克，紫草100克。

2.3 Other therapies

(1) Chinese patent medicine: ① *Notoginseng Tablets* (San Qi Pian). Take 3 to 4 tablets each time, for 3 times per day, or *Notoginseng Powder* (San Qi Fen): Take 2 grams each time, after infused with water, used for ecchymona and pain. ② *Yunnan White Drug* (Yun Nan Bai Yao): Take 1g each time, for 3 times per day, used for ecchymoma and pain. ③ *Red Trauma Pills* (Hong Shang Wan). Take 5 grams each time, for 3 times per day, used for ecchymoma and pain. ④ *Anti-Bruise Powder* (Qi Li San). Take 1 to 2 grams each time, for twice per day, used for ecchymoma and pain. ⑤ *Bone-Setting Purple Gold Elixir* (Zheng Gu Zi Jin Dan).

2.3 其他疗法

(1) 中成药：①三七片，每服3～4片，每日3次；或三七粉，每次2克，开水冲服。用于瘀肿疼痛。②云南白药，每服1克，每日3次。用于瘀肿疼痛。③红伤丸，每服5克，每日3次。用于瘀肿疼痛。④七厘散，每服1～2克，每日2次。用于瘀肿疼痛。⑤正骨紫金丹，每服2～5克，每日2次。用于鼻骨骨折。

Take 2 to 5 grams each time, for twice per day, used for nose bone fracture.

(2) External therapies: ① Ecchymoma and pain, in the initial stage of injury (within 24 hours), it is advisable to apply cold compress, in order to stop bleeding and prevent stagnant blood from dispersion. After 48 hours, it is advisable to use hot compress, in order to activate blood, disperse blood stasis, diminish swelling and stop pain, or decoct the herbal dregs left over after oral administration again to take liquid for wet hot compress, and it is also advisable to herbal products for activating blood, circulating qi, expelling blood stasis and stopping pain topically, such as *Ten Thousand-Flower Oil* (Wan Hua You), *Jade Dragon Oil* (Yu Long You), etc. It is also advisable to apply *Golden Yellow Powder* (Jin Huang San) for topical application, but it is prohibited to rub forcefully, in order to avoid causing bleeding again. ② Injury of skin and flesh: it is just needed to clean the wound and apply some medications to stop bleeding and stop pain, such as *Safflower Oil* (Hong Hua You), *Lucky Golden Yellow Powder* (Ru Yi Jin Huang San) or *Ten Thousand-Flower Oil* (Wan Hua You). If the wound is big and deep, it is necessary to do debridement and suturing. ③ For fracture of the nose bone, it is necessary to do the reduction of bone fracture.

（2）外治法：①瘀肿疼痛，受伤初期(24 小时以内)，宜冷敷，利于止血或防止瘀血扩散。48 小时后，可改用热敷，以活血散瘀，消肿止痛；或用内服中药渣再煎，取药汁湿热敷，也可外涂活血行气祛瘀止痛药，如万花油、玉龙油等，亦可用金黄散调敷，但忌用力揉擦，以防止再度出血。②皮肉受损，轻者只需清洁创口，涂以止血止痛药物，如红花油、如意金黄散或万花油。若伤口较深或较长，应予清创缝合。③鼻骨骨折者，行骨折复位。

Postnasal drip syndrome

鼻后滴漏综合征

It refers to secretions caused by nose-sinus or nasopharyngeal diseases, flowing back to the throat

鼻后滴漏综合征是指鼻-鼻窦或鼻咽部疾病引起分泌

and even into the glottis or trachea, characterized mainly by the clinical symptoms of cough, profuse sputum, and sensation of foreign body in the throat.

物倒流至咽喉部，甚至流入声门或气管，以咳嗽、痰多、咽异物感等为主要临床表现的综合征。

1 Diagnostic essentials

1 诊断要点

1.1 Paroxysmal or persistent cough, mainly in the daytime.

1.1 阵发性或持续性咳嗽，以白天为主。

1.2 Accompanied by backflow of the nasal secretions, itching sensation, sensation of foreign body in the throat, and frequent clearing the throat in most patients.

1.2 多数患者伴有鼻内分泌物倒流，咽部发痒，异物感，常频繁清嗓。

1.3 Possible nasal itching, nasal obstruction, nasal discharge, and sneezing, seldom hoarse voice, and even cough induced by speaking.

1.3 可有鼻痒、鼻塞、流鼻涕、打喷嚏等症状，声音嘶哑少见，甚至讲话也会诱发咳嗽。

1.4 Mostly accompanied by the history of deviation of the nasal septum, allergic rhinitis, chronic nasosinusitis, nasopharyngitis, and adenoidal hypertrophy.

1.4 多有鼻中隔偏曲，过敏性鼻炎，慢性鼻-鼻窦炎，鼻咽炎，腺样体肥大等病史。

1.5 Deviation of the nasal septum, swollen inferior nasal concha, polyp-like change in the middle nasal concha, increased secretions of the nasal passage, and thickened nasopharyngeal mucosa present in the inspections.

1.5 检查可见鼻中隔偏曲，下鼻甲肿大，中鼻甲息变，中鼻道息肉，鼻道分泌物增多，鼻咽黏膜肿胀增厚等。

2 Therapeutic methods

2 治疗方法

2.1 Therapentic principle

2.1 治疗原则

Clinically, it can be divided into the five patterns: pattern of invasion of pathogenic wind and cold, pattern of invasion of pathogenic wind and heat, pattern of upward accumulation of phlegm and dampness, pattern of upward disturbance of phlegm and heat, and pattern of deficiency in the lung and kidney. The treatment is mainly applied to

鼻后滴漏综合征临床可分为风寒外袭、风热外袭、痰湿上壅、痰热上泛、肺肾亏虚5型。初期治疗以祛风为主，日久以理气化痰、补肺益肾为法。

expel wind in the initial stage and to regulate qi, dissolve phlegm, replenish the lung and benefit the kidney in the course of the time.

2.2 Treatment based on syndrome differentiation

(1) **Pattern of invasion of pathogenic wind and cold**

Main symptoms: Fever, headache, aversion to cold, no sweating, nasal obstruction, profuse nasal discharge, white sputum, sneezing, frequent cough, itching sensation in the throat, low voice, thin and white tongue coating, superficial and tense pulse

Therapeutic method: To promote the lung for its spreading ability, dredge the aperture and stop cough.

Herbal formulas and drugs: *Pepperweed Seed and Jujube Lung-Cleaning Decoction* (Ting Li Da Zao Xie Fei Tang) plus *Almond and Perilla Powder* (Xing Su San) (modified). Semen Descurainiae (Ting Li Zi) 9g, *Fructus Ziziphi Jujubae* (Da Zao) 4 pieces, *Semen Armeniacae Amarum* (Ku Xing Ren) 9g, *Folium Penillae* (Zi Su Ye) 9g, Exocarpium Citri Grandis (Ju Hong) 6g, *Rhizoma Pinelliae* (Ban Xia) 6g, *Sclerotium Poria* (Fu Ling) 9g, *Radix Glycyrrhizae Praeparata* (Zhi Gan Cao) 6g, *Radix Peucedani* (Qian Hu) 9g, *Fructus Aurantii* (Zhi Ke) 9g, *Radix Platycodi* (Jie Geng) 6g, and *Rhizoma Zingiberis Recens* (Sheng Jiang) 6g. For profuse nasal discharge, add *Fructus Xanthii* (Cang Er Zi) 10g, and *Radix Angelicae Dahuricae* (Bai Zhi) 10g. For serious cough, add *Flos Inulae* (Xuan Fu Hua) 3g, and *Radix Aster tatarici* (Zi Yuan) 3g. For cough and shortness of breath, take out *Folium Penillae* (Zi Su Ye) and add *Herba Ephedrae* (Ma

2.2 辨证论治

(1) **风寒外袭**

主症:发热头痛,恶寒无汗,鼻塞,多涕痰白,喷嚏、咳嗽频作,喉痒声重,苔薄白,脉浮紧。

治法:宣肺散寒,通窍止咳。

方药:葶苈大枣泻肺汤合杏苏散加减。葶苈子9克,大枣4枚,杏仁9克,紫苏叶9克,橘红6克,半夏6克,茯苓9克,炙甘草6克,前胡9克,枳壳9克,桔梗6克,生姜6克。如涕多明显,加苍耳子10克、白芷10克;咳嗽甚,加旋覆花3克、紫苑3克;咳而气急,去紫苏加麻黄5克、苏子5克;表邪甚,加防风10克、羌活10克;气虚者,加党参10克。

Huang) 5g, and *Fructus Perillae* (Zi Su Zi) 5g. For serous exogenous pathogens, add *Radix Ledebouriellae* (Fang Feng) 10g, and *Rhizoma seu Radix Notopterygii* (Qiang Huo) 10g. For qi deficiency, add *Radix Codonopsis Pilosulae* (Dang Shen) 10g.

(2) **Pattern of invasion of pathogenic wind and heat**

(2) 风热外袭

Main symptoms: Profuse nasal discharge, in white or slight yellow color, red nasal mucosa, turbid nasal discharge in the nasal passage, cough, tenacious sputum, difficult expectoration, dry mouth, sore throat, fever, sweating, aversion to wind, headache, thin and yellow tongue coating, superficial and rapid pulse.

主症：涕多，质白或略黄，鼻膜潮红，鼻道浊涕，咳嗽痰稠，咯痰不爽，口干咽痛，发热，汗出恶风，头痛，苔薄黄，脉浮数。

Therapeutic method: To expel wind, clear away heat, promote the lung for its spreading ability and dissolve phlegm.

治法：疏风清热，宣肺化痰。

Herbal formulas and drugs: *Mulberry and Chrysanthemum Drink* (Sang Ju Yin) (modified). *Folium Mori* (Sang Ye) 9g, *Flos Chrysanthemi* (Ju Hua) 9g, *Semen Armeniacae Amarum* (Ku Xing Ren) 9g, *Radix Platycodi* (Jie Geng) 9g, *Fructus Forsythiae* (Lian Qiao) 9g, *Herba Menthae* (Bo He) 6g, *Rhizoma Phragmitis* (Lu Gen) 9g, and *Radix Glycyrrhizae* (Gan Cao) 6g. For profuse nasal discharge, add *Fructus Xanthii* (Cang Er Zi) 10g, and *Radix Angelicae Dahuricae* (Bai Zhi) 10g. For serious cough, add *Herba Houttuyniae* (Yu Xing Cao) 15g, Folium Eriobotryae (Pi Pa Ye) 15g. *Bulbus Fritillariae Thumbergii* (Zhe Bei Mu) 10g, and *Herba Ardisiae Japonicae* (Zi Jin Niu) 30g. For serous pathogenic heat, feverish sensation and thirst, add *Radix Scutellariae* (Huang Qin) 6g, *Rhizoma Anemarrhenae* (Zhi Mu) 3g, *Fructus Trichosanthis*

方药：桑菊饮加减。桑叶 9 克，菊花 9 克，杏仁 9 克，桔梗 6 克，连翘 9 克，薄荷 6 克，芦根 9 克，甘草 6 克。若涕多明显，加苍耳子 10 克、白芷 10 克；咳嗽甚，加鱼腥草 15 克、枇杷叶 15 克、浙贝母 10 克、紫金牛 30 克；热邪较甚，身热口渴，加黄芩 6 克、知母 3 克、瓜蒌 3 克；咽痛明显，加射干 9 克；风热伤络，加白茅根 30 克、藕节 15 克。

(Gua Lou) 3g. For obvious sore throat, add *Rhizoma Belamecandae* (She Gan) 9g. For damage of collaterals by wind and heat, add *Rhizoma Imperatae* (Bai Mao Gen) 30g, and *Nodus Nelumbinis Rhizomatis* (Ou Jie) 15g.

(3) **Pattern of upward accumulation of phlegm and dampness**

(3) **痰热上壅**

Main symptoms: White and turbid or slight yellow profuse nasal discharge, cough with profuse tenacious sputum, stuffy sensation in the chest and epigastric region, rattling sound at night, poor appetite, lassitude in the four limbs, loose stool, thin and greasy tongue coating, soft and rolling pulse.

主症：涕多白浊或略黄，咳嗽多黏痰，胸脘作闷，夜间痰声辘辘，纳差，四肢乏力，大便溏稀，苔薄腻，脉濡滑。

Therapeutic method: To strengthen the spleen, dry up dampness, regulate qi and dissolve phlegm.

治法：健脾燥湿，理气化痰。

Herbal formulas and drugs: *Double Vintage Decoction* (Er Chen Tang) (modified). *Rhizoma Pinelliae* (Ban Xia) 15g, *Pericarpium Citri Tangerinae* (Chen Pi) 10g, *Sclerotium Poria* (Fu Ling) 12g, and *Radix Glycyrrhizae Praeparata* (Zhi Gan Cao) 3g. For profuse nasal discharge, add *Radix Linderae* (Wu Yao) 6g, *Fructus Alpinae Oxyphyllae* (Yi Zhi Ren) 9g. For serious phlegm and dampness, add *Rhizoma Atractylodis* (Cang Zhu) 9g, *Cortex Magnoliae Officinalis* (Hou Pu) 6g, *Semen Coicis* (Yi Yi Ren) 30g, and *Semen Armeniacae Amarum* (Ku Xing Ren) 10g. For phlegm in cold nature, add *Rhizoma Zingiberis* (Gan Jiang) 6g, and *Herba Asari* (Xi Xin) 3g.

方药：二陈汤加减。半夏 15 克，陈皮 10 克，茯苓 12 克，炙甘草 33。如涕多明显，加乌药 6 克、益智仁 9 克；痰湿重，加苍术 9 克、厚朴 6 克、薏苡仁 30 克、杏仁 10 克；若为寒痰，加干姜 6 克、细辛 3 克。

(4) **Pattern of upward disturbance of phlegm and heat**

(4) **痰热上泛**

Main symptoms: Profuse yellow turbid phlegm, couth with tenacious sputum, or sputum with blood, stuffy sensation in the chest, fever, thirst, dry

主症：痰多黄浊，咳嗽痰稠，或痰中带血，胸闷，发热口渴，口干苦，唇红面赤，咽

mouth and bitter taste in the mouth, red lips, flushed cheeks, sore throat, dry stool, brown urine, thin and greasy tongue coating, rolling and rapid pulse.

痛,大便干燥,小便色黄,苔薄腻,脉滑数。

Therapeutic method: To clear away heat, clean the lung, promote expectoration and stop nasal discharge.

治法:清热肃肺,豁痰止涕。

Herbal formulas and drugs: *Metal-Clarifying and Phlegm-Dissolving Decoction* (Qing Jin Hua Tan Tang) (modified). *Radix Scutellariae* (Huang Qin) 12g, *Fructus Gardeniae* (Zhi Zi) 12g, *Rhizoma Anemarrhenae* (Zhi Mu) 15g, *Cortex Mori Radicis* (Sang Bai Pi) 15g, *Semen Trichosanthis* (Gua Lou Zi) 15g, *Bulbus Fritillariae Cirrhosae* (Chuan Bei Mu) 9g, *Radix Ophiopogonis* (Mai Dong) 9g, *Exocarpium Citri Grandis* (Ju Hong) 9g, *Sclerotium Poria* (Fu Ling) 9g, *Radix Platycodi* (Jie Geng) 9g, and *Radix Glycyrrhizae* (Gan Cao) 3g. For profuse nasal discharge, add *Fructus Xanthii* (Cang Er Zi) 10g, and *Radix Angelicae Dahuricae* (Bai Zhi) 10g. For abundant accumulation of heat in the lung, cough, panting, strong feverish sensation and thirst, take out *Radix Platycodi* (Jie Geng) and *Pericarpium Citri Tangerinae* (Chen Pi) add *Flos Lonicerae* (Jin Yin Hua) 15g, *Herba Houttuyniae* (Yu Xing Cao) 15g, *Gypsum Fibrosum* (Shi Gao) 3g, and *Semen Descurainiae* (Ting Li Zi) 10g.

方药:清金化痰汤加减。黄芩 12 克,山栀子 12 克,知母 15 克,桑白皮 15 克,瓜蒌仁 15 克,贝母 9 克,麦门冬 9 克,橘红 9 克,茯苓 9 克,桔梗 9 克,甘草 3 克。如涕多明显,加苍耳子 10 克、白芷 10 克;肺热壅盛,咳喘,壮热口渴,去桔梗、陈皮,加金银花 15 克、鱼腥草 15 克、石膏 3 克、葶苈子 10 克。

(5) **Pattern of deficiency in the lung and kidney**

(5) **肺肾亏虚**

Main symptoms: Profuse, white and turbid nasal discharge, in persistent condition, frequent cough, clear and thin sputum and saliva, stuffy chest and panting, aggravated by cold, dizziness, palpitation, aversion to cold, heavy sensation in the limbs, soreness and weakness in the low back,

主症:涕多白浊,绵绵不断,咳嗽频发,痰涎清稀,胸闷气喘,遇寒加重,头眩心悸,畏寒肢重,腰酸困倦乏力,动则汗出,咳甚时二便失禁或小便不利,苔白润,脉沉

sweating by exertion, incontinence of urine and feces or difficult urination in serious cough, white and moist tongue coating, deep and rolling pulse.

滑。

Therapeutic method: To replenish the kidney, accept qi, warm up the lung and stop nasal discharge.

治法：补肾纳气，温肺止涕。

Herbal formulas and drugs: *True Warrior Decoction* (Zhen Wu Tang) plus *Stream-Reducing Pills* (Suo Quan Wan) (modified). *Sclerotium Poria* (Fu Ling) 9g, *Radix Paeoniae* (Shao Yao) 9g, *Rhizoma Atractylodis Macrocephalae* (Bai Zhu) 6g, *Rhizoma Zingiberis Recens* (Sheng Jiang) 9g, *Radix Aconiti Praeparata* (Fu Zi) 9g, *Radix Linderae* (Wu Yao) 6g, and *Fructus Alpinae Oxyphyllae* (Yi Zhi Ren) 9g. For serious cough, add *Herba Asari* (Xi Xin) 3g, and *Fructus Schisandrae* (Wu Wei Zi) 9g. For stuffy sensation in the chest and hypochondriac region, add *Semen Sinapis Albae* (Bai Jie Zi) 6g. and Flos Inulae (Xuan Fu Hua) 3g. For shortness of breath, add *Radix Codonopsis Pilosulae* (Dang Shen) 10g. For loose stool, add *Rhizoma Zingiberis* (Gan Jiang) 6g.

方药：真武汤合缩泉丸加减。茯苓 9 克，芍药 9 克，白术 6 克，生姜 9 克，附子 9 克，乌药 6 克，益智仁 9 克。如咳甚，加细辛 3 克、五味子 9 克；胸胁满闷，加白芥子 6 克、旋覆花 3 克；气短，加党参 10 克；大便稀溏，加干姜 6 克。

2.3 Other therapies

Please refer to other nose and sinus diseases and adopt the corresponding therapeutic methods.

2.3 其他疗法

参照其他鼻-鼻窦疾病，采取相应的治疗方法。

Chapter 3 Laryngopharyngeal Diseases

第3章 咽喉科疾病

Acute tonsillitis

急性扁桃体炎

It refers to acute non-specific inflammation of the palatine tonsil, often accompanied by inflammation of the pharyngeal mucous membrane and lymphatic tissues. It is a commonly seen disease in the throat. The main pathogenic bacterium is beta hemolytic streptococcus. It mainly occurs in children and young adults and easily occurs in the spring and autumn.

急性扁桃体炎为腭扁桃体的急性非特异性炎症，常伴有不同程度的咽黏膜和淋巴组织炎症，是一种很常见的咽部疾病。主要致病菌为乙型溶血性链球菌，多发生于儿童及青年，春、秋两季易发。

1 Diagnostic essentials

1 诊断要点

1.1 Acute onset, accompanied by the symptoms of aversion to cold, fever, and sore throat.

1.1 起病急，可有畏寒发热，咽痛为主要症状。

1.2 Diffuse congestion in the pharyngeal mucous membrane, worse in the tonsil and two palates, swollen palatine tonsil with yellow and white pus spots on the surface, yellow and white or white dot and bean dreg-like exudates in the recess, possible forming pseudomembrane, but not over the scope of the tonsil, easy to wipe off and not easy to bleed.

1.2 咽部黏膜呈弥漫性充血，以扁桃体及两腭弓最严重。腭扁桃体肿大，表面可见黄白色脓点、隐窝口有黄白色或白色点状豆渣样渗出物，可连片形成假膜，不超过扁桃体范围，易拭去，不易出血。

1.3 Swollen submandibular lymphatic nodes, obvious tenderness.

1.3 颌下淋巴结肿大，压痛明显。

1.4 Elevated white blood cell count, and elevated neutrophil count.

1.5 It is necessary to differentiate it from pharyngeal diphtheria, Vincent's angina and angina induced by some blood diseases.

2 Therapeutic methods

2.1 Therapeutic principles

The pathological position of acute tonsillitis is in the throat, lung and stomach. It is caused by infection of exogenous pathogenic wind and heat, the internal accumulation of heat in the lung and stomach, and association of internal and external toxins, attacking the throat upward. The commonly seen patterns of acute tonsillitis include pattern of invasion of pathogenic wind and heat into the lung, pattern of heat abundance in the lung and stomach. The treatment is mainly given to expel wind and clear away heat.

2.2 Treatment based on syndrome differentiation

(1) **Pattern of invasion of pathogenic wind and heat into the lung**

Main symptoms: Sore throat, pain aggravated in swallowing and cough, dry throat, burning sensation, possible general symptoms of fever, aversion to cold, headache, tiredness in the limbs, productive cough, and congestion in the palate and tonsil, red tongue margin and tip, thin and white or slight yellow tongue coating, superficial and rapid pulse.

Therapeutic method: To expel wind, clear away heat, diminish swelling and benefit the throat.

Herbal formulas and drugs: *Wind-Expelling and Heat-Eliminating Decoction* (Shu Feng Qing Re Tang) (modified). *Herba Schizonepetae* (Jing Jie)

1.4 查血白细胞总数升高，中性粒细胞增高。

1.5 注意与咽白喉、奋森咽峡炎及某些血液病引起的咽峡炎等疾病鉴别。

2 治疗方法

2.1 治疗原则

急性扁桃体炎病位在咽、肺、胃，其发生为外感风热邪毒，内有肺胃郁热，内外邪毒交结，上攻咽喉所致。急性扁桃体炎常见证型有风热犯肺、肺胃热盛等证。治疗以疏风清热为主。

2.2 辨证论治

（1）**风热犯肺**

主症：咽痛，吞咽或咳嗽时疼痛加剧，咽干灼热。全身可见发热恶寒，头痛，肢体倦怠，咳嗽有痰。检查见腭舌弓及扁桃体充血。舌边尖红，苔薄白或微黄，脉浮数。

治法：疏风清热，消肿利咽。

方药：疏风清热汤加减。荆芥 6 克，防风 6 克，金银花 10 克，连翘 10 克，黄芩 6 克，

6g, *Radix Ledebouriellae* (Fang Feng) 6g, *Flos Lonicerae* (Jin Yin Hua) 10g, *Fructus Forsythiae* (Lian Qiao) 10g, *Radix Scutellariae* (Huang Qin) 6g, *Radix Paeoniae Rubra* (Chi Shao) 6g, *Radix Scrophulariae* (Xuan Shen) 10g, *Bulbus Fritillariae Thumbergii* (Zhe Bei Mu) 10g, *Radix Trichosanthis* (Tian Hua Fen) 10g, *Cortex Mori Radicis* (Sang Bai Pi) 10g, *Fructus Arctii* (Niu Bang Zi) 10g, *Radix Platycodi* (Jie Geng) 6g, and *Radix Glycyrrhizae* (Gan Cao) 3g. For serious swollen tonsil, add Radix Isatidis (Ban Lan Gen) 15g, and *Folium Isatidis* (Da Qing Ye) 15g. For constipation, add *Fructus Trichosanthis* (Gua Lou) 20g, or *Rhizoma Rhei Cruda* (Sheng Da Huang) 5g.

赤芍药6克，玄参10克，浙贝母10克，天花粉10克，桑白皮10克，牛蒡子10克，桔梗6克，甘草3克。若扁桃体红肿甚，加板蓝根15克、大青叶15克；大便干结，加全瓜蒌20克，或用生大黄5克。

(2) **Pattern of heat abundance in the lung and stomach**

(2) **肺胃热盛**

Main symptoms: Serious sore throat, radiating to the ear and submandibular region, difficult swallow, with obstructive sensation, possible general symptoms of fever, thirst with preference of drinks, cough, yellow and tenacious sputum, foul breath, constipation, brown urine, obvious swollen tonsil, with yellow and white pus dots on the surface, pseudomembrane in patch, and even swollen pharyngeal isthmus, swollen submandibular lymphatic nodes, obvious tenderness, red tongue, yellow and thick tongue coating, floody and rapid pulse.

主症：咽痛剧烈，可向耳根及颌下放射，吞咽困难，有堵塞感。全身可有发热，口渴引饮，咳嗽痰稠黄，口臭，大便秘结，小便黄。检查扁桃体红肿明显，表面有黄白色脓点，伪膜可连成片状，甚或咽峡红肿，颌下有淋巴结肿大，压痛明显。舌质红赤，苔黄厚，脉洪大而数。

Therapeutic method: To clear away heat, resolve toxin, benefit the throat, and diminish swelling.

治法：清热解毒，利咽消肿。

Herbal formulas and drugs: ① *Throat-Clarifying and Diaphragm-Benefiting Decoction* (Qing Yan Li Ge Tang) (modified). *Rhizoma Rhei Cruda*

方药：①清咽利膈汤加减。生大黄5克，黄芩6克，蒲公英15克，金银花10克，

(Sheng Da Huang) 5g, *Radix Scutellariae* (Huang Qin) 6g, *Herba Taraxaci* (Pu Gong Ying) 15g, *Flos Lonicerae* (Jin Yin Hua) 10g, *Fructus Forsythiae* (Lian Qiao) 10g, *Bulbus Fritillariae Thumbergii* (Zhe Bei Mu) 10g, *Calyx et Fructus Physalis* (Gua Jin Deng) 15g, *Rhizoma Belamecandae* (She Gan) 5g, *Bombyx Batryticatus* (Bai Jiang Can) 10g, Pericarpium Trichosanthis (Gua Lou Pi) 10g, and *Radix Glycyrrhizae* (Gan Cao) 3g. For profuse sputum in the throat, add *Gypsum Fibrosum* (Shi Gao) (Decoct first) 20g, *Concretio Siliceae Bambusae* (Tian Zhu Huang) 6g. For excessive pseudomembrane, add *Lasiosphaera Seu Calvatia* (Ma Bo) 3g. ② *Universal Salvation Detoxifying Drink* (Pu Ji Xiao Du Yin). *Radix Scutellariae* (Huang Qin) 15g, *Rhizoma Coptidis* (Huang Lian) 15g, *Pericarpium Citri Tangerinae* (Chen Pi) 6g, *Radix Glycyrrhizae* (Gan Cao) 6g, *Radix Scrophulariae* (Xuan Shen) 6g, *Radix Bupleuri* (Chai Hu) 6g, *Radix Platycodi* (Jie Geng) 6g, *Fructus Forsythiae* (Lian Qiao) 3g, *Radix Isatidis* (Ban Lan Gen) 3g, *Lasiosphaera Seu Calvatia* (Ma Bo) 3g, *Fructus Arctii* (Niu Bang Zi) 3g, *Herba Menthae* (Bo He) 3g, *Bombyx Batryticatus* (Bai Jiang Can) 2g, and *Rhizoma Cimicifugae* (Sheng Ma) 2g.

2.3 Other therapies

(1) Chinese patent medicine: ① Swelling and Pain Easing Capsules, Take two capsules each time, for 3 times per day, used for pattern of invasion of pathogenic wind and heat in the lung. ② *Heat-Clarifying and Aperture-Opening Granules* (Qing Kai Ling Chong Ji), Take 1 to 2 packets each time, for 3 times per day, used for pattern of abundant heat in the lung and stomach. ③ *Isatis Granules* (Ban

连翘 10 克,浙贝母 10 克,挂金灯 15 克,射干 5 克,白僵蚕 10 克,瓜蒌皮 10 克,生甘草 3 克。若咽喉痰多,加石膏(先煎)20 克、天竺黄 6 克;伪膜多,加马勃 3 克。②普济消毒饮。黄芩 15 克,黄连 15 克,陈皮 6 克,甘草 6 克,玄参 6 克,柴胡 6 克,桔梗 6 克,连翘 3 克,板蓝根 3 克,马勃 3 克,牛蒡子 3 克,薄荷 3 克,僵蚕 2 克,升麻 2 克。

2.3 其他疗法

(1)中成药:①肿痛安胶囊,每服 2 粒,每日 3 次。用于风热犯肺证。②清开灵冲剂,每服 1～2 包,每日 3 次。用于肺胃热盛证。③板蓝根冲剂,每服 1～2 包,每日 3 次。六神丸、一清胶囊、万应胶囊、清咽滴丸、疏风解毒颗

Lan Gen Chong Ji), Take 1 to 2 packets, for 3 times per day. *Six Divine Pills* (Liu Shen Wan), *All Clarifying Capsules* (Yi Qing Jiao Nang), *Throat-Clearing Dropping Pills* (Qing Yan Di Wan), *Wind-Expelling and Toxin-Resolving Granules* (Shu Feng Jie Du Jiao Nang) can all be used for acute tonsillitis.

粒等，急性扁桃体炎均可应用。

(2) Simple and proved formulas: ① *Decoct Flos Chrysanthemi Indici* (Ye Ju Hua) 30g, *Herba Hedyotis Diffusae* (Bai Hua She She Cao) 30g, *Herba Elephantopi* (Ku Di Dan) 30g, *Herba Centellae Asiaticae* (Ji Xue Cao) 30g, and *Rhizoma Imperatae* (Bai Mao Gen) 30g. with water for oral administration, for twice per day. ② *Decoct Radix Sophorae Subprostratae* (Shan Dou Gen) 30g, and *Calyx et Fructus Physalis* (Gua Jin Deng) with water for oral administration, for twice per day.

（2）单验方：①野菊花30克，白花蛇舌草30克，苦地胆30克，积雪草30克，白茅根30克，水煎服，每日2次。②山豆根30克，锦灯笼30克，水煎服，每日2次。

(3) External therapies: *Tin-Type Powder* (Xi Lei San), *Borneol and Borax Powder* (Bing Peng San), and *Pearl and Bezoar Powder* (Zhu Huang San) in clearing away heat, resolving toxin, expelling the decay and diminishing swelling can be blown to the surface of the tonsil, once per 1 to 2 h. It is also advisable to rinse the mouth with *Mouth-Washing Formula* (Shu Kou Fang) or water prepared with *Herba Schizonepetae* (Jing Jie) and *Flos Chrysanthemi* (Ju Hua) to clean the oral cavity, in the effects to expel wind, clear away heat, resolve toxin and diminish swelling. It is also advisable to take *Iron Flute Pills* (Tie Di Wan) or *Throat-Moistening Pills* (Run Hou Wan) to clear away heat and moisten dryness.

（3）外治法：锡类散、冰硼散、珠黄散等清热解毒、祛腐消肿之品吹于扁桃体表面，每1～2小时1次；也可用漱口方或荆芥、菊花煎水含漱，以清洁口腔，有疏风清热、解毒消肿止痛作用；亦可含服铁笛丸或润喉丸以清热润燥。

Chronic tonsillitis

慢性扁桃体炎

It refers to the chronic inflammation of the palatine tonsil, mostly caused by the repeated seizure of acute tonsillitis or obstructed drainage of the tonsil crypt and infection of bacteria in the crypt, with streptococci and staphylococci.

慢性扁桃体炎是腭扁桃体的慢性炎症，多因急性扁桃体炎反复发作或因扁桃体隐窝引流不畅，窝内细菌、病毒滋生感染所致，链球菌和葡萄球菌为其主要致病菌。

1 Diagnostic essentials

1 诊断要点

1.1 Frequently history of acute seizures, no obvious subjective symptoms in the ordinary times, often discomfort in the throat or foul breath, various abnormal sensations of foreign body in the throat, pricking pain, paroxysmal cough, possible difficult breathing and swallowing due to over enlarged tonsil, aphasia, headache, lassitude, low-grade fever, and digestive disturbance.

1.1 常有急性发作病史，平时多无明显自觉症状。咽部经常不适或有口臭，可有咽异物感、刺痛感、阵发性咳嗽或各种感觉异常。如扁桃体过于肥大可有呼吸、吞咽困难，言语含糊不清。亦可有头痛、乏力、低热和消化障碍等。

1.2 Chronic congestion in the tonsil and palatoglossal arch, different size in tonsil, mostly shrunk, scared and uneven and adhered with surrounding tissues in adults, yellow or white cheese-like stuffs present in the mouth of the crypt by pressing the palatoglossal arch, swollen submandibular lymphatic nodes.

1.2 检查可见扁桃体和腭舌弓呈慢性充血，扁桃体大小不定，成人多缩小，有瘢痕、凹凸不平，与周围组织有粘连。挤压腭舌弓时隐窝口有时可见黄、白色干酪样点状物溢出。颌下淋巴结常肿大。

1.3 It is necessary to differentiate it from physiological hypertrophy of the tonsil, tonsil keratosis and tonsil tumors.

1.3 应与扁桃体生理性肥大，扁桃体角化病及扁桃体肿瘤等相鉴别。

2 Therapeutic methods

2 治疗方法

2.1 Therapeutic principles

2.1 治疗原则

Chronic tonsillitis is mostly caused by upward flaming of deficient fire, due to deficiency in the

慢性扁桃体炎为肺、肾等脏腑虚损，虚火上炎所致。

lung and kidney. The treatment is mainly applied to nourish yin, and to clear away heat as well.

治疗以养阴为主,佐以清热。

2.2 Treatment based on syndrome differentiation

2.2 辨证论治

(1) **Pattern of insufficiency of lung yin**

(1) 肺阴不足

Main symptoms: Dry and uncomfortable, slight painful and slight itching sensation in the throat, dry cough without sputum or with scanty tenacious sputum, possibly accompanied by afternoon feverish sensation, feverish sensation in the chest, palms and soles, weak voice, enlarged and red tonsil, or with yellow and white pus spots on the surface, red tongue, scanty tongue coating, thready and rapid pulse.

主症:咽部干燥不适,微痛,微痒,干咳无痰或痰少而黏。可伴午后颧红、手足心热,讲话乏力。检查见扁桃体肥大,潮红,表面或有黄白色脓点。舌质红,少苔,脉细数。

Therapeutic method: To nourish yin, clarify the lung, produce body fluid and moisten dryness.

治法:养阴清肺,生津润燥。

Herbal formulas and drugs: ① *Yin-Nourishing and Lung-Cleaning Decoction* (Yang Yin Qing Fei Tang) (modified). *Radix Scrophulariae* (Xuan Shen) 10g, *Radix Rehmanniae Cruda* (Sheng Di Huang) (fresh) 10g, *Bulbus Lilii* (Bai He) 5g, *Rhizoma Imperatae* (Bai Mao Gen) 10g, *Rhizoma Phragmitis* (Lu Gen) 30g, *Herba Menthae* (Bo He) (decoct later) 6g, *Fructus Arctii* (Niu Bang Zi) 10g, *Flos Lonicerae* (Jin Yin Hua) 10g, *Fructus Forsythiae* (Lian Qiao) 10g, *Radix Platycodi* (Jie Geng) 6g, *Radix Trichosanthis* (Tian Hua Fen) 10g, and *Radix Glycyrrhizae* (Gan Cao) 3g. ② Sweet Dew Drink (Gan Lu Yin). *Radix Rehmanniae Praeparata* (Shu Di Huang) 15g, *Radix Rehmanniae Cruda* (Sheng Di Huang) 12g, *Radix Ophiopogonis* (Mai Dong) 10g, *Tuber Asparagi* (Tian Men Dong) 10g, *Herba Dendrobii* (Shi Hu) 10g, *Folium Eriobotryae* (Pi Pa Ye) 9g, *Fructus Aurantii* (Zhi Ke) 6g, *Herba Artemisiae Scopariae*

方药:①养阴清肺汤加减。玄参 10 克,生地黄 10 克,百合 10 克,白茅根 10 克,芦根 30 克,薄荷(后下)6 克,牛蒡子 10 克,金银花 10 克,连翘 10 克,桔梗 6 克,天花粉 10 克,生甘草 3 克。②甘露饮。熟地 15 克,生地 12 克,麦冬 10 克,天冬 10 克,石斛 10 克,枇杷叶 9 克,枳壳 6 克,茵陈 10 克,黄芩 6 克,甘草 6 克。

(Yin Chen) 10g, *Radix Scutellariae* (Huang Qin) 6g, and *Radix Glycyrrhizae* (Gan Cao) 6g.

(2) **Pattern of kidney yin deficiency**

Main symptoms: Dry, uncomfortable and slight painful sensation in the throat, difficult swallow, dry mouth without preference for drinks, possibly accompanied by the general symptoms of dizziness, blurred vision, tinnitus, deafness, soreness and weakness of low back and knee, vexation due to deficiency, insomnia, red colour in the tonsil and palatoglossal arch, yellow and white cheese-like secretions in the mouth of the crypt, red tongue, scanty tongue coating, thready and rapid pulse.

Therapeutic method: To nourish yin, reduce fire, clean and benefit the throat.

Herbal formulas and drugs: *Anemarrhena, Phellodendron, and Rehmannia Pills* (Zhi Bai Di Huang Wan) (modified). *Rhizoma Anemarrhenae* (Zhi Mu) 10g, *Cortex Phellodendri* (Huang Bo) 10g, *Radix Rehmanniae Praeparata* (Shu Di Huang) 10g, *Fructus Corni* (Shan Zhu Yu) 10g, *Radix Scrophulariae* (Xuan Shen) 10g, *Radix Ophiopogonis* (Mai Dong) 10g, *Herba Dendrobii* (Shi Hu) 10g, *Cortex Moutan Radicis* (Mu Dan Pi) 6g, *Rhizoma Alismatis* (Ze Xie) 6g, *Radix Platycodi* (Jie Geng) 6g, and *Radix Glycyrrhizae* (Gan Cao) 3g. For low spirit, cold sensation in the hands and feet, loose stool, pale tongue and white tongue coating present in chronic tonsillitis, it is advisable to replenish the kidney and support yang by using *Aconite and Cinnamon and Eight Ingredient Pills* (Fu Gui Ba Wei Wan). If deficiency of qi and blood is present, it is advisable to use *Eight Jewel Decoction* (Ba Zhen Tang) plus *Platycodon and Liquorice*

(2) **肾阴虚损**

主症:咽喉干燥不适,微痛,哽咽不利,口干不喜多饮。全身可伴有头昏眼花,耳鸣、耳聋,腰酸膝软,虚烦失眠。检查见扁桃体及腭弓潮红,隐窝口有黄白色干酪样分泌物。舌质红,少苔,脉细数。

治法:滋阴降火,清利咽喉。

方药:知柏地黄汤加减。知母 10 克,黄柏 10 克,熟地黄 10 克,山萸肉 10 克,玄参 10 克,麦门冬 10 克,石斛 10 克,牡丹皮 6 克,泽泻 6 克,桔梗 6 克,甘草 3 克。若慢性扁桃体炎如症见精神疲倦、手足冷、大便溏泄、舌淡苔白者,宜用补肾扶阳之法,可用附桂八味丸;如症见气虚血弱者,可用八珍汤合桔梗甘草汤,以气血双补、利咽祛痰;如症见纳差、脘腹胀闷、便溏者,可选用参苓白术散以健脾益气。

Decoction (Jie Geng Gan Cao Tang), in order to replenish both qi and blood, and benefit the throat and dissipate phlegm. If poor appetite, distending and stuffy sensation in the abdominal and epigastric region, and loose stool are present, it is advisable to use *Ginseng, Poria and Atractylodes Powder* (Shen Ling Bai Zhu San) to strengthen the spleen and benefit qi.

2.3 Other therapies

(1) Simple and proved formula: Grind *Flos Lonicerae* (Jin Yin Hua), *Radix Scrophulariae* (Xuan Shen), *Fructus Terminalinae Xchebulae Immaturi* (Zang Qing Guo), in equal propotion, into powder and infuse with water, for rinsing the mouth frequently.

(2) Sublingual administrating method: *Throat-Clearing Dropping Pills* (Qing Yan Di Wan), Take 4 pills in the mouth, for 3 times per day.

2.3 其他疗法

（1）单验方：金银花、玄参、藏青果等分研末泡水，不拘次数含嗽。

（2）含化法：清咽滴丸，每次 4 丸含化，每日 3 次。

Adenoid hypertrophy

Under the normal physiological circumstances, the adenoid is biggest at the age of 6 to 7 and gradually shrinks after 10 years old. If the adenoid becomes hypertrophic and induces the corresponding symptoms, it is termed adenoid hypertrophy. This diseases mostly occurs in the children at the age of 3 to 5 and is seldom in the adults. The pathological hypertrophy of the adenoid can occur due to the repeated autologous stimulation from the inflammation of the nasopharynx and its nearby positions or adenoid. It belongs to the scope of "snoring sleep" in Chinese medicine.

腺样体肥大

正常生理情况下，腺样体 6～7 岁时最大，10 岁后逐渐萎缩。若腺样体增生并引起相应的症状，称为腺样体肥大。本病多发生于 3～5 岁儿童，成人罕见。鼻咽部及其毗邻部位或腺样体自身的炎症反复刺激，使腺样体发生病理性增生。属中医学"鼾眠"范畴。

1 Diagnostic essentials

1.1 Nasal obstruction, nasal discharge, nasal obstructive twang in speaking, snoring in sleep, often complicated with rhinitis, nasosinusitis.

1.2 Distending and stuffy sensation in the ear, hearing loss, tinnitus.

1.3 Frequent paroxysmal cough, but scanty sputum, easy to induce bronchitis.

1.4 Adenoidal face present in severe condition: Because of long-term respiration by opening the mouth, the skull development is impacted, leading to lengthened maxillary bone, elevated palatine elevated, odontoloxia, malocclusion, protrusion of upper incisor, thickened lips, dropped lower jaw, and dull expression.

1.5 Possible nightmare, screaming, odontoprisis, enuresis crowing convulsion or asthma during sleep, and malnutrition, slow response and poor concentration present in long-term duration.

1.6 Inspection

Inspections show adenoidal face, elevated and narrow hard palate, protrusion of red cloddy stuff in the posterior wall in the roof of the nasopharynx, palpable soft lymph lump, and also hypertrophic tonsil.

1.7 X-ray radiography or CT scan of the nasopharynx is beneficial to the diagnosis.

2 Therapeutic methods

2.1 Therapeutic principles

The nose is an external indicator of the lung and the throat is a door of the lung. In children, the liver is often superabound and the lung, spleen and

1 诊断要点

1.1 鼻塞、流涕，说话时带鼻塞性鼻音，睡时打鼾。常并发鼻炎、鼻窦炎。

1.2 可有耳闷胀感、听力下降、耳鸣。

1.3 常见阵咳但少痰，易引发支气管炎。

1.4 严重者出现腺样体面容：因长期张口呼吸，影响颅骨发育，上颌骨变长，腭骨高拱，牙列不齐，咬合不良，上切牙突出，唇厚，下颌下垂，表情淡漠。

1.5 可有睡眠时噩梦、惊叫、磨牙、遗尿、喘鸣性痉挛或哮喘。病程久者可营养不良，反应迟钝，注意力不集中。

1.6 检查

腺样体面容，硬腭高而窄；鼻咽顶后壁红色团块状物隆起，触诊可及柔软的淋巴组织团块。扁桃体亦可肥大。

1.7 鼻咽 X 线侧位拍片或 CT 扫描，有助于诊断。

2 治疗方法

2.1 治疗原则

鼻为肺窍，咽为肺之门户。小儿肝常有余，肺、脾、肾常显不足。治疗以益气养

kidney are often insufficient. The treatment is mainly given to benefit qi, nourish yin, regulate qi and disperse blood stasis.

阴、理气化瘀为主。

2.2 Treatment based on syndrome differentiation

(1) Pattern of qi deficiency in the lung and spleen, and accumulation of turbid phlegm

Main symptoms: Nasal obstruction, white nasal discharge, white and tenacious sputum, soft adenoid, low spirit, lassitude, pale complexion, dull expression, abdominal distension, poor appetite, susceptible to cold, snoring at night, pale and swollen tongue with teeth marks, thready and feeble pulse.

Therapeutic method: To benefit qi, strengthen the spleen, dissolve phlegm and disperse accumulation.

Herbal formulas and drugs: *Jade Wind-Barrier Powder* (Yu Ping Feng San) plus *Double Vintage Decoction* (Er Chen Tang)(modified). *Radix Astragali* (Huang Qi) 6g, *Radix Codonopsis Pilosulae* (Dang Shen) 6g, *Radix Pseudostellariae* (Tai Zi Shen) 9g, *Rhizoma Atractylodis Macrocephalae* (Bai Zhu) 6g, *Radix Ledebouriellae* (Fang Feng) 4.5g, *Rhizoma Pinelliae* (Ban Xia) 6g, *Pericarpium Citri Tangerinae* (Chen Pi) 6g, *Radix Bupleuri* (Chai Hu) 6g, *Rhizoma Cimicifugae* (Sheng Ma) 6g, *Bulbus Fritillariae Thumbergii* (Zhe Bei Mu) 9g, *Bombyx Batryticatus* (Jiang Can) 3g, *Radix Codonopsis Lanceolatae* (Shan Hai Lou) 12g, *Sclerotium Poria* (Fu Ling) 3g, and *Radix Glycyrrhizae* (Gan Cao) 3g. For abdominal distension and poor appetite, add *Fructus Crataegi* (Shan Zha) 6g, *Fructus Amomi* (Sha Ren) 2.4g, *Endothelium Corneum Gigeriae Galli* (Ji Nei Jin) 5g, *Fructus Oryzae Germinatus* (Gu Ya) 6g, and *Fructus Hordei Germinatus*

2.2 辨证论治

(1) 肺脾气虚，痰浊凝滞

主症：鼻塞，涕色白，咯痰白黏，腺样体触之较软，神疲乏力，面色苍白，表情淡漠，腹胀纳呆，易感冒，夜间打鼾，舌淡胖，有齿痕，脉细无力。

治法：益气健脾，化痰散结。

方药：玉屏风散合二陈汤加味。黄芪6克，党参6克，太子参9克，炒白术6克，防风4.5克，半夏6克，陈皮6克，柴胡6克，升麻6克，浙贝母9克，僵蚕3克，山海螺12克，茯苓3克，甘草3克。若腹胀纳呆、不思饮食者，加山楂6克、砂仁2.4克、鸡内金5克、谷芽6克、麦芽6克；鼻塞重、涕白者，加细辛3克、白芷6克、辛夷花6克。

(Mai Ya) 6g. For serious nasal obstruction and white nasal discharge, add *Herba Asari* (Xi Xin) 3g, *Radix Angelicae Dahuricae* (Bai Zhi) 6g. and *Flos Magnoliae Liliflorae* (Xin Yi Hua) 6g.

(2) **Pattern of yin deficiency in the lung and kidney**

Main symptoms: Nasal obstruction, yellow and white nasal discharge, snoring at night, dry and uncomfortable sensation in the throat, lingering hypertrophic adenoid, swollen tonsil, accompanied by headache, poor memory, restless sleep, continuous snoring, profuse sweating, teeth grinding, red tongue, scanty tongue coating, thready and feeble pulse.

Therapeutic method: To nourish yin, replenish the lung, reinforce the kidney and fill up essence.

Herbal formulas and drugs: *Rehmannia Decoction with Six Ingredients* (Liu Wei Di Huang Tang) (modified). *Radix Rehmanniae Cruda* (Sheng Di Huang) 9g, *Rhizoma Dioscoreae* (Shan Yao) 12g, *Herba Dendrobii* (Shi Hu) 6g, *Sclerotium Poria* (Fu Ling) 9g, *Cortex Moutan Radicis* (Mu Dan Pi) 6g, *Radix Scrophulariae* (Xuan Shen) 6g, *Radix Ophiopogonis* (Mai Dong) 6g, *Radix Platycodi* (Jie Geng) 4.5g, *Bulbus Lilii* (Bai He) 9g, *Semen Zizyphi Spinosae* (Suan Zao Ren) 9g, *Bulbus Fritillariae Cirrhosae* (Chuan Bei Mu) 9g, *Cortex Lycii Radicis* (Di Gu Pi) 6g, *Radix Codonopsis Lanceolatae* (Shan Hai Lou) 12g. For serious nasal obstruction, add *Radix Angelicae Dahuricae* (Bai Zhi) 6g, *Herba Asari* (Xi Xin) 3g. and *Flos Magnoliae Liliflorae* (Xin Yi Hua) 6g. For poor memory, add *Fructus Alpinae Oxyphyllae* (Yi Zhi Ren) 6g, *Fructus Ligustri Lucidi* (Nü Zhen Zi) 6g, and *Fructus Lycii* (Gou Qi Zi)

(2) **肺肾阴虚**

主症：鼻塞，涕黄白，夜间打鼾，喉咙部干燥不适，腺样体肥大久而不消，扁桃体肿大，兼见头痛，健忘，夜卧不安，夜寐鼾声持续不断，多汗，磨牙，舌红少苔，脉细无力。

治法：滋阴补肺，补肾填精。

方药：六味地黄汤加减。生地黄 9 克，怀山药 12 克，石斛 6 克，茯苓 9 克，牡丹皮 6 克，玄参 6 克，麦冬 6 克，桔梗 4.5 克，百合 9 克，炒酸枣仁 9 克，川贝母 9 克，地骨皮 6 克，山海螺 12 克。若鼻塞重者，加白芷 6 克、细辛 3 克、辛夷花 6 克；健忘者，加益智仁 6 克、女贞子 6 克、枸杞子 12 克；头痛者，加川芎 6 克、杭菊花 6 克。

12g. For headache, add *Rhizoma Ligustici Chuanxiong* (Chuan Xiong) 6g, and *Flos Chrysanthemi* (Ju Hua) 6g.

(3) **Pattern of qi stagnation and blood stasis**

Main symptoms: Obvious nasal obstruction, hypertrophic adenoid, hard and lingering in nature, snoring at night, difficult respiration, often breathing with open mouth, and even suffocated condition, or accompanied by stuffy and distending sensation in the ear, hearing loss, dark red tongue or with ecchymosis, and choppy pulse.

Therapeutic method: To activate blood, disperse blood stasis, dissipate accumulation and diminish swelling.

Herbal formulas and drugs: *Epiglottis Blood Stasis-Dissipating Decoction* (Hui Yan Zhu Yu Tang) (modified). *Radix Paeoniae Rubra* (Chi Shao) 9g, *Radix Rehmanniae Cruda* (Sheng Di Huang) 9g, *Rhizoma Ligustici Chuanxiong* (Chuan Xiong) 9g, *Radix Salviae Miltiorrhizae* (Dan Shen) 6g, *Radix Bupleuri* (Chai Hu) 6g, *Radix Platycodi* (Jie Geng) 6g, *Fructus Aurantii* (Zhi Ke) 4. 5g, *Spina Gleditsiae* (Zao Jiao Ci) 3g, Radix Codonopsis Lanceolatae (Shan Hai Lou) 12g, *Bombyx Batryticatus* (Bai Jiang Can) 3g, and *Radix Glycyrrhizae* (Gan Cao) 3g. For profuse sputum, add *Bulbus Fritillariae Thumbergii* (Zhe Bei Mu) 6g, *Radix Scrophulariae* (Xuan Shen) 6g, *Radix Trichosanthis* (Tian Hua Fen) 6g. For effusion in the ear, add *Rhizoma Alismatis* (Ze Xie) 6g, *Sclerotium Poria* (Fu Ling) 6g. For yellow nasal discharge, add *Radix Scutellariae* (Huang Qin) 3g, and *Fructus Forsythiae* (Lian Qiao) 10g.

(3) **气滞血瘀**

主症:鼻塞明显,腺样体肿大,质硬难消,日久不愈,夜间打鼾,呼吸困难,常张口呼吸,甚则憋气、窒息状,或伴耳中闷胀,听力下降,舌质暗红或有瘀斑,脉涩。

治法:活血化瘀,散结消肿。

方药:会厌逐瘀汤加减。赤芍 9 克,生地黄 9 克,川芎 6 克,丹参 6 克,柴胡 6 克,桔梗 6 克,枳壳 4.5 克,皂角刺 3 克,山海螺 12 克,僵蚕 3 克,甘草 3 克。若咯痰量多者,加浙贝母 6 克、玄参 6 克、天花粉 6 克;有中耳积液者,加泽泻 6 克、茯苓 6 克;涕黄者,加黄芩 3 克、连翘 10 克。

2.3 Other therapies

(1) External therapies: Please refer to "chronic rhinitis".

(2) Sublingual administrating method: It is advisable to select *Throat Lozenge* (Run Hou Pian), *Sarcandra Thorat Tablets* (Cao Shan Hu Han Pian), *Cydiodine Buccal Tablets* (Hua Su Pian), and take in the mouth for several times per day.

2.3 其他疗法

（1）外治法：参阅"慢性鼻炎"。

（2）含服法：可选用润喉丸、草珊瑚含片、华素片等，每日口含数次。

Acute pharyngitis

急性咽炎

It refers to acute inflammation of the pharyngeal mucosa and submucous tissues, mostly involving the lymphatic tissues of the pharynx. It can occur individually and also secondarily to acute rhinitis or acute tonsillitis. It is mostly seen in the autumn and winter or in the juncture of winter and spring and is related to viral or bacterial infection. The commonly seen viruses include Coxsackie virus, adenovirus, parainfluenza virus, rhinovirus, influenza virus, and bacteria of beta hemolytic streptococcus, staphylococcus, and streptococcus pneumoniae.

急性咽炎是咽部黏膜、黏膜下组织的急性炎症，多累及咽部淋巴组织。可单独发生，亦常继发于急性鼻炎或急性扁桃体炎。秋冬季及冬春季之交多见，与病毒或细菌感染有感，常见的病毒有柯萨奇病毒、腺病毒、副流感病毒、鼻病毒、流感病毒，细菌有乙型溶血性链球菌、葡萄球菌、肺炎双球菌等。

1 Diagnostic essentials

1.1 Acute onset, dry, burning hot and slight painful sensation in the throat at the beginning, more obvious in swallowing food, discomfort in swallowing, cough, hoarse voice, hearing loss, accompanied by the general symptoms of fever, headache, poor appetite, dry mouth, aching pain in the four limbs, possible high fever, nausea and vomiting in infants.

1.2 In inspection are present acute diffuse conges-

1 诊断要点

1.1 起病较急，初起咽部干燥灼热、微痛，吞咽时明显。可有吞咽不适、咳嗽、声嘶、听力减退等；全身可有发热、头痛、食欲不振、口干、四肢酸痛，在幼儿可有高热寒战、恶心、呕吐等。

1.2 检查可见口咽部黏膜

tion and tumefaction in the mucosa of the oral pharynx, in deep red color, worse in the lateral wall of the oral pharynx, and congestion and edema in the uvula, soft palate and tonsil, tumefaction and congestion of the lymphoid follicle at the posterior wall of the pharynx, and also tumefaction in the nasopharyngeal and laryngopharynx, and tumefaction and tenderness in the submaxillary lymph nodes.

呈急性弥漫性充血、肿胀，呈深红色，以口咽外侧壁为甚。悬雍垂、软腭及扁桃体充血、水肿，咽后壁淋巴滤泡肿大、充血，鼻咽及喉咽部亦可红肿。颌下淋巴结肿大有压痛。

1.3 It is necessary to differentiate it from the premonitory symptoms of acute infectious diseases, such as measles, scarlet fever, influenza, and infectious mononucleosis, and from hematologic angina, such as angina of granulocytopenia, and angina of lymphocytic leukemia.

1.3 应与麻疹、猩红热、流行型感冒、传染性单核细胞增多症等急性传染病的前驱症状相区别，与急性粒细胞减少性咽峡炎、淋巴细胞白血病咽峡炎等血液病性咽峡炎相鉴别。

2 Therapeutic methods

2 治疗方法

2.1 Therapeutic principles

2.1 治疗原则

The pathological position of acute pharyngitis is in the throat, but it is related to the lung and stomach. It can be caused by invasion of pathogenic wind and heat toxin into the throat, or leading to internal production of heat, and accumulation in the lung and stomach. The treatment is mainly applied to clear away heat from the lung and stomach.

急性咽炎病位在咽，与肺、胃相关。风热邪毒外袭咽喉，或化火入里，蕴结肺胃而致病。治疗以清肺胃之热为主。

2.2 Treatment based on syndrome differentiation

2.2 辨证论治

(1) **Pattern of invasion of wind and heat into the lung**

(1) 风热犯肺

Main symptoms: Painful, burning hot, dry and uncomfortable or obstructive sensation in the throat, possibly accompanied by the general symptoms of aversion to cold, fever, slight thirst, aching pain in the whole body, lassitude, and congestion and tumefaction in the pharyngeal mucosa, red

主症：咽痛、灼热、干燥不适，或有梗阻感。全身可有恶寒、发热，口微渴，周身酸痛，乏力。检查见咽黏膜充血、肿胀。舌边尖红，苔薄白，脉浮数。

tongue margin and tip, thin and white tongue coating, superficial and rapid pulse.

Therapeutic method: To expel wind, promote the lung for its spreading ability, clear away heat and benefit the throat.

治法:疏风宣肺,清热利咽。

Herbal formulas and drugs: ① *Mulberry and Chrysanthemum Drink* (Sang Ju Yin)(modified): *Folium Mori* (Sang Ye) 10g, *Flos Chrysanthemi* (Ju Hua) 10g, *Fructus Forsythiae* (Lian Qiao) 10g, Radix Isatidis (Ban Lan Gen) 15g, *Radix Ledebouriellae* (Fang Feng) 6g, *Radix Platycodi* (Jie Geng) 6g, *Herba Menthae* (Bo He) (decoct later) 6g, *Rhizoma Belamecandae* (She Gan) 5g, *Radix Glycyrrhizae* (Gan Cao) 3g, and *Rhizoma Phragmitis* (Lu Gen) 30g. For serious sore throat and tumefaction of pharyngeal mucosa, add *Radix Scutellariae* (Huang Qin) 6g, and *Herba Taraxaci* (Pu Gong Ying) 15g. For constipation, add *Rhizoma Rhei Cruda* (Sheng Da Huang) 5g. ② *Wind-Expelling and Heat-Eliminating Decoction* (Shu Feng Qing Re Tang). Please refer to "acute tonsillitis".

方药:①桑菊饮加减。桑叶10克,菊花10克,连翘10克,板蓝根15克,防风6克,桔梗6克,薄荷(后下)6克,射干5克,甘草3克,芦根30克。若咽痛、咽黏膜红肿甚,加黄芩6克、蒲公英15克;大便干结,加生大黄5克。②疏风清热汤。见"急性扁桃体炎"。

(2) **Pattern of heat abundance in the lung and stomach**

(2) **肺胃热盛**

Main symptoms: Obvious sore throat and swallowing pain, even difficult swallow, fever, no aversion to cold, thirst with preference for drinks, constipation, scanty and brown urine, fresh red or deep red pharyngeal mucosa, retropharyngeal folliculosis, tumefaction in the lateral pharyngeal bands, red tongue, yellow and greasy tongue coating, rolling and rapid pulse.

主症:咽痛,吞咽痛明显,甚则吞咽困难。发热,不恶寒,口渴多饮,大便干结,小便短赤。检查见咽黏膜鲜红或深红,咽后壁淋巴滤泡增生,咽侧索红肿。舌质红,苔黄腻,脉滑数。

Therapeutic method: To clear away heat, discharge fire, diminish swelling and benefit the throat.

治法:清热泻火,消肿利咽。

Herbal formulas and drugs: Throat-Clarifying and Diaphragm-Benefiting Decoction (Qing Yan Li Ge Tang)(modified). *Rhizoma Rhei Cruda* (Sheng Da Huang) 5g, *Natrii Sulfas Exsiccatus* (Xuan Ming Fen) 10g, *Radix Scutellariae* (Huang Qin) 6g, *Gypsum Fibrosum* (Shi Gao) (Decoct first) 20g, *Radix Angelicae Dahuricae* (Bai Zhi) 6g, *Fructus Forsythiae* (Lian Qiao) 10g, *Flos Lonicerae* (Jin Yin Hua) 10g, *Radix Platycodi* (Jie Geng) 6g, *Radix Trichosanthis* (Tian Hua Fen) 10g, and *Radix Glycyrrhizae* (Gan Cao) 3g. For serious pathogenic heat, add *Fructus Trichosanthis* (Gua Lou) 10g, *Radix Peucedani* (Qian Hu) 10g, *Radix Stemonae* (Bai Bu) 10g, *Caulis Bambusae in Taeniam* (Zhu Ru) 10g, *Rhizoma Belamecandae* (She Gan) 5g, *Semen Armeniacae Amarum* (Ku Xing Ren) 10g, and *Concretio Siliceae Bambusae* (Tian Zhu Huang) 6g.

方药：清咽利膈汤加减。生大黄5克，玄明粉10克，黄芩6克，生石膏（先煎）20克，白芷6克，连翘10克，金银花10克，桔梗6克，甘草3克。若热邪甚，酌情加瓜蒌10克、前胡10克、百部10克，竹茹10克、射干5克、杏仁10克、天竺黄6克。

2.3 Other therapies

(1) Chinese patent medicine: ① *Double Coptis Oral Liquid* (Shuang Huang Lian Kou Fu Ye), Take two ampoules each time, for 3 times per day, used to various pattern of acute pharyngitis. ② *Six Divine Pills* (Liu Shen Wan), *All Clarifying Capsules* (Yi Qing Jiao Nang), *Throat-Clearing Dropping Pills* (Qing Yan Di Wan), *Wind-Expelling and Toxin-Resolving Granules* (Shu Feng Jie Du Jiao Nang) can all be used for acute pharyngitis.

(2) Simple and proved formulas: ① Decoct fresh *Herba Commlinae* (Ya Zhi Cao) 10g. with water for oral administration, for twice per day. ② *Decoct Radix Isatidis* (Ban Lan Gen) 30g, *Herba Physalis Peruvianae* (Deng Long Cao) 30g. with water for oral administration, one dose per day, and take twice per day. ③ *Decoct Radix Achyranthis*

2.3 其他疗法

（1）中成药：①双黄连口服液，每次服用2支，每日3次。用于急性咽炎各证型。②六神丸、一清胶囊、万应胶囊、清咽滴丸、疏风解毒颗粒等，急性咽炎均可应用

（2）单验方：①鲜鸭跖草10克，水煎，每日1剂，煎服2次。②板蓝根30克，灯笼草30克，水煎，每日1剂，煎服2次。③土牛膝30克，挂金灯15克，每日1剂，煎服2次。

Bidentatae (Tu Niu Xi) 30g, and *Calyx et Fructus Physalis* (Gua Jin Deng) 15g. with water for oral administration, one dose per day, and take twice per day.

(3) External therapies: ① Grind Borax (Peng Sha) 3g, *Borneolum Syntheticum* (Bing Pian) 3g, *and Radix Ardisiae crispae* (Ba Zhua Jin Long) 6g. into powder and blow proper amount into the throat. ② *Blow Universal Swelling-Diminishing Powder* (Tong Yong Xiao Zhong San) into the throat, for once every 2 to 3 h.

（3）外治法：①硼砂 3 克，冰片 3 克，八爪金龙 6 克，共研为末，每次适量吹咽。②通用消肿散吹咽，每2～3小时 1 次。

Chronic pharyngitis

慢 性 咽 炎

It refers to chronic inflammation of the pharyngeal mucosa, submucosal and lymphatic tissues, mostly caused by repeated seizure of acute inflammation or prolonged illness and stimulation from lesions of the nearby organs. The diffuse inflammation is often a part of chronic inflammation of the upper respiratory tract. The limited inflammation is mostly inflammation of the pharyngeal lymphatic tissues. This disease is very common and mostly seen in the adults, characterized by long duration, intractable symptoms, repeated seizure and difficult cure. Clinically, it is divided into simple, hypertrophic and dry types.

慢性咽炎是咽黏膜、黏膜下及淋巴组织的慢性炎症，多因急性炎症反复发作或病程迁延，以及邻近器官病灶刺激引起。弥漫性炎症常为上呼吸道慢性炎症的一部分，局限性炎症多为咽部淋巴组织炎症。本病极为常见，多见于成年人。病程长，症状顽固，反复发作及不易治愈是其特点。临床分单纯性、肥厚性和干燥性三型。

1 Diagnostic essentials

1.1 Long duration and repeated seizures.

1.2 There are various uncomfortable sensation in the throat, such as dry, itching, burning hot, slight

1 诊断要点

1.1 病程长，反复发作。

1.2 咽部有各种不适感觉，如干燥、发痒、灼热、微痛、咳

painful sensation, cough, and sensation of foreign body and stimulation, sensitiveness in the throat, easy nausea, more or less secretions, but tenacious on the posterior wall of the pharynx, seldom hoarse voice, tinnitus, and hearing loss.

嗽、异物感或刺激感等，咽部敏感易作呕，分泌物或多或少，但粘稠附于咽后壁。少有声嘶、耳鸣、听力障碍等。

1.3 The inspections can show dark red congestion in the mucous membrane of the pharyngeal part (posterior wall of the pharynx, border of the soft palate, palatine arch, tonsil), net-like hemangiectasis in the posterior wall of the pharynx, scattered or cloddy hypertrophy of the lymphatic follicles, with yellow and white small dots and tenacious pus or thick and tenacious secretions on the surface, and even atrophy and thinning of the mucous membrane coated with deep gray or brown crust, and congestion and tumefaction of the lateral pharyngeal bands. The lesion can involve the nasopharynx and laryngopharynx.

1.3 检查可见咽部（咽后壁、软腭边缘、腭弓、扁桃体）黏膜充血呈暗红色，咽后壁血管扩张呈网，淋巴滤泡散在或团块状增生，表面有黄白色小点及黏脓或稠厚分泌物，甚或黏膜萎缩变薄被覆深灰色或棕褐色痂皮等，咽侧索常充血肿胀。病变可延伸至鼻咽及喉咽。

1.4 For those with sensation of foreign body in the throat, it is necessary to differentiate it from the diseases of nasal cavity and sinus, diseases of the upper digestive tract and upper respiratory tract and cervical spondylopathy, and from tumors in the laryngopharyngeal part and esophagus. It is also necessary to differentiate it from tuberculosis, syphilis and lupus.

1.4 对咽部异物感者，需排除鼻腔、鼻窦疾病，上消化道、下呼吸道疾病和颈椎病，尤其是喉咽部及食管肿瘤；还应与咽部结核、梅毒及狼疮鉴别。

2 Therapeutic methods

2 治疗方法

2.1 Therapeutic principles

2.1 治疗原则

The pathological position of chronic pharyngitis is in the throat, but it is related to the lung, spleen and kidney. Long-term deficiency in the lung and kidney and insufficiency of yin body fluid will lead to malnutrition in the throat. If the spleen fails to

慢性咽炎病位在咽，与肺、脾、肾三脏有关，久病肺肾亏虚，阴液不足，咽喉失于濡养；脾失健运，难化精微，津液难以上承，咽喉干枯失

perform its transportation, it is unable to transform and transport the essential stuffs and body fluid upward, the throat will be dry. If yin is insufficient, yang is surplus, burning body fluid into phlegm, and hence leading to accumulation of phlegm and heat in the throat. The commonly seen patterns include pattern of yin deficiency in the lung and kidney, pattern of qi deficiency in the lung and spleen, and pattern of internal accumulation of phlegm and heat. The treatment is mainly given to benefit qi, nourish yin, clear away heat and dissolve phlegm.

容;阴不足则阳有余,灼津为痰,痰热蕴结咽喉,均可致病。常见证型有肺肾阴虚、肺脾气虚、痰热内蕴等。治疗以益气养阴、清热化痰为主。

2.2 Treatment based on syndrome differentiation

(1) **Pattern of yin deficiency in the lung and kidney**

Main symptoms: Dry, burning hot or painful sensation in the throat, in long duration, aggravated by fatigue, cold and long speaking, itching sensation in the throat, cough, scanty sputum, difficult to cough up, frequent clearing voice, dark red and dry or atrophic mucous membrane in the throat, flushed cheeks in the afternoon, vexation due to deficiency, poor sleep, soreness and weakness in the low back and knee, feverish sensation in the hand and foot, red tongue, scanty tongue coating, thready and rapid pulse.

Therapeutic method: To nourish and replenish the lung and kidney, nourish yin and produce body fluid.

Herbal formulas and drugs: *Lily Metal-Consolidating Decoction* (Bai He Gu Jin Tang) (modified). *Bulbus Lilii* (Bai He) 10g, *Radix Rehmanniae Cruda* (Sheng Di Huang) 10g, *Radix Scrophulariae* (Xuan Shen) 10g, *Herba Dendrobii* (Shi Hu) 10g, *Radix Trichosanthis* (Tian Hua Fen) 10g, *Radix*

2.2 辨证论治

(1) **肺肾阴虚**

主症:咽喉干燥,灼热,或疼痛,日久不愈,每因劳累、受凉、言多后症状加重。咽部作痒而咳,痰少,不易咯出,常有"吭、喀"清嗓习惯。检查见咽部黏膜暗红、干燥,或有萎缩。午后颧红、虚烦少寐、腰膝酸软、手足心热。舌红少苔,脉细数。

治法:滋补肺肾,养阴生津。

方药:百合固金汤加减。百合10克,生地黄10克,玄参10克,石斛10克,天花粉10克,白芍药6克,桔梗6克,甘草3克。若咽后壁淋巴滤泡增生,加香附6克、郁

Paeoniae Albae (Bai Shao) 6g, *Radix Platycodi* (Jie Geng) 6g, and *Radix Glycyrrhizae* (Gan Cao) 3g. For proliferation of lymphatic follicles at the posterior wall of the pharynx, add *Rhizoma Cyperi* (Xiang Fu) 6g, *Radix Curcumae* (Yu Jin) 6g, and Flos Albiziae (He Huan Hua) 10g. For lassitude in the whole body, shortness of breath, reluctance in speaking, and panting with exertion, add *Rhizoma Dioscoreae* (Shan Yao) 10g, *Rhizoma Atractylodis Macrocephalae* (Bai Zhu) 10g, and *Radix Astragali* (Huang Qi) 10g. For slight redness and serious dryness in the throat, constipation, fire hyperactivity due to yin deficiency, it is advisable to use *Anemarrhena, Phellodendron, and Rehmannia Pills* (Zhi Bai Di Huang Wan) (modified).

金6克、合欢花10克；全身乏力、少气懒言、动则气喘者，加山药10克、白术10克、黄芪10克；若咽喉微红、干燥较甚、大便秘结者为阴虚火旺，方用知柏地黄汤加减。

(2) **Pattern of qi deficiency in the lung and spleen**

(2) **肺脾气虚**

Main symptoms: Dry, painful or foreign body sensation in the throat, in long duration, aggravated by fatigue, tenacious sputum in the throat, in scanty volume, shortness of breath, reluctance in speaking, tiredness, lassitude, poor appetite, loose stool, tumefaction in the mucous membrane of the pharyngeal part, in pale color, proliferation of lymphatic follicles at the posterior wall of the pharynx, pale and swollen tongue, with teeth marks, white tongue coating, thready and feeble pulse.

主症：咽喉干燥、疼痛，或咽中有异物感，日久不愈，劳累后症状加重。咽部黏痰，量不多。全身有少气懒言、倦怠乏力、纳呆便溏等症。检查见咽部黏膜肿胀，颜色偏淡，咽后壁淋巴滤泡增生。舌淡胖，边有齿印，苔白，脉细弱。

Therapeutic method: To replenish and benefit the lung and spleen, diminish swelling and promote the throat.

治法：补益肺脾，消肿利咽。

Herbal formulas and drugs: *Center-Supplementing Qi-Boosting Decoction* (Bu Zhong Yi Qi Tang) (modified). *Radix Pseudostellariae* (Tai Zi Shen) 10g, *Rhizoma Atractylodis Macrocephalae* (Bai Zhu) 10g, *Sclerotium Poria* (Fu Ling) 10g,

方药：补中益气汤加减。太仓参10克，白术10克，茯苓10克，山药10克，白扁豆10克，陈皮6克，葛根10克，桔梗6克，甘草3克。若咽干

Rhizoma Dioscoreae (Shan Yao) 10g, *Semen Dolichoris Album* (Bai Bian Dou) 10g, *Pericarpium Citri Tangerinae* (Chen Pi) 6g, *Radix Puerariae* (Ge Gen) 10g, *Radix Platycodi* (Jie Geng) 6g, and *Radix Glycyrrhizae* (Gan Cao) 3g. For serious dry throat, add *Herba Dendrobii* (Shi Hu) 10g, *Bulbus Lilii* (Bai He) 10g, and *Rhizoma Polygonati* (Huang Jing) 10g. For deficiency of yin blood, manifested by pale and lustrousless lips, dizziness and blurred vision, it is advisable to use *Four Agents Decoction* (Si Wu Tang) plus *Radix Polygoni Multiflori* (He Shou Wu) 10g, *Colla Corii Asini* (E Jiao) 10g, and *Radix Ophiopogonis* (Mai Dong) 10g.

甚,加石斛10克、百合10克、黄精10克;若阴血亏虚,症见唇淡无华、头晕目眩者,用四物汤加何首乌10克、阿胶10克、麦门冬10克。

(3) **Pattern of internal accumulation of phlegm and heat**

(3) **痰热内蕴**

Main symptoms: Burning hot, painful or foreign body sensation in the throat, profuse sputum in the throat, in yellow or white color, difficult to cough up clearly, often serious cough, thirst, constipation, brown urine, deep red mucous membrane of the pharynx, proliferation of lymphatic follicles at the posterior wall of the pharynx, obvious tumefaction in the lateral pharyngeal bands, red tongue yellow and greasy tongue coating, rolling and rapid pulse.

主症:咽喉灼热、疼痛,或有异物感。咽中痰多,色黄或白,不易咯吐干净,常常剧咳。口渴,大便干燥,小便色黄。检查咽黏膜深红,咽后壁淋巴滤泡增生,咽侧索红肿较明显。舌质红,苔黄腻,脉滑数。

Therapeutic method: To clear away heat, discharge fire, dissolve phlegm and promote the throat.

治法:清热泻火,化痰利咽。

Herbal formulas and drugs: *Qi-Clarifying and Phlegm-Dissolving Pills* (Qing Qi Hua Tan Wan) (modified). *Radix Scutellariae* (Huang Qin) 6g, *Flos Lonicerae* (Jin Yin Hua) 6g, *Cortex Mori Radicis* (Sang Bai Pi) 10g, *Bulbus Fritillariae Thumbergii* (Zhe Bei Mu) 10g, Pericarpium Trichosanthis

方药:清气化痰丸加减。黄芩6克,金银花6克,桑白皮10克,浙贝母10克,瓜蒌皮10克,竹茹10克,天竺黄6克,桔梗6克,甘草3克。若咽干,咽黏膜暗红、干燥,

(Gua Lou Pi) 10g, *Caulis Bambusae in Taeniam* (Zhu Ru) 6g, *Radix Platycodi* (Jie Geng) 6g, and *Radix Glycyrrhizae* (Gan Cao) 3g. For dry throat, dark red and dry pharyngeal mucosa, add *Herba Dendrobii* (Shi Hu) 10g, *Radix Trichosanthis* (Tian Hua Fen) 10g, and *Radix Scrophulariae* (Xuan Shen) 10g. For shortness of breath, reluctance in speaking, tiredness, and lassitude, add *Radix Pseudostellariae* (Tai Zi Shen) 10g, *Rhizoma Atractylodis Macrocephalae* (Bai Zhu) 10g, *Rhizoma Dioscoreae* (Shan Yao) 10g, and *Sclerotium Poria* (Fu Ling) 10g.

加石斛10克、天花粉10克、玄参10克；少气懒言、倦怠乏力者，加太子参10克、白术10克、山药10克、茯苓10克。

2.3 Other therapies

(1) Chinese patent medicine: ① *Figwort, Ophiopogon, Liquorice and Platycodon Granules* (Xuan Mai Gan Ju Ke Li), Take 1 to 2 packets each time, for three times per day. Besides, *Throat-Clarifying and Promoting Granules* (Qing Hou Li Yan Ke Li) can be used for chronic pharyngitis in pattern of yin deficiency in the lung and kidney. ② *Center-Supplementing Qi-Boosting Pills* (Bu Zhong Yi Qi Wan), Take 5g each time, for 3 times per day, appropriate for chronic pharyngitis in pattern of qi deficiency in the lung and spleen. ③ *Natural Indigo and Scutellaria Phlegm-Dissolving Pills* (Dai Qin Hua Tan Wan), Take 5g each time, for three times per day, appropriate for chronic pharyngitis in pattern of internal accumulation of phlegm and heat.

(2) Simple and proved formulas: ① Decoct *Rhizoma Tinosporae sagittatae* (Jin Guo Lan) 10g. with water for oral administration or mouthwash, for one dose per day. ② Decoct *Fructus Terminaliae Chebulae* (He Zi) 10g, *Fructus Mume* (Wu Mei) 10g, and *Radix*

2.3 其他疗法

(1) 中成药：①玄参甘桔颗粒，每服1～2包，每日3次。另有清喉利咽颗粒等，用于慢性咽炎肺肾阴虚证。②补中益气丸，每服5克，每日3次。用于慢性咽炎肺脾气虚证。③黛芩化痰丸，每服5克，每日3次，用于慢性咽炎痰热内蕴证。

(2) 单验方：①金果榄10克，水煎内服或含漱，每日1剂。②诃子10克，乌梅10克，甘草10克，水煎服，每日2剂。

Glycyrrhizae (Gan Cao) 10g. with water for oral administration, for two doses per day.

(3) External therapies: It is advisable to use the powder-blowing, mouth-rinsing and sublingual administrative method, please refer to "acute and chronic tonsillitis".

(3) 外治法：可用吹药、含漱、含服等法，可参考"急慢性扁桃体炎"。

Peritonsillar abscess

扁桃体周脓肿

It refers to suppurative inflammation of the peritonsillar interstice. Before the formation of abscess, it is peritonsillitis. Its pathogenic bacteria are similar to those in tonsillitis, including staphylococcus aureus, beta hemolytic streptococcus, and swine streptococcus viridians, etc. It usually occurs on one side and is mostly seen in young adults.

扁桃体周脓肿为扁桃体周围间隙内的化脓性炎症。在脓肿为形成之前，成为扁桃体周炎，其致病菌与扁桃体炎相同，有金黄色葡萄球菌、乙型溶血性链球菌、甲型草绿色链球菌等。好发于一侧，多见于青壮年。

1 Diagnostic essentials

1.1 First, sore throat, aggravation in swallowing and fever, 2 to 3 d later, sore throat focused on one side and gradually aggravated, radiating to the ear of the same side, foul breath, salivation, aphasia, difficult to open the mouth, often accompanied by lymph node pain in the neck.

1.2 In the inspections present are face of acute and serious illness, suffering expression, stiffness in the neck, limitation in turning the head and opening the mouth, obvious protrusion of the local lesion, tumefaction and protrusion of the palatine arch and soft palate of the sick side, deviation of edematous uvula to the opposite side, with the tonsil covered and pushed inferiorly.

1 诊断要点

1.1 先有咽痛，吞咽时加重，发热等。2～3 日后，咽痛偏于一侧，逐渐加剧，并向同侧耳部放射。口臭，流涎，语音含糊，张口困难，常伴有颈部淋巴结肿痛。

1.2 检查见急性重病容，表情痛苦，颈部僵直，转头及张口受限。病变局部隆起明显，病侧腭弓及软腭红肿突出，悬雍垂水肿偏向对侧，扁桃体被遮盖且被推向下方。

1.3 Pus is present by puncture on the most obvious protrusion.

2 Therapeutic methods

2.1 Therapeutic principles

Peritonsillar abscess is divided into the initial, middle and later stage, respectively similar to pattern of invasion of wind and heat into the lung, pattern of heat abundance in the lung and stomach, and pattern of retention of pathogens due to yin deficiency. Suppuration is not formed in the initial stage. Suppuration is formed in the middle stage. Suppuration is already ruptured in the later stage. Before suppuration in the initial stage, the treatment is mainly given to clear away heat and diminish swelling. When the suppuration is formed in the middle stage, the treatment is mainly given to dissolve pus and resolve toxin. When suppuration is ruptured in the later stage, the treatment is mainly given to nourish yin and clear away heat.

2.2 Treatment based on syndrome differentiation

(1) **Pattern of invasion of wind and heat into the lung**

Main symptoms: Fever, aversion to cold, sore throat, aggravated in swallowing, obvious congestion in the palatine arch of one side, red tongue thin and white or slight yellow tongue coating, superficial and rapid pulse.

Therapeutic method: To expel wind, clear away heat, resolve toxin and diminish swelling.

Herbal formulas and drugs: *Five Ingredients Detoxifying Drink* (Wu Wei Xiao Du Yin) (modified). *Flos Lonicerae* (Jin Yin Hua) 10g, *Flos Chrysanthemi* (Ju Hua) 10g, *Herba Taraxaci* (Pu Gong Ying)

1.3 隆起最明显处穿刺有脓。

2 治疗方法

2.1 治疗原则

扁桃体周脓肿分初期、中期、后期,分别相当于辨证分型之风热犯肺、肺胃热盛、阴虚邪恋证。初期脓未成,中期脓已成,后期脓已溃,治法各异。初期脓未成,治法以清热消肿为主;中期脓已成,治法以化脓解毒为主;后期脓已溃,治法以养阴清热为主。

2.2 辨证论治

(1) 风热犯肺

主症:发热,恶寒,咽痛,吞咽时加剧。检查可见一侧腭舌弓充血明显。舌质红,苔薄白或微黄,脉浮数。

治法:疏风清热,解毒消肿。

方药:五味消毒饮加减。金银花 10 克,菊花 10 克,蒲公英 15 克,紫花地丁 10 克,天葵子 10 克,荆芥 6 克,防风

15g, *Herba Violae* (Zi Hua Di Ding) 10g, Radix *Semiaquilegiae Adoxoidis* (Tian Kui Zi) 10g, *Herba Schizonepetae* (Jing Jie) 6g, *Radix Ledebouriellae* (Fang Feng) 6g, *Radix Angelicae Dahuricae* (Bai Zhi) 6g, *Radix Platycodi* (Jie Geng) 6g, and *Radix Glycyrrhizae* (Gan Cao) 3g. For accumulation of wind and heat in the throat, qi stagnation and blood stasis, add *Radix Angelicae Sinensis* (tail) (Dang Gui Wei) 10g, *Radix Paeoniae Rubra* (Chi Shao) 6g, *Squama Manitis* (Chuan Shan Jia) 10g, and *Myrrha* (Mo Yao) 10g. For profuse saliva in the mouth, add *Bulbus Fritillariae Thumbergii* (Zhe Bei Mu) 10g, and *Bombyx Batryticatus* (Bai Jiang Can) 10g.

6克,白芷6克,桔梗6克,甘草3克。若风热搏结咽喉,气滞血瘀,加当归尾10克、赤芍药6克、穿山甲10克、没药10克;口中痰涎较多,加浙贝母10克、白僵蚕10克。

(2) **Pattern of heat abundance in the lung and stomach**

(2) **肺胃热盛**

Main symptoms: High fever, serious sore throat, difficulty in swallowing, profuse saliva in the mouth, difficulty in opening the mouth, aphasia, headache, foul breath, stuffy sensation in the chest and abdomen, constipation, brown urine, obvious tumefaction and protrusion of the superior palatoglossal arch, tumefaction of soft palate and uvula of the same side, deviating to the opposite side, with the tonsil covered and pushed backward and inferiorly, red tongue, yellow and thick or greasy tongue coating, floody, rapid and forceful pulse.

主症:高热,咽痛剧烈,吞咽困难,口中唾液潴留,张口困难,语音含糊。头痛,口臭,胸闷腹胀,大便干结,小便黄。检查见腭舌弓上方红肿隆起明显,同侧软腭及悬雍垂红肿,向对侧偏斜,扁桃体被遮盖推向后下方。舌质红,苔黄厚或腻,脉洪数有力。

Therapeutic method: To clear away heat, discharge fire, dissipate toxin and diminish swelling.

治法:清热泻火,托毒消肿。

Herbal formulas and drugs: *Throat-Clarifying and Diaphragm-Benefiting Decoction* (Qing Yan Li Ge Tang) (modified). *Radix Scutellariae* (Huang Qin) 10g, *Fructus Forsythiae* (Lian Qiao) 10g,

方药:清咽利膈汤加减。黄芩10克,连翘10克,牛蒡子10克,防风6克,石膏(先煎)20克,荆芥6克,金银花

Fructus Arctii (Niu Bang Zi) 10g, *Radix Ledebouriellae* (Fang Feng) 6g, *Gypsum Fibrosum* (Shi Gao) (Decoct first) 20g, *Herba Schizonepetae* (Jing Jie) 6g, *Flos Lonicerae* (Jin Yin Hua) 10g, *Rhizoma Rhei Cruda* (Sheng Da Huang) 5g, *Fructus Gardeniae* (Zhi Zi) 10g, and *Herba Menthae* (Bo He) (Decoct later) 6g.

10克，生大黄5克，山栀子10克，薄荷(后下)6克。

If abundant phlegm and heat gushes upward to the throat or abscess is ruptured, with the pus flowing out and blocking the air passage, the respiration will be difficult. Therefore, for abundant accumulation of phlegm and saliva, it is advisable to add *Bombyx Batryticatus* (Bai Jiang Can) 10g, *Arisaema cum Bile* (Dan Nan Xing) 6g, and *Bulbus Fritillariae Thumbergii* (Zhe Bei Mu) 10g. For formation of suppuration, add *Radix Angelicae Sinensis* (Dang Gui) 10g, *Radix Paeoniae Rubra* (Chi Shao) 6g, *Resina Olibani* (Ru Xiang) 10g, *Myrrha* (Mo Yao) 10g.

若壮热烦躁、神昏谵语、舌红绛少苔，症见热入营血，宜清营凉血解毒，可用犀角地黄汤，选加安宫牛黄丸或紫雪丹以开窍安神。若痰热壅盛上涌咽喉或痈肿破裂，脓液溢出阻塞气道，可使呼吸困难。故痰涎壅盛者，加白僵蚕10克、胆南星6克、浙贝母10克；脓已成者，加当归10克、赤芍药6克、乳香10克、没药10克。

(3) **Pattern of retention of pathogens due to yin deficiency**

(3) **阴虚邪恋**

Main symptoms: Alleviated fever and sore throat, alleviated difficulty in opening the mouth and swallowing, thirst, brown urine, constipation, alleviated protrusion of tumefaction in the superior palatoglossal arch, discharge of pus, red tongue, thin and scanty tongue coating, thready and rapid pulse.

主症：发热及咽痛减轻，张口困难及吞咽困难症状缓解，口渴尿黄，大便干。检查见腭舌弓上方红肿隆起减轻，有脓液排出。舌质红，苔薄少，脉细数。

Therapeutic method: To nourish yin, support the constitution, clear away heat and benefit the throat.

治法：养阴扶正，清热利咽。

Herbal formulas and drugs: *Adenophora and Ophiopogon Decoction* (Sha Shen Mai Dong Tang) plus *Five Ingredients Detoxifying Drink* (Wu Wei Xi-

方药：沙参麦冬汤合五味消毒饮加减。南沙参10克，麦门冬10克，玉竹10克，

ao Du Yin) (modified). *Radix Adenophorae* (Nan Sha Shen) 10g, *Radix Ophiopogonis* (Mai Dong) 10g, *Rhizoma Polygonati Odorati* (Yu Zhu) 10g, *Radix Glycyrrhizae* (Gan Cao) 3g, *Folium Mori* (Sang Ye) 10g, *Semen Dolichoris* (Bian Dou) 10g, *Radix Trichosanthis* (Tian Hua Fen) 10g, *Flos Lonicerae* (Jin Yin Hua) 10g, *Herba Taraxaci* (Pu Gong Ying) 15g, *Flos Chrysanthemi Indici* (Ye Ju Hua) 10g, *Herba Violae* (Zi Hua Di Ding) 10g, *Radix Semiaquilegiae Adoxoidis* (Tian Kui Zi) 10g. For local redness, swelling, heat and pain due to retention of residual pathogens, add *Radix Platycodi* (Jie Geng) 6g, and *Bulbus Fritillariae Thumbergii* (Zhe Bei Mu) 10g. For profuse sweating, lassitude, dry mouth, red tongue and scanty body fluid due to deficient constitution, add *Radix Codonopsis Pilosulae* (Dang Shen) 10g, *Radix Scrophulariae* (Xuan Shen) 10g, *Rhizoma Atractylodis Macrocephalae* (Bai Zhu) 10g, and *Rhizoma Dioscoreae* (Shan Yao) 10g.

生甘草 3 克,桑叶 10 克,生扁豆 10 克,天花粉 10 克,金银花 10 克,蒲公英 15 克,野菊花 10 克,紫花地丁 10 克,天葵子 10 克。若余邪残存,局部红肿热痛,加桔梗 6 克、浙贝母 10 克;若体虚多汗、乏力、口干、舌红少津,加党参 10 克、玄参 10 克、白术 10 克、山药 10 克。

2.3 Other therapies

(1) Chinese patent medicine: ① *Honeysuckle and Scutellaria Granules* (Yin Huang Ke Li), Take 1 to 2 packets, each time, for 3 times per day, used for peritonsillar abscess in pattern of invasion of wind and heat into the lung. ② Mo Family Clarifying and Calming Pills (Mo Jia Qing Ning Wan), Take 6 grams each time, for once per day, used for peritonsillar abscess complicated with constipation.

(2) Simple and proved formulas: ① *Soak Radix Sophorae Subprostratae* (Shan Dou Gen) 30g, into proper amount of vinegar and have its juice in the mouth, for one dose per day. ② Pound fresh *Radix Achyranthis Bidentatae* (Tu Niu Xi) 60g, to get its

2.3 其他疗法

(1) 中成药:①银黄颗粒,每服 1～2 包,每日 3 次。用于扁桃体周脓肿风热犯肺证。②莫家清宁丸,每服 6 克,每日 1 次。用于扁桃体周脓肿症见大便干结者。

(2) 单验方:①山豆根 30 克浸入适量醋中,口噙咽汁,每日 1 剂。②鲜土牛膝根 60 克,捣汁徐徐咽下,每日 1 剂。③薄荷 5 克,半边莲

juice and swallow the juice slowly down, for one dose per day. ③ Pound *Herba Menthae* (Bo He) 5g, and *Herba Lobeliae Chinensis* (Ban Bian Lian) 10g, and decoct with water for oral administration, for two doses per day.

10 克，捣烂水煎服，每日 2 剂。

(3) External therapies

(3) 外治法

1) Blow herbal powder: Blow *Borneol and Borax Powder* (Bing Peng San), *Borneol and Musk Powder* (Bing She San), and *Universal Swelling-Diminishing Powder* (Tong Yong Xiao Zhong San) into the sick area, for 6 to 7 times per day, in the effects to reduce heat, resolve toxin, remove the decay and diminish swelling.

1) 吹药：用冰硼散、冰麝散，通用消肿散等吹患部，每日 6～7 次，有消热解毒，清腐消肿的作用。

2) Mouthwash: *Rinse the mouth with Mouthwash Formula* (Shu Kou Fang) [*Herba Schizonepetae* (Jing Jie) 6g, *Radix Ledebouriellae* (Fang Feng) 6g, *Herba Menthae* (Bo He) 6g, *Radix Glycyrrhizae* (Gan Cao) 6g, *Flos Lonicerae* (Jin Yin Hua) 9g, *Fructus Forsythiae* (Lian Qiao) 10g, decoct with water].

2) 含漱：可用漱口方(荆芥 6 克，防风 6 克，薄荷 6 克，甘草 6 克，金银花 9 克，连翘 9 克，水煎液)漱口。

3) Topical application: For submaxillary lymph node enlargement, it is advisable to apply *Lucky Golden Yellow Powder* (Ru Yi Jin Huang San), *Purple Gold Ingot* (Zi Jin Ding) externally, and also to smash *Folium Hibisci Mutabilis* (Fu Rong Ye) for topical application.

3) 外敷法：颔下淋巴结肿大者，可用如意金黄散外敷，紫金锭外搽；亦可用木芙蓉叶，捣烂外敷。

Nasopharyngeal carcinoma

鼻咽癌

It is one of the frequently occurring tumors in China. The incidence rate is highest in Guangdong province, and in turns Guangxi, Hunan, and Fujian province (region). It is mostly seen in the males, at

鼻咽癌为中国多发肿瘤之一，发病率广东省最高，其次为广西、湖南、福建等省(区)。鼻咽癌多见于男性，

the age of 50 to 54, with the ratio between the males and females in about 2 to 3∶1. This disease is characterized by phenomenon of family cluster. Its occurrence may be related to the environmental, viral infection and hereditary factors. It often occurs in the posterior wall of the nasopharyngeal roof, and then lateral wall, anterior wall in turns and bottom and can be presented with five shapes of nodular, cauliflower, infiltrating, ulcerative and submucosal type. Pathologically, it can be divided into anaplastic carcinoma, poorly differentiated carcinoma, and high differentiation carcinoma. It belongs to the scope of "nasopharyngeal carcinoma" and "withered complexion" in Chinese medicine.

50～54岁年龄组高发,男女比例约2～3∶1,本病有家族聚集现象,其发生可能与环境、病毒感染和遗传因素等有关。多发于鼻咽顶后壁,其次为侧壁,前壁和底壁极少。可呈结节型、菜花型、浸润型、溃疡型及黏膜下型五种形态。病理学分为未分化癌、低分化癌和较高分化癌。属中医学"颃颡癌""失荣"范畴。

1 Diagnostic essentials

1 诊断要点

1.1 The common symptoms include nasal discharge with blood or nasal bleeding, tinnitus or hearing loss, nasal obstruction, headache, diplopia, hypopsia, limited motion of eyeball, and lump in the upper neck. This disease should be considered, if there are auricular and nasal symptoms, in particular nasal discharge with blood, tinnitus and hearing loss continuously for over two weeks, accompanied by headache of same side, gradually enlarged, hard and immobile painless lump in the neck, diplopia, and motor impairment of the eyeballs.

1.1 常见症状有涕中带血或鼻出血,耳鸣或听力下降,鼻塞,头痛,复视,视力减退,眼球活动受限及颈上部包块等。凡有耳鼻症状,特别是涕中带血、耳鸣和听力减退,持续2周以上,且伴有同侧头痛者,颈部无痛性肿块逐渐增大且质硬不易活动者,复视或眼球运动障碍者,均应考虑本病。

1.2 If solitary nodular or asymmetrical submucosal protuberance or ulceration in the nasopharyngeal membrane is present in the endoscopy of the nasopharyngeal part, it should be suspected and biopsy is needed.

1.2 鼻咽部内镜检查见鼻咽黏膜孤立性结节或不对称黏膜下隆起或溃疡者,均应怀疑并作活组织检查。

1.3 The positive rate of IgA/VCA in the serological test of EB virus of nasopharyngeal carcinoma

1.3 鼻咽癌EB病毒血清学检测 IgA/VCA 阳性率达

reaches 93%.

93%。

1.4 X-ray radiography or CT scan can indicate nasopharyngeal carcinoma and its scope, determine if there are bone destruction in the skull base, involvement of adjacent tissues of the nasopharynx, and metastasis in the lymph nodes of the neck, lung and skeleton.

1.4 X线或CT检查可提示鼻咽部肿瘤及范围，确定颅底骨质有无破坏，鼻咽邻近组织有无侵犯，颈部淋巴结及肺部、骨骼有无转移。

1.5 The diagnosis can be confirmed by transoral or transnasal biopsy tissue pathological test.

1.5 经口或经鼻活检组织病理学检查可明确诊断。

2 Therapeutic methods

2 治疗方法

2.1 Therapeutic principles

2.1 治疗原则

Nasopharyngeal carcinoma is complicated etiologically and may be related to emotional disturbance, invasion of pathogenic factors, improper food ingestion and bad habits. In pathogenesis, it is mainly related to dysfunction of the internal organs, leading to qi stagnation, blood stasis, accumulation of phlegm, long-term accumulation turning into fire, and hence retention of fire toxin inside the body, consumption of qi, injury of yin, gradual decline of qi and blood, and consumption of constitutional energy. The treatment is mainly applied to benefit qi and nourish yin.

鼻咽癌病因复杂，与情志不遂、邪毒外犯、饮食所伤、不良嗜好等因素有关。其主要病机为脏腑功能失常，致气滞血瘀痰凝，痞塞日久化为火毒，困于体内，耗气伤阴，气血渐衰，正气耗竭。治疗以益气养阴为法。

2.2 Treatment based on syndrome differentiation

2.2 辨证论治

(1) **Pattern of accumulation of phlegm and blood stasis**

(1) **痰瘀互结**

Main symptoms: Nasal obstruction, nasal discharge with blood streak, or no obvious symptoms, nodular lump, in slight red or dark red color, and enlarged lymph nodes in the neck present in the inspection, thin and white or white and greasy tongue coating, normal tongue or with purple shadow.

主症：鼻塞，涕带血丝，或无明显症状。检查见鼻咽部有结节肿块，色淡红或暗红，颈部可有淋巴结肿大。舌苔薄白或白腻，舌质如常或有紫气。

Therapeutic method: To circulate qi, disperse

治法：行气化瘀，消痰软

blood stasis, eliminate phlegm and soften the hard.

Herbal formulas and drugs: Double Vintage Decoction (Er Chen Tang) plus *Aperture-Opening and Blood-Activating Decoction* (Tong Qiao Huo Xue Tang) (modified). *Pericarpium Citri Tangerinae* (Chen Pi) 6g, *Rhizoma Pinelliae* (Ban Xia) 6g, *Radix Paeoniae Rubra* (Chi Shao) 6g, *Rhizoma Ligustici Chuanxiong* (Chuan Xiong) 5g, *Semen Persicae* (Tao Ren) 10g, *Flos Carthami* (Hong Hua) 10g, *Herba Selaginella doederleinii* (Shi Shang Bai) 10g, *Arisaema cum Bile* (Dan Nan Xing) 6g, *Pseudobulbus Cremastrae seu Pleiones* (Shan Ci Gu) 10g, *Bryozoatum* (Hai Fu Shi) 20g, and *Lasiosphaera Seu Calvatia* (Ma Bo) 3g. For accompanying stuffy chest, irritability and full and distending sensation in the hypochondriac region, add *Radix Bupleuri* (Chai Hu) 6g, *Rhizoma Cyperi* (Xiang Fu) 10g, *Radix Curcumae* (Yu Jin) 10g, and *Fructus Gardeniae* (Zhi Zi) 10g. For abundance of turbid phlegm, accompanied by nausea, stuffy chest, and greasy tongue coating, add *Sclerotium Poria* (Fu Ling) 10g, *Bulbus Fritillariae Thumbergii* (Zhe Bei Mu) 10g, *Herba Agastachis* (Huo Xiang) 10g, *Caulis Bambusae in Taeniam* (Zhu Ru) 10g. For profuse nasal bleeding, take out herbal drugs to activate blood and disperse blood stasis, and add *Herba Agrimoniae* (Xian He Cao) 10g, *Caumen Biotae* (Ce Bai Ye) 10g, *Radix Sanguisorbae Carbonisastus* (Di Yu Tan) 10g, *Fructus Gardeniae* (Zhi Zi) 10g. For headache, comparatively large lymph nodes in the neck, add *Scorpio* (Quan Xie) 10g, *Scolopendra subspinipes* (Wu Gong) 10g, *Rhizoma Zedoariae* (E Zhu) 10g, and *Nidus Vespae* (Lu Feng Fang) 10g.

坚。

方药：二陈汤合通窍活血汤加减。陈皮6克，半夏6克，赤芍药6克，川芎5克，桃仁10克，红花10克，石上柏10克，胆南星6克，山慈菇10克，海浮石20克，马勃3克。若伴胸闷烦躁、胁肋满胀，加柴胡6克、香附10克、郁金10克、山栀子10克；痰浊偏盛，伴呕恶、胸闷、苔腻，加茯苓10克、象贝母10克、藿香10克、竹茹10克；涕血多，去活血化瘀之品，加仙鹤草10克、侧柏叶10克、白茅根10克、地榆炭10克、山栀子10克；若头痛、颈部淋巴结较大者，加全蝎10克、蜈蚣10克、莪术10克、蜂房10克。

(2) Pattern of accumulation of fire and toxin

(2) 火毒蕴结

Main symptoms: Nasal obstruction, epistaxis, or yellow and tenacious nasal discharge with blood streak, irritability, easy anger, poor sleep, serious headache, tinnitus, distending sensation in the eyes, dry mouth, bitter taste in the mouth, nasopharyngeal lump in cauliflower shape, rupture and blood oozing, covered with much secretion, red tongue, wiry and rolling or wiry and rapid pulse.

Therapeutic method: To discharge fire, resolve toxin, diminish swelling and soften the hard.

Herbal formulas and drugs: *Qi-Clarifying and Phlegm-Dissolving Pills* (Qing Qi Hua Tan Wan) plus *Bupleurum Liver-Clarifying Decoction* (Chai Hu Qing Gan Tang) (modified). *Pericarpium Citri Tangerinae* (Chen Pi) 6g, *Radix Scutellariae* (Huang Qin) 10g, *Arisaema cum Bile* (Dan Nan Xing) 6g, *Radix Rehmanniae Cruda* (Sheng Di Huang) 10g, *Semen Trichosanthis* (Gua Lou Zi) 10g, *Radix Bupleuri* (Chai Hu) 6g, *Fructus Aurantii* (Zhi Ke) 6g, *Rhizoma Paridis* (Zhong Lou) 10g, *Spica Prunellae* (Xia Ku Cao) 10g, *Fructus Gardeniae* (Zhi Zi) 10g, *Radix Sophorae Subprostratae* (Shan Dou Gen) 10g, and *Herba Solani Nigri* (Long Kui) 10g. For bleeding in profuse volume, add *Radix Sanguisorbae* (Di Yu) 10g, *Radix Arnebiae seu Lithospermi* (Zi Cao) 10g, *Herba Ecliptae* (Han Lian Cao) 10g, and *Herba Agrimoniae* (Xian He Cao) 10g. For serious headache, add *Concha Haliotidis* (Shi Jue Ming) 10g, *Herba Leonuri* (Yi Mu Cao) 10g, *Radix Achyranthis Bidentatae* (Niu Xi) 10g, and *Cornu Naemorhedi* (Shan Yang Jiao) 10g. For abdominal distention and constipation, add *Rhizoma Rhei Cruda* (Sheng Da Huang) 5g. For dry nose, dry mouth and obvious

主症：鼻塞，鼻衄或涕黄稠带血丝，烦躁易怒，夜寐难眠，头痛较剧，耳鸣目胀，口干口苦。检查见鼻咽部肿物呈菜花状，溃烂渗血，被覆有较多分泌物。舌质红赤，脉弦滑或弦数。

治法：泻火解毒，消肿软坚。

方药：清气化痰丸合柴胡清肝汤加减。陈皮 6 克，黄芩 10 克，胆南星 6 克，生地黄 10 克，瓜蒌仁 10 克，柴胡 6 克，枳壳 6 克，重楼 10 克，夏枯草 10 克，山栀子 10 克，山豆根 10 克，龙葵 10 克。若出血量多，加地榆 10 克、紫草根 10 克、旱莲草 10 克、仙鹤草 10 克；头痛较剧，加石决明 10 克、益母草 10 克、牛膝 10 克、山羊角 10 克；腹胀便结，加生大黄 5 克；鼻干、口干、舌赤明显，加天花粉 10 克、麦门冬 10 克、玄参 10 克、南沙参 10 克；神疲乏力，加太子参 10 克、西洋参 10 克、白术 10 克。

red tongue, add *Radix Trichosanthis* (Tian Hua Fen) 10g, *Radix Ophiopogonis* (Mai Dong) 10g, *Radix Scrophulariae* (Xuan Shen) 10g, and *Radix Adenophorae* (Nan Sha Shen) 10g. For low spirit and lassitude, add *Radix Pseudostellariae* (Tai Zi Shen) 10g, *Radix Panacis Quinquefolii* (Xi Yang Shen) 10g, and *Rhizoma Atractylodis Macrocephalae* (Bai Zhu) 10g.

(3) **Pattern of pathogen preponderance and constitution decline**

(3) **邪盛正衰**

Main symptoms: Headache, nasal obstruction, dirty and stinky nasal discharge, dark and turbid blood, dizziness, blurred vision, deviated mouth and eye, shortness of breath, reluctance in speaking, or aphasia, tinnitus, deafness, pale complexion, low spirit, poor appetite, distending sensation in the epigastric and hypochondriac region, hard and large lump in the neck, pale tongue, white or gray and greasy tongue coating, thready and feeble pulse.

主症：头痛鼻塞，鼻涕污秽，恶臭，血暗浊，头晕目眩或视力模糊，口眼歪斜，气短懒言或语謇，耳鸣耳聋，面色苍白，精神萎靡，恶食纳减，脘胀胁痞，颈部包块坚大。舌质淡，苔白或灰腻，脉细弱。

Therapeutic method: To strengthen the spleen, replenish the kidney, resolve toxin and disperse accumulation.

治法：健脾补肾，解毒散结。

Herbal formulas and drugs: *Angelica Splenic Decoction* (Gui Pi Tang) plus *Wheat Flavor Rehamnnia Pills* (Mai Wei Di Huang Wan) (modified). *Radix Astragali* (Huang Qi) 10g, *Radix Codonopsis Pilosulae* (Dang Shen) 10g, *Rhizoma Atractylodis Macrocephalae* (Bai Zhu) 10g, *Radix Angelicae Sinensis* (Dang Gui) 10g, *Radix Ophiopogonis* (Mai Dong) 10g, *Fructus Schisandrae* (Wu Wei Zi) 10g, *Rhizoma Dioscoreae* (Shan Yao) 10g, *Sclerotium Poria* (Fu Ling) 10g, *Fructus Lycii* (Gou Qi Zi) 10g, *Radix Rehmanniae Praeparata* (Shu Di Huang)

方药：归脾汤合麦味地黄丸加减。黄芪 10 克，党参 10 克，白术 10 克，当归 10 克，麦门冬 10 克，五味子 10 克，山药 10 克，茯苓 10 克，枸杞子 10 克，熟地黄 10 克，山萸肉 10 克，薏苡仁 10 克。若头昏目眩、耳鸣腰酸，加肉苁蓉 10 克、巴戟天 10 克、淫羊藿 10 克、龟甲 10 克；便溏纳减、腹胀，加白豆蔻 10 克、砂

10g, *Fructus Corni* (Shan Zhu Yu) 10g, and *Semen Coicis* (Yi Yi Ren) 10g. For dizziness, blurred vision, tinnitus, soreness and weakness in the low back, add *Herba Cistanchis* (Rou Cong Rong) 10g, *Radix Morindae Officinalis* (Ba Ji Tian) 10g, *Epimedium davidii* (Yin Yang Huo) 10g, and *Plastrum Testudinis* (Gui Ban) 10g. For loose stool, poor appetite, and abdominal distension, add *Semen Amomi Cardamomi* (Bai Dou Kou) 10g, and *Fructus Amomi* (Sha Ren) 6g. For symptoms of heat toxin, add *Flos Chrysanthemi Indici* (Ye Ju Hua) 10g, *Herba Hedyotis Diffusae* (Bai Hua She She Cao) 30g, *Radix Sophorae Subprostratae* (Shan Dou Gen) 10g, and *Rhizoma Paridis* (Zhong Lou) 10g. For red tongue with scanty tongue coating, add *Radix Adenophorae* (Nan Sha Shen) 10g, *Herba Dendrobii* (Shi Hu) 10g, and *Rhizoma Anemarrhenae* (Zhi Mu) 10g.

仁 6 克;有热毒症状,加野菊花 10 克、白花蛇舌草 30 克、山豆根 10 克、重楼 10 克;咽干、舌红少苔,加南沙参 10 克、石斛 10 克、知母 10 克。

2.3 Other therapies

Simple and proved formulas: ① Decoct *Herba Scutellariae Barbatae* (Ban Zhi Lian) 30g, and *Herba Hedyotis Diffusae* (Bai Hua She She Cao) 60g, with water as drinking tea, for one dose per day. ② Decoct fresh *Semen Fagopyri esculenti* (Qiao Mai) 30g, fresh *Radix Stephaniae Tetrandrae* (Han Fang Ji) 30g, fresh *Radix Achyranthis Bidentatae* (Tu Niu Xi) 30g, with water for oral administration, for one dose per day. ③ Decoct *Radix Arnebiae seu Lithospermi* (Zi Cao) 30g, with water for oral administration, for one dose per day.

2.3 其他疗法

单验方:①半枝莲 30 克,白花蛇舌草 60 克,水煎当茶饮,每日 1 剂;②鲜野荞麦 30 克,鲜汉防己 30 克,鲜土牛膝 30 克,水煎,每日 1 剂服用;③紫草根 30 克,水煎,每日 1 剂服用。

Acute epiglottitis

急性会厌炎

It is also termed acute supraglottic pharyngitis

急性会厌炎又名急性声

and refers to acute infectious disease of the epiglottis, characterized clinically by serious sore throat, difficulty in swallowing, difficulty in respiration, and even suffocation. It frequently occurs in young adults and is mostly seen in autumn and spring. The main pathogenic bacteria include hemophilus influenzae, hemolytic streptococci, staphylococcus, and streptococcus pneumoniae, etc. It can also be caused by viral infection. The mucous membrane on the epiglottis is flaccid and easy to become swelling in inflammation. In serious condition, the epiglottis can be swollen like a ball. In fewer cases, abscess can be formed. It belongs to the scope of "acute sore throat" in Chinese medicine.

门上喉炎，是以会厌为主的急性感染性疾病。临床主要表现为咽喉剧烈疼痛、吞咽困难、呼吸困难，甚至窒息。好发于青壮年，以冬秋，秋春季节交替时为多见。主要致病菌有流感嗜血杆菌、溶血性链球菌、葡萄球菌、肺炎双球菌等，也可夹杂病毒感染。会厌舌面黏膜松弛，炎症时易于肿胀，严重者会厌肿大如球状，少数可形成脓肿。属中医学"急喉风"范畴。

1 Diagnostic essentials

1.1 Acute onset, quick development, mainly manifested by sore throat, swallowing pain, difficulty in swallowing, aphasia, without hoarse voice in most condition, difficult respiration and even suffocation in severe cases.

1.2 Fever, aversion to cold, suffering expression

1.3 Tumefaction in the epiglottis is worse on the tongue surface, mostly in a ball shape, with yellow and white pus dots on the surface. The vocal area is difficult to be observed. There are inspiratory dyspnea, signs of "three concaves", cyanosis and irritability, etc.

1.4 White blood cell count and neutrophil are elevated. The enlarged epiglottis and shrunk laryngopharynx can be seen in X-ray radiography of the throat.

1 诊断要点

1.1 起病急，进展快，以咽痛、吞咽痛、吞咽困难、言语不清为主要表现，多无声音嘶哑。严重者可有呼吸困难，甚至窒息。

1.2 发热畏寒，表情痛苦。

1.3 会厌红肿以舌面为甚，多呈球形，表面或可见黄白色脓点。声门区难于窥清。或有吸气性呼吸困难、"三凹"征、紫绀及烦躁等。

1.4 化验白细胞总数及中性粒细胞升高。喉部X线侧位片，可见会厌增大，喉咽腔缩小。

2 Therapeutic methods

2.1 Therapeutic principles

Because acute epiglottitis is in the throat, an important pathway for respiration, it is necessary to prevent frequent migration and constant change of pathogenic wind. White swelling of the epiglottis can easily block the air passage, leading to critical pattern of suffocation. Therefore, in the administration of Western medications for resisting inflammation and diminishing swelling, the treatment is mainly given to expel wind, clear away heat, dissolve phlegm. It is necessary to observe carefully, and to carry out immediately tracheotomy if the air passage is blocked.

2.2 Treatment based on syndrome differentiation

(1) Pattern of invasion of wind and heat

Main symptoms: Sore throat, difficulty in swallowing, obstructive sensation in the throat, aversion to cold, fever, a little bit thirst, congestion and tumefaction in the epiglottis, poor mobility in the epiglottis, red tongue margin and tip, thin and white tongue coating, superficial and rapid pulse.

Therapeutic method: To expel wind, dissipate heat, promote the lung for its spreading ability and benefit the throat.

Herbal formulas and drugs: *Lonicera and Forsythia Powder* (Yin Qiao San) (modified). *Flos Lonicerae* (Jin Yin Hua) 10g, *Fructus Forsythiae* (Lian Qiao) 10g, Radix Isatidis (Ban Lan Gen) 10g, *Herba Schizonepetae* (Jing Jie) 10g, *Radix Ledebouriellae* (Fang Feng) 10g, *Bombyx Batryticatus* (Bai Jiang Can) 10g, *Radix Platycodi* (Jie Geng) 6g, *Herba Menthae* (Bo He) (Decoct later)

2 治疗方法

2.1 治疗原则

由于急性会厌炎病位在喉，为呼吸要道，须防风邪善行数变，会厌白肿者容易致气道阻塞，陷入窒息危证。故治疗在西药抗炎消肿同时，祛风清热化痰，密切观察，有气道阻塞时及时气管切开。

2.2 辨证论治

(1) 风热外袭

主症：咽痛、吞咽困难、咽喉有阻塞感，恶寒发热，口微渴。检查见会厌充血肿胀，会厌活动度差。舌边尖红，苔薄白，脉浮数。

治法：疏风散热，宣肺利喉。

方药：银翘散加减。金银花 10 克，连翘 10 克，板蓝根 10 克，荆芥 10 克，防风 10 克，白僵蚕 10 克，桔梗 6 克，薄荷(后下)6 克，射干 6 克，甘草 3 克。

6g, *Rhizoma Belamecandae* (She Gan) 6g, and *Radix Glycyrrhizae* (Gan Cao) 3g.

(2) **Pattern of pathogenic wind with phlegm**

Main symptoms: Sore throat, difficulty in swallowing, obstructive and uncomfortable sensation in the throat, obstructive respiration, rattling sound in the throat, aversion to cold, fever, no thirst, serious congestion and edeman in the epiglottis, or in semi-ball shape, slight red tongue, greasy tongue coating, rolling pulse.

Therapeutic method: To expel wind, dissolve phlegm, diminish swelling and benefit the throat.

Herbal formulas and drugs: Six Ingredients Decoction (Liu Wei Tang) (modified). *Herba Schizonepetae* (Jing Jie) 10g, *Radix Ledebouriellae* (Fang Feng) 10g, *Bombyx Batryticatus* (Bai Jiang Can) 10g, *Radix Angelicae Dahuricae* (Bai Zhi) 10g, *Rhizoma Pinelliae* Preparata (Zhi Ban Xia) 10g, *Herba Menthae* (Bo He) (Decoct later) 6g, *Radix Platycodi* (Jie Geng) 6g, *Concretio Siliceae Bambusae* (Tian Zhu Huang) 6g, *Rhizoma Belamecandae* (She Gan) 5g, powder of *Bulbus Fritillariae Cirrhosae* (Chuan Bei Mu) (Take seperately) 3g, and *Radix Glycyrrhizae* (Gan Cao) 3g.

2.3 Other therapies

External therapies by herbal drugs: ① Blow *Borneol and Borax Powder* (Bing Peng San) to the throat, 0.1 to 0.2g, each time, for 5 to 6 times per day. ② Decoct *Herba Menthae* (Bo He) with water and inhale its steam while it is still hot. Flavor of herbal liquid is cool and refreshing, fragrant and able to benefit the throat, diminish swelling and dredge the aperture.

(2) **风邪挟痰**

主症：咽痛、吞咽困难，喉部阻塞不舒，呼吸不畅，喉间有痰鸣声。恶寒、发热，口不渴。检查见会厌充血，水肿较甚，或呈半球形。舌质淡红，苔腻，脉滑。

治法：祛风化痰，消肿利喉。

方药：六味汤加味。荆芥 10 克，防风 10 克，白僵蚕 10 克，白芷 10 克，制半夏 10 克，薄荷（后下）6 克，桔梗 6 克，天竺黄 6 克，射干 5 克，川贝母粉（另吞）3 克，甘草 3 克。

2.3 其他疗法

药物外治：①冰硼散吹撒于咽部，每次 0.1～0.2 克，每日 5～6 次；②薄荷煎水，乘热吸入其蒸气，药液气味清凉，芳香，可利喉消肿通窍。

Acute laryngitis

急性喉炎

It refers to acute non-specific inflammation of the laryngeal mucosa. It frequently occurs in the winter and spring. The incidence rate is high in the males and the pathological condition is worse in children. It is mostly caused by infection of influenza virus, Coxsackie virus, streptococcus pneumoniae, streptococcus, staphylococcus aureus, when the immunity is lower in the whole body. Dust, harmful gas stimulation, inappropriate voice, traumatic injury, over tobacco and liquor are often the inducing factors. It belongs to the scope of "acute sore throat" and "sudden aphonia" in Chinese medicine.

急性喉炎是喉黏膜的急性非特异性炎症。多发于冬、春两季，男性发病率较高，儿童病情多较严重。多为全身抵抗力低下时，遭受流感病毒、柯萨奇病毒以及肺炎球菌、链球菌、金黄色葡萄球菌等感染。粉尘、有害气体刺激，用声不当或过度，外伤，烟酒过度等也是常见诱因。属中医学"急喉瘖""暴喑"范畴。

1 Diagnostic essentials

1 诊断要点

1.1 Uncomfortable, dry and foreign body sensation in the throat, hoarse voice, dry cough, or coughing up tenacious and purulent secretions, possible dyspnea in children, fever, aversion to cold, discomfort in the whole body, possibly accompanied by the symptoms of infection of the upper respiratory tract.

1.1 喉部疼痛不适、干燥、异物感，声音嘶哑，干咳或咳出黏脓性分泌物，小儿可有呼吸困难。可有发热、恶寒及全身不适等症状，也可伴有上呼吸道感染症状。

1.2 Diffuse congestion and tumefaction in the laryngeal mucosa, congestion in the vocal cord, but normal mobility, barking cough, and inspiratory dyspnea in children.

1.2 喉黏膜弥漫性充血肿胀，声带充血，但运动正常。小儿可有犬吠样咳嗽，吸气性呼吸困难。

1.3 It is necessary to differentiate it from laryngeal diphtheria, laryngeal tuberculosis, and allergic laryngeal edema.

1.3 应排除喉白喉、喉结核、变应性喉水肿等疾病。

2 Therapeutic methods

2 治疗方法

2.1 Therapeutic principles

2.1 治疗原则

Acute laryngitis is mostly caused by invasion of

急性喉炎多因风寒或风

pathogenic wind and cold or pathogenic wind and heat into the lung, blocking the lung qi and disorder in closure and opening of the glottis. The treatment is mainly given to expel wind and promote the lung for its spreading ability.

热邪毒侵袭肺金,使肺气壅遏不宣,声门开合不利。治疗以祛风宣肺为主。

2.2 Treatment based on syndrome differentiation

(1) Pattern of invasion of wind and heat

Main symptoms: Hoarse voice, dry throat, cough due to itching, low and coarse voice, difficult phonation, or burning hot and pain in the throat, accompanied by fever, slight aversion to cold, slight sweating, headache, tiredness in the limbs, slight red tongue margin, thin and white tongue coating, superficial and rapid pulse.

Therapeutic method: To expel wind, clear away heat, promote the lung for its spreading ability and promote phonation.

Herbal formulas and drugs: *Wind-Expelling and Heat-Clarifying Decoction* (Shu Feng Qing Re Tang) (modified). *Flos Lonicerae* (Jin Yin Hua) 10g, *Folium Mori* (Sang Ye) 10g, *Fructus Arctii* (Niu Bang Zi) 10g, *Radix Scrophulariae* (Xuan Shen) 10g, *Bulbus Fritillariae Thumbergii* (Zhe Bei Mu) 10g, *Radix Scutellariae* (Huang Qin) 6g, *Radix Paeoniae Rubra* (Chi Shao) 6g, *Radix Platycodi* (Jie Geng) 6g, *Herba Menthae* (Bo He) (Decoct later) 6g, *Semen Oroxyli* (Mu Hu Die) 5g, and *Radix Glycyrrhizae* (Gan Cao) 3g. For abundant accumulation of pathogenic heat, and heat abundance in the stomach, it is necessary to discharge heat, resolve toxin, benefit the throat and promote phonation, by using *Throat-Clarifying and Diaphragm-Benefiting Decoction* (Qing Yan Li Ge Tang) plus *Periostracum Cicadae* (Chan Tui) 5g, and *Semen Sterculiae*,

2.2 辨证论治

(1) 风热外袭

主症:声音嘶哑,喉内干燥,痒咳,音低而粗,发声不利,或喉内灼热疼痛。伴发热,微恶寒,微有出汗,头痛,肢体倦怠。舌边微红,苔薄白,脉浮数。

治法:疏风清热,宣肺开音。

方药:疏风清热汤加减。金银花 10 克,桑叶 10 克,牛蒡子 10 克,玄参 10 克,浙贝母 10 克,黄芩 6 克,赤芍药 6 克,桔梗 6 克,薄荷(后下)6 克,木蝴蝶 5 克,甘草 3 克。若邪热壅盛、胃腑热盛,宜泄热解毒、利喉开音,可选用清咽利膈汤加蝉蜕 5 克、胖大海 10 克;若邪热传里,去荆芥、防风;若痰多、声带红肿甚,加天竺黄 6 克、瓜蒌 10 克、前胡 6 克、竹茹 10 克。

Lychnophorae (Pang Da Hai) 10g. For inward transmission of pathogenic heat, take out *Herba Schizonepetae* (Jing Jie) and *Radix Ledebouriellae* (Fang Feng). For profuse sputum, and swollen vocal cord, add *Concretio Siliceae Bambusae* (Tian Zhu Huang) 6g, *Fructus Trichosanthis* (Gua Lou) 10g, *Radix Peucedani* (Qian Hu) 6g, and *Caulis Bambusae in Taeniam* (Zhu Ru) 6g.

(2) **Pattern of invasion of wind and cold**

Main symptoms: After catching wind, cold and rains, hoarse voice, low voice, slight sore throat, or slight dry sensation in the throat, no desire for drinks, cough with thin sputum, easy to cough up, or nasal obstruction, clear and thin nasal discharge, non-obvious fever, thin and white tongue coating, superficial and tense pulse.

Therapeutic method: To expel wind, disperse cold, promote the lung for its spreading ability and promote phonation.

Herbal formulas and drugs: *Six Ingredients Decoction* (Liu Wei Tang) (modified). *Herba Schizonepetae* (Jing Jie) 10g, *Radix Ledebouriellae* (Fang Feng) 6g, *Radix Platycodi* (Jie Geng) 6g, *Herba Menthae* (Bo He) (Decoct later) 6g, Folium Penillae (Zi Su Ye) 10g, *Semen Armeniacae Amarum* (Ku Xing Ren) 10g, *Bombyx Batryticatus* (Bai Jiang Can) 10g, *Periostracum Cicadae* (Chan Tui) 5g, *Semen Oroxyli* (Mu Hu Die) 5g, and *Radix Glycyrrhizae* (Gan Cao) 3g. For cough and profuse sputum, add *Rhizoma Pinelliae* Preparata (Fa Ban Xia) 6g, and *Rhizoma Cynanchi Stauntonii* (Bai Qian) 6g.

2.3 Other therapies

(1) Chinese patent medicine: HUANG's Voice

(2) **风寒外袭**

主症：感受风寒淋雨之后，声音嘶哑，发声低沉，咽喉微痛，或有轻微干燥感，不欲饮水，咳嗽有痰稀，易于咯出，或有鼻塞，流涕清稀，或有恶寒，发热不著。舌苔薄白，脉浮紧。

治法：疏风散寒，宣肺开音。

方药：六味汤加减。荆芥 10 克，防风 6 克，桔梗 6 克，薄荷（后下）6 克，紫苏叶 10 克，杏仁 10 克，白僵蚕 10 克，蝉蜕 5 克，木蝴蝶 5 克，甘草 3 克。若咳嗽痰多，加法半夏 6 克、白前 6 克。

2.3 其他疗法

（1）中成药：黄氏响声

Pills (Huang Shi Xiang Sheng Wan), Take 5 grams each time, for three times per day, used for acute laryngitis in pattern of invasion of wind and heat.

(2) Simple and proved formulas: ① Decoct *Herba Andrographis* (Chuan Xin Lian) 15g, *Flos Chrysanthemi Indici* (Ye Ju Hua) 15g, *Herba seu Radix Solidaginis* (Yi Zhi Huang Hua) 15g, *Herba Elephantopi* (Ku Di Dan) 15g, *Radix Achyranthis Bidentatae* (Tu Niu Xi) 30g, and *Herba Emiliae Sonchifoiae* (Yang Ti Cao) 30g, with water, one dose per day, for taking in 3 times. ② Decoct *Herba Menthae* (Bo He), *Herba Schizonepetae* (Jing Jie), *Radix Platycodi* (Jie Geng) and *Semen Sterculiae, Lychnophorae* (Pang Da Hai), each in proper amount, with water for oral administration, for one dose per day.

(3) External therapies: ① Blow herbal powder. It is advisable to blow *Borneol and Borax Powder* (Bing Peng San), and *Pearl and Bezoar Powder* (Zhu Huang San) to the throat, for 5 to 6 times per day, in order to clear away heat, diminish swelling, dissolve phlegm and benefit the throat. ② Take pills in the mouth. Keep proper amount of *Six Divine Pills* (Liu Shen Wan) or *Throat Lozenge* (Run Hou Pian) in the mouth, for 3 to 4 times per day, in order to resolve toxin, diminish swelling, stop pain and benefit the throat. ③ Inhale steam. Decoct proper amount of *Herba Menthae* (Bo He), *Herba Agastachis* (Huo Xiang), *Herba Eupatorii* (Pei Lan), *Flos Lonicerae* (Jin Yin Hua), *Flos Chrysanthemi* (Ju Hua) or *Folium Penillae* (Zi Su Ye), and *Bulbus Allii Fistulosi* (Cong Bai) with water and inhale its steam, for twice per day, in order to dredge the aperture by fragrance, expel wind, clear away

丸，每服 5 克，每日 3 次。用于急性喉炎风热外袭证。

（2）单验方：①穿心莲 15 克，野菊花 15 克，佛手柑 15 克，一枝黄花 15 克，苦地胆 15 克，土牛膝根 30 克，羊蹄草 30 克，水煎，每日 1 剂，分 3 次服用。②薄荷、荆芥、桔梗、胖大海各适量，水煎，每日 1 剂口服。

（3）外治法：①吹药。可用冰硼散、珠黄散等药吹喉，每日 5～6 次，以清热消肿，化痰利喉。②含法。六神丸或润喉丸，适量含服，每日 3～4 次，以解毒消肿，止痛利喉。③蒸汽吸入法。可用薄荷，藿香，佩兰，金银花，菊花或紫苏叶，葱白等药适量煎水作蒸汽吸入，每日 2 次，有芳香通窍，疏风清热或散寒之功。

heat or disperse cold.

Chronic laryngitis

It refers to chronic inflammatory lesion of the laryngeal mucosa, possibly involving the submucosa and intrinsic laryngeal muscle. It is related to improper treatment of acute laryngitis, widespread influence of adjacent inflammation, various physical and chemical stimulations, over phonation and improper phonation, gastroesophageal reflux, and infection of helicobacter pylori. It is divides into simple, hypertrophic and atrophic type. It belongs to the scope of "chronic sore throat" in Chinese medicine.

1 Diagnostic essentials

1.1 There is a history of contact and exposure to susceptible factor.

1.2 There are slow duration, easy repetition, hoarse voice, dry cough or cough with tenacious sputum, uncomfortable, burning and dry sensation and pricking pain in the throat, and even expectoration with blood and stinky crust.

1.3 Inspections

Diffuse congestion and tumefaction in the laryngeal mucosa, pink or deep red colour in the two vocal cords, with stria vascularis parallel to the free edge of the vocal cord, dull or uneven border of the vocal cord, or cleft in opening and closing the vocal cord, often with tenacious fluid and wiredrawing phenomenon on the surface of the vocal cord, or even shine of laryngeal mucosa, black brown or

慢性喉炎

慢性喉炎是喉黏膜的慢性炎性病变，可波及黏膜下层和喉内肌。与急性喉炎治疗不当、邻近炎症蔓延影响、各种物理化学刺激、用声过度、用声不当、胃食管反流、幽门螺杆菌感染等有关。分单纯性、肥厚性和萎缩性三型。属中医学“慢喉喑”范畴。

1 诊断要点

1.1 具有易感因素接触暴露史。

1.2 病程缓慢，易反复。可有声嘶、干咳或咳嗽痰黏、喉部不适感、烧灼感、干燥感、刺痛等。甚或咳痰带血和臭味痂皮。

1.3 检查

喉黏膜弥漫性充血、肿胀；双声带呈粉红色或深红色，表面有血管纹与声带游离缘平行；声带边缘变钝，或表面不平，闭合时可出现裂隙；声带表面常有黏液附着，有拉丝现象，甚或喉黏膜光亮，喉腔可见黑褐色或绿色

green scabs noticeable in the laryngeal cavity. The partial vocal cord is covered by hypertrophic ventricular bands. The movement of the vocal cord is normal.

结痂；室带肥厚可遮盖部分声带；声带活动正常。

1.4 It is necessary to differentiate it from laryngeal tuberculosis, pachydermia laryngis, and early laryngeal tumor.

1.4 应与喉结核、喉厚皮病、早期喉肿瘤等疾病鉴别。

2 Therapeutic methods

2 治疗方法

2.1 Therapeutic principles

2.1 治疗原则

The voice comes from the lung but is rooted in the kidney. The lung dominates qi. The spleen is the resource of qi. The kidney is a root of qi. If the kidney essence is sufficient, qi will be vigorous in the lung and spleen and the voice will be sonorous. Deficiency of qi and yin in the lung, spleen and kidney, accompanied by accumulation of phlegm, blood stasis and qi stagnation, can cause chronic laryngitis. The treatment is mainly given to benefit qi, and to regulate qi, dissolve phlegm and disperse accumulation additionally.

声音出于肺而根于肾，肺主气，脾为气之源，肾为气之根，肾精充沛，肺脾气旺，则声音洪亮；肺、脾、肾气阴两虚，伴痰瘀气滞，声门开阖乏力，可致慢性喉炎。治疗以益气为主，辅以理气化痰消瘀。

2.2 Treatment based on syndrome differentiation

2.2 辨证论治

(1) **Pattern of yin deficiency in the lung and kidney**

(1) **肺肾阴虚**

Main symptoms: Lingering hoarse voice, easy fatigue after speaking, symptoms aggravated after fatigue and long speaking, slight painful and uncomfortable and dry sensation in the throat, cough due to itching, with little sputum, often clearing voice, slight tumefaction in the vocal cord, with slightly thickened border, or flushed cheeks and red lips, vexation due to deficiency, poor sleep, soreness and weakness of the low back and knee, feverish sensation in the palms and soles, red tongue,

主症：声音嘶哑，日久不愈，讲话易疲劳，每因劳累、多言之后症状加重。喉部微感疼痛不适，干燥，痒咳痰少，不易咯出，常有“吭、咯”清嗓习惯。检查可见声带微红肿，边缘稍增厚。或有颧红唇赤，虚烦少寐，腰膝酸软，手足心热等症状。舌红少苔，脉细数。

scanty tongue coating, thready and rapid pulse.

Therapeutic method: To replenish the lung and kidney, benefit the throat and promote phonation.

治法:滋补肺肾,利喉开音。

Herbal formulas and drugs: *Lily Metal-Consolidating Decoction* (Bai He Gu Jin Tang) (modified). Bulbus Lilii (Bai He) 10g, *Radix Rehmanniae Cruda* (Sheng Di Huang) 10g, *Radix Rehmanniae Praeparata* (Shu Di Huang) 10g, *Radix Ophiopogonis* (Mai Dong) 10g, *Radix Scrophulariae* (Xuan Shen) 10g, *Radix Angelicae Sinensis* (Dang Gui) 10g, *Radix Paeoniae Albae* (Bai Shao) 6g, *Radix Platycodi* (Jie Geng) 6g, and *Radix Glycyrrhizae* (Gan Cao) 3g. For dry and itching in the throat, cough, it is advisable to use Sweet Dew Drink (Gan Lu Yin). For dry and painful sensation in the throat, flushed cheeks, red lips, and feverish sensation in the palms and soles, add *Cortex Phellodendri* (Huang Bo) 10g, and *Rhizoma Anemarrhenae* (Zhi Mu) 10g.

方药:百合固金汤加减。百合 10 克,生地黄 10 克,熟地黄 10 克,麦门冬 10 克,玄参 10 克,当归 10 克,白芍药 6 克,桔梗 6 克,甘草 3 克。若咽喉干痒、咳嗽,宜用甘露饮;若咽喉干痛、颧红唇赤、手足心热,加黄柏 10 克、知母 10 克。

(2) **Pattern of qi deficiency in the lung and spleen**

(2) **肺脾气虚**

Main symptoms: Lingering hoarse voice, aggravated after fatigue, worse in the mornings, low voice, speaking with effort, unable to speak for long time, light colour in the laryngeal mucosa, flaccid and feeble vocal cord, with poor closure and opening, accompanied by the general symptoms of shortness of breath, reluctance in speaking, lassitude, poor appetite, loose stool, pale and swollen tongue, white tongue coating, thready and feeble pulse.

主症:声音嘶哑日久,疲劳后加重,上午明显,语言低微,讲话费力,不能持久。检查喉部黏膜色淡,声带松弛无力,闭合不良。全身可有少气懒言,倦怠乏力,纳呆便溏等症。舌淡胖,苔白,脉细弱。

Therapeutic method: To replenish and benefit the lung and spleen, benefit the throat and promote phonation.

治法:补益肺脾,利喉开音。

Herbal formulas and drugs: Center-Supplementing Qi-Boosting Decoction (Bu Zhong Yi Qi Tang)

方药:补中益气汤加减。黄芪 10 克,党参 10 克,白术

(modified). *Radix Astragali* (Huang Qi) 10g, *Radix Codonopsis Pilosulae* (Dang Shen) 10g, *Rhizoma Atractylodis Macrocephalae* (Bai Zhu) 10g, *Sclerotium Poria* (Fu Ling) 10g, *Rhizoma Cimicifugae* (Sheng Ma) 3g, *Radix Puerariae* (Ge Gen) 10g, *Fructus Terminaliae Chebulae* (He Zi) 10g, *Rhizoma Acori Graminei* (Shi Chang Pu) 3g, *Radix Platycodi* (Jie Geng) 6g, and *Radix Glycyrrhizae* (Gan Cao) 3g. For profuse sputum, add *Rhizoma Pinelliae Preparata* (Fa Ban Xia) 10g, *Sclerotium Poria* (Fu Ling) 10g, and *Semen Dolichoris Album* (Bai Bian Dou), 10g.

10克,茯苓10克,升麻3克,葛根10克,诃子10克,石菖蒲3克,桔梗6克,甘草3克。若痰多,加法半夏6克、茯苓10克、白扁豆10克;声带松弛,加五味子10克、补骨脂10克、胡桃肉10克。

(3) **Pattern of qi stagnation, blood stasis and phlegm accumulation**

(3) **气滞血瘀痰凝**

Main symptoms: Lingering hoarse voice, speaking with effort, discomfort in the throat, foreign body sensation in the throat, frequently clearing voice, hypertrophy in the vocal cord and ventricle, or vocal nodules, vocal polyp, with tenacious sputum glued on the vocal cord, possible no general symptoms, or stuffy chest, cough and expectoration, dark red tongue, thin and white tongue coating, choppy pulse.

主症:声音嘶哑日久,讲话费力,喉内不适,有异物感,常作"吭、喀"清嗓。检查见声带、室带肥厚,或有声带小结、息肉,常有黏痰附于声带上。可无全身症状,或有胸闷、咳嗽咯痰等。舌暗红,苔薄白,脉涩。

Therapeutic method: To circulate qi, activate blood, dissolve phlegm and promote phonation.

治法:行气活血,化痰开音。

Herbal formulas and drugs: *Epiglottis Blood Stasis-Dissipating Decoction* (Hui Yan Zhu Yu Tang)(modified). *Semen Persicae* (Tao Ren) 10g, *Flos Carthami* (Hong Hua) 6g, *Radix Angelicae Sinensis* (Dang Gui) 10g, *Radix Paeoniae Rubra* (Chi Shao) 6g, *Radix Rehmanniae Cruda* (Sheng Di Huang) 10g, *Radix Bupleuri* (Chai Hu) 6g, *Bulbus Fritillariae Thumbergii* (Zhe Bei Mu) 10g, *Radix Platycodi* (Jie Geng) 6g, and *Radix Glycyrrhizae*

方药:会厌逐瘀汤加减。桃仁10克,红花6克,当归10克,赤芍药6克,生地黄10克,柴胡6克,浙贝母10克,桔梗6克,甘草3克。若气滞血瘀为主,加三棱10克、莪术10克、枳壳6克;气滞痰凝为主,加海藻10克、昆布10克、瓦楞子20克、海浮石20

(Gan Cao) 3g. For qi stagnation and blood stasis in predominance, add *Rhizoma Sparganii Stoloniferi* (San Leng) 10g, *Rhizoma Zedoariae* (E Zhu) 10g, and *Fructus Aurantii* (Zhi Ke) 6g. For qi stagnation and phlegm accumulation in predominance, add *Sargassum* (Hai Zao) 10g, *Thallus Laminariae seu Eckloniae* (Kun Bu) 10g, *Concha Arcae* (Wa Leng Zi) 20g, and *Bryozoatum* (Hai Fu Shi) 20g.

克。

2.3 Other therapies

(1) **Chinese patent medicine:** ① *Figwort, Ophiopogon, Liquorice and Platycodon Granules* (Xuan Mai Gan Ju Ke Li), Take 1 to 2 packets each time, for 3 times per day, used for chronic laryngitis in pattern of yin deficiency in the lung and kidney. ② *Center-Supplementing Qi-Boosting Pills* (Bu Zhong Yi Qi Wan), Take 5 grams each time, for three times per day, used for chronic laryngitis in pattern qi deficiency in the lung and spleen. ③ *Huang's Voice Pills* (Huang Shi Xiang Sheng Wan), Take 5 grams each time, for three times per day. It is also advisable to use *Golden Voice Phonation Pills* (Jin Sang Kai Yin Wan), and *Golden Voice Accumulation-Dispersing Pills* (Jin Sang San Jie Wan), for chronic laryngitis in pattern of qi stagnation and phlegm accumulation.

2.3 其他疗法

（1）**中成药：**①玄麦甘桔颗粒，每服1～2包，每日3次。用于慢性喉炎肺肾阴虚证。②补中益气丸，每服5克，每日3次。用于慢性喉炎肺脾气虚证。③黄氏响声丸，每服5克，每日3次。亦可用金嗓开音丸、金嗓散结丸等，用于慢性喉炎气滞痰凝证。

(2) **Simple and proved formulas:** ① Decoct *Cortex Lycii Radicis* (Di Gu Pi) 20g, *Radix Adenophorae* (Nan Sha Shen) 10g, and *Radix Ophiopogonis* (Mai Dong) 20g, with water for oral administration, for one dose per day. ② Decoct *Fructus Terminaliae Chebulae* (He Zi) 10g, *Radix Astragali* (Huang Qi) 10g, and *Rhizoma Acori Graminei* (Shi Chang Pu) 3g, with water for oral administration, for one dose per day. ③ Decoct *Radix Salviae Miltiorrhizae*

（2）**单验方：**①地骨皮20克，南沙参10克，麦门冬20克，水煎服，每日1剂。②诃子10克，黄芪10克，石菖蒲5克，水煎，每日1剂。③丹参5克，玉竹10克，麦门冬10克，青果2个，水煎服，每日1剂。④桔梗10克，甘草10克，木蝴蝶10克，金黄榄

(Dan Shen) 5g, *Rhizoma Polygonati Odorati* (Yu Zhu) 10g, and *Radix Ophiopogonis* (Mai Dong) 10g, and *Fructus Canarii* (Qing Guo) 2 pieces, with water for oral administration, for one dose per day. ④ Decoct *Radix Platycodi* (Jie Geng) 10g, *Radix Glycyrrhizae* (Gan Cao) 10g, *Semen Oroxyli* (Mu Hu Die) 10g, *Rhizoma Tinosporae sagittatae* (Jin Guo Lan) 10g, with water for oral administration, for one dose per day.

10 克，水煎服，每日 1 剂。

(3) **External therapies:** ① Take pills in the mouth. *Iron Flute Pills* (Tie Di Wan), keep one pill in the mouth, for twice per day. ② Inhale steam. It is advisable to choose *Radix Rehmanniae Cruda* (Sheng Di Huang), *Radix Ophiopogonis* (Mai Dong), and *Radix Scrophulariae* (Xuan Shen) for pattern of yin deficiency, to choose *Rhizoma Atractylodis Macrocephalae* (Bai Zhu) and *Fructus Terminaliae Chebulae* (He Zi) for pattern of qi deficiency, and to choose *Flos Carthami* (Hong Hua), *Radix Angelicae Sinensis* (Dang Gui) and *Rhizoma Ligustici Chuanxiong* (Chuan Xiong) for pattern of qi stagnation and blood stasis. All herbal drugs are decocted with water for inhaling hot steam, or herbal decoction is atomized by a ultrasonic atomizer for inhalation, for twice per day.

(3) **外治法：**①含法。铁笛丸，每次 1 丸含服，每日 2 次。②蒸汽吸入法。阴虚证可选用生地黄、麦门冬、玄参；气虚证可选用白术、诃子；气滞血瘀痰凝证可选用红花、当归、川芎。将药物水煎热雾吸入，或水煎液用超声雾化器作雾化吸入，每日 2 次。

Pharyngeal paraesthesia

咽异感症

It refers to a paresthetic disease manifested by a sensation of foreign body in the throat, unable to cough up and to swallow down, without organic lesion under the objective inspection. It frequently occurs in women at the age of 30 to 50. It belongs to

咽异感症是以咽喉如有物梗阻，咯之不出，咽之不下，客观检查未见器质性病变的一种感觉异常性疾病。好发于 30～50 岁妇女。属

the scope of "plum seen sensation" in Chinese medicine.

中医学"梅核气"范畴。

1 Diagnostic essentials

1 诊断要点

1.1 There are sensation of foreign body in the throat, unable to cough up and to swallow down, or move upward or downward, or immobile, no impact on food ingestion, burning or uncomfortable sensation in the throat, possibly accompanied by belching, stuffy chest, and worry, anxiety and stressful mode during seizure, alleviated sometimes and aggravated sometimes, without any rule.

1.1 咽部梗阻感，咳之不出，咽之不下，或上下移动，或固定不动，不影响进食；咽部烧灼或不适感觉；可伴有嗳气、胸闷。发作常伴有焦虑、急躁和紧张情绪，症状时轻时重，无一定规律。

1.2 It is necessary to check the nasopharynx, oropharynx, laryngopharynx and neck, and to check the organic lesions in the laryngopharynx, esophagus and neck by endoscopy, and B-ultrasonic and imageological inspection.

1.2 仔细检查鼻咽、口咽、喉咽、颈部等，必要时内镜、B超及影像学检查喉咽、食管、颈部等处器质性病变。

2 Therapeutic methods

2 治疗方法

2.1 Therapeutic principles

2.1 治疗原则

Its occurrence is related to liver qi stagnation and accumulation of phlegm and qi. Therefore, the treatment is mainly applied to soothe the liver, relieve stagnation, regulate qi and dissolve phlegm.

咽异感症发生与肝郁气滞和痰气交阻有关，故治疗以疏肝解郁、理气化痰为主。

2.2 Treatment based on syndrome differentiation

2.2 辨证论治

(1) **Pattern of liver qi stagnation**

Main symptoms: Sensation of foreign body in the throat, like plum seed, or like lump, unable to swallow down and to cough up, intolerable suffocating sensation, but no impact in food ingestion, often accompanied by emotional depression, worries, doubtfulness, stuffy and distending sensation in the chest and hypochondriac region, vexation, easy anger, frequent sighing, or distending and full sensation in the epigastric and abdominal region, wiry

(1) **肝郁气滞**

主症：咽喉内有异物感，或如梅核，或如肿物，吞之不下，吐之不出，甚则窒闷难忍，但不碍饮食。常有精神抑郁，多虑多疑，胸闷胁胀，心烦郁怒，善太息，或脘腹胀满等。脉弦。

pulse.

Therapeutic method: To soothe the liver, regulate qi, relieve stagnation and disperse accumulation.

治法:疏肝理气,解郁散结。

Herbal formulas and drugs: *Free Wanderer Powder* (Xiao Yao San) (modified). *Radix Bupleuri* (Chai Hu) 10g, *Radix Paeoniae Albae* (Bai Shao) 6g, *Rhizoma Pinelliae* (Ban Xia) 6g, *Rhizoma Corydalis* (Yan Hu Suo) 10g, *Caulis Bambusae in Taeniam* (Zhu Ru) 10g, *Radix Scutellariae* (Huang Qin) 10g, *Fructus Aurantii* (Zhi Ke) 10g, *Radix Aucklandiae* (Mu Xiang) 6g, and *Lignum Aquilariae Resinatum* (Chen Xiang) 6g.

方药:逍遥散加减。柴胡10克,白芍药6克,半夏6克,延胡索10克,竹茹10克,黄芩10克,枳壳10克,木香6克,沉香6克。

(2) **Pattern of accumulation of phlegm and qi**

(2) **痰气交阻**

Main symptoms: Sputum-like sensation in the throat, profuse sputum in the throat, unable to cough up, or cough with thin and white sputum, tiredness in the limbs, lassitude, poor appetite, distending and full sensation in the epigastric and abdominal region, swollen tongue, white and greasy tongue coating, rolling pulse.

主症:咽喉有痰状异物感,喉内痰多,咯吐不出,或有咳痰稀白,肢倦乏力,纳呆,脘腹胀满。舌胖,苔白腻,脉滑。

Therapeutic method: To regulate qi, dissolve phlegm, relieve stagnation and disperse accumulation.

治法:理气化痰,解郁散结。

Herbal formulas and drugs: *Pinellia and Magnolia Decoction* (Ban Xia Hou Pu Tang) (modified). *Rhizoma Pinelliae* (Ban Xia) 10g, *Cortex Magnoliae Officinalis* (Hou Pu) 10g, *Sclerotium Poria* (Fu Ling) 10g, *Bulbus Fritillariae Cirrhosae* (Chuan Bei Mu) 3g, *Pericarpium Citri Tangerinae* (Chen Pi) 6g, *Radix Platycodi* (Jie Geng) 6g, and *Radix Glycyrrhizae* (Gan Cao) 3g. For fatigue and profuse sputum, add *Radix Codonopsis Pilosulae* (Dang Shen) 10g, and *Rhizoma Atractylodis Macrocepha-*

方药:半夏厚朴汤加减。半夏10克,厚朴10克,伏苓10克,川贝母3克,陈皮6克,桔梗6克,甘草3克。若疲乏、痰多,加党参10克、白术6克。

lae (Bai Zhu) 6g.

2.3 Other therapies

(1) **Chinese patent medicine:** ① *Free Wanderer Pills* (Xiao Yao Wan), Take 6 grams each times orally, for 3 times per day, used for various patterns of pharyngeal paraesthesia. ② *Stagnancy-Relieving Pills* (Yue Ju Wan), Take 6 grams each times orally, for three times per day, used for various patterns of pharyngeal paraesthesia.

(2) **Simple and proved formulas:** ① Decoct *Fructus Hordei Germinatus* (Mai Ya) 30g, with water as drinking tea, and drink frequently every day. ② Make tea with *Flos Citri Sarcodactylis* (Fo Shou Hua) 10g, and *Flos Mume* (Lu Mei Hua), and drink frequently every day.

2.3 其他疗法

（1）**中成药:**①逍遥丸，每服6克，每日3次口服。治疗咽异感症各证型。②越鞠丸，每服6克，每日3次口服。治疗咽异感症各证。

（2）**单验方①炒麦芽30克，煎汤代茶，每日多次饮用。②佛手花10克，绿梅花6克，泡茶，每日多次饮用。**

Hysterial aphonia

It refers to psychogenic aphonia, or termed neurosis aphonia, and is a manifestation of neurosis in the throat, characterized by sudden aphonia and quick recovery. It is mostly seen in women and is mostly related to emotional stimulation, such as anger, excitement, terror, melancholy, and sadness. It belongs to the scope of "sudden aphonia" in Chinese medicine.

1 Diagnostic essentials

1.1 Sudden aphonia, or only whispered voice, normal phonation in cough or crying or laughing, possible depression, slow action, sleeping disturbance, gastrointestinal dysfunction, and pharyngeal paraesthesia.

癔病性失音

癔病性失音也称心因性失音，或称神经症性失音，是神经官能症在喉部的表现。突然失音，可能又很快恢复。多见于女性，多数与精神受刺激，如发怒、激动、恐怖、忧虑、悲伤等有关。属中医学"暴喑"范畴。

1 诊断要点

1.1 突然失音，或仅发耳语声。咳嗽或哭笑时发声如常。可有情绪低落，动作缓慢，睡眠障碍。可有胃肠功能紊乱，咽异感症等。

1.2 Low sensation in the throat

1.3 In the inspection are present incomplete closure of the vocal cord in phonation, in abduction or only slight vibration of the vocal cord, and closure of the vocal cord in cough, crying and laughing.

1.4 It is necessary to exclude tumor in the larynx, pharynx and neck and other organic lesions in the whole body.

2 Therapeutic methods

2.1 Therapeutic principles

Hysterial aphonia is related to liver qi stagnation and malnutrition of the spirit and mind. Therefore, the treatment is mainly applied to soothe the liver, relieve stagnation, and nourish the heart and promote phonation.

2.2 Treatment based on syndrome differentiation

(1) **Pattern of liver qi stagnation**

Main symptoms: Sudden aphonia, but normal sound in cough, crying and laughing, emotional stimulation and fluctuation before onset, impatience and easy anger, distending and full sensation in the epigastric and hypochondriac region, frequent belching, thin and white tongue coating, wiry pulse.

Therapeutic method: To soothe the liver, regulate qi, relieve stagnation and promote phonation.

Herbal formulas and drugs: *Free Wanderer Powder* (Xiao Yao San) (modified). *Radix Bupleuri* (Chai Hu) 10g, *Radix Paeoniae Albae* (Bai Shao) 6g, *Pericarpium Citri Reticulatae Viride* (Qing Pi) 6g, *Rhizoma Corydalis* (Yan Hu Suo) 10g, *Caulis Bambusae in Taeniam* (Zhu Ru) 10g, *Radix Platycodi* (Jie Geng) 10g, *Periostracum Cicadae* (Chan

1.2 喉部感觉减退。

1.3 检查见发音时声带不闭合,位于外展位或仅见声带微微颤动。咳嗽、哭笑时,声带闭合。

1.4 应注意排除喉、咽部、颈部肿瘤及全身其他器质性病变。

2 治疗方法

2.1 治疗原则

癔病性失音与肝郁气滞和心神失养有关,故治疗以疏肝解郁、养心开音为主。

2.2 辨证论治

(1) **肝郁气滞**

主症:突然失音,但咳嗽及哭笑声如常。发病前多有精神刺激,情绪波动史,平时急躁易怒,胸胁胀满,嗳气频频。舌苔薄白,脉弦。

治法:疏肝理气,解郁开音。

方药:逍遥散加减。柴胡10克,白芍药6克,青皮6克,延胡索10克,竹茹10克,桔梗10克,蝉蜕3克,甘草3克。

Tui) 3g, and *Radix Glycyrrhizae* (Gan Cao) 3g.

(2) **Pattern of malnutrition of spirit and mind**

Main symptoms: Sudden aphonia, sorrow and desire to weep, normal phonation in crying and laughing, speaking like whisper, vexation, insomnia, poor appetite, lustrousless complexion, slight red tongue, thin and white tongue coating, thready and feeble pulse.

Therapeutic method: To benefit qi, nourish the heart, calm the mind and promote phonation.

Herbal formulas and drugs: *Liquorice, Wheat and Jujube Decoction* (Gan Mai Da Zao Tang) (modified). *Radix Glycyrrhizae* (Gan Cao) 5g, *Fructus Tritici Levis* (Fu Xiao Mai) 15g, *Fructus Ziziphi Jujubae* (Da Zao) 10 pieces, *Radix Codonopsis Pilosulae* (Dang Shen) 10g, *Radix Paeoniae Albae* (Bai Shao) 10g, *Radix Angelicae Sinensis* (Dang Gui) 10g, *Flos Carthami* (Hong Hua) 6g, and *Rhizoma Acori Graminei* (Shi Chang Pu) 3g. For poor sleep, add *Radix Polygoni Multiflori* (He Shou Wu) 10g, and *Cortex Alibiziae* (He Huan Pi) 10g.

2.3 Other therapies

(1) Chinese patent medicine: *Free Wanderer Pills* (Xiao Yao Wan), Take 6 grams each times orally, for three times per day, appropriate for pattern of liver qi stagnation.

(2) Simple and proved formulas: ① Decoct *Fructus Hordei Germinatus* (Mai Ya) 30g, with water as drinking tea, and drink frequently every day, appropriate for pattern of malnutrition of the heart and mind. ② Make tea with *Flos Citri Sarcodactylis* (Fo Shou Hua) 10g, and *Flos Mume* (Lu Mei Hua), and drink frequently every day, appropriate for va-

(2) **心神失养**

主症：突然失音，悲伤欲哭，哭笑时可正常发音，讲话如耳语，心烦失眠，食少，面色不华。舌淡红，苔薄白，脉细弱。

治法：益气养心，安神开音。

方药：甘麦大枣汤加减。甘草5克，浮小麦15克，大枣10枚，党参10克，白芍药10克，当归10克，红花6克，石菖蒲3克。若夜寐差，加制何首乌10克、合欢皮10克。

2.3 其他疗法

(1) 中成药：逍遥丸，每次6克，每日3次口服。适用于肝气郁结证。

(2) 单验方：①炒麦芽30克，煎汤代茶，每日多次饮用。适用于心神失养证。②佛手花、绿梅花各6克，泡茶，每日多次饮用。适用于癔病性失音各证。

rious patterns of hysterial aphonia.

Laryngeal cough

It refers to a disease characterized by intolerable itching sensation in the throat, paroxysmal or spasmodic cough. It is a specific type in various patterns of cough. The pathological position is above the glottis and starts from aperture of larynx. Once cough occurs, it will last for several minutes to dozen of minutes, and even several hours, with nasal discharge and tears in severe condition, possibly accompanied by dry throat, itching and burning sensation in the throat, no sputum or scanty tenacious sputum difficult to cough up in most conditions. It will last for several months or years. It is mostly seen in adults and easily occurs in the autumn and winter.

1 Diagnostic essentials

1.1 Dry and itching throat, continuous irritating cough, possibly accompanied by burning pain and foreign body sensation in the throat, cough often relieved by drinking water.

1.2 Mostly there is a history of inflammation of the upper respiratory tract, such as common cold, nasosinusitis, and pharyngitis.

1.3 In the inspection are present chronic congestion of the pharynx, scattered proliferation of lymphatic follicles at the posterior wall of the pharynx, hypertrophic lateral pharyngeal bands, in dim and dark or fresh red color, or dry shine in the surface of the mucous membrane.

喉源性咳嗽

喉源性咳嗽是以咽喉内奇痒难忍，阵发性或痉挛性咳嗽为特点的疾病。喉源性咳嗽是诸多咳嗽证中的特殊类型，其病位在声门以上，起点在喉口，不咳则已，一旦咳嗽，则持续数分钟到数十分钟，甚至数小时，严重者涕泪皆流，可伴有咽干，咽痒，咽部灼热，大多无痰或少量痰液黏稠难出咳出，常数月甚至经年不愈。成人多见，秋冬季易发。

1 诊断要点

1.1 咽干发痒，呛咳不断。可伴咽部灼痛，异物感等症。饮水常可缓解咳嗽。

1.2 多有上呼吸道炎症病史，如感冒、鼻-鼻窦炎、咽炎等。

1.3 检查可见咽部慢性充血，咽后壁淋巴滤泡散在性增生，咽侧索肥厚，色晦暗或红艳，或黏膜表面干而发亮等。

1.4 It is necessary to differentiate it from bronchial asthma, pulmonary and cardiac cough.

1.4 需与支气管炎、肺源性和心源性咳嗽相鉴别。

2 Therapeutic methods

2 治疗方法

2.1 Therapeutic principles

2.1 治疗原则

Laryngeal cough is related to injury of body fluid by pathogenic wind and dryness, and malnutrition of the throat. Dryness produces wind. Wind will lead to itching. Itching will result in cough. The treatment is mainly given to replenish and benefit the spleen and lung, nourish yin and clear away heat.

喉源性咳嗽为风燥伤及津液,咽喉失于濡养。干生燥,燥生风,风生痒,痒则咳。治疗以补益脾肺、养阴清热为法。

2.2 Treatment based on syndrome differentiation

2.2 辨证论治

(1) **Pattern of blockage of pathogens in the lung meridian**

(1) **邪困肺经**

Main symptoms: Cough due to itching in the throat, scanty sputum in white color, difficult expectoration, dry throat with preference for drinks, sensitive to cold wind, pale tongue, thin and white tongue coating, superficial pulse.

主症:喉痒而咳,痰少色白,咯痰不爽,咽干喜热饮,对寒风刺激较敏感。舌淡,苔薄白,脉浮。

Therapeutic method: To descend qi, stop itching, stop cough and dissolve phlegm.

治法:降气止痒,止咳化痰。

Herbal formulas and drugs: *Three Disobedience Decoction* (San Ao Tang) (modified). *Herba Ephedrae* (Ma Huang) 3g, *Semen Armeniacae Amarum* (Ku Xing Ren) 10g, and *Radix Glycyrrhizae* (Gan Cao) 3g, *Rhizoma Zingiberis Recens* (Sheng Jiang) 10g, *Lumbricus* (Di Long) 10g, *Periostracum Cicadae* (Chan Tui) 10g, *Radix Platycodi* (Jie Geng) 10g, *Caulis Perillae* (Su Geng) 10g, and *Fructus Perillae* (Zi Su Zi) 10g.

方药:三拗汤加减。麻黄3克,杏仁10克,甘草3克,生姜10克,干地龙10克,蝉蜕10克,桔梗6克,苏梗10克,苏子10克。

(2) **Pattern of abundance of internal fire**

(2) **内火独盛**

Main symptoms: Itching in the throat, dry cough, burning pain relieved by drinking water, red

主症:喉痒干咳、灼痛而饮水则舒。舌红,苔薄白,脉

tongue, thin and white tongue coating, thready and rapid pulse.

细数。

Therapeutic method: To clear away heat, cool blood, nourish yin and stop itching.

治法：清热凉血，滋阴止痒。

Herbal formulas and drugs: *Heat-Abducting Powder* (Dao Chi San) (modified). *Radix Rehmanniae Cruda* (Sheng Di Huang) 15g, *Folium Phyllostachydis Henonis* (Zhu Ye) 10g, *Medulla Junci* (Deng Xin Cao) 9g, *Rhizoma Phragmitis* (Lu Gen) 20g, *Rhizoma Imperatae* (Bai Mao Gen) 30g, *Radix Rubiae* (Qian Cao) 15g, *Radix Arnebiae seu Lithospermi* (Zi Cao) 15g, and *Herba Ecliptae* (Han Lian Cao) 15g,

方药：导赤散加减。生地15克，竹叶10克，灯心草9克，芦根20克，茅根30克，茜草15克，紫草15克，旱莲草15克。

(3) **Pattern of stomach fire and kidney deficiency**

(3) **胃火肾虚**

Main symptoms: Dry cough due to itching in the throat, difficult cough, dry throat with preference for cold drinks, accompanied by foul breath, nausea, or occasional loose teeth, gum bleeding, brown urine, constipation, red tongue, thin and yellow tongue coating, rolling and excessive pulse.

主症：喉痒干咳，咳而不爽，咽干喜凉饮，伴口秽泛恶，偶或牙龈松动，牙齿出血，尿黄便干，舌红，苔薄黄，脉滑实。

Therapeutic method: To clear away heat, discharge fire, nourish yin and benefit the throat.

治法：清热泻火，养阴利咽。

Herbal formulas and drugs: *Jade Lady Decoction* (Yu Nu Jian) (modified). *Radix Rehmanniae Praeparata* (Shu Di Huang) 15g, *Radix Rehmanniae Cruda* (Sheng Di Huang) 15g, *Gypsum Fibrosum* (Shi Gao) 20g, *Radix Ophiopogonis* (Mai Dong) 12g, *Radix Achyranthis Bidentatae* (Niu Xi) 10g, *Rhizoma Phragmitis* (Lu Gen) 12g, *Radix Adenophorae* (Nan Sha Shen) 15g, *Semen Armeniacae Amarum* (Ku Xing Ren) 12g, and *Lasiosphaera Seu Calvatia* (Ma Bo) 10g.

方药：玉女煎加减。熟地15克，生地15克，生石膏20克，麦冬12克，炒牛膝10克，芦根12克，沙参15克，杏仁12克，马勃10克。

(4) **Pattern of depletion of body fluid**

(4) **津液亏损**

Main symptoms: Frequent cough due to itching

主症：喉痒频咳，咽干钝

in the throat, dry throat with dull pain, relieved by drinking water, subjective sensation of foreign body in the throat, accompanied by dry nose, dry eyes, dry skin, constipation, red tongue with cracks, thin tongue coating, thready or normal pulse.

痛,饮水得解,自觉咽喉部有异物感。伴鼻干目涩,皮肤干燥,大便干结,舌红有裂纹,苔薄,脉细或平。

Therapeutic method: To nourish yin, moisten dryness, clarify the throat and benefit the throat.

治法:滋阴润燥,清喉利咽。

Herbal formulas and drugs: *Humor-Increasing Decoction* (Zeng Ye Tang) (modified). *Radix Rehmanniae Cruda* (Sheng Di Huang) 15g, *Radix Ophiopogonis* (Mai Dong) 15g, *Radix Scrophulariae* (Xuan Shen) 10g, *Radix Adenophorae* (Nan Sha Shen) 10g, *Radix Platycodi* (Jie Geng) 10g, and *Radix Glycyrrhizae* (Gan Cao) 6g.

方药:增液汤加减。生地 15 克,麦冬 10 克,玄参 10 克,沙参 10 克,桔梗 10 克,甘草 6 克。

(5) **Pattern of spleen decline and earth weakness**

(5) **脾衰土弱**

Main symptoms: Cough due to itching in the throat, drinking frequently for moistening the throat, with sputum glued in the throat, frequently clearing the throat, relieved after expectoration, occasional stuffy sensation in the chest and epigastric region, low spirit, lassitude, clear urine, or constipation, pale and swollen tongue, white and greasy tongue coating, soft and thready pulse.

主症:喉痒作咳、多饮求润,咽喉有痰附着,频频清嗓,咯痰得爽。时感胸闷脘痞,神疲乏力,便清或干而不爽,舌淡胖,苔白腻,脉濡细。

Therapeutic method: To strengthen the spleen, remove dampness, dissolve phlegm and stop cough.

治法:健脾利湿,化痰止咳。

Herbal formulas and drugs: *Ginseng, Poria and Atractylodes Powder* (Shen Ling Bai Zhu San)(modified). *Radix Pseudostellariae* (Tai Zi Shen) 15g, *Rhizoma Atractylodis Macrocephalae* (Bai Zhu) 12g, *Sclerotium Poria* (Fu Ling) 15g, *Semen Dolichoris Album* (Bai Bian Dou), 15g, *Rhizoma Dioscoreae* (Shan Yao) 15g, *Bulbus Lilii* (Bai He) 12g, *Semen Armeniacae Amarum* (Ku Xing Ren) 10g, *Pericarpium Citri Tangerinae* (Chen Pi) 10g,

方药:参苓白术散加减。太子参 15 克,白术 12 克,茯苓 15 克,白扁豆 15 克,山药 15 克,百合 12 克,杏仁 10 克,陈皮 10 克,升麻 10 克,桔梗 10 克,甘草 6 克。

Rhizoma Cimicifugae (Sheng Ma) 10g, *Radix Platycodi* (Jie Geng) 10g, and *Radix Glycyrrhizae* (Gan Cao) 6g.

2.3 Other therapies

(1) Chinese patent medicine: *Throat-Clarifying and Promoting Granules* (Qing Hou Li Yan Ke Li), Take 5 grams each time orally, for 3 times per day, appropriate for cough caused by infection of exogenous wind and heat. *Golden Fruit Drinks* (Jin Guo Yin), Take 15 m. each time, for 3 times per day, appropriate for cough induced by yin deficiency and internal heat.

(2) Buccal medications: *Throat-Clearing Dropping Pills* (Qing Yan Di Wan), *Cydiodine Buccal Tablets* (Hua Su Pian), and *Watermelon Frost Throat Tablets* (Xi Gua Shuang Run Hou Pian) are appropriate for various patterns of laryngeal cough.

2.3 其他疗法

（1）中成药：清喉利咽颗粒，每次5克，每日3次口服，适用于外感风热引起的咳嗽。金果饮，每次15毫升，每日3次口服，适用于阴虚内热引起的咳嗽。

（2）含化药：清咽滴丸、华素片、西瓜霜润喉片等，适用于喉源性咳嗽各证型。

Shanghai Pujiang Education Press (Former Shanghai University of Traditional Medicine Press)
1550 Haigang Ave, Shanghai, P.R.China 201306

图书在版编目(CIP)数据

中医眼耳鼻咽喉科学:英汉对照/黄平,缪晚虹,张治军主编. —上海:上海浦江教育出版社有限公司,2018.12
(精编实用中医文库/陈凯先,李其忠,何星海总主编)
ISBN 978-7-81121-588-5

Ⅰ.①中… Ⅱ.①黄… ②缪… ③张… Ⅲ.①中医五官科学—英、汉
Ⅳ.①R276

中国版本图书馆 CIP 数据核字(2018)第300707号

上海浦江教育出版社出版
社址:上海海港大道 1550 号上海海事大学校内　　邮政编码:201306
分社:上海蔡伦路 1200 号上海中医药大学内　　邮政编码:201203
电话:(021)38284910(12)(发行)　38284923(总编室)　38284910(传真)
E-mail:cbs@shmtu. edu. cn　URL:http://www. pujiangpress. cn
上海盛通时代印刷有限公司印装　上海浦江教育出版社发行
幅面尺寸:170 mm×240 mm　印张:31. 5　字数:600 千字
2018 年 12 月第 1 版　2019 年 4 月第 1 次印刷
责任编辑:黄　健　封面设计:赵宏义
定价:128. 00 元